MALE HYPOGONADISM

CONTEMPORARY ENDOCRINOLOGY

P. Michael Conn, SERIES EDITOR

MALE HYPOGONADISM

BASIC, CLINICAL, AND THERAPEUTIC PRINCIPLES

Edited by

STEPHEN J. WINTERS, MD

Chief, Division of Endocrinology, Metabolism and Diabetes,
Department of Medicine, University of Louisville, Louisville, KY

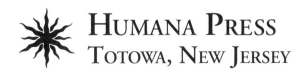

© 2004 Humana Press Inc.
999 Riverview Drive, Suite 208
Totowa, New Jersey 07512
www.humanapress.com

The content and opinions expressed in this book are the sole work of the authors and editors, who have warranted due diligence in the creation and issuance of their work. The publisher, editors, and authors are not responsible for errors or omissions or for any consequences arising from the information or opinions presented in this book and make no warranty, express or implied, with respect to its contents.

Due diligence has been taken by the publishers, editors, and authors of this book to assure the accuracy of the information published and to describe generally accepted practices. The contributors herein have carefully checked to ensure that the drug selections and dosages set forth in this text are accurate and in accord with the standards accepted at the time of publication. Notwithstanding, since new research, changes in government regulations, and knowledge from clinical experience relating to drug therapy and drug reactions constantly occur, the reader is advised to check the product information provided by the manufacturer of each drug for any change in dosages or for additional warnings and contraindications. This is of utmost importance when the recommended drug herein is a new or infrequently used drug. It is the responsibility of the treating physician to determine dosages and treatment strategies for individual patients. Further, it is the responsibility of the health care provider to ascertain the Food and Drug Administration status of each drug or device used in their clinical practice. The publishers, editors, and authors are not responsible for errors or omissions or for any consequences from the application of the information presented in this book and make no warranty, express or implied, with respect to the contents in this publication.

This publication is printed on acid-free paper. ∞

ANSI Z39.48-1984 (American National Standards Institute) Permanence of Paper for Printed Library Materials.

Production Editor: Robin B. Weisberg.
Cover illustration: From Fig. 1 in Chapter 9, "Klinefelter's Syndome," by John K. Amory and William J. Bremner.
Cover design by Patricia F. Cleary.

For additional copies, pricing for bulk purchases, and/or information about other Humana titles,
contact Humana at the above address or at any of the following numbers: Tel: 973-256-1699;
Fax: 973-256-8341; E-mail: humana@humanapr.com or visit our website at http://humanapress.com

Printed in the United States of America. 10 9 8 7 6 5 4 3 2 1

1-59259-727-0 (e-book)

Library of Congress Cataloging-in-Publication Data

Male hypogonadism : basic, clinical, and therapeutic principles / edited by Stephen J. Winters.
    p. ; cm. -- (Contemporary endocrinology)
Includes bibliographical references and index.
  ISBN 1-58829-131-6 (alk. paper)
  1. Hypogonadism. 2. Generative organs, Male--Diseases.
  [DNLM: 1. Hypogonadism. 2. Genital Diseases, Male. WK 900 M245 2004]
I. Winters, Stephen J. II. Series: Contemporary endocrinology (Totowa, N.J.)
  RC898.M345 2004
  616.6'8--dc21
                                                    2003013034

PREFACE

Recent advances in cellular and molecular biology have markedly increased our understanding of normal and abnormal hypothalamic–pituitary–testicular function. Like other volumes in the *Contemporary Endocrinology* series, the goal of *Male Hypogonadism: Basic, Clinical, and Therapeutic Principles* is to link current knowledge of basic biology to the practice of medicine. The development of new methods for testosterone replacement has substantially increased the number of men who are seeking to determine whether they are hypogonadal, and who are using testosterone replacement therapy, thus mandating a broader understanding of testosterone deficiency.

The chapters of this book were contributed by authors from around the world, and from various scientific and clinical disciplines, who have devoted their careers to the study of the physiology and pathophysiology of the male. Thus, this comprehensive and focused volume is intended for a wide audience encompassing both basic scientists and practicing clinicians. Its scope will provide a wealth of information for students and fellows as well.

Chapters 1–3 review the neuroendocrine regulation of testicular function and provide an overview of Leydig cell steroidogenesis and the normal spermatogenic process in primates. The causes of gonadotropin deficiency and testicular failure are described in Chapters 4–10. The impact of chronic illness on testicular function is the focus of Chapters 11–13. Chapter 14 describes the endocrine mechanism for the decline in testicular function with aging. Chapter 15 summarizes the data supporting an impact of environmental factors on testicular function, whereas Chapters 16 and 17 discuss the testicular consequences of exercise and obesity. Finally, Chapters 18 and 19 provide an overview of androgen replacement therapy and an approach to stimulating spermatogenesis in gonadotropin-deficient men.

I wish to thank the contributors who spent many hours researching, pondering, and preparing their chapters, which collectively are exceedingly informative and clearly presented.

Stephen J. Winters, MD

CONTENTS

CONTRIBUTORS

JOHN K. AMORY, MD • *Department of Medicine, University of Washington, Seattle, WA*

SHALENDER BHASIN, MD • *Department of Medicine, UCLA School of Medicine, Division of Endocrinology, Metabolism, and Molecular Medicine, Charles R. Drew University of Medicine and Science, Los Angeles, CA*

WILLIAM J. BREMNER, MD, PhD • *Department of Medicine, University of Washington, Seattle, WA*

ANNAMARIA COLAO, MD, PhD • *Department of Molecular and Clinical Endocrinology and Oncology, "Federico II" University of Naples, Naples, Italy*

MICHAEL T. COUGHLIN, MA • *Department of Critical Care Medicine, University of Pittsburgh School of Medicine, Pittsburgh, PA*

WILLIAM F. CROWLEY, MD • *Reproductive Endocrine Unit, National Center for Infertility Research, Department of Medicine, Massachusetts General Hospital, Boston, MA*

ALAN C. DALKIN, MD • *Division of Endocrinology, Department of Medicine, University of Virginia, Charlottesville, VA*

MARION DEPENBUSCH, MD • *Institute of Reproductive Medicine of the University, Münster, Germany*

MICHELE DE ROSA, MD • *Department of Molecular and Clinical Endocrinology and Oncology, "Federico II" University of Naples, Italy*

JENNIFER DOBRIDGE, MA • *Department of Exercise and Sport Science, University of North Carolina, Chapel Hill, NC*

QIANG DONG, MD, PhD • *Department of Urology, West China Hospital of Sichuan University, Chengdu, P.R. China*

LEO DUNKEL, MD • *Division of Pediatric Endocrinology, Hospital for Children and Adolescents, Helsinki, Finland*

ANTHONY C. HACKNEY, PhD, FACSM • *Department of Exercise and Sport Science, Department of Nutrition, School of Public Health, and Department of Cell-Molecular Physiology, School of Medicine, University of North Carolina, Chapel Hill, NC*

DAVID J. HANDELSMAN, MB BS, PhD • *ANZAC Research Institute, University of Sydney, Sydney, Australia*

MATTHEW P. HARDY, PhD • *Center for Biomedical Research, Population Council and the Rockefeller University, New York, NY*

AD R. M. M. HERMUS, PhD, MD • *Department of Endocrinology, University Medical Center Nijmegen, Nijmegen, The Netherlands*

SIMON J. HOWELL, MD, MRCP • *Department of Endocrinology, Christie Hospital NHS Trust, Manchester, United Kingdom*

ILPO T. HUHTANIEMI, MD, PhD • *Institute of Reproductive and Developmental Biology, Imperial College London, Faculty of Medicine, London, United Kingdom*

ALI IRANMANESH, MD • *Endocrine Section, Medical Service, Salem Veterans Affairs Medical Center, Salem, VA*

DANIEL KEENAN, PhD • *Department of Statistics, University of Virginia, Charlottesville, VA*

BARRY A. KOGAN, MD • *Division of Urology, Albany Medical College, Albany, NY*

PETER A. LEE, MD, PhD • *Department of Pediatrics, Penn State College of Medicine, The Milton S. Hershey Medical Center, Hershey, PA*

PETER Y. LIU, MB BS, PhD • *Department of Andrology, Concord Hospital, ANZAC Research Institute, University of Sydney, Sydney , Australia*

GAETANO LOMBARDI, MD • *Department of Molecular and Clinical Endocrinology and Oncology, "Federico II" University of Naples, Italy*

GARY R. MARSHALL, PhD • *Department of Medicine, Division of Endocrinology and Metabolism, University of Pittsburgh School of Medicine, Pittsburgh, PA*

EBERHARD NIESCHLAG, MD • *Institute of Reproductive Medicine of the University of Münster, Münster, Germany*

BARTO J. OTTEN, MD, PhD • *Department of Pediatric Endocrinology, University Medical Center Nijmegen, Nijmegen, The Netherlands*

NELLY PITTELOUD, MD • *Reproductive Endocrine Unit, Department of Medicine, National Center for Infertility Research, Massachusetts General Hospital, Boston, MA*

STEPHEN M. SHALET, MD, FRCP • *Department of Endocrinology, Christie Hospital NHS Trust, Manchester, United Kingdom*

RICHARD M. SHARPE, PhD • *MRC Human Reproductive Sciences Unit, Centre for Reproductive Biology, University of Edinburgh, Edinburgh, United Kingdom*

NIKE M. M. L. STIKKELBROECK, PhD, MD • *Department of Pediatric Endocrinology, University Medical Center Nijmegen, Nijmegen, The Netherlands*

RONALD S. SWERDLOFF, MD • *Division of Endocrinology, Department of Medicine, Harbor-UCLA Medical Center and Research and Education Institute, Torrance, CA*

JOHANNES D. VELDHUIS, MD • *Endocrine Research Unit, Mayo Clinic and Foundation, Rochester, MN*

GIOVANNI VITALE, MD • *Department of Molecular and Clinical Endocrinology and Oncology, "Federico II" University of Naples, Italy*

CHRISTINA WANG, MD • *Division of Endocrinology, Department of Medicine, Harbor-UCLA Medical Center and Research and Education Institute, Torrance, CA*

STEPHEN J. WINTERS, MD • *Division of Endocrinology, Metabolism and Diabetes, Department of Medicine, University of Louisville, Louisville, KY*

JOSEPH M. ZMUDA, PhD • *Department of Epidemiology, Graduate School of Public Health, University of Pittsburgh, Pittsburgh, PA*

1

Neuroendocrine Control of Testicular Function

Stephen J. Winters, MD and Alan C. Dalkin, MD

CONTENTS

OVERVIEW

The proximate regulator of testicular function is gonadotropin-releasing hormone (GnRH), which is produced in neurons scattered throughout the anterior hypothalamus. When it reaches the anterior pituitary, GnRH stimulates the synthesis and secretion of the pituitary gonadotropic hormones, luteinizing hormone (LH), and follicle-stimulating hormone (FSH). LH and FSH are released into the circulation in bursts and activate G protein-coupled receptors (GPCRs) on Leydig and Sertoli cells, respectively, that stimulate testosterone production and spermatogenesis. The system is tightly regulated and is maintained at a proper set point by the negative feedback effects of testicular steroids and inhibin-B. Testicular function is also influenced by multiple internal and external environmental factors.

From: *Male Hypogonadism:*
Basic, Clinical, and Therapeutic Principles
Edited by: S. J. Winters © Humana Press Inc., Totowa, NJ

GnRH SYNTHESIS AND SECRETION

GnRH is the proximate regulator of reproduction. GnRH, a C-terminal amidated decapeptide (pGlu-His-Trp-Ser-Tyr-Gly-Leu-Arg-Pro-Gly-NH2), is found in a small number of neurons that are located diffusely throughout the anterior hypothalamus in primates *(1)*. GnRH neurons send axons through subventricular and periventricular pathways to terminate in the capillary space within the median eminence. GnRH from these axons enters the capillaries and is transported in the hypothalamic portal blood to the cells of the anterior pituitary.

Many factors influence the amount of GnRH that is secreted. GnRH mRNA levels are determined by the transcription rate of the pro-GnRH gene, which is controlled by the POU-homeodomain protein, Oct-1, adhesion-related kinase (Ark), and retinoid-X receptors, among other factors *(2)*. Studies in GT1-7 cells, a GnRH-producing murine neuronal cell line, suggest that mRNA stability also plays an important role in maintaining GnRH gene expression. GnRH mRNA levels increase in the hypothalamus of adult male monkeys after bilateral orchidectomy *(3)*, indicating that the testis secretes endocrine hormones, presumably testosterone, that suppress GnRH gene expression. GnRH mRNA transcription produces a pro-GnRH precursor, and yet another control level in GnRH neurons involves the posttranslational processing of the inactive precursor to the active decapeptide. Subsequent to its secretion, peptidases in the median eminence inactivate and thereby further regulate the GnRH concentration.

GnRH, like most hypophysiotropic peptides, is released into the portal blood in bursts. The average GnRH concentration in hypothalamic portal blood (in rams) is approx 20 pg/mL (0.02 nM), and levels in conscious sheep ranged from nadir values of less than 5 pg/mL to pulse peak values of approx 30 pg/ml *(4)*. In those studies, the amplitudes of GnRH pulses in intact, castrated, and testosterone-replaced rams were roughly equivalent; by contrast, GnRH pulse frequency was higher in castrates than in intact animals, and was reduced by testosterone replacement. The implication of those observations is that GnRH secretion rises with testosterone deficiency, primarily because GnRH pulse frequency is accelerated.

GnRH pulse frequency is controlled by the "GnRH pulse generator," the term used to describe the highly synchronized firing of GnRH neurons in the mediobasal hypothalamus (MBH). The belief that changes in cell membrane potentials predispose to bursts of GnRH release is based on the finding that bursts of electrical activity in the MBH in the nonhuman primate coincide with LH secretion pulses *(5)*. The coincident firing of multiple GnRH-expressing neurons may reflect communication by gap junctions, through interneurons, or second messengers. The identification of GnRH-receptors on GnRH neurons and the observation that adding GnRH to GnRH neuronal cultures depresses GnRH pulsatile release provide a possible framework for intraneuronal communication by GnRH *(6)*. Experiments using various 5′ deletion constructs of the GnRH promoter-luciferase vector suggest that episodic GnRH gene expression is a promoter-dependent event that is mediated by Oct-1 *(7)*.

As shown in Fig. 1, GnRH release is influenced by multiple neurotransmitters, including glutamate, γ-aminobutyric acid (GABA), neuropeptide Y, opiates, dopamine, norepinephrine, cyclic adenosine monophosphate (cAMP), and nitric oxide *(8)*. The presence of receptors on GnRH neurons for most of these substances implies that they directly influence GnRH neurons. *N*-methyl-D-aspartate (NMDA) receptors that medi-

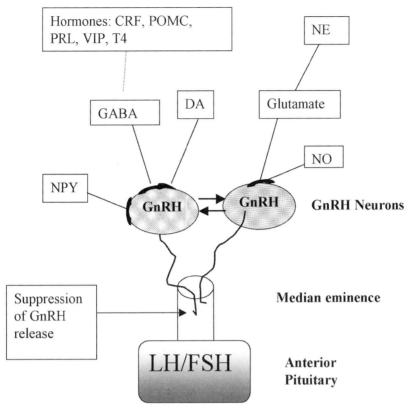

Fig. 1. Diagram showing activation of gonadotropin-releasing hormone (GnRH) neurons by neuro-transmitters and the relationship to the anterior pituitary.

ate glutamate GnRH activation may involve the nitric oxide signaling pathway. Neuro-transmitters with receptors that are not expressed on GnRH neurons may regulate GnRH via synaptic connections between GnRH neurons and other interneurons. GnRH secretion regulation may also occur directly on neuronal axon terminals that abut on capillaries in the median eminence.

A second form of GnRH, GnRH-2 *(9,10)* that was initially identified in nonverte-brates, is also found in the primate brain *(11)*. GnRH-2 activates a unique GnRH-II receptor *(12)* but this receptor is not expressed in humans *(13)*. Thus, the significance of GnRH-2 in humans is not yet known.

GONADOTROPHS AND GnRH RECEPTORS

Gonadotrophs account for 6–10% of the cells of the normal anterior pituitary *(14)*. Gonadotrophs may be small and round or larger and ovoid and are difficult to identify by morphological criteria. Instead, immunostaining, using specific antibodies for LH-β and FSH-β proteins, is used to identify gonadotrophs. In primates *(15)*, as in rodents *(14)*, the majority of gonadotrophs are bihormonal, i.e., they express both LH-β and FSH-β subunit genes. A small fraction of cells express LH or FSH selectively, and

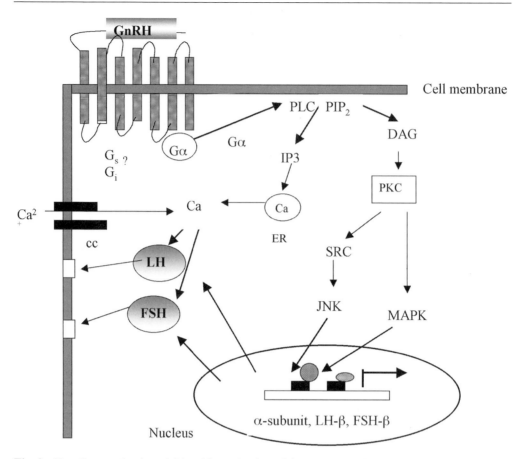

Fig. 2. Signaling mechanisms initiated by activation of the gonadotropin-releasing hormone (GnRH) receptor stimulate gonadortopin synthesis and secretion.

some gonadotrophs produce growth hormones, as well as the gonadotropic hormones. However, the biological significance of these observations remains unclear.

GnRH activates gonadotrophs through both short-term and long-term mechanisms that are illustrated in Fig. 2. After reaching the pituitary, GnRH binds to and activates a cell-surface G protein-coupled receptor (GnRH-R) *(16)*. This receptor is a structurally unique member of the seven-transmembrane G protein-linked receptor family that lacks the long C-terminal intracellular tail that is typical of most GPCRs. This tail is important in the rapid desensitization of other GPCRs, whereas downregulation of the GnRH receptor by GnRH is a relatively delayed event occurring over hours rather than minutes. GnRH binding to its receptor facilitates binding of a G protein to the receptor's third intracellular loop. The bound G protein exchanges guanosine 5′-diphosphate (GDP) for guanosine 5′-triphosphate (GTP) and dissociates into its constituent α and $\beta\gamma$ subunits. The α-subunits are unique to each G protein, whereas the β- and γ-subunits of the different G proteins are similar. The dissociated G protein α-subunit activates downstream signaling pathways *(17)*. Gqα, the major G protein that associates with the GnRH-R, activates membrane-associated phospholipase C to hydrolyze membrane phosphoinositides and increases intracellular inositol phosphates (Ips), including inositol triphosphate $(I_{1,4,5})P3$. IP3 rapidly mobilizes calcium from intracellular stores, and voltage-gated calcium channels open, after which extracellular calcium enters the cell *(17)*. The rise in intracellular free calcium is primarily responsible for the immediate LH and FSH release *(18)*. GnRH receptors may also interact with other G proteins.

The long-term stimulatory effects of GnRH are to increase transcription of the genes for the gonadotropin subunits and for the GnRH receptor. These effects occur primarily through liberation of membrane diacylglycerol (DAG) that, in turn, activates protein kinase C (PKC). The subsequent phosphorylation of subfamilies of mitogen-activated protein kinases (MAP kinases), including members of the Extracellular Signal-regulated Kinase (ERK) and JNK families, initiates nuclear translocation of proteins that bind directly to the 5′ regulatory regions of the gonadotropin subunit and the GnRH-receptor genes or serve as cofactors for promoter activation *(19)*. Increased intracellular calcium also contributes to the transcriptional GnRH effects *(20)*.

GnRH receptors are upregulated by pulsatile GnRH *(21)*. Accordingly, when pulsatile GnRH secretion increases, as in castration or primary testicular failure, GnRH receptors increase. Gonadotrophs become more responsive to GnRH, and the LH response to GnRH stimulation is amplified *(22)*. With continuous GnRH treatment, on the other hand, GnRH receptors decline, followed by a suppression of LH-β and FSH-β mRNAs. This 'homologous desensitization" of the GnRH-R is regulated by several serine-threonine protein kinases, including protein kinase A (PKA) and PKC, as well as by G protein-coupled receptor kinases (GRKs). GnRH receptors also decline with GnRH deficiency.

THE GONADOTROPIC HORMONES

LH and FSH are members of the glycoprotein family of hormones, which also includes thyroid-stimulating hormone (TSH) and human chorionic gonadotropin (hCG). These heterodimers are composed of a common α-subunit and unique β-subunits. The subunits have oligosaccharide chains that are associated with asparagine residues. Each subunit is encoded by a unique gene that is found on a separate chromosome: the human α-subunit gene is on 6p21.1–23, LH-β is on 19q13.3, and FSH-β is on 11p13 (see Chapter 6).

LH and FSH production is directly influenced by the level of the gonadotropin subunit mRNAs. This relationship is especially strong for FSH-β mRNA and FSH secretion. Each of the gonadotropin subunit mRNAs is increased by GnRH, and stimulation of the β-subunit genes by GnRH is primarily transcriptional. Complexes of transcription factors, including SF-1, EGR-1, and SP1, are activators of the LHβ-subunit gene *(23)*, whereas the AP1 proteins fos/jun are important for upregulation of FSH-β transcription by GnRH *(24)*. GnRH stimulation must be pulsatile for LH-β and FSH-β mRNA levels to increase. Transcriptional regulatory proteins that control α-subunit expression include cAMP response element-binding protein (CREB), MAP kinase/ERK1, and GATA-binding proteins *(25)*. α-Subunit gene expression is increased robustly by both pulsatile and continuous GnRH, and GnRH not only stimulates α-subunit transcription but also prolongs the half-life of the α-subunit mRNA *(26)*. Thus, the requirements for α-subunit mRNA upregulation by GnRH are less stringent than those for the β-subunit genes. These factors partly explain why α-subunit is synthesized in excess of β-subunits and why β-subunits are rate limiting for gonadotropin synthesis.

Proteins that are destined for secretion are synthesized on ribosomes that are bound to the endoplasmic reticulum. During the translational process, preformed oligosaccharide chains are linked to the side chain amino group of asparagines on the gonadotropin subunits. As translation continues, sugar moieties are trimmed and the subunits change configuration, allowing for their combination. A region of the β-subunit, termed the "seatbelt," wraps around the α-subunit loop 2 *(27)*. Dimeric LH and FSH are segregated in the endoplasmic reticulum (er) and transferred to the Golgi, where they are concentrated in secretory granules. These protein-rich vesicles subsequently fuse with the plasma membrane after GnRH stimulation. This process is termed "exocytosis." There is evidence that FSH-containing granules are also exported directly to the plasma membrane, independent of GnRH pulsatile stimulation. This mode of secretion allows for FSH secretion between pulses. Gonadotrophs also secrete uncombined α-subunit, both in pulsatile fashion and continuously.

PULSATILE GONADOTROPIN SECRETION

Experiments in ovariectomized rhesus monkeys rendered gonadotropin deficient with hypothalamic lesions led to the proposal that an intermittent pattern of GnRH secretion was necessary for normal LH secretion *(28)*. In those animals, GnRH administered in pulses stimulated LH secretion, but GnRH administered continuously was much less effective. The pulsatile nature of LH secretion was subsequently established in all species, including man *(29)*. Accordingly, LH secretion is stimulated when GnRH is administered in pulses to patients who are gonadotropin deficient but not when GnRH is administered continuously *(30)*. An understanding of these physiological principles led to the use of pulsatile GnRH as a treatment to stimulate fertility and to the development of long-acting GnRH analogs that produce a biochemical gonadectomy as a treatment for patients with prostate cancer and other androgen-dependent disorders *(31)*.

With current assays, GnRH is undetectable in the peripheral circulation. Therefore, GnRH secretion cannot be studied directly in humans. Instead, changes in circulating LH levels are used as a surrogate marker for GnRH pulse generator activity. LH secretion is determined by the frequency, amplitude, and duration of its secretory pulses. Presumably because of its longer circulating half-life, FSH pulses are less clearly defined in peripheral blood than are LH pulses. FSH pulses are clearly evident in jugular blood (in ewes) where clearance effects are minimized *(32)*.

Cultured pituitary cells that are perifused with GnRH pulses are a powerful model, yielding important information on GnRH actions and other factors that regulate gonadotropin secretion under controlled conditions. Using this experimental approach, shown in Fig. 3, episodes of LH, as well as FSH secretion, are distinct and short lived, with a rapid upstroke and abrupt termination. LH pulse amplitude is directly proportional to the GnRH dose administered, and the median duration of an LH pulse approx 25 min.

In contrast to the regularity of LH pulses produced by a constant dose of GnRH in vitro, Fig. 4 illustrates that LH pulses in the peripheral circulation in man vary in amplitude and that interpulse intervals are inconstant. LH pulses in vivo are also characterized by a less rapid upstroke and a slower decline from the peak than are pulses in vitro. This

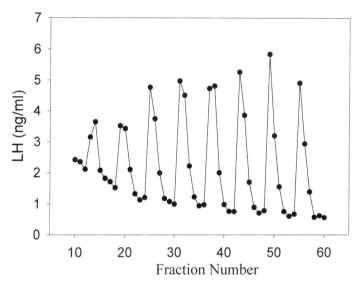

Fig. 3. Secretion of luteinizing hormone (LH) by pituitary cells from adult male primates perifused with pulses of gonadotropin-releasing hormone (GnRH). Pulses of GnRH (2.5 nM) were applied to the cells every 1 hr for 2 min. Fractions of the column effluent were collected every 10 min, and LH was measured in the media by immunoassay. (Data from ref. *56.*)

presumably reflects dilution of secreted hormone by plasma in the general circulation and the influence of LH clearance by the liver and kidney. Whether LH is released in the basal interval between GnRH-initiated secretory episodes has been debated, but this mode of secretion is small and is probably not biologically important.

Hormone pulse detection has been standardized by the development of computer algorithms *(33)*. Using this approach, objective assessment of the frequency and amplitude characteristics of hormone pulses has been possible. LH secretion pulses occur throughout the day and night in normal adult men. However, estimates of the LH frequency (GnRH) pulses in men have varied based on the intensity and duration of the blood sampling protocol, the assay used to measure LH, and the algorithm used to identify pulses. Most investigators have proposed an average frequency of 1 LH pulse every 1–2 h for normal men, but, interestingly, there is a large between-individual variation *(34)*. Because of variability in pulse amplitude and frequency, the distinction between true and artifactual pulses is difficult. One approach is to coanalyze LH and uncombined α-subunit pulses *(34),* because α-subunit is released into the circulation by GnRH, together with LH and FSH (*see* Fig. 4). According to this logic, concordant LH and α-subunit fluctuations presumably reflect true GnRH pulsatile signals. There is generally a positive relationship between LH pulse amplitude and the preceding interpulse interval, in part because a longer interval allows for the circulating level to decline to a lower baseline value.

In addition to moment-to-moment pulsatile pattern of LH secretion, there is a diurnal rhythm in circulating LH, as well as testosterone levels, in pubertal boys with increased LH pulsatile amplitude during sleep and increased testosterone levels in the early morning hours *(35)*. Although there is a diurnal variation in plasma testosterone in adults, there is no clear diurnal rhythm for LH in most adult men *(36),* implying that the diurnal variation in testosterone levels in men is only partly

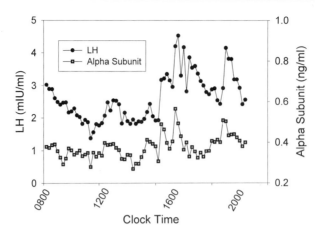

Fig. 4. Circulating luteinizing hormone (LH) and α-subunit levels in a normal adult man. Blood samples were drawn every 10 min for 12 h beginning at 0800 h and measured for LH using Nichols Allegro LH 2-site assay and a specific assay double antibody immunoassay for α-subunit.

LH controlled. The diurnal testosterone variation in men is disrupted by fragmented sleep *(37),* but the mechanism for this alteration has not been established. The diurnal variation in testosterone is blunted in older men *(38)* and in young men with testicular failure *(39).*

LH CONTROL OF TESTOSTERONE SYNTHESIS

Testosterone, a C19 3-keto, 17β-hydroxy Δ4 steroid, is synthesized from cholesterol through a series of cytochrome P450- and dehydrogenase-dependent enzymatic reactions *(40).* The conversion of cholesterol to pregnenolone occurs within mitochondria and is catalyzed by P450scc, the cytochrome P450 side-chain cleavage enzyme. Pregnenolone exits the mitochondria and can be converted to testosterone by two alternative routes that are referred to as the Δ^4-pathway or the Δ^5-pathway, based on whether the steroid intermediates are 3-keto, Δ^4 steroids (Δ^4) or 3-hydroxy, Δ^5 steroids (Δ^5). Classical experiments using human testicular microsomes incubated with radiolabeled steroids revealed that the Δ^5-pathway predominates in the human testis. In that pathway, C17 hydroxylation of pregnenolone to form 17α-hydroxypregnenolone is followed by cleavage of the C17-C20 bond of 17α-hydroxypregnenolone to produce dehydroepiandrosterone (DHEA). Oxidation of the 3β-hydroxy group and isomerization of the C5-C6 double bond of DHEA by 3β-hydroxysteroid dehydrogenase/Δ^5–Δ^4 isomerase (3βHSD) forms androstenedione. The C17 keto group of androstenedione is oxidized to a hydroxyl group by 17β-hydroxysteroid dehydrogenase (17β HSD) producing testosterone (*see* Chapter 2).

In the Δ^4-pathway that predominates in rodents, pregnenolone is metabolized to progesterone by 3βHSD. Progesterone is hydroxylated at C17 to produce 17α-hydroxyprogesterone, followed by cleavage of the C17-C20 bond of 17α-hydroxyprogesterone to produce androstenedione. Cytochrome P450c17 catalyzes both reactions. Finally, the C17 keto group of androstenedione is oxidized to a hydroxy group by 17β HSD to produce testosterone.

LH stimulates testosterone biosynthesis in Leydig cells through a G protein-associated seven-transmembrane receptor *(41)*. LH binding to the receptor initiates a signaling cascade by activating Gs that stimulate adenylate cyclase activity and increase intracellular cAMP levels to activate cAMP-dependent protein kinase A (PKA). cAMP-dependent PKA stimulates testosterone synthesis in at least two ways. An acute response, within minutes of hormonal stimulation, is characterized by an increase in cholesterol transport into the mitochondria and is mediated by the steroidogenic acute regulatory (StAR) protein *(42)*. StAR functions at the mitochondrial outer membrane, but how it regulates cholesterol transport is not known. The chronic response to LH, which requires several hours, involves transcriptional activation of the genes encoding the steroidogenic enzymes of the testosterone biosynthetic pathway, P450scc, P450c17, 3βHSD, and 17βHSD.

Other factors that stimulate testosterone synthesis directly include PRL, GH, T3, PACAP, VIP, and inhibin, whereas glucocorticoids, estradiol, activin, AVP, CRF, and IL-1 reduce testosterone production by Leydig cells. Although controversial for many years, recent experiments with recombinant FSH suggest that FSH is not an important regulator of Leydig cell function *(43,44)*. However, unidentified Sertoli cell proteins regulated by the FSH receptor may stimulate testosterone biosynthesis.

The blood production rate of testosterone in normal adult men has been estimated to range from 5000 to 7500 µg/24 h *(45)*, and levels of total testosterone in normal men range from 250 to 1000 ng/dL (10–40 nmol/L) in most assays. The testosterone level in adult men declines by more than 95% if the testes are removed. The remainder of the testosterone is derived from androstenedione and DHEA production by the adrenal cortex.

ESTROGENS IN MALES

Normal men produce approx 40 µg of estradiol and 60 µg of estrone per day. Estradiol is produced from testosterone and estrone from androstenedione, by aromatase P450, the product of the CYP19 gene *(46)*. This microsomal enzyme oxidizes the C19 angular methyl group to produce a phenolic A ring. Aromatase mRNA is expressed in adult Leydig cells, where it is activated by LH/hCG *(47)*. However, most of the estrogen in men is derived from aromatase in adipose and skin stromal cells, aortic smooth muscle cells, kidney, skeletal cells, and the brain. The promoter sequences of the extragonadal and testicular and P450 aromatase genes are distinct and tissue specific, resulting from differential splicing, but the translated protein is the same in all tissues. The factors that regulate extratesticular aromatase are not well understood.

Exogenous estrogens suppress testosterone production and disrupt spermatogenesis by reducing GnRH secretion and decreasing responsiveness to GnRH *(48)*. It is now known that there are two forms of the ER that are encoded by separate genes and play a role in reproduction *(49)*. These genes have been designated ER-α and ER-β. ER-α is the dominant form in the pituitary and hypothalamus, whereas ER-α and ER-β are both found in the testis, prostate, and epididymis *(50)*. Clinical findings in an adult man with an inactivating mutation of the ER-α and in two men with mutations of the CYP19 aromatase gene (reviewed *51*), together with results from mice in which estrogen receptors *(49)* or aromatase *(52)* have been "knocked-out," have enhanced understanding of the importance of estradiol in the neuroendocrine control of testicular function, as described

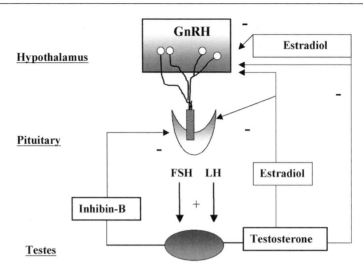

Fig. 5. Diagram of the negative feedback control of gonadotropin secretion by testicular hormones.

in the section on testicular control of gonadotropin secretion. Dilatation and atrophy of the seminiferous tubules are also found in ER-α-deficient mice, implying an effect of estrogen to regulate the efferent ductules of the testis. Aromatase-deficient mice although fertile in early life, develop infertility. Thus, estradiol is essential for male fertility.

TESTICULAR CONTROL OF GONADOTROPIN SECRETION

Gonadotropin secretion, although upregulated by GnRH, is maintained at physiological levels through testicular negative feedback mechanisms summarized in Fig. 5. Accordingly, plasma LH and FSH levels decrease after testosterone or estradiol administration and rise when negative feedback is disrupted by castration.

The process of negative feedback control of LH and FSH by gonadal steroids in males is partly species-specific. There is considerable evidence in primates that androgens suppress LH synthesis and secretion primarily through an action on the GnRH pulse generator. For example, LH pulse frequency and amplitude are elevated in castrated primates, and are suppressed by testosterone replacement *(53)*. Furthermore, when male rhesus monkeys were rendered gonadotropin deficient with radiofrequency lesions and stimulated with GnRH pulses, LH secretion increased little after bilateral orchidectomy, until GnRH pulse frequency was increased *(54)*. In addition, expression of the mRNAs for GnRH *(3)*, as well as pituitary GnRH-receptors, and the gonadotropin subunit genes are increased in orchidectomized monkeys *(55)*. Moreover, when pituitary cells from adult male monkeys were stimulated with GnRH pulses, no inhibition of GnRH-induced LH secretion by testosterone or DHT occurred. In pituitary cells from rats, on the other hand, the gonadotroph is a direct site of testosterone-negative feedback control, because GnRH-stimulated LH pulses were suppressed in amplitude by testosterone and α-subunit gene expression was reduced *(56)*.

GnRH-deficient men represent a human model to examine the effects of testicular steroids on the hypothalamus and pituitary. When such patients were treated with fixed

Table 1
Hormone Levels in a Man With a Mutation of the Estrogen Receptorα
and Two Men Deficient in Aromatase

Age (yr)	Testosterone (ng/dL)	Estradiol (pg/mL)	Luteinizing Hormone (mIU/mL)	Follicle-Stimulating Hormone (mIU/mL)	Reference
28	445	119	37 (2.0–20)	33 (2.0–15)	Smith et al. (57)
24	2015	<7	26.1 (2.0–9.9)	28.3 (5.0–9.9)	Morishina et al. (58)
31	523	<10	5.6 (1.4–8.9)	17.1 (1.7–6.9)	Carini et al. (59)

Luteinizing hormone and follicle-stimulating hormone levels in parentheses are the normal ranges reported in those references.

GnRH doses (57), testosterone suppressed LH secretion less than in normal men, implying that testosterone controls GnRH secretion. Moreover, suppression by testosterone was blocked by the aromatase inhibitor testolactone (57), and in separate experiments, dihydrotestosterone had no effect (58). Together, these data imply that the pituitary effect of testosterone to inhibit LH was through bioconversion to estradiol.

Whether it is testosterone and/or the estradiol derived from testosterone by aromatase in the central nervous system or in peripheral tissues that controls LH secretion is of considerable interest. The finding that dihydrotestosterone (DHT), a nonaromatizable androgen, decreases LH pulse frequency strongly supports a role for androgens in the regulation of the GnRH pulse generator. Furthermore, LH pulse frequency is increased in patients with nonfunctional androgen receptors (AR) in the complete androgen insensitivity syndrome, indicating that AR signaling regulates GnRH pulse frequency (59).

Estradiol also plays an important physiological role in the negative feedback control of gonadotropin secretion in men. This control mechanism was suggested by pharmacological studies using the estrogen antagonist clomiphene (60) or the aromatase inhibitor testolactone (61). When those drugs were administered to normal men, circulating LH and FSH levels rose, together with plasma testosterone concentrations. More recently, as shown in Table 1, gonadotropin and testosterone levels increased in a man with an inactivating mutation of the estrogen receptor-α (62) and in two men with mutations in the aromatase gene (63,64). In these models, even though androgen levels were increased, estrogen blockade or deficiency was associated with increased gonadotropin secretion. Moreover, in one man with aromatase deficiency, estrogen treatment suppressed serum gonadotropin levels. The finding that clomiphene increased LH pulse frequency (60) indicated that the negative feedback action of estradiol was partly at the level of the GnRH pulse generator. This finding was recently confirmed and extended using the aromatase inhibitors anastrazole (65). Estradiol treatment also decreases the LH response to GnRH stimulation in men (66) and in primate pituitary cells perifused with GnRH pulses, (56) indicating an additional direct negative effect on the pituitary gland.

GnRH neurons appear by autoradiography and immunocytochemistry to lack both androgen and estrogen receptors. Thus, the mechanism for their effect on GnRH neurons is believed to involve transsynaptic or neuronal-glial interactions or nongenomic membrane effects.

INHIBIN, ACTIVIN, AND FSH

There are both similarities and differences in how FSH secretion is regulated when compared to LH. The synthesis and secretion of LH as well as FSH is stimulated by GnRH and suppressed by gonadal steroid hormones through GnRH suppression. However, two paracrine factors, pituitary activin and follistatin, and testicular inhibin-B selectively regulate FSH secretion by regulating FSH-β gene expression *(67)*. Because of these unique control mechanisms for FSH, LH and FSH secretion are sometimes dissociated.

Activin, a member of the TGF-β family of growth factors, stimulates FSH-β mRNA transcription and prolongs FSH-β mRNA half-life *(68–70)*. Activin is a dimeric peptide composed of two similar subunits that were designated as β-subunits because the identification of activin followed the cloning of inhibin, an α-β heterodimer. There are at least four forms the β subunit: $β_A$, $β_B$, $β_C$, and $β_D$. The pituitary expresses $β_B$, and activin-B ($β_Bβ_B$) is the predominate form in the pituitary, whereas most other tissues produce activin-A. Activin functions in neural and mesodermal morphogenesis, wound healing, vascular remodeling, and inflammation, as well as in reproduction *(71–74)*.

In the process of activin signaling (*see* Fig. 6), a series of events, including the activation of intracellular messengers, is involved. Initially, the activin ligand binds to a specific type II receptor subunit, either ActRII or IIB *(75–77)*. Subsequent to ligand binding, the type II subunit pairs with a type I receptor subunit (either ActRI or IB) and forms a heteromeric complex at the cell surface *(78–80)*. It is believed that the serine/threonine kinase of the type II subunit is responsible for phosphorylation of the type I subunit, thereby initiating postreceptor signaling/phosphorylation (see *81* for review). Although several potential postreceptor targets have been proposed, the best characterized family involved in activin signaling includes the mothers against dpp-related (Smad) proteins (see *81–83* for reviews).

The initial family member, MAD, was identified in *Drosophila* and was downstream to the BMP receptor (also a member of the TGF-β family) *(84)*. Thereafter, the mammalian Smads were identified *(85–92)*. In relation to the activin response system, Smad-2 and Smad-3 are primarily involved, partnering with Smad-4 (also known as DPC4) to convey the postreceptor signal to the nucleus *(85–89)*. The Smad-2 gene product, when overexpressed in *Xenopus* ectodermal explants, induces mesodermal differentiation similar to activin *(85,90)*. Yet, both Smad-2 and Smad-3 associate with activin receptors (and TGF-β receptors for the Smad-3), whereby after activin/activin receptor binding, they undergo phosphorylation and then translocation from cytoplasm to nucleus *(81,87,89,91)*.

Activin actions may use the signaling Smads in a tissue-specific fashion. In the rat ovary, Smad-2 mRNA and protein expression are significantly higher and may vary with follicular development when compared with Smad-3 mRNA, which was expressed at a low, constant level *(92)*. A nuclear target for Smad-2 is likely in mammals in light of data obtained in *Xenopus,* where Smad-2 is involved in the activin-mediated activation of the MIX.2 gene via binding to FAST-1 (a winged-helix DNA-binding protein now known as FoxH1) *(93)*. In addition, a second forkhead domain protein, FAST2, may play a role in the transduction of activin signals to the nucleus *(94)*. Smad-2 expression is also likely to be under physiologic regulation, with protein content increasing in granulosa cells during follicular development and Smad-2 protein and mRNA concentrations increasing with TGF-β treatment *(95)*.

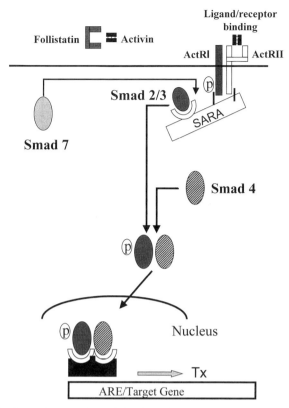

Fig. 6. A diagram for activin signaling through Smad proteins.

As noted previously, Smad-2 mediated actions likely involve association with Smad-4 and the formation of hetero-oligomers *(86)*. Smad-4 is essential for activin signaling, because transfection of a constitutively active Smad-4 construct alone can induce activin-like effects, whereas cellular expression of Smad-2 alone does not confer responsiveness *(86)*. Furthermore, the Smad-2/3 binding to Smad-4 may represent an additional regulatory site in light of data suggesting the presence of "inhibitory" Smads. Smad-6 and -7 do not contain a C-terminal region required for phosphorylation and, therefore, their activation is not regulated by kinases *(89,96)*. Data regarding physiologic regulation of the inhibitory Smads' gene or protein expression are currently lacking, but TGF-β can rapidly (30–60 min) induce Smad-7 mRNA expression in COS cells *(97)*. Therefore, alteration in Smad-7 (or Smad-6) could represent an important mechanism in modulating activin action.

Activin actions are antagonized by follistatin that binds to and neutralizes the bioactivity of activin, as well as by inhibin that competes with activin for binding to the activin receptor *(98)*. Inhibin is an antagonist of activin because it fails to initiate intracellular SMAD signaling. Betaglycan, a membrane proteoglycan, functions as an accessory receptor binding protein for inhibin, as well as for TGF-β, and functions in inhibin suppression of activin signaling *(99)*. Follistatin is structurally unrelated to activin and inhibin but, like activin, is found in all tissues examined. In the rat pituitary gland, follistatin is upregulated by activin, GnRH, and pituitary adenylate cyclase-activating polypeptide (PACAP) and is suppressed by testosterone and by follistatin, no doubt through binding to activin. In primate pituitary cultures, on the other hand, GnRH is ineffective, and testosterone, as well as activin, increases follistatin expression (100). Pituitary follistatin influences the FSH and LH response to castration. Follistatin expression increases after orchidectomy in adult male rats (101), and there is a reciprocal relationship over time between follistatin and FSH-β gene expression, implying that follistatin attenuates the FSH castration response in that species. In male primates, including man, by contrast, the follistatin mRNA level is unaffected by bilateral orchidectomy and FSH-β mRNA increases approx 50-fold (55). Thus, follistatin functions as a brake on FSH production in male rodents but not in primates.

Inhibin is produced by Sertoli cells and by fetal Leydig cells and plays a fundamental role in the selective regulation of FSH (102). Inhibin may also be an intragonadal regulator, but that function of inhibin is less well understood. The term inhibin was first applied in 1932 (103) to the aqueous extract of bull testis that prevented the development of castration cells within the anterior pituitary and was distinguished from androitin, which was present in the ether extract and stimulated prostate growth, and is now known as testosterone.

Inhibin is a heterodimer of an α-subunit and one of two β-subunits, β_A and β_B. Of these, only the β_B subunit is expressed by the testis, and, therefore, testicular inhibin is inhibin B. The inhibin α-subunit gene is upregulated by FSH, whereas the factors regulating the β_B subunit gene are not well understood. The level of inhibin/activin β_B mRNA in the rat testis is unaffected by hypophysectomy or by FSH treatment (103a). Transcription factors of the GATA-binding protein family regulate both the inhibin β- and the α-subunit promoters (104). Control of inhibin β_B by a germ cell factor is suggested by the decline in plasma inhibin-B levels, but not inhibin-α subunit levels, that follow destruction of germ cells by cancer chemotherapy (105).

Because inhibin suppresses FSH secretion (106), plasma inhibin-B and FSH concentrations are inversely related in normal men and are more strongly correlated inversely when values from men with primary testicular failure are included in the analysis (107). The relationship between circulating inhibin-B and FSH in normal men differs from that between serum LH and testosterone, which is bidirectional. Consequently, there is no correlation between circulating LH and testosterone among normal men. The different relationships between plasma LH with testosterone compared to FSH with inhibin-B levels was clearly demonstrated in experiments conducted by Ramaswamy et al. (108). These investigators removed one testis from adult male rhesus monkeys, after which the plasma levels of both testosterone and inhibin B decreased. However, the decline in testosterone was brief and was restored to normal by a rise in LH, whereas inhibin-B levels remained at approx 50% of baseline values for up to 6 wk, even though FSH levels rose. Similarly, Anawalt et al. (107) found that large FSH doses were required to increase circulating inhibin B levels in normal men. Thus, LH and testosterone form a classical feed-forward/feedback loop in adults, whereas inhibin-B controls FSH but is less dependent on FSH stimulation. Inhibin-B levels increase during the neonatal phase of development and again at puberty. Although plasma LH and FSH levels rise at these developmental stages, the number of Sertoli cells also increases. Furthermore, studies in adult monkeys showed a strong positive correlation between circulating inhibin-B levels and Sertoli cell number (109).

Thus, circulating inhibin-B reflects the number and function of Sertoli cells and is less dependent on FSH stimulation.

FSH activates a G protein-associated seven-transmembrane Sertoli cell receptor *(110)*. The activated receptor stimulates adenylate cyclase and increases intracellular cAMP levels. Numerous Sertoli cell genes are activated by cAMP, most often through cAMP-dependent PKA, with subsequent phosphorylation of the CREB transcription factor. The role of FSH in spermatogenesis is, however, a matter of controversy (*see* Chapter 6). The classical view was that FSH stimulates spermatogenesis and that LH stimulated testosterone production. However, spermatogenesis is qualitatively maintained by testosterone alone in hypophysectomized rats or in rats immunized against GnRH. More recently, men with an inactivating mutation of the FSH-R gene were identified in Finland. The testes of the five homozygous men were reduced in size and the sperm count and or motility was reduced, but two men were fertile *(111)*. Moreover, an FSH-β-deficient mouse was developed, and was likewise fertile *(112)*, implying that FSH is not essential for male fertility. On the other hand, spermatogenesis is not quantitatively normal in these models, and FSH acts synergistically with testosterone in rodents or with hCG in men, implying a role for FSH receptor activation in spermatogenesis. Species differences in the progression of undifferentiated spermatogonia and in the production of FSH independent of GnRH, may explain why FSH is less important in rodents than in primates.

Activin, inhibin, and follistatin may also act locally in the testes to regulate reproductive function. Activin receptor gene expression has been detected in Sertoli cells, primary spermatocytes and round spermatids, and radiolabeled activin-A binding has been demonstrated in the latter cell types *(113–115)*. Both proposed inhibin receptors, betaglycan and InhBP/p120, are present in rat Ledig cells *(99,116)*, and betaglycan is expressed in germ cells *(117)*. In general, activin treatment reduces hCG-driven Leydig cell production of androgens *(118)*, whereas inhibin action can prevent activin effects *(118)* and stimulates testosterone release in some *(119)*, but not all *(120)*, studies. In terms of actions on gamete production, activin and inhibin have opposing actions with activin-stimulating *(121)* and inhibin-reducing *(122,123)* spermatogenesis. Thus, the balance of activin and inhibin (and potentially follistatin), directly in the testes, may affect both endocrine signals via altered testosterone production, as well as gamete maturation.

NEUROENDOCRINE MECHANISMS FOR
THE DIFFERENTIAL CONTROL OF FSH AND LH

In addition to the selective regulation of FSH-β mRNA levels by pituitary activin and follistatin and by testicular inhibin-B, there may be other mechanisms for the differential secretion of FSH and LH. Results from studies in rats *(124)* and rat pituitary cell cultures *(125)* revealed that the frequency of GnRH pulses regulates LH-β and FSH-β mRNA levels differently, with rapid GnRH pulse frequencies (every 15–30 min) favoring LH-β over FSH-β gene expression. This difference may be partly due to upregulation of follistatin mRNA levels by rapid GnRH pulse frequencies *(125)*, with subsequent blockade by follistatin of activin-stimulated FSH-β gene expression. Although this mechanism is applicable to rats, its importance in men is less well established. For example, in men with congenital hypogonadotropic hypogonadism (e.g., Kallmann syndrome) who were treated long-term with pulsatile GnRH, increasing the frequency of GnRH stimulation from every 2 h to every 30 min for 7 d increased serum LH levels threefold, but FSH levels rose by 50% *(126)*. These findings are consistent with the greater rise in LH than in FSH secretion when normal men are administered a GnRH bolus. In a second study in a similar population of men, increasing the GnRH pulse frequency from every 1.5 h to every 0.5 h suppressed plasma FSH, but plasma LH levels were unchanged *(127)*. In both studies, changes in testosterone, estradiol, and inhibin-B levels as a consequence of increased GnRH may have influenced the results. PACAP is a neuropeptide that stimulates α-subunit transcription and lengthens LH-β mRNA transcripts and presumably prolongs half-life but suppresses FSH-β mRNA levels by stimulating follistatin transcription *(128)*. These observations in vitro suggest that PACAP could play a role in the differential production of FSH and LH. A third idea is that increasing the frequency of GnRH pulses modifies GnRH-receptor signaling pathways and thereby regulates FSH-β and LH-β gene expression differently *(129)*.

CONCLUSION

This chapter provides background information on the normal function of the hypothalamic–pituitary–testicular unit in men. The recent growth of understanding of this system through the application molecular and cellular methods is impressive. In the following chapters, conditions that disrupt these normal processes are discussed.

REFERENCES

1. Goldsmith PC, Song T, Kim EJ, Boggan JE. Location of the neuroendocrine gonadotropin-releasing hormone neurons in the monkey hypothalamus by retrograde tracing and immunostaining. J Neuroendocrinol 1990;2:157–168.
2. Kepa JK, Spaulding AJ, Jacobsen BM, et al. Structure of the distal human gonadotropin releasing hormone (hGnrh) gene promoter and functional analysis in Gt1-7 neuronal cells. Nucleic Acids Res 1996;24:3614–3620.
3. El Majdoubi M, Sahu A, Plant TM. Changes in hypothalamic gene expression associated with the arrest of pulsatile gonadotropin-releasing hormone release during infancy in the agonadal male rhesus monkey *(Macaca mulatta)*. Endocrinology 2000;141:3273–3277.
4. Caraty A, Locatelli A. Effect of time after castration on secretion of LHRH and LH in the ram. J Reprod Fertil 1988;82:263–269.
5. Knobil E. The electrophysiology of the GnRH pulse generator in the rhesus monkey. J Steroid Biochem 1989;33:669–671.
6. Krsmanovic LZ, Martinez-Fuentes AJ, Arora KK, et al. Local regulation of gonadotroph function by pituitary gonadotropin-releasing hormone. Endocrinology 2000;141:1187–1195.
7. Vazquez-Martinez R, Leclerc GM, Wierman ME, Boockfor FR. Episodic activation of the rat GnRH promoter: role of the homeoprotein oct-1. Mol Endocrinol 2002;16:2093–2100.
8. Urbanski HF, Kohama SG, Garyfallou VT. Mechanisms mediating the response of GnRH neurones to excitatory amino acids. Rev Reprod 1996;1:173–181.
9. White RB, Eisen JA, Kasten TL, Fernald RD. Second gene for gonadotropin-releasing hormone in humans. Proc Natl Acad Sci USA 1998;95:305–309.
10. Sherwood NM, Lovejoy DA, Coe IR. Origin of mammalian gonadotropin-releasing hormones. Endocr Rev 1993;14:241–254.
11. Lescheid DW, Terasawa E, Abler LA, et al. A second form of gonadotropin-releasing hormone (GnRH) with characteristics of chicken GnRH-II is present in the primate brain. Endocrinology 1997;138:5618–5629.
12. Neill JD, Duck LW, Sellers JC, Musgrove LC. A gonadotropin-releasing hormone (GnRH) receptor specific for GnRH II in primates. Biochem Biophys Res Comm 2001;282:1012–1018.

13. van Biljon W, Wykes S, Scherer S, Krawetz SA, Hapgood J. Type II gonadotropin-releasing hormone receptor transcripts in human sperm. Biol Reprod 2002;67:1741–1749.
14. Childs GV. Division of labor among gonadotropes. Vitam Horm 1995;50:215–286.
15. Okada Y, Fujii Y, Moore JP, Jr., Winters SJ. Androgen receptors in gonadotrophs in pituitary cultures from adult male monkeys and rats. Endocrinology 2003;144:267–273.
16. Shacham S, Harris D, Ben-Shlomo H, et al. Mechanism of GnRH receptor signaling on gonadotropin release and gene expression in pituitary gonadotrophs. Vitam Horm 2001;63:63–90.
17. Stojilkovic SS, Reinhart J, Catt KJ. Gonadotropin-releasing hormone receptors: structure and signal transduction pathways. Endocr Rev 1994;15:462–499.
18. Conn PM, Janovick JA, Stanislaus D, Kuphal D, Jennes L. Molecular and cellular bases of gonadotropin-releasing hormone action in the pituitary and central nervous system. Vitam Horm 1995;50:151–214.
19. Weck J, Anderson AC, Jenkins S, Fallest PC, Shupnik MA. Divergent and composite gonadotropin-releasing hormone-responsive elements in the rat luteinizing hormone subunit genes. Mol Endocrinol 2000;14:472–485.
20. Haisenleder DJ, Yasin M, Marshall JC. Gonadotropin subunit and gonadotropin-releasing hormone receptor gene expression are regulated by alterations in the frequency of calcium pulsatile signals. Endocrinology 1997;138:5227–5230.
21. Kaiser UB, Jakubowiak A, Steinberger A, Chin WW. Regulation of rat pituitary gonadotropin-releasing hormone receptor mRNA levels in vivo and in vitro. Endocrinology 1993;133:931–934.
22. Clayton RN, Catt KJ. Gonadotropin-releasing hormone receptors: characterization, physiological regulation, and relationship to reproductive function. Endocr Rev 1981;2:186–209.
23. Kaiser UB, Halvorson LM, Chen MT. Sp1, steroidogenic factor 1 (SF-1), and early growth response protein 1 (egr-1) binding sites form a tripartite gonadotropin-releasing hormone response element in the rat luteinizing hormone-beta gene promoter: an integral role for SF-1. Mol Endocrinol 2000;14:1235–1245.
24. Strahl BD, Huang HJ, Sebastian J, Ghosh BR, Miller WL. Transcriptional activation of the ovine follicle-stimulating hormone beta-subunit gene by gonadotropin-releasing hormone: involvement of two activating protein-1-binding sites and protein kinase C. Endocrinology 1998;139:4455–4465.
25. Maurer RA, Kim KE, Schoderbek WE, Roberson MS, Glenn DJ. Regulation of glycoprotein hormone alpha-subunit gene expression. Recent Prog Horm Res 1999;54:455–484.
26. Chedrese PJ, Kay TW, Jameson JL. Gonadotropin-releasing hormone stimulates glycoprotein hormone alpha-subunit messenger ribonucleic acid (mRNA) levels in alpha T3 cells by increasing transcription and mRNA stability. Endocrinology 1994;134:2475–2481.
27. Xing Y, Williams C, Campbell RK, et al. Threading of a glycosylated protein loop through a protein hole: implications for combination of human chorionic gonadotropin subunits. Protein Sci 2001;10:226–235.
28. Belchetz PE, Plant TM, Nakai Y, Keogh EJ, Knobil E. Hypophysial responses to continuous and intermittent delivery of hypopthalamic gonadotropin-releasing hormone. Science 1978;202:631–633.
29. Nankin HR, Troen P. Repetitive luteinizing hormone elevations in serum of normal men. J Clin Endocrinol Metab 1971;33:558–560.
30. Crowley WF, Jr., McArthur JW. Simulation of the normal menstrual cycle in Kallman's syndrome by pulsatile administration of luteinizing hormone-releasing hormone (LHRH). J Clin Endocrinol Metab 1980;51:173–175.
31. Labrie F. Endocrine therapy for prostate cancer. Endocrinol Metab Clin North Am 1991;20:845–872.
32. Padmanabhan V, McFadden K, Mauger DT, Karsch FJ, Midgley AR, Jr. Neuroendocrine control of follicle-stimulating hormone (FSH) secretion. I. Direct evidence for separate episodic and basal components of FSH secretion. Endocrinology 1997;138:424–432.
33. Veldhuis JD, Johnson ML. Testing pulse detection algorithms with simulations of episodically pulsatile substrate, metabolite, or hormone release. Methods Enzymol 1994;240:377–415.
34. Spratt DI, Carr DB, Merriam GR, Scully RE, Rao PN, Crowley WF, Jr. The spectrum of abnormal patterns of gonadotropin-releasing hormone secretion in men with idiopathic hypogonadotropic hypogonadism: clinical and laboratory correlations. J Clin Endocrinol Metab 1987;64:283–291.
35. Boyar RM, Rosenfeld RS, Kapen S, et al. Human puberty. Simultaneous augmented secretion of luteinizing hormone and testosterone during sleep. J Clin Invest 1974;54:609–618.
36. Tenover JS, Matsumoto AM, Clifton DK, Bremner WJ. Age-related alterations in the circadian rhythms of pulsatile luteinizing hormone and testosterone secretion in healthy men. J Gerontol 1988;43:M163–M169.

37. Luboshitzky R, Zabari Z, Shen-Orr Z, Herer P, Lavie P. Disruption of the nocturnal testosterone rhythm by sleep fragmentation in normal men. J Clin Endocrinol Metab 2001;86:1134–1139.

38. Bremner WJ, Vitiello MV, Prinz PN. Loss of circadian rhythmicity in blood testosterone levels with aging in normal men. J Clin Endocrinol Metab 1983;56:1278–1281.

39. Winters SJ. Diurnal rhythm of testosterone and luteinizing hormone in hypogonadal men. J Androl 1991;12:185–190.

40. Payne AH, Youngblood GL. Regulation of expression of steroidogenic enzymes in Leydig cells. Biol Reprod 1995;52:217–225.

41. Dufau ML. The luteinizing hormone receptor. Annu Rev Physiol 1998;60:461–496.

42. Stocco DM. StAR protein and the regulation of steroid hormone biosynthesis. Annu Rev Physiol 2001;63:193–213.

43. Mannaerts B, de Leeuw R, Geelen J, et al. Comparative in vitro and in vivo studies on the biological characteristics of recombinant human follicle-stimulating hormone. Endocrinology 1991;129:2623–2630.

44. Majumdar SS, Winters SJ, Plant TM. A study of the relative roles of follicle-stimulating hormone and luteinizing hormone in the regulation of testicular inhibin secretion in the rhesus monkey *(Macaca mulatta)*. Endocrinology 1997;138:1363–1373.

45. Vierhapper H, Nowotny P, Waldhausl W. Production rates of testosterone in patients with Cushing's syndrome. Metabolism 2000;49:229–231.

46. Jones ME, Simpson ER. Oestrogens in male reproduction. Baillieres Best Pract Res Clin Endocrinol Metab 2000;14:505–516.

47. Brodie A, Inkster S, Yue W. Aromatase expression in the human male. Mol Cell Endocrinol 2001;178:23–28.

48. Simpson ER, Davis SR. Minireview: aromatase and the regulation of estrogen biosynthesis—some new perspectives. Endocrinology 2001;142:4589–4594.

49. Couse JF, Curtis Hewitt S, Korach KS. Receptor null mice reveal contrasting roles for estrogen receptor alpha and beta in reproductive tissues. J Steroid Biochem Mol Biol 2000;74:287–296.

50. Couse JF, Lindzey J, Grandien K, Gustafsson JA, Korach KS. Tissue distribution and quantitative analysis of estrogen receptor-alpha (ERalpha) and estrogen receptor-beta (ERbeta) messenger ribonucleic acid in the wild-type and ERalpha-knockout mouse. Endocrinology 1997;138:4613–4621.

51. Grumbach MM, Auchus RJ. Estrogen: consequences and implications of human mutations in synthesis and action. J Clin Endocrinol Metab 1999;84:4677–4694.

52. Robertson KM, O'Donnell L, Jones ME, et al. Impairment of spermatogenesis in mice lacking a functional aromatase (cyp 19) gene. Proc Natl Acad Sci USA 1999;96:7986–7991.

53. Plant TM. Effects of orchidectomy and testosterone replacement treatment on pulsatile luteinizing hormone secretion in the adult rhesus monkey *(Macaca mulatta)*. Endocrinology 1982;110:1905–1913.

54. Plant TM, Dubey AK. Evidence from the rhesus monkey *(Macaca mulatta)* for the view that negative feedback control of luteinizing hormone secretion by the testis is mediated by a deceleration of hypothalamic gonadotropin-releasing hormone pulse frequency. Endocrinology 1984;115:2145–2153.

55. Winters SJ, Kawakami S, Sahu A, Plant TM. Pituitary follistatin and activin gene expression, and the testicular regulation of FSH in the adult Rhesus monkey *(Macaca mulatta)*. Endocrinology 2001;142:2874–2848.

56. Kawakami S, Winters SJ. Regulation of lutenizing hormone secretion and subunit messenger ribonucleic acid expression by gonadal steroids in perifused pituitary cells from male monkeys and rats. Endocrinology 1999;140:3587–3593.

57. Finkelstein JS, Whitcomb RW, O'Dea LS, Longcope C, Schoenfeld DA, Crowley WF, Jr. Sex steroid control of gonadotropin secretion in the human male. I. Effects of testosterone administration in normal and gonadotropin-releasing hormone-deficient men. J Clin Endocrinol Metab 1991;73:609–620.

58. Bagatell CJ, Dahl KD, Bremner WJ. The direct pituitary effect of testosterone to inhibit gonadotropin secretion in men is partially mediated by aromatization to estradiol. J Androl 1994;15:15–21.

59. Naftolin F, Pujol-Amat P, Corker CS, et al. Gonadotropins and gonadal steroids in androgen insensitivity (testicular feminization) syndrome: effects of castration and sex steroid administration. Am J Obstet Gynecol 1983;147:491–496.

60. Winters SJ, Troen P. Evidence for a role of endogenous estrogen in the hypothalamic control of gonadotropin secretion in men. J Clin Endocrinol Metab 1985;61:842–845.

61. Marynick SP, Loriaux DL, Sherins RJ, Pita JC, Jr., Lipsett MB. Evidence that testosterone can suppress pituitary gonadotropin secretion independently of peripheral aromatization. J Clin Endocrinol Metab 1979;49:396–398.

62. Smith EP, Boyd J, Frank GR, et al. Estrogen resistance caused by a mutation in the estrogen-receptor gene in a man. N Engl J Med 1994;331:1056–1061.

63. Morishima A, Grumbach MM, Simpson ER, Fisher C, Qin K. Aromatase deficiency in male and female siblings caused by a novel mutation and the physiological role of estrogens. J Clin Endocrinol Metab 1995;80:3689–3698.

64. Carani C, Qin K, Simoni M, et al. Effect of testosterone and estradiol in a man with aromatase deficiency. N Engl J Med 1997;337:91–95.

65. Hayes FJ, Seminara SB, Decruz S, Boepple PA, Crowley WF, Jr. Aromatase inhibition in the human male reveals a hypothalamic site of estrogen feedback. J Clin Endocrinol Metab 2000;85:3027–3035.

66. Santen RJ, Bardin CW. Episodic luteinizing hormone secretion in man. Pulse analysis, clinical interpretation, physiologic mechanisms. J Clin Invest 1973;52:2617–2628.

67. Mather JP, Moore A, Li RH. Activins, inhibins, and follistatins: further thoughts on a growing family of regulators. Proc Soc Exp Biol Med 1997;215:209–222.

68. Carroll RS, Corrigan AZ, Vale W, Chin WW. Activin stabilizes follicle-stimulating hormone-beta messenger ribonucleic acid levels. Endocrinology 1991;129:1721–1726.

69. Weiss J, Guendner MJ, Halvorson LM, Jameson JL. Transcriptional activation of the follicle-stimulating hormone beta-subunit gene by activin. Endocrinology 1995;136:1885–1891.

70. Suszko MI, Lo DJ, Suh H, Camper SA, Woodruff TK. Regulation of the rat follicle-stimulating hormone beta-subunit promoter by activin. Mol Endocrinol 2003;17:318–332.

71. McDowell N, Gurdon JB. Activin as a morphogen in Xenopus mesoderm induction. Sem Cell Dev Biol 1999;10:311–317.

72. Munz B, Tretter YP, Hertel M, Engelhardt F, Alzheimer C, Werner S. The roles of activins in repair processes of the skin and the brain. Mol Cell Endocrinol 2001;180:169–177.

73. Phillips DJ, Jones KL, Scheerlinck JY, Hedger MP, de Kretser DM. Evidence for activin A and follistatin involvement in the systemic inflammatory response. Mol Cell Endocrinol 2001;180:155–162.

74. Plendl J. Angiogenesis and vascular regression in the ovary. Anat Histol Embryol 2000;29:257–266.

75. Pangas SA, Woodruff TK. Activin signal transduction pathways. Trends Endocrinol Metab 2000;11:309–314.

76. Mathews LS, Vale WW. Expression cloning of an activin receptor, a predicted transmembrane serine kinase. Cell 1991;65:973–982.

77. Mathews LS, Vale WW, Kintner CR. Cloning of a second type of activin receptor and functional characterization in Xenopus embryos. Science 1992;255:1702–1705.

78. Tsuchida K, Lewis KA, Mathews LS, Vale WW. Molecular characterization of rat transforming growth factor-beta type II receptor. Biochem Biophys Res Comm 1993;191:790–795.

79. Attisano L, Carcamo J, Ventura F, Weis FM, Massague J, Wrana JL. Identification of human activin and TGF beta type I receptors that form heteromeric kinase complexes with type II receptors. Cell 1993;75:671–680.

80. Wrana JL, Attisano L, Wieser R, Ventura F, Massague J. Mechanism of activation of the TGF-beta receptor. Nature 1994;370:341–347.

81. Attisano L, Wrana JL. Signal transduction by members of the transforming growth factor-beta superfamily. Cytokine Growth Factor Rev 1996;7:327–339.

82. Kawabata M, Imamura T, Inoue H, et al. Intracellular signaling of the TGF-beta superfamily by Smad proteins. Ann N Y Acad Sci 1999;886:73–82.

83. Derynck R, Zhang Y, Feng XH. Smads: transcriptional activators of TGF-beta responses. Cell 1998;95:737–740.

84. Hoodless PA, Haerry T, Abdollah S, et al. MADR1, a MAD-related protein that functions in BMP2 signaling pathways. Cell 1996;85:489–500.

85. Baker JC, Harland RM. A novel mesoderm inducer, Madr2, functions in the activin signal transduction pathway. Genes Dev 1996;10:1880–1889.

86. Lagna G, Hata A, Hemmati-Brivanlou A, Massague J. Partnership between DPC4 and SMAD proteins in TGF-beta signalling pathways. Nature 1996;383:832–836.

87. Macias-Silva M, Abdollah S, Hoodless PA, Pirone R, Attisano L, Wrana JL. MADR2 is a substrate of the TGFbeta receptor and its phosphorylation is required for nuclear accumulation and signaling. Cell 1996;87:1215–1224.

88. Wu RY, Zhang Y, Feng XH, Derynck R. Heteromeric and homomeric interactions correlate with signaling activity and functional cooperativity of Smad3 and Smad4/DPC4. Mol Cell Biol 1997;17:2521–2528.

89. Lebrun JJ, Takabe K, Chen Y, Vale W. Roles of pathway-specific and inhibitory Smads in activin receptor signaling. Mol Endocrinol 1999;13:15–23.

90. Graff JM, Bansal A, Melton DA. Xenopus Mad proteins transduce distinct subsets of signals for the TGF beta superfamily. Cell 1996;85:479–487.

91. Nakao A, Roijer E, Imamura T, et al. Identification of Smad2, a human Mad-related protein in the transforming growth factor beta signaling pathway. J Biol Chem 1997;272:2896–28900.

92. Drummond AE, Le MT, Ethier JF, Dyson M, Findlay JK. Expression and localization of activin receptors, Smads, and beta glycan to the postnatal rat ovary. Endocrinology 2002;143:1423–1433.

93. Chen X, Rubock MJ, Whitman M. A transcriptional partner for MAD proteins in TGF-beta signalling. Nature 1996;383:691–696.

94. Labbe E, Silvestri C, Hoodless PA, Wrana JL, Attisano L. Smad2 and Smad3 positively and negatively regulate TGF beta-dependent transcription through the forkhead DNA-binding protein FAST2. Mol Cell 1998;2:109–120.

95. Li M, Li J, Hoodless PA, et al. Mothers against decapentaplegic-related protein 2 expression in avian granulosa cells is up-regulated by transforming growth factor beta during ovarian follicular development. Endocrinology 1997;138:3659–3665.

96. Hayashi H, Abdollah S, Qiu Y, et al. The MAD-related protein Smad7 associates with the TGFbeta receptor and functions as an antagonist of TGFbeta signaling. Cell 1997;89:1165–1173.

97. Nakao A, Afrakhte M, Moren A, et al. Identification of Smad7, a TGFbeta-inducible antagonist of TGF-beta signalling. Nature 1997;389:631–635.

98. DePaolo LV. Inhibins, activins, and follistatins: the saga continues. Proc Soc Exp Biol Med 1997;214:328–339.

99. Lewis KA, Gray PC, Blount AL, et al. Betaglycan binds inhibin and can mediate functional antagonism of activin signalling. Nature 2000;404:411–414.

100. Kawakami S, Fujii Y, Okada Y, Winters SJ. Paracrine regulation of FSH by follistatin in folliculostellate cell-enriched primate pituitary cell cultures. Endocrinology 2002;143:2250–2258.

101. Kaiser UB, Chin WW. Regulation of follistatin messenger ribonucleic acid levels in the rat pituitary. J Clin Invest 1993;91:2523–2531.

102. Burger HG, Robertson DM. Editorial: inhibin in the male—progress at last. Endocrinology 1997;138:1361–1362.

103. McCullagh D. Dual endocrine activity of the testes. Science 1932;76:19–20.

103a. Krummen LA, Toppari J, Kim WH, et al. Regulation of testicular inhibin subunit messenger ribonucleic acid levels in vivo: effects of hypophysectomy and selective follicle-stimulating hormone replacement. Endocrinology 1989;125:1630–1637.

104. Feng ZM, Wu AZ, Zhang Z, Chen CL. GATA-1 and GATA-4 transactivate inhibin/activin beta-B-subunit gene transcription in testicular cells. Mol Endocrinol 2000;14:1820–1835.

105. Wallace EM, Groome NP, Riley SC, Parker AC, Wu FC. Effects of chemotherapy-induced testicular damage on inhibin, gonadotropin, and testosterone secretion: a prospective longitudinal study. J Clin Endocrinol Metab 1997;82:3111–3115.

106. Carroll RS, Corrigan AZ, Gharib SD, Vale W, Chin WW. Inhibin, activin, and follistatin: regulation of follicle-stimulating hormone messenger ribonucleic acid levels. Mol Endocrinol 1989;3:1969–1976.

107. Anawalt BD, Bebb RA, Matsumoto AM, et al. Serum inhibin B levels reflect Sertoli cell function in normal men and men with testicular dysfunction. J Clin Endocrinol Metab 1996;81:3341–3345.

108. Ramaswamy S, Marshall GR, McNeilly AS, Plant TM. Dynamics of the follicle-stimulating hormone (FSH)-inhibin B feedback loop and its role in regulating spermatogenesis in the adult male rhesus monkey *(Macaca mulatta)* as revealed by unilateral orchidectomy. Endocrinology 2000;141:18–27.

109. Ramaswamy S, Marshall GR, McNeilly AS, Plant TM. Evidence that in a physiological setting Sertoli cell number is the major determinant of circulating concentrations of inhibin B in the adult male rhesus monkey *(Macaca mulatta)*. J Androl 1999;20:430–434.

110. Simoni M, Gromoll J, Nieschlag E. The follicle-stimulating hormone receptor: biochemistry, molecular biology, physiology, and pathophysiology. Endocr Rev 1997;18:739–773.

111. Tapanainen JS, Vaskivuo T, Aittomaki K, Huhtaniemi IT. Inactivating FSH receptor mutations and gonadal dysfunction. Mol Cell Endocrinol 1998;145:129–135.

112. Kumar TR, Wang Y, Lu N, Matzuk MM. Follicle stimulating hormone is required for ovarian follicle maturation but not male fertility. Nat Genet 1997;15:201–204.

113. de Winter JP, Themmen AP, Hoogerbrugge JW, Klaij IA, Grootegoed JA, de Jong FH. Activin receptor mRNA expression in rat testicular cell types. Mol Cell Endocrinol 1992;83:R1–R8.

114. Kaipia A, Parvinen M, Toppari J. Localization of activin receptor (ActR-IIB2) mRNA in the rat seminiferous epithelium. Endocrinology 1993;132:477–479.

115. Krummen LA, Moore A, Woodruff TK, et al. Localization of inhibin and activin binding sites in the testis during development by in situ ligand binding. Biol Reprod 1994;50:734–744.

116. Chong H, Pangas SA, Bernard DJ, et al. Structure and expression of a membrane component of the inhibin receptor system. Endocrinology 2000;141:2600–2607.

117. MacConell LA, Leal AM, Vale WW. The distribution of betaglycan protein and mRNA in rat brain, pituitary, and gonads: implications for a role for betaglycan in inhibin-mediated reproductive functions. Endocrinology 2002;143:1066–1075.

118. Lin T, Calkins JK, Morris PL, Vale W, Bardin CW. Regulation of Leydig cell function in primary culture by inhibin and activin. Endocrinology 1989;125:2134–2140.

119. Hsueh AJ, Dahl KD, Vaughan J, et al. Heterodimers and homodimers of inhibin subunits have different paracrine action in the modulation of luteinizing hormone-stimulated androgen biosynthesis. Proc Natl Acad Sci USA 1987;84:5082–5086.

120. Risbridger GP, Clements J, Robertson DM, et al. Immuno- and bioactive inhibin and inhibin alpha-subunit expression in rat Leydig cell cultures. Mol Cell Endocrinol 1989;66:119–122.

121. Mather JP, Attie KM, Woodruff TK, Rice GC, Phillips DM. Activin stimulates spermatogonial proliferation in germ-Sertoli cell cocultures from immature rat testis. Endocrinology 1990;127:3206–3214.

122. van Dissel-Emiliani FM, Grootenhuis AJ, de Jong FH, de Rooij DG. Inhibin reduces spermatogonial numbers in testes of adult mice and Chinese hamsters. Endocrinology 1989;125:1899–1903.

123. Hakovirta H, Kaipia A, Soder O, Parvinen M. Effects of activin-A, inhibin-A, and transforming growth factor-beta 1 on stage-specific deoxyribonucleic acid synthesis during rat seminiferous epithelial cycle. Endocrinology 1993;133:1664–1668.

124. Kirk SE, Dalkin AC, Yasin M, Haisenleder DJ, Marshall JC. Gonadotropin-releasing hormone pulse frequency regulates expression of pituitary follistatin messenger ribonucleic acid: a mechanism for differential gonadotrope function. Endocrinology 1994;135:876–880.

125. Besecke LM, Guendner MJ, Schneyer AL, Bauer-Dantoin AC, Jameson JL, Weiss J. Gonadotropin-releasing hormone regulates follicle-stimulating hormone-beta gene expression through an activin/follistatin autocrine or paracrine loop. Endocrinology 1996;137:3667–3673.

126. Spratt DI, Finkelstein JS, Butler JP, Badger TM, Crowley WF, Jr. Effects of increasing the frequency of low doses of gonadotropin-releasing hormone (GnRH) on gonadotropin secretion in GnRH-deficient men. J Clin Endocrinol Metab 1987;64:1179–1186.

127. Gross KM, Matsumoto AM, Berger RE, Bremner WJ. Increased frequency of pulsatile luteinizing hormone-releasing hormone administration selectively decreases follicle-stimulating hormone levels in men with idiopathic azoospermia. Fertil Steril 1986;45:392–396.

128. Tsujii T, Ishizaka K, Winters SJ. Effects of pituitary adenylate cyclase-activating polypeptide on gonadotropin secretion and subunit messenger ribonucleic acids in perifused rat pituitary cells. Endocrinology 1994;135:826–833.

129. Kaiser UB, Sabbagh E, Katzenellenbogen RA, Conn PM, Chin WW. A mechanism for the differential regulation of gonadotropin subunit gene expression by gonadotropin-releasing hormone. Proc Natl Acad Sci USA 1995;92:12280–12284.

2 Leydig Cell Function in Man

Qiang Dong, MD, PhD
and Matthew P. Hardy, PhD

CONTENTS

INTRODUCTION

In humans, as in all mammalian males, Leydig cells are the main source of the androgenic hormone, testosterone, which is essential for male sexual differentiation, gamete production and maturation, and development of secondary sexual characteristics. In this chapter, the development, steroidogenic function, and regulation of human Leydig cells are summarized. Clinical aspects of androgen secretion and pathology related to Leydig cells are also reviewed. The information presented is based, in part, on studies conducted in laboratory animals because of the larger database available for these species.

LEYDIG CELL DEVELOPMENT

Leydig cells were first described by the German histologist Franz Leydig in 1850 *(1)*. In all mammalian species, Leydig cells are located in the interstitial compartment of the testis, between and surrounding the seminiferous tubules *(2)*. Human Leydig cells are epithelioid and ovoid or polygonal. Other cytological features include eosinophilic cytoplasm, euchromatic round eccentric nuclei with a peripheral distribution of heterochromatin, and conspicuous nucleolus. The predominant cytoplasmic organelle is the smooth endoplasmic reticulum (SER), which is characteristically more abundant in steroidogenic cells when compared to other cell types. Mitochondria and lipid droplets are also numerous in Leydig cells and play a role in steroidogenesis that is discussed later in this

From: *Male Hypogonadism:*
Basic, Clinical, and Therapeutic Principles
Edited by: S. J. Winters © Humana Press Inc., Totowa, NJ

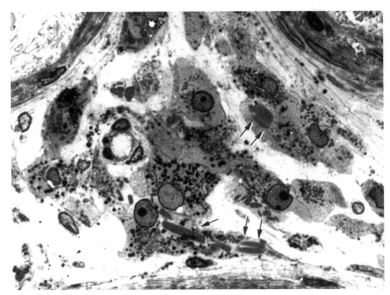

Fig. 1. Testicular interstitial space of an adult man (original image magnification × 7,000). This semithin plastic section shows mature Leydig cells surrounding a capillary. In humans, Leydig cells are embedded in a loose connective tissue. The arrows point to Reinke crystals in the cytoplasm of Leydig cells. (Photo supplied by Dr. Hector Chemes, from ref. *13,* with the publisher's permission.)

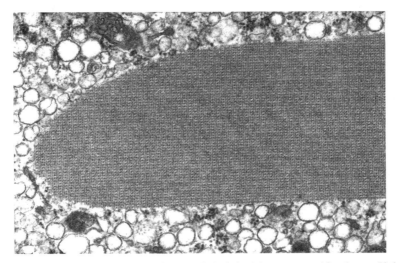

Fig. 2. A Reinke crystal. This electron micrograph (original image magnification × 50,000) shows the highly ordered lattice of filaments within these crystals. (Photo supplied by Dr. Hector Chemes, from ref. *13,* with permission from the publisher.)

chapter *(3,4)*. Reinke crystals are observed exclusively in human Leydig cells and are believed to be indicative of diminished steroidogenic capacity during aging *(5–7)*. Human Leydig cell structure and Reinke crystals are shown in Figs. 1 and 2.

In humans, blood levels of testosterone peak three times during development *(8)*. The first peak occurs at 12–14 wk of gestation, during the fetal differentiation of Leydig cells *(9)*. Testosterone levels then decline and are low for the remainder of gestation and the early neonatal period. A second peak at 2 mo postpartum is associated with renewed Leydig cell proliferation. Leydig cells then atrophy a second time, and, for the next decade, the interstitium is populated by steroidogenically inactive precursor cells. The adult generation of Leydig cells differentiates pubertally and is complete by 12 to 13 yr of age. Serum levels of testosterone average 6 ng/mL during adulthood (10). Finally, there is a decline in testosterone secretion with aging, which varies in its age of onset. The age-related testosterone decrease is caused primarily by gradual atrophy and loss of adult Leydig cells and also by declines in steroidogenic capacity (11). The fetal, neonatal, and adult epochs of testosterone secretion are associated with three separate waves of increases and declines in Leydig cell numbers (12).

Fetal Leydig Cells

Until recently, the precursors of Leydig cells were believed to be of mesenchymal origin and derived from cells in the mesonephros (primitive kidney) (14–16). However, recent tissue recombination studies do not support the hypothesis that precursor cells migrate into the interstitium from the mesonephros, and ontogeny from the embryonic neural crest has been suggested (17). By the sixth week of gestation, seminiferous cord formation within the gonadal blastema simultaneously creates the outer interstitial compartment (18). Fetal Leydig cells become identifiable in this compartment among the undifferentiated mesenchymal cells at 8 wk of gestation (19). Then, Leydig cell numbers increase continuously and reach a maximum by 14 to 15 wk, when they fill the space between the cords and comprise more than half the volume of the fetal testis. Although testosterone is first detectable in the testis as early as 6 to 7 wk of gestation (20), the sharp increment in the numbers of fetal Leydig cells is accompanied by further rises in androgen concentrations in testicular tissue, blood, and amniotic fluid, which reach a maximum at week 15 (21). After the 16th wk of gestation, the numbers of fetal Leydig cells, serum testosterone concentrations, and testicular mRNA levels for at least two of the testosterone biosynthetic enzymes, P450scc and P45017α, decline (21–23). At birth, the total number of Leydig cells per testis is 60% lower compared to the prenatal peak, and the remaining Leydig cells are half the size (21).

Neonatal Leydig Cells

Just after birth, the number of Leydig cells again increases to a peak at 2 to 3 mo of age, contributing to a second surge in plasma testosterone levels. At this stage, Leydig cells contain abundant SER membranes and mitochondria, as well as varying amounts of lipid droplets (4,24–27). In the neonatal testis, fetal Leydig cells persist through at least 3 mo after birth. Postnatal increase in the number of these cells most likely results from recruitment of interstitial precursor cells. After this increase, neonatal Leydig cell numbers regress rapidly to a nadir by the end of the first year. The neonatal period is relatively brief, extending only through the first year of life (28,29).

After the first year and continuing for a decade, Leydig cells are in a state of prepubertal quiescence. During this phase, well-differentiated Leydig cells are absent from the interstitial space. In their place are partially differentiated Leydig cells and primitive fibroblastic cells. At this stage, Leydig cells are dispersed in a loose connective tissue matrix and contain elongated nuclei with scarcely visible cytoplasm. It has been proposed that these partially differentiated Leydig cells and primitive fibroblasts are precursors of adult Leydig cells (13,25,30–32).

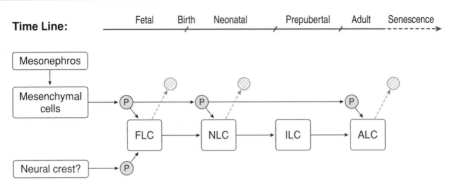

Fig. 3. Human Leydig cell development. FLC, fetal Leydig cells; NLC, neonatal Leydig cells; ILC, immature Leydig cells; ALC, adult Leydig cells, P, fibroblastic precursors of Leydig cells. The cross-hatched circles indicate degeneration of FLC, NLC, and ALC. The far left-hand column of the compartments represents stem cells, including mesonephros-derived mesenchyme and/or neural crest. The time line shows the developmental period: fetal (from 8 wk gestation to birth), neonatal (first year of life), prepubertal (from second year to approx 10 yr of life), and adult (from approx 13 yr old onward). According to the hypothesized ontogeny, mesonephros-derived mesenchymal cells, or possibly neural crest, supply precursors for FLC. After birth, NLC arise from redifferentiation of FLC and new differentiation from mesenchymal cell precursors. After the first year of life, NLC regress to the partially differentiated ILC. ILC are then present through childhood. Starting at approx 10 yr of age, ILC and mesenchymal precursors again differentiate, maturing into ALC. With senescence, Leydig cells begin to lose full steroidogenic function and, as indicated, atrophy.

Adult Leydig Cells

The precursor cells for adult Leydig cells begin their transformation at approx 10 yr of age, and differentiation is complete by 13 yr of age *(33)*. During puberty, the number of adult Leydig cells increases and reaches a maximum of 5×10^8 per testis in the early 20s *(25)*. At this time, a third peak in testosterone concentrations occurs. Thereafter, Leydig cell numbers gradually decrease by 50% in men aged 60 yr and older *(34)*. Between ages 20 and 60 yr, there is an equilibrium in the numbers of Leydig cells, which comprise approx 4% of the volume of the mature testis *(14)*. The overall scheme of human Leydig cell development is summarized in Fig. 3.

STEROIDOGENIC FUNCTION OF LEYDIG CELLS

The primary function of Leydig cells is to synthesize and secrete androgenic steroids. The process of androgen biosynthesis requires the activities of four enzymes: cytochrome P450 cholesterol side chain cleavage enzyme (P450scc), 3β-hydroxysteroid dehydrogenase/Δ^{5-4} isomerase (3β-HSD), cytochrome P450 17α-hydroxylase (P45017α), and 17β–hydroxysteroid dehydrogenase (17β-HSD) *(35)*. Leydig cells are the only cells in the testis containing P450scc and 3β-HSD. Thus, Leydig cells are the sole testicular location for the first two steps in steroidogenesis converting cholesterol, the substrate for all steroid hormones, to pregnenolone and pregnenolone to progesterone *(36–38)*. Thereafter, with the catalytic activities of P45017α and 17β-HSD, steroidogenesis proceeds to the ultimate product, testosterone *(39)*. The synthetic process involves three hydroxylations (at carbons 17, 20, and 22), two cleavages (at carbons

20–22 and 17–20), two dehydrogenations (3β,17β), and one Δ^{5-4} isomerization (the steroidogenic pathway is shown in Fig. 4).

Conversion of Cholesterol to Pregnenolone

In all species, the first step in androgen biosynthesis is the conversion of cholesterol to pregnenolone, which is catalyzed by P450scc located in the inner mitochondrial membrane. This reaction also requires a mitochondrial electron transfer system, consisting of adrenodoxin and adrenodoxin reductase, to convey electrons from NAPDH to P450scc *(40)*. The P450scc enzyme catalyzes three sequential oxidation reactions of cholesterol, with each reaction requiring 1 molecule of O_2 and one molecule of nicotinamide adenine dinucleotide phosphate (NAPDH). The first reaction is hydroxylation at C_{22}, followed by hydroxylation at C_{20} to yield (20,22) R-hydroxycholesterol, which is cleaved between C_{20} and C_{22} to yield the C_{21} steroid pregnenolone and isocaproaldehyde *(41,42)*. Isocaproaldehyde is unstable and quickly oxidized to isocaproic acid *(43)*.

The rate-limiting step in the synthesis of steroid hormones is not the first enzymatic reaction catalyzed by P450scc but rather the transport of precursor cholesterol from intracellular sources to the inner mitochondrial membrane and subsequent loading of cholesterol into the catalytic site of P450scc *(44,45)*. Hydrophobic cholesterol cannot traverse the aqueous intermembrane space of mitochondria and reach the P450scc rapidly enough by simple diffusion to support acute steroid synthesis *(46)*. Thus, cholesterol is mobilized by carrier proteins. Both steroidogenic acute response (StAR) protein and peripheral benzodiazepine receptor (PBR) are believed to participate in cholesterol delivery to the mitochondria, with StAR being primarily involved in gonadotropin-stimulated transfer.

Cholesterol, the raw material for steroidogenesis, is obtained from (1) lipoprotein in circulation, with low-density lipoprotein (LDL) being the primary source in humans; (2) *de novo* synthesis from acetate in the SER; and (3) free cholesterol liberated by cholesterol esterase from less directly available esters in lipid droplets *(47)*.

Conversion of Δ^5-3β-Hydroxysteroids to Δ^4-3-Ketosteroids

After cholesterol side-chain cleavage, two different pathways (Δ^5 and Δ^4) have been identified, which are defined by the position of one of the double bonds in the steroid molecule. In the Δ^4 pathway, pregnenolone, which has a double bond between carbons 5 and 6 of the steroid backbone, is converted to progesterone, which has a double bond between carbons 4 and 5. An isomerization reaction shifts the position of the double bond from between carbons 5 and 6 to between carbons 4 and 5. In the Δ^5 pathway, Δ^5 to Δ^4 isomerization does not occur until the last step, in which androstenediol is converted to testosterone. The intermediates of the two pathways are Δ^5-3β-hydroxysteroids and Δ^4-3-ketosteroids, respectively. The conversion of Δ^5-3β-hydroxysteroids to Δ^4-3-ketosteroids is accomplished by 3β-HSD enzyme, which uses NAD^+ as a cofactor, sequentially catalyzing a 3β dehydrogenation and isomerization *(48)*. The 3β-HSD enzymes can act on three Δ^5 intermediates, pregnenolone, 17α-hydroxypregnenolone, and dehydroepiandrosterone, converting them, respectively, to the Δ^4 steroids progesterone, 17α-hydroxyprogesterone, and androstenedione. The predominant Δ^5 to Δ^4 conversion occurs most commonly with either pregnenolone or dehydroepiandrosterone as substrates rather than 17α-hydroxypregnenolone. Whether the Δ^5- or Δ^4-pathway is followed from pregnenolone to

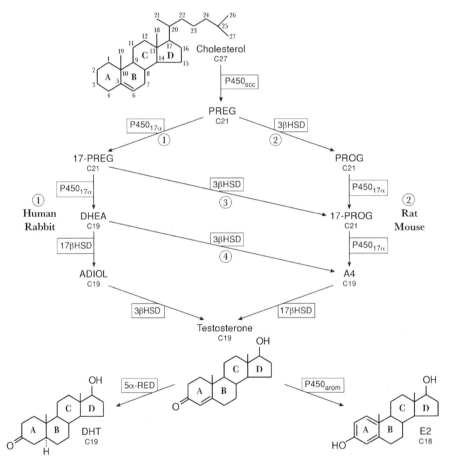

Fig. 4. Pathway of testosterone biosynthesis. Of the four possible biosynthetic pathways, the first or Δ^5 predominates in the rabbit and human, whereas the second or Δ^4 predominates in rodents. CHOL, cholesterol; PREG, pregnenolone; 17-PREG, 17-hydroxypregnenolone; DHEA, dehydroepiandrosterone; ADIOL, androstenediol; PROG, progesterone; 17-PROG, 17-hydroxyprogesterone; A4, androstenedione;T, testosterone; DHT, dehydrotestosterone; E_2 17β-estradiol.

testosterone depends on the species and developmental status of the Leydig cell. In humans, the Δ^5 pathway is predominant *(49–52)*. Mammalian 3β-HSDs comprise a large family of enzymes *(53,54)*. In the human branch of this family, two genes encode two corresponding, type I and II, 3β-HSD enzymes. Both types dehydrogenate 3β-hydroxysteroids and isomerize C_{21} and C_{19} steroids. Type I 3β-HSD is exclusively present in placenta and skin, whereas type II is the predominant form expressed in the adrenal, ovary, and testis. In the testis, type II 3β-HSD activity is localized exclusively in Leydig cells *(37,55)*.

Conversion of C_{21} Steroids into C_{19} Steroids

Conversion of C_{21} to C_{19} requires two steps, 17α-hydroxylation and cleavage of the C_{17-20} bond, both of which are catalyzed by a single enzyme, the cytochrome P450 17α-hydroxylase/C_{17-20} lyase (P45017α). This enzyme catalyzes the bioconversion of pregnenolone and progesterone to the C_{19} steroids, dehydroepiandrosterone and androstenedione, respectively *(56,57)*. In this two-step reaction, 17α-hydroxypregnenolone or 17α-hydroxyprogesterone exist as transient intermediates that are rapidly converted to dehydroepiandrosterone or androstenedione. The substrate preference and reaction velocities of P45017α differ, depending on the species and tissue source. In humans, P45017α has a higher affinity for 17α-hydroxypregnenolone, with dehydroepiandrosterone as the end product, and fails to show detectable C_{17-20} lyase activity with 17α-hydroxyprogesterone as substrate to generate androstenedione *(58,59)*. In contrast, rat P45017α readily cleaves the Δ^4-C_{21} 17α-hydroxypregnenolone and Δ^5-C_{21} 17α-hydroxyprogesterone to dehydroepiandrosterone and androstenedione, respectively. Guinea pig P45017α also has a high affinity for Δ^4-C_{21} steroids, *(54)*, and both species contrast with the human, where the Δ^5 pathway predominates

Conversion of Dehydroepiandrosterone to Testosterone

The microsomal enzyme 17β-hydroxysteroid dehydrogenase (17β-HSD) catalyzes the interconversion of dehydroepiandrosterone and androstenediol, or androstenedione and testosterone. The 17β-dehydrogenase reaction is reversible, in contrast to the previous reactions in testosterone biosynthesis *(60)*. Following the Δ^5 pathway in humans, the C_{19} product, dehydroepiandrosterone, is converted to androstenediol by 17β-HSD, and then androstenediol is converted to testosterone by 3β-HSD. In the Δ^4 pathway occurring in rodents, 17β-HSD uses androstenedione as substrate to produce testosterone *(61)*. Testosterone is the principle steroid end product secreted by adult Leydig cells, but it can be further metabolized to 17β-estradiol (E_2) and dehydrotestosterone (DHT) before secretion.

Conversion of Testosterone to E_2

Aromatization of testosterone is catalyzed by the microsomal enzyme, cytochrome P450 aromatase (P450arom). Once substrate binding occurs, there is a sequential hydroxylation, oxidation, and removal of the C_{19} carbon, followed by aromatization of the A ring of the steroid. The entire aromatase reaction uses three molecules of oxygen and three electrons donated by NADPH *(62–64)*. In the testis, aromatase activity is detectable in Leydig cells, Sertoli cells, and germ cells *(65–69)*. The relative contributions of each of these testicular cell types to testicular aromatase activity varies with age and between species *(70)*. In the rat and mouse, germ cells are a significant site of activity during adulthood *(68)*. Sertoli cells contribute to testicular aromatase activity only in immature animals *(71)*. However, in humans, Leydig cells are the only source of testicular estrogens at all ages *(39)*. Sertoli cell cultures from juvenile monkeys expressed follicle-stimulating hormone (FSH) driven aromatase *(72)*.

Conversion of Testosterone to DHT

DHT, a more potent androgen than testosterone, is produced in a reaction catalyzed by the 5α-reductase enzyme. This conversion generally occurs in androgenic target tissues, such as the prostate gland, but 5α-reductase activity is high in Leydig cells prepubertally. Two isoforms of 5α-reductase, type I and type II, have been identified. The type II isoform is found in human prostate tissue and in Leydig cells *(73,74)*.

Testosterone Secretion

The first step of androgen biosynthesis, catalyzed by P450scc, occurs in Leydig cell mitochondria, and subsequent steps occur in the SER. After synthesis, testosterone, which is lipophilic, moves out of the Leydig cell by passive diffusion, down a concentration gradient. There is no evidence of packaging testosterone into secretory granules *(8)*. In the testis, testosterone diffuses freely into the interstitial space and associates in rodents with androgen-binding protein (ABP) produced by Sertoli cells *(75,76)* as a transport vehicle to the seminiferous tubules and epididymis.

Testosterone enters the testicular blood capillaries that are immediately adjacent to Leydig cells. Once a part of the systemic circulation, secreted testosterone binds to plasma proteins and is present in both bound and unbound forms. In humans, more than 95% of testosterone is complexed with proteins, both the high-affinity ($K_D = 1$ nM) sex hormone-binding globulin (SHBG) and the low-affinity ($K_D = 1000$ nM) albumin (Alb). The proportion of testosterone that is unbound or loosely bound represents the biologically active fraction, which freely diffuses from capillaries into cells. In contrast, the SHBG-bound fraction is believed to act as a reservoir for the steroid.

SHBG is a plasma protein synthesized and secreted by the liver. As its name suggests, SHBG has the ability to bind androgens and estrogens and the capacity to regulate the free concentrations of the steroids that bind to it. SHBG also participates in signal transduction for sex steroids at the cell membrane. SHBG binds with high affinity to a specific membrane receptor (R_{SHBG}) in prostate stromal and epithelial cells, wherein the SHBG / R_{SHBG} complex forms. Once an appropriate steroid, e.g., 3α-androstanediol or estradiol, binds to this complex, an increase of intracellular cyclic adenosine monophosphate (cAMP) occurs and intracellular signal transduction is initiated. Moreover, SHBG not only is a plasma protein secreted by the liver but also is expressed in the prostate tissue itself, specifically by prostate stromal and epithelial cells *(77)*. (*See* Chapter 17.) The process of testosterone secretion and regulation of Leydig cell function are illustrated in Fig. 5.

REGULATION OF LEYDIG CELL FUNCTION

Steroidogenesis in adult Leydig cells is controlled by the pituitary gonadotropic hormones. Of the two gonadotropins, luteinizing hormone (LH) is the main stimulus for androgen biosynthesis. LH signal transduction is initiated on binding of the hormone to specific receptors on the Leydig cell surface. The receptor for LH (LH-R) belongs to a superfamily of G protein-coupled receptor (GPCR) *(78)*.

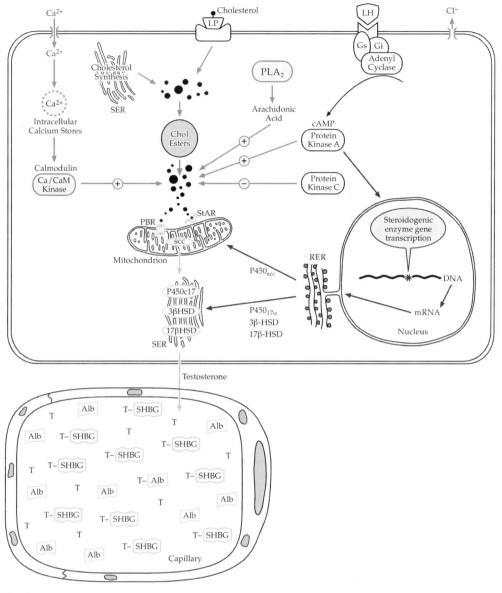

Fig. 5. Acute regulation of Leydig cell steroidogenesis by luteinizing hormone (LH). The complex of LH and LHRs triggers adenylate cyclase-mediated increases cytoplasmic cyclic adenosine monophosphate (cAMP) levels. Activation of protein kinase A and cholesterol esterase results in cholesterol mobilization from extracellular lipoprotein (low-density lipoprotein) and intercellular sources (including *de novo* synthesis) in the smooth endoplasmic reticulum (SER) and released from lipid droplet stores. Cholesterol moves across the outer to the inner membrane of the mitochondrion via shuttle proteins steroidogenic acute response (StAR) and peripheral benzodiazepine receptor (PBR). Cholesterol side-chain cleavage enzyme catalyzes the initial step in steroid biosynthesis. The subsequent steps are catalyzed by P45017α, 3βHSD, and 17βHSD in the SER. The ultimate product, testosterone, moves out of the Leydig cell down a concentration gradient and is carried to androgen-responsive tissues by androgen-binding protein (rodents) and sex hormone-binding globulin (SHBG) (humans). The response to LH also involves an increased cytoplasmic calcium, synthesis of arachidomic acid, and efflux of chloride ions. The mechanism of Ca^{2+} action involves a calcium/calmodulin (Ca/CaM) protein kinase. Activation of phospholipase A_2 (PLA$_2$) produces arachidonic acid (AA), which has a stimulatory effect on cholesterol mobilization to mitochondria. (Courtesy of P.N. Schlegel and M.P. Hardy (2002) *[79]* with the publisher's permission.)

Acute Effects of LH

Two types of responses to LH are seen in Leydig cells. The acute response triggers a rapid production of steroid within minutes *(46)*. In the acute LH signal transduction process, LH-Rs interact with intracytoplasmic adenylate cyclase to form the second messenger adenosine 3',5'-cAMP. A sharp increase in cytoplasmic cAMP levels elicits a cascade of events leading to testosterone synthesis, including increased translocation of cholesterol from the cytosol to the inner mitochondrial membrane, conversion of cholesterol to pregnenolone, and, ultimately, transformation of steroid intermediates into testosterone. In addition to stimulating cAMP formation, LH acts on other intracellular signaling systems, including release of calcium from internal stores, synthesis of arachidonic acid (AA) and its metabolites from membrane phospholipid, and efflux of chloride ions, which have all been linked to the steroidogenic process *(80)*.

The acute response of Leydig cells to LH does not require new transcription of mRNA *(81)*. However, carrier proteins are required in the cholesterol translocation process for the rapid steroid production in the acute response. StAR is a 30-kDa molecular weight cholesterol transporter, and blockade of its synthesis by cycloheximide prevents the LH-induced increase in testosterone biosynthesis *(82)*. Transient transfection of COS-1 cells with the cDNA for StAR increases the conversion of cholesterol to pregnenolone. StAR gene mutations result in the pathological condition of congenital lipoid adrenal hyperplasia (lipoid CAH), in which patients are unable to convert cholesterol to pregnenolone. This confirms a cholesterol-shuttling role for StAR protein in steroidogenesis *(46,83,84)*. StAR protein biochemistry, as it is currently understood, may not completely account for transfer of cholesterol across mitochondrial membranes *(85)*. Another candidate protein for cholesterol trafficking is the mitochondrial PBR, which is an 18-kDa integral outer mitochondrial membrane phosphoprotein that has a high affinity for cholesterol binding *(86)*. PBR expression decreases are correlated with the decreased steroid synthesis *(87)*. PBR plays a role in the maintenance of the basal pool of mitochondrial cholesterol *(88)*. It has been postulated that PBR functions in cholesterol transport in steroidogenic tissues by mediating the entry, distribution, and/or availability of cholesterol within mitochondria *(87,89)*. Recently, it was proposed by West et al. that PBR associates with StAR and that the two proteins may work in tandem at the outer mitochondrial membrane *(90)*.

Chronic Effects of LH

LH also has long-term trophic effects on Leydig cells, requiring both transcription and increased translation of proteins. Chronic stimulation by LH is required for maintenance of Leydig cell steroidogenic enzyme levels and to support the steroidogenic organelle aparatus, including mitochondrial membrane potential and SER volume.

Inhibition of LH action can be achieved by hypophysectomy *(91–93)*, suppression of gonadotropins through steroid administration *(94–96)*, and neutralization of LH or LH-releasing hormone (GnRH) by specific antibodies *(97)*. LH blockade eliminates the chronic effects of this hormone, causing Leydig cell atrophy and loss of cellular volume, SER, steroidogenic enzyme activities (particularly P-450$17\alpha$ and P-450scc), LH receptor numbers, and the ability to secrete testosterone in response to LH *(91,95)*. In LH-deprived rats, Leydig cell structure and function are restored by LH replacement

(93,94,96). Similarly, daily injections of LH to the hypogonadal mouse markedly increase steroidogenic enzyme activities *(98)*.

In addition to LH, FSH and local cell-cell interactions participate in the regulation to Leydig cells. FSH regulatory control of Leydig cells is based on the correlation between serum FSH levels and the steroidogenic response of Leydig cells to LH during sexual maturation in humans. Because FSH-R are present only in the Sertoli cells, FSH acts on Leydig cells indirectly through Sertoli cell-secreted factors *(99,100)*. Huhtaniemi and colleagues (*see* Chapter 6), in a study of FSHβ And FSH-R knockout mice, recently demonstrated FSH signaling involvement in Leydig cell development. LH alone is sufficient for normal postnatal development of Leydig cells only if FSH-R are present. In the absence of LH, FSH stimulates Leydig cell steroidogenesis *(101)*. Sertoli cells may also modulate Leydig cell numbers via paracrine interactions *(14,102,103)*. Several factors produced by Sertoli cells, including insulin-like growth factor (IGF) 1, epidermal growth factor (EGF)-α, transforming growth factor (TGF)-α, and TGF-β, inhibin, and activin, influence Leydig cells. TGF-β is believed to be a strong inhibitor of Leydig cell steroidogenesis, whereas IGF-1 is a stimulator. EGF-α and TGF-α stimulate steroidogenesis during adulthood but may inhibit differentiation of immature Leydig cells. Germ cells, through their interactions with Sertoli cells, are believed to affect Leydig cells indirectly *(81)*.

CLINICAL ASPECTS

Aging of Leydig Cells

Reproductive function declines as men grow older. An age-associated decline in plasma testosterone concentration occurs even in healthy men *(104,105)*, although there is considerable variation in the age of onset *(106)*. The level of testosterone in the blood stream declines on average by 1.2% each year for men over 40 yr of age. Because SHBG rises, the level of free (bioavailable) testosterone in the blood decreases more with age compared to total testosterone *(106,107)*. Because clearance of testosterone does not rise with age, it is reasonable to deduce that the age-related decreases in androgen concentrations result from decreased Leydig cell androgen production *(108,109)*.

Age-related declines in testosterone could be caused by decreased Leydig cell numbers and atrophy of their structure and/or reduced steroidogenic ability. Leydig cell numbers are inversely correlated with age, decreasing 44% by age 58 compared to 32-yr-old men *(34)*. Leydig cell numbers decline because of degeneration rather than dedifferentiation *(110)*. In addition, aged Leydig cells contain cytoplasmic or intranuclear crystalline inclusions, lipofuscin granules, diminished SER, and smaller and fewer mitochondria compared to young men *(7,111–113)*. Older men with higher serum LH and low serum testosterone levels also have a large number of abnormal Leydig cells, suggesting that Leydig cell structural changes are related to changes in steroidogenic function *(112)*. Age-related declines in steroidogenesis are caused by a global reduction in steroidogenic enzyme gene expression and by decreases in the rate of cholesterol transfer to mitochondria *(114–117)*. In fact, the senescence of Leydig cells is involved at all aspects of the steroidogenic process, from LH binding to the steroidogenic reactions in the SER. Zirkin and colleagues report that reactive oxygen, produced as a by-product of steroidogenesis itself, may be responsible for age-related reductions testosterone production *(118)*.

Therefore, unless Leydig stem cells can be recruited to restore the Leydig cell numbers, age-related declines in testosterone levels are unavoidable. The endocrine changes with aging in men are reviewed more thoroughly in Chapter 14.

Leydig Cell Tumors

Testicular tumors occur at a rate of 2 cases per 100,000 men and constitute 1% of all tumors in men. Leydig cell tumors (LCTs) account for 1 to 3% of testicular tumors [119]. LCTs were first identified by Sacchi in 1895 [120]. Although they are rare gonadal stromal tumors, LCTs may occur at any age and represent approx 40% of all non-germ cell testicular tumors [121]. Most LCTs are unilateral; only 3% are bilateral [121].

LCTs are found at all ages from 2 to 90 yr, with a peak occurrence in the fifth decade of life. In boys, these tumors typically occur between the ages of 4 and 10 yr and account for approx 10% of cases of precocious puberty [122]. They are uniformly benign hormonally active tumors that present with macrogenitosomia (a syndrome that is characterized by precocious enlargement of the genitals), including an enlarged phallus and/or prostate, and premature growth of pubic hair [120]. Adult men with LCTs often present with a painless testicular mass, usually associated with gynecomastia, infertility, decreased libido, and other feminizing features. Gynecomastia is bilateral in 90% of the cases [123,124].

LCTs secrete both androgenically and estrogenically active steroids. Unlike normal Leydig cells, androgen secretion by the tumor is in independent of pituitary control. LCTs have an abnormally high aromatase activity and secrete E_2 [125]. The resulting elevated E_2 and decreased, or low-normal T values cause gynecomastia and infertility [126]. This alteration in the T/E_2 ratio, together with suppressed LH secretion, may be useful for clinical diagnosis.

Macroscopically, the lesions are generally small, yellow to brown, well circumscribed, and rarely hemorrhagic or necrotic. Microscopically, they consist of uniformly polyhedral packed cells with round and slightly eccentric nuclei, and eosinophilic granular cytoplasm with lipoid vacuoles, lipofuscin granules, and occasionally, Reinke's crystals [127].

Most LCTs are benign, but approx 10% are malignant [128]. Large size, extensive necrosis, gross or microscopic evidence of infiltration, invasion of blood vessels, and excessive mitotic activity are all features that suggest malignancy. However, the presence of metastases, most often to pelvic lymph nodes and bone, is the only reliable criterion of malignancy. The appearance of metastases may be delayed for as many as 9 yr [129].

Inguinal orchidectomy is the treatment of choice for benign tumors. Recent reports have cited testis-sparing enucleation as an alternative treatment for benign lesions in children, especially those with bilateral tumors [130,131]. Testis-sparing surgery is also an option for children with the clinical and biochemical findings typical of LCTs and an ultrasonographically defined encapsulated intratesticular mass. In cases managed by enucleation, local relapse remains a possibility, even when specimen margins are free of tumor cells and uniformly benign [120]. Malignant LCTs are radioresistant and chemoresistant and have a poor prognosis. The mean survival time after surgery for patients with malignant LCTs is approx 3 yr [127].

Leydig cell hyperplasia (LCH) shares the same clinical presentation as LCTs, including painful gynecomastia and decreased libido in adults, precocious puberty in children,

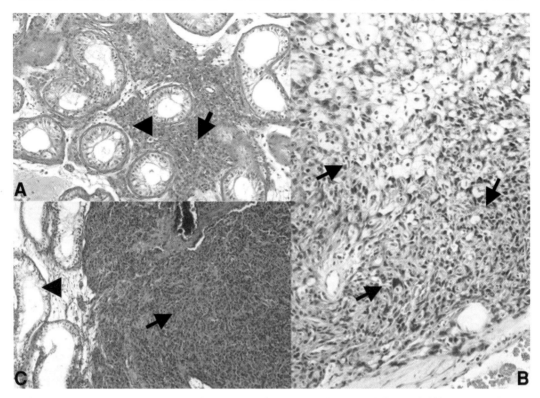

Fig. 6. Benign and malignant Leydig cell tumors (LCTs). The upper left panel, **(A)** an example of Leydig cell hyperplasia (LCH), is seen with an increased number of Leydig cells and an intertubular growth pattern (original image magnification × 200). The lower left panel, **(C)** is a benign LCT with a loss of normal tubules and peripheral compression of adjacent seminiferous tubules (original image magnification × 100). In the right panel, **(B)** a malignant LCT is shown with significant nuclear atypia and an invasive border (original image magnification × 300). (Photos supplied by Drs. Cathy Naughton and Peter Humphrey of Washington University School of Medicine.)

and complaints of infertility or even palpable testicular masses. However, histological features help to distinguish LCH from normal Leydig cells and benign LCTs. Hyperplastic Leydig cells are arranged in diffuse, multifocal, small nodules and lack cytological atypia, frequent mitoses, necrosis, and vascular invasion. Hyperplastic Leydig cells usually infiltrate between seminiferous tubules, whereas benign LCTs form nodules that compress surrounding tubules. LCTs grow as nodules, efface normal testicular architecture, with loss of seminiferous tubules, and compress the adjacent tissue. Most LCH cases are multifocal and bilateral *(132)*. Figure 6 shows the histological appearance of benign and malignant LCTs, as well as LCH.

Leydig Cells as a Target for Male Contraception

Current approaches to fertility control are predominantly targeted to women. However, men have traditionally and historically played an important role in contraception. Thus, until the second half of the 20th century, periodic abstinence, coitus interruptus, condoms, and vasectomy, all of which are male-directed or male-oriented methods, were the only means for couples to limit family size. However, all of these methods are associated with limited effectiveness, lower acceptability, and partial irreversibility. Therefore, protracted efforts have been made to develop an endocrine male contraceptive regimen. Although our limited understanding of the complex regulatory mechanisms underlying normal spermatogenesis makes it difficult to identify specific testicular targets for pharmacological disruption, both T and FSH are required for complete spermatogenesis in humans. Therefore, to suppress spermatogenesis, the pituitary gonadotropic stimulus is inhibited, thereby abrogating Leydig cell steroidogenesis and nullifying FSH simultaneously. The consequent depletion of intratesticular testosterone and loss of FSH action result in a collapse of spermatogenesis without affecting stem cells. Maintenance of the spermatogonial stem cell population ensures that hormonal suppression of spermatogenesis is reversible. Because testosterone is necessary for spermatogenesis (133), Leydig cells represent an obvious target for hormonal contraception.

Hormonal contraception targets Leydig cells, suppressing their androgenic function. How much testosterone is needed for normal spermatogenesis in humans remains to be determined. In rats, intratesticular testosterone concentrations as low as 5% of normal support the complete spermatogenic process, whereas in the nonhuman primate, testicular androgen levels of 30% of baseline do not prevent complete suppression of germ cell development (134,135). Therefore, testosterone levels must be reduced below a threshold for successful interruption of spermatogenesis. In primates, however, the selective suppression of Leydig cell testosterone production is not sufficient to accomplish the goal of fertility regulation, and the additional inhibition of FSH secretion is necessary (136). One effective approach may be to suppress both LH and FSH secretion and, simultaneously, supply androgen to avoid peripheral androgen deficiency (137).

Leydig Cell Toxicology

Several agents have been identified as Leydig cell toxicants, including ethanol, ethane 1,2 dimethanesulphonate (EDS), 2,3,7,8 tetrachlorodibenzo-p-dioxin (TCCD), and steroid hormone receptor antagonists. These toxicants can damage Leydig cells in three ways: overstimulation or inhibition of steroidogenesis, induction of tumor formation, and promotion of cell death. Leydig cells are vulnerable to several toxins through direct actions and/or by disruption of the hypothalamic–pituitary axis.

Toxicants, such as ethanol, interfere with Leydig cell steroidogenesis by interfering with LH secretion, LH receptor binding, intracellular signal transduction pathways, and steroidogenic enzyme activities. Ethanol, for example, decreases LH secretion and reduces LH receptor binding and intracellular cyclic guanosine 5′-monophosphate (GMP) levels. Hence, chronic alcohol abuse causes declines in testosterone levels (138–140). Tumor formation and cell death are also observed after toxicant exposures. Carcinogenesis is considered to be a consequence of multiple insults to the genome. Necrosis and apoptosis have both been implicated in the process of toxicant-related Leydig cell death, with ethylene dimethanesulfonate exposure as the experimental paradigm (141).

SUMMARY

Leydig cells represent the endocrine proportion of the testis. In all mammalian males, Leydig cells are the main site of testosterone synthesis and secretion and are, thus, essential for male reproductive function. Developmentally, human Leydig cells appear in three separate stages: fetal, neonatal, and pubertal. Each of these stages underlies a corresponding epoch of testosterone secretion in the male lifespan.

Testosterone is synthesized from cholesterol in a series of reactions catalyzed by four enzymes. The first enzyme, P450scc, converts cholesterol to pregnenolone and is located in the inner mitochondrial membrane. Therefore, movement of cholesterol from the Leydig cell cytosol into the mitochondria is the rate-limiting step and is performed by the carrier proteins StAR and PBR. The three other biosynthetic enzymes, 3β-HSD, P450$17\alpha$, and 17β-HSD, are situated in the SER. Testosterone can be metabolized into other steroids, DHT and E_2, primarily by two enzymes: 5α-reductase and P450arom. The Δ^5 and Δ^4 steroidogenic pathways are followed in Leydig cells, with one preferred over the other depending on the species and developmental status. In humans, the Δ^5 pathway from 17α-hydroxypregnenolone to dehydroepiandrosterone is predominant.

Development of steroidogenesis in Leydig cells is regulated by the pituitary gonadotropic hormone LH. FSH and cell–cell interactions in the testis also participate in this regulatory process. Decreased numbers and atrophy of cytological structure, as well as reduced steroidogenic ability, occur during Leydig cell aging, lowering testosterone secretion in older men. LCTs have a low incidence in humans, constituting only 1–3% of testicular neoplasms, with the highest incidence being for men in their 50s. Because testosterone is necessary for spermatogenesis, Leydig cells are a target for male hormonal contraception. Control of male fertility through suppression of Leydig cells will require identifying a level of intratesticular androgen concentration that is sufficient for spermatogenesis while maintaining libido and skeletal muscle mass in the periphery. Studies of reproductive toxicants have shown that disruption of Leydig cell steroidogenic function cannot be ignored as a causative factor.

ACKNOWLEDGMENTS

Support from the National Institutes of Health (HD 32588) facilitated the preparation of this chapter. The authors are also grateful to Dr. Hector Chemes of the Buenos Aires Children's Hospital and Drs. Cathy Naughton and Peter Humphrey of the Washington University School of Medicine, who provided photos of Leydig cell histology. The illustrations were drawn by Evan Read at the Population Council.

REFERENCES

1. Glees P. Leydig, Franz von. In: Gillispie CC, ed. Dictionary of Scientific Biology. Charles Scribner's Sons, New York, 1973, pp. 301–303.
2. Schulze C. Sertoli cells and Leydig cells in man. Adv Anat Embryol Cell Biol 1984;88:1–104.
3. Christensen AK. Leydig cells. In: Greep RO, Astwood EB, eds. Handbook of Physiology. Vol. V. American Physiological Society, Washington DC, 1975, pp. 57–94.
4. Huhtaniemi I, Pelliniemi LJ. Fetal Leydig cells: cellular origin, morphology, life span, and special functional features. Proc Soc Exp Biol Med 1992;201:125–140.
5. Irby DC, Kerr JB, Risbridger GP, de Kretser D. Seasonally and experimentally induced changes in testicular function of the Australian bush rat (Rattus fuscipes). J Reprod Fertil 1984;70:657–666.
6. Kerr JB, Abbenhuis DC, Irby DC. Crystalloid formation in rat Leydig cells. An ultrastructural and hormonal study. Cell Tiss Res 1986;245:91–100.
7. Mori H, Fukunishi R, Fujii M, Hataji K, Shiraishi T, Matsumoto K. Steroidogenical analysis of Reinke crystalloids in human Leydig cells. Pathol Anat 1978;380:1–10.

8. Bardin CW, Hardy MP, Catterall JF. Androgens. In: Adashi E, ed. Reproductive Endocrinology, Surgery, and Technology. Lippincott-Rauen Publishers, Philadelphia, 1995, pp. 505–525.

9. Muller J, Skakkebaek NE. The prenatal and postnatal development of the testis. Baillieres Clin Endocrinol Metab 1992;6:251–271.

10. Carlstrom K, Eriksson A, Stege R, Rannevik G. Relationship between serum testosterone and sex hormone-binding globulin in adult men with intact or absent gonadal function. Int J Androl 1990;13:67–73.

11. Paniagua R, Nistal M, Saez FJ, Fraile B. Ultrastructure of the aging human testis. J Electron Microsc Tech 1991;19:241–260.

12. Prince FP. Ultrastructural evidence of mature Leydig cells and Leydig cell regression in the neonatal human testis. Anat Rec 1990;228:405–417.

13. Chemes HE. Leydig cell development in humans. In: Payne AH, Hardy MP, Russell L, eds. The Leydig Cell. Cache River Press, Viena IL, 1996, pp. 175–201.

14. de Kretser DM, Kerr JB. The cytology of the testis. In: Ernst K, Neil JD, eds. The Physiology of Reproduction. Vol. 1. Raven, New York, 1994, pp. 1177–1290.

15. Wartenberg H. Human testicular development and the role of the mesonephros in the origin of a dual Sertoli cell system. Andrologia 1978;10:1–21.

16. Wartenberg H. Differentiation and development of the testes. In: Burger H, de Kretser D, eds. Comprehensive Endocrinology, the Testis. Raven, New York, 1981, pp. 39–80.

17. Schulze W, Davidoff MS, Holstein AF. Are Leydig cells of neural origin? Substance P-like immunoreactivity in human testicular tissue. Acta Endocrinol (Copenh) 1987;115:373–377.

18. Gondos B. Development and differentiation of the testis and male reproductive tract. In: Steinberger A, Steinberger E, eds. Testicular Development, Structure, and Function. Vol. 3. Raven, New York, 1980, p. 20.

19. Voutilainen R. Differentiation of the fetal gonad. Horm Res 1992;38:66–71.

20. Tapanainen J, Kellokumpu-Lehtinen P, Pelliniemi L, Huhtaniemi I. Age-related changes in endogenous steroids of human fetal testis during early and midpregnancy. J Clin Endocrinol Metab 1981;52:98–102.

21. Reyes FI, Winter JSD, Faiman C. Endocrinology of the fetal testis. In: Bergur H, de Kretser DM, eds. The Testis. Raven, New York, 1989, pp. 119–142.

22. Zondek LH, Zondek T. Fetal hilar cells and Leydig cells in early pregnancy. Biol Neonate 1975;30:193–199.

23. Voutilainen R, Miller WL. Developmental expression of genes for the stereoidogenic enzymes P450scc (20,22-desmolase), P450c17 (17 a-hydroxylase/17,20-lyase), and P450c21 (21-hydroxylase) in the human fetus. J Clin Endocrinol Metab 1986;63:1145–1150.

24. Nistal M, Paniagua R. Testicular and Epididymal Pathology. Thieme-Stratton Inc., New York, 1984.

25. Nistal M, Paniagua R, Regadera J, Santamaria L, Amat P. A quantitative morphological study of human Leydig cells from birth to adulthood. Cell Tissue Res 1986;246:229–236.

26. Pelliniemi LJ, Niei M. Fine structure of the human foetal testis. I. The interstitial tissue. Z Zellforsch Mikrosk Anat 1969;99:507–522.

27. Mancini RE, Vilar O, Lavieri JC, Abbenhuis DC, Heinrich JJ. Development of Leydig cells in normal human testis: a cytological, cytochemical and quantitative study. Am J Anat 1963;112:203–214.

28. Forest MG, Cathiard AM, Bertrand JA. Evidence of testicular activity in early infancy. J Clin Endocrinol Metab 1973;37:148–151.

29. Fouquet JP, Meusy-Dessolle N, Dang DC. Relationships between Leydig cell morphometry and plasma testosterone during postnatal development of the monkey, *Macaca fascicularis.* Reprod Nutr Dev 1984;24:281–296.

30. Prince FP. Ultrastructure of immature Leydig cells in the human prepubertal testis. Anat Rec 1984;209:165–176.

31. Chemes H, Cigorraga S, Bergada C, Schteingart H, Rey R, Pellizzari E. Isolation of human Leydig cell mesenchymal precursors from patients with the androgen insensitivity syndrome: testosterone production and response to human chorionic gonadotropin stimulation in culture. Biol Reprod 1992;46:793–801.

32. Chemes HE, Gottlieb SE, Pasqualini T, Domenichini E, Rivarola MA, Bergada C. Response to acute hCG stimulation and steroidogenic potential of Leydig cell fibroblastic precursors in humans. J Androl 1985;6:102–112.

33. Hardy MP, Zirkin BR, Leydig cell function. In: Lipshultz LI, Howards SS, eds. Infertility in the Male. Mosby-Year Book, St. Louis, MO, 1997, pp. 59–70.

34. Neaves WB, Johnson L, Porter JC, Parker CR, Jr., Petty CS. Leydig cell numbers, daily sperm production, and serum gonadotropin levels in aging men. J Clin Endocrinol Metab 1984;59:756–763.

35. Hall PF. Testicular steroid synthesis. In: Knobil E, Neill JD, eds. The Physiology of Reproduction. Raven, New York, 1994, pp. 1335–1362.

36. Rouiller V, Gangnerau MN, Vayssiere JL, Picon R. Cholesterol side-chain cleavage activity in rat fetal gonads: a limiting step for ovarian steroidogenesis. Mol Cell Endocrinol 1990;72:111–120.

37. Dupont E, Zhao HF, Rheaume E, et al. Localization of 3β-hydroxysteroid dehydrogenase/Δ^5-Δ^4 isomerase in rat gonads and adrenal glands by immunocytochemistry and in situ hybridization. Endocrinology 1990;127:1394–1403.

38. Pelletier G, Dupont E, Simard J, Luu-The V, Belanger A, Labrie F. Ontogeny and subcellular localization of 3 b-hydroxysteroid dehydrogenase (3β-HSD) in the human and rat adrenal, ovary and testis. J Steroid Biochem Mol Biol 1992;43:451–467.

39. Payne AH, Kelch RP, Musich SS, Halpern ME. Intratesticular site of aromatization in the human. J Clin Endocrinol Metab 1976;42:1081–1087.

40. Simpson ER. Cholesterol side-chain cleavage, cytochrome P450, and the control of steroidogenesis. Mol Cell Endocrinol 1979;13:213–227.

41. Boyd GS, Simpson ER. Studies on the conversion of cholestrol to pregnenolone in bovine adrenal mitochondria. In: Mckern KW, ed. Functions of the Adrenal cortex. Vol. 1. Appleton-Century-Crofts, New York, 1968, pp. 49–76.

42. Burstein S, Gut M. Intermediates in the conversion of cholesterol to pregnenolone: kinetics and mechanism. Steroids 1976;28:115–131.

43. Schulster D, Burstein S, Cooke BA. Biosynthesis of steroid hormone. In: Schulze C, Burstein S, Cooke BA, eds. Molecular Endocrinology of the Steroid Hormones. John Wiley & Sons, London, 1976, pp. 44–74.

44. Black SM, Harikrishna JA, Szklarz GD, Miller WL. The mitochondrial environment is required for activity of the cholesterol side-chain cleavage enzyme, cytochrome P450scc. Proc Natl Acad Sci USA 1994;91:7247–7251.

45. Farkash Y, Timberg R, Orly J. Preparation of antiserum to rat cytochrome P-450 cholesterol side chain cleavage, and its use for ultrastructural localization of the immunoreactive enzyme by protein A-gold technique. Endocrinology 1986;118:1353–1365.

46. Stocco DM, Clark BJ. Regulation of the acute production of steroids in steroidogenic cells. Endocr Rev 1996;17:221–244.

47. Freeman DA, Rommerts FFG. Regulation of Leydig Cell cholesterol transport. In: Payne AH, Hardy MP, Russell LD, eds. The Leydig Cell. Cache River, New York, 1996, pp. 232–236.

48. de Launoit Y, Simard J, Durocher F, Labrie F. Androgenic 17β-hydroxysteroid dehydrogenase activity of expressed rat type I 3β-hydroxysteroid dehydrogenase/Δ^5-Δ^4 isomerase. Endocrinology 1992;130:553–555.

49. Rajfer J, Sikka SC, Swerdloff RS. Lack of a direct effect of gonadotropin hormone-releasing hormone agonist on human testicular steroidogenesis. J Clin Endocrinol Metab 1987;64:62–67.

50. Rey R, Campo S, Ayuso S, Nagle C, Chemes H. Testicular steroidogenesis in the Cebus monkey throughout postnatal development. Biol Reprod 1995;52:997–1002.

51. Preslock JP. In vitro steroidogenesis in subhuman primates. In: Steinberger E, Steinberger A, eds. Testicular Development, Structure, and Function. Raven, New York, 1980, pp. 249–268.

52. Preslock JP, Steinberger E. Testicular steroidogenesis in the common marmoset, Callithrix jacchus. Biol Reprod 1977;17:289–293.

53. Labrie F, Simard J, Luu-The V, et al. Structure and tissue-specific expression of 3β-hydroxysteroid dehydrogenase/5-ene-4-ene isomerase genes in human and rat classical and peripheral steroidogenic tissues. J Steroid Biochem Mol Biol 1992;41:421–435.

54. Tremblay Y, Fleury A, Beaudoin C, Vallee M, Belanger A. Molecular cloning and expression of guinea pig cytochrome P450c17 cDNA (steroid 17α-hydroxylase/17,20 lyase): tissue distribution, regulation, and substrate specificity of the expressed enzyme. DNA Cell Biol 1994;13:1199–1212.

55. Dupont E, Labrie F, Luu-The V, Pelletier G. Ontogeny of 3β-hydroxysteroid dehydrogenase/Δ^5-Δ^4 isomerase (3β-HSD) in rat testis as studied by immunocytochemistry. Anat Embryol (Berl) 1993;187:583–589.

56. Hauffa BP, Miller WL, Grumbach MM, Conte FA, Kaplan SL. Congenital adrenal hyperplasia due to deficient cholesterol side-chain cleavage activity (20, 22-desmolase) in a patient treated for 18 years. Clin Endocrinol (Oxf) 1985;23:481–493.

57. Hall PF. Cytochrome P-450 C21scc: one enzyme with two actions: hydroxylase and lyase. J Steroid Biochem Mol Biol 1991;40:527–532.

58. Pang S, Yang X, Wang M, et al. Inherited congenital adrenal hyperplasia in the rabbit: absent cholesterol side-chain cleavage cytochrome P450 gene expression. Endocrinology 1992;131:181–186.

59. Fevold HR, Lorence MC, McCarthy JL, et al. Rat P450(17 a) from testis: characterization of a full-length cDNA encoding a unique steroid hydroxylase capable of catalyzing both delta 4- and delta 5-steroid-17,20-lyase reactions. Mol Endocrinol 1989;3:968–975.

60. Payne AH, O' Shaughnessy PJ. Structure, function and regulation of steroidogenic enzymes in the Leydig cell. In: Payne AH, Hardy MP, Zirkin BR, eds. The Leydig Cell. Cahce River, New York, 1996, p. 260.

61. Hardy MP, Gelber SJ, Zhou ZF, et al. Hormonal control of Leydig cell differentiation. Ann N Y Acad Sci 1991;637:152–163.

62. Fishman J, Goto J. Mechanism of estrogen biosynthesis. Participation of multiple enzyme sites in placental aromatase hydroxylations. J Biol Chem 1981;256:4466–4471.

63. Thompson EA, Jr., Siiteri PK. Utilization of oxygen and reduced nicotinamide adenine dinucleotide phosphate by human placental microsomes during aromatization of androstenedione. J Biol Chem 1974;249:5364–5372.

64. Thompson EA, Jr., Siiteri PK. The involvement of human placental microsomal cytochrome P-450 in aromatization. J Biol Chem 1974;249:5373–5378.

65. Raeside JI, Lobb DK. Metabolism of androstenedione by Sertoli cell enriched preparations and purified Leydig cells from boar testes in relation to estrogen formation. J Steroid Biochem 1984;20:1267–1272.

66. Raeside JI, Renaud RL. Estrogen and androgen production by purified Leydig cells of mature boars. Biol Reprod 1983;28:727–733.

67. Canick JA, Makris A, Gunsalus GL, Ryan KJ. Testicular aromatization in immature rats: localization and stimulation after gonadotropin administration in vivo. Endocrinology 1979;104:285–288.

68. Dorrington JH, Fritz IB, Armstrong DT. Control of testicular estrogen synthesis. Biol Reprod 1978;18:55–64.

69. Nitta H, Bunick D, Hess RA, et al. Germ cells of the mouse testis express P450 aromatase. Endocrinology 1993;132:1396–1401.

70. Rommerts FF, de Jong FH, Brinkmann AO, van der Molen HJ. Development and cellular localization of rat testicular aromatase activity. J Reprod Fertil 1982;65:281–288.

71. Dorrington JH, Khan SA. Steroid production, metabolism, and release by Sertoli cells. In: Russell L, Griswold M, eds. The Sertoli Cell. Cache River, Clearwater, FL, 1993, pp. 537–549.

72. Majumdar SS, Winters SJ, Plant TM. Procedures for the isolation and culture of Sertoli cells from the testes of infant, juvenile, and adult rhesus monkeys (Macaca mulatta). Biol Reprod 1998;58:633–640.

73. Andersson S, Russell DW. Structural and biochemical properties of cloned and expressed human and rat steroid 5 a-reductases. Proc Natl Acad Sci USA 1990;87:3640–3644.

74. Andersson S, Bishop RW, Russell DW. Expression cloning and regulation of steroid 5 a-reductase, an enzyme essential for male sexual differentiation. J Biol Chem 1989;264:16249–16255.

75. Gunsalus GL, Bardin CW. Sertoli-germ cell interactions as determinants of bidirectional secretion of androgen-binding protein. Ann N Y Acad Sci 1991;637:322–326.

76. Gunsalus GL, Larrea F, Musto NA, Becker RR, Mather JP, Bardin CW. Androgen binding protein as a marker for Sertoli cell function. J Steroid Biochem 1981;15:99–106.

77. Hryb DJ, Nakhla AM, Kahn SM, et al. Sex hormone-binding globulin in the human prostate is locally synthesized and may act as an autocrine/paracrine effector. J Biol Chem 2002;277:26618–26622.

78. McFarland KC, Sprengel R, Phillips HS, et al. Lutropin-choriogonadotropin receptor: an unusual member of the G protein-coupled receptor family. Science 1989;245:494–499.

79. Schlegel PN, Hardy MP. Male Reproductive Physiology. In: Partin K, Peters N, eds. Campbell's Urology. Vol. 2. Saunders, Philadelphia, 2002, pp. 1437–1474.

80. Cooke BA, Choi MC, Dirami G, Lopez-Ruiz MP, West AP. Control of steroidogenesis in Leydig cells. J Steroid Biochem Mol Biol 1992;43:445–449.

81. Saez JM. Leydig cells: endocrine, paracrine, and autocrine regulation. Endocr Rev 1994;15:574–626.

82. Luo L, Chen H, Stocco DM, Zirkin BR. Leydig cell protein synthesis and steroidogenesis in response to acute stimulation by luteinizing hormone in rats. Biol Reprod 1998;59:263–270.

83. Lin D, Sugawara T, Strauss JF, 3rd, et al. Role of steroidogenic acute regulatory protein in adrenal and gonadal steroidogenesis. Science 1995;267:1828–1831.

84. Sugawara T, Lin D, Holt JA, et al. Structure of the human steroidogenic acute regulatory protein (StAR) gene: StAR stimulates mitochondrial cholesterol 27-hydroxylase activity. Biochemistry 1995;34:12506–12512.

85. Christenson LK, Strauss JF. Steroidogenic acute regulatory protein (StAR) and the intramitochondrial translocation of cholesterol. Biochim Biophys Acta 2000;1529:175–187.

86. Li H, Papadopoulos V. Peripheral-type benzodiazepine receptor function in cholesterol transport. Identification of a putative cholesterol recognition/interaction amino acid sequence and consensus pattern. Endocrinology 1998;139:4991–4997.

87. Papadopoulos V, Amri H, Li H, Boujrad N, Vidic B, Garnier M. Targeted disruption of the peripheral-type benzodiazepine receptor gene inhibits steroidogenesis in the R2C Leydig tumor cell line. J Biol Chem 1997;272:32129–32135.

88. Krueger KE, Papadopoulos V. Peripheral-type benzodiazepine receptors mediate translocation of cholesterol from outer to inner mitochondrial membranes in adrenocortical cells. J Biol Chem 1990;265:15015–15022.

89. Papadopoulos V, Amri H, Boujrad N, et al. Peripheral benzodiazepine receptor in cholesterol transport and steroidogenesis. Steroids 1997;62:21–28.

90. West LA, Horvat RD, Roess DA, Barisas BG, Juengel JL, Niswender GD. Steroidogenic acute regulatory protein and peripheral-type benzodiazepine receptor associate at the mitochondrial membrane. Endocrinology 2001;142:502–505.

91. Swerdloff RS, Heber D. Endocrine control of testicular function from birth to puberty. In: HB, D Kretser, eds. The Testis. Raven, New York, 1981, pp. 108–126.

92. Mori H, Christensen AK. Morphometric analysis of Leydig cells in the normal rat testis. J Cell Biol 1980;84:340–354.

93. Teerds KJ, Closset J, Rommerts FF, et al. Effects of pure FSH and LH preparations on the number and function of Leydig cells in immature hypophysectomized rats. J Endocrinol 1989;120:97–106.

94. Russell LD, Corbin TJ, Ren HP, Amador A, Bartke A, Ghosh S. Structural changes in rat Leydig cells posthypophysectomy: a morphometric and endocrine study. Endocrinology 1992;131:498–508.

95. Keeney DS, Mendis-Handagama SM, Zirkin BR, Ewing LL. Effect of long-term deprivation of luteinizing hormone on Leydig cell volume, Leydig cell number, and steroidogenic capacity of the rat testis. Endocrinology 1988;123:2906–2915.

96. Wing TY, Ewing LL, Zegeye B, Zirkin BR. Restoration effects of exogenous luteinizing hormone on the testicular steroidogenesis and Leydig cell ultrastructure. Endocrinology 1985;117:1779–1787.

97. Awoniyi CA, Santulli R, Chandrashekar V, Schanbacher BD, Zirkin BR. Quantitative restoration of advanced spermatogenic cells in adult male rats made azoospermic by active immunization against luteinizing hormone or gonadotropin-releasing hormone. Endocrinology 1989;125:1303–1309.

98. O'Shaughnessy PJ. Steroidogenic enzyme activity in the hypogonadal (hpg) mouse testis and effect of treatment with luteinizing hormone. J Steroid Biochem Mol Biol 1991;39:921–928.

99. Orth J, Christensen AK. Localization of 125I-labeled FSH in the testes of hypophysectomized rats by autoradiography at the light and electron microscope levels. Endocrinology 1977;101:262–278.

100. Bardin CW. The Sertoli cell. In: Knobil E, ed. The physiology of reproduction. Vol. 2. Raven, New York, 1988.

101. Baker PJ, Abel MH, Charlton HM, Huhtaniemi IT, O'Shaughnessy PJ. Failure of normal Leydig cell development in FSH receptor deficient mice but not in FSHβ-deficient mice. Endocrinology, 2003;144:138–145.

102. Feig LA, Bellve AR, Erickson NH, Klagsbrun M. Sertoli cells contain a mitogenic polypeptide. Proc Natl Acad Sci USA 1980;77:4774–4778.

103. Ewing L, Keeney D. Leydig cells: structure and function. In: Desjardins C, Ewing LL, eds. Cell and Molecular Biology of the Testis. Oxford University Press, New York, 1993, pp. 137–165.

104. Belanger A, Candas B, Dupont A, et al. Changes in serum concentrations of conjugated and unconjugated steroids in 40- to 80-year-old men. J Clin Endocrinol Metab 1994;79:1086–1090.

105. Dabbs JM, Jr. Age and seasonal variation in serum testosterone concentration among men. Chronobiol Int 1990;7:245–249.

106. Gray A, Feldman HA, McKinlay JB, Longcope C. Age, disease, and changing sex hormone levels in middle-aged men: results of the Massachusetts Male Aging Study. J Clin Endocrinol Metab 1991;73:1016–1025.

107. Harman SM, Tsitouras PD. Reproductive hormones in aging men. I. Measurement of sex steroids, basal luteinizing hormone, and Leydig cell response to human chorionic gonadotropin. J Clin Endocrinol Metab 1980;51:35–40.

108. Vermeulen A, Rubens R, Verdonck L. Testosterone secretion and metabolism in male senescence. J Clin Endocrinol Metab 1972;34:730–735.

109. Baker HW, Burger HG, de Kretser DM, et al. Changes in the pituitary-testicular system with age. Clin Endocrinol (Oxf) 1976;5:349–372.

110. Neaves WB, Johnson L, Petty CS. Age-related change in numbers of other interstitial cells in testes of adult men: evidence bearing on the fate of Leydig cells lost with increasing age. Biol Reprod 1985;33:259–269.

111. Mori H, Hiromoto N, Nakahara M, Shiraishi T. Stereological analysis of Leydig cell ultrastructure in aged humans. J Clin Endocrinol Metab 1982;55:634–641.

112. Paniagua R, Amat P, Nistal M, Martin A. Ultrastructure of Leydig cells in human ageing testes. J Anat 1986;146:173–183.

113. Nistal M, Codesal J, Paniagua R. Multinucleate spermatids in aging human testes. Arch Androl 1986;16:125–129.

114. Giusti G, Gonnelli P, Borrelli D, et al. Age-related secretion of androstenedione, testosterone and dihydrotestosterone by the human testis. Exp Gerontol 1975;10:241–245.

115. Piotti LE, Ghiringhelli F, Magrini U. Apropos of the testicular function of the aged: histochemical and biological observations. Rev Fr Endocrinol Clin 1967;8:479–491.

116. Purifoy FE, Koopmans LH, Mayes DM. Age differences in serum androgen levels in normal adult males. Hum Biol 1981;53:499–511.

117. Serio M, Gonnelli P, Borrelli D, et al. Human testicular secretion with increasing age. J Steroid Biochem 1979;11:893–897.

118. Zirkin BR, Chen H. Regulation of Leydig cell steroidogenic function during aging. Biol Reprod 2000;63:977–981.

119. Mottola A, di Cello V, Saltutti C, Bianchi S. Leydig cell tumor of the testis. Therapeutic and anatomopathologic clinical study of 2 new cases. Arch Esp Urol 1989;42:433–435.

120. Rich MA, Keating MA. Leydig cell tumors and tumors associated with congenital adrenal hyperplasia. Urol Clin North Am 2000;27:519–528.

121. Cortez JC, Kaplan GW. Gonadal stromal tumors, gonadoblastomas, epidermoid cysts, and secondary tumors of the testis in children. Urol Clin North Am 1993;20:15–26.

122. Ducharme JR, Collu R. Pubertal development: normal, precocious and delayed. Clin Endocrinol Metab 1982;11:57–87.

123. Fallick ML, Lin WW, Lipshultz LI. Leydig cell tumors presenting as azoospermia. J Urol 1999;161:1571–1572.

124. Kondoh N, Koh E, Nakamura M, et al. Bilateral Leydig cell tumors and male infertility: case report. Urol Int 1991;46:104–106.

125. Sasano H, Nakashima N, Matsuzaki O, et al. Testicular sex cord-stromal lesions: immunohistochemical analysis of cytokeratin, vimentin and steroidogenic enzymes. Virchows Arch A Pathol Anat Histopathol 1992;421:163–169.

126. Kuhn JM, Duranteau L, Rieu MA, Lahlou N, Roger M, Luton JP. Evidence of oestradiol-induced changes in gonadotrophin secretion in men with feminizing Leydig cell tumours. Eur J Endocrinol 1994;131:160–166.

127. Ritchie JP. Neoplasms of the testis. In: Walsh P, Reitik A, Vaughan E, Wein A, eds. Campell's Urology. WB Saunders, Philadelphia, 1992, pp. 1222–1263.

128. Grem JL, Robins HI, Wilson KS, Gilchrist K, Trump DL. Metastatic Leydig cell tumor of the testis. Report of three cases and review of the literature. Cancer 1986;58:2116–2119.

129. Mellor SG, McCutchan JD. Gynaecomastia and occult Leydig cell tumour of the testis. Br J Urol 1989;63:420–422.

130. Konrad D, Schoenle EJ. Ten-year follow-up in a boy with Leydig cell tumor after selective surgery. Horm Res 1999;51:96–100.

131. Rushton HG, Belman AB. Testis-sparing surgery for benign lesions of the prepubertal testis. Urol Clin North Am 1993;20:27–37.

132. Naughton CK, Nadler RB, Basler JW, Humphrey PA. Leydig cell hyperplasia. Br J Urol 1998;81:282–289.

133. Marshall GR, Jockenhovel F, Ludecke D, Nieschlag E. Maintenance of complete but quantitatively reduced spermatogenesis in hypophysectomized monkeys by testosterone alone. Acta Endocrinol (Copenh) 1986;113:424–431.

134. Bartlett JM, Weinbauer GF, Nieschlag E. Differential effects of FSH and testosterone on the maintenance of spermatogenesis in the adult hypophysectomized rat. J Endocrinol 1989;121:49–58.

135. Weinbauer GF, Gockeler E, Nieschlag E. Testosterone prevents complete suppression of spermatogenesis in the gonadotropin-releasing hormone antagonist-treated nonhuman primate *(Macaca fascicularis)*. J Clin Endocrinol Metab 1988;67:284–290.
136. Wickings EJ, Nieschlag E. The effects of active immunization with testosterone on pituitary-gonadal feedback in the male rhesus monkey *(Macaca mulatta)*. Biol Reprod 1978;18:602–607.
137. Weinbauer GF, Nieschlag E. The Leydig Cell as a Target for Male Contraception. The Leydig Cell. Cache River, New York, 1996, pp. 640–649.
138. Adams ML, Forman JB, Kalicki JM, Meyer ER, Sewing B, Cicero TJ. Antagonism of alcohol-induced suppression of rat testosterone secretion by an inhibitor of nitric oxide synthase. Alcohol Clin Exp Res 1993;17:660–664.
139. Pajarinen JT, Karhunen PJ. Spermatogenic arrest and Sertoli cell-only syndrome—common alcohol-induced disorders of the human testis. Int J Androl 1994;17:292–299.
140. Van Thiel DH, Gavaler JS. Hypothalamic-pituitary-gonadal function in liver disease with particular attention to the endocrine effects of chronic alcohol abuse. Prog Liver Dis 1986;8:273–282.
141. Morris ID. Leydig cell toxicology. In: Payne AH, Hardy MP, Russell LD, eds. The Leydig Cell. Cache River, New York, 1996, pp. 575–585.

3 Spermatogenesis and Its Regulation in Higher Primates

Gary R. Marshall, PhD

CONTENTS

INTRODUCTION

Spermatogenesis is the series of processes occurring in the testis that results in the production of highly differentiated haploid spermatozoa from undifferentiated diploid spermatogonia. The purpose of this chapter is to review spermatogenesis and its hormonal regulation in higher primates; that is, species chiefly classified in the suborder Catarrhini.[1] Although many basic concepts concerning spermatogenesis have resulted from experimental studies of rodent species, the suitability of these species for investigating all aspects of spermatogenesis and generalizing those results to primates, including man, must be considered with caution. This note of caution derives from observations indicating fundamental differences between the two phylogenic orders in development, cellular events of spermatogenesis, and hormonal regu-

---

[1] Romer (1) defined the higher primates, Catarrhini, to comprise four families, namely, Anthropoidea, Cercopithecidae (Old-World Monkeys), Siimidae (manlike apes), and Hominidae (human). More recently, Hill (2) has revised the taxonomy of primates in his seminal work, *The Primates,* and has modified Romer's definition of higher primates into Platyrrhini (New-World primates) and Catarrhini (Old-World primates). The Catarrhini are divided further into two superfamilies, Cercopithecidea (Old-World monkeys) and Homonoidea (Old-World apes and man). In addition, the Old-World monkeys and the Hominoidea are more closely related to one another than either is related to the New-World monkeys.

From: *Male Hypogonadism:*
Basic, Clinical, and Therapeutic Principles
Edited by: S. J. Winters © Humana Press Inc., Totowa, NJ

lation of spermatogenesis. This should not be surprising. Although species of both orders have adapted successfully in many different environments, essentially spreading throughout the world, rodents' and primates' adaptive strategies are fundamentally different. Rodents have remained small animals throughout their evolutionary history, growing and maturing rapidly, usually in a few months, and reproducing frequently with large numbers of offspring in each litter. Rodents produce large populations of offspring, with diverse genotypes on which selective adaptation may operate (3). In contrast, primates have become larger during their evolutionary history, growing and maturing slowly usually for years, and reproducing infrequently, with only one or two offspring per pregnancy (4). Primates have produced small populations of individuals, with less genetic diversity on which selective adaptation may operate. Primates, perhaps because of their arboreal origin, have highly developed nervous systems, allowing these species to be more inquisitive, exploring new environmental niches, and learning rather than genetically adapting to novel habitats.

Although spermatogenesis is generally similar between these two orders, many details are remarkably different, and perhaps these differences accommodate the diverse strategies of adaptation. Three types of germ cells, namely, spermatogonia, spermatocytes, and spermatids, and one somatic cell type, the Sertoli cells, that provide the structural support of and nutrients to the germ cells, comprise the epithelium of the seminiferous tubule of the mammalian testis. Perhaps the most remarkable difference between spermatogenesis in rodents and primates was identified in an early observation by a pioneer of reproductive biology. Smith (5) observed that surgical ablation of the pituitary gland of adult primates led to a more complete regression of the seminiferous epithelium than this surgery in rodents. In the former species, only Sertoli cells and stem spermatogonia remain after hypophysectomy, whereas in the rat, spermatogenesis was arrested during spermiogenesis (6–9). This difference is not likely to result from incomplete ablation of the rodent pituitary, as suggested by Smith (5), because chemical hypophysectomy in rats using a gonadotropin-releasing hormone-receptor (GnRH-R) antagonist, that dramatically suppresses gonadotropin secretion (10–12), similarly arrested spermatogenesis during spermiogenesis. Moreover, GnRH antagonist treatment of intact adult monkeys also causes regression of the seminiferous epithelium identical to that produced by hypophysectomy (10–12). In primates, the gonadotropic hormones are obligatory for development of differentiated spermatogonia, spermatocytes, and spermatids, whereas in rodents, a limited number of spermatids may be produced in the absence of a gonadotropin drive. The second major difference is that the mechanism of stem cell renewal is fundamentally dissimilar between rodents and higher primates (13). Third, the morphology of the various types of germ cells and the temporal relationships are more alike in the Cercopithecadea and Hominadea than other species (13).

ANATOMY OF THE MALE REPRODUCTIVE TRACT

The gross anatomy of the reproductive system of male primates encompasses two of the cardinal characteristics of the order primate.[2] Hill (2) stated that the testes, although

---

[2] According to Hill (2), Mivart stated in 1873 the characteristics of primates: "unguiculate, claviculate placental mammals, with orbits encircled by bone; three kinds of teeth, at least, at one time in life; brain always a posterior lobe and calcarine fissure; innermost digit of at least one pair of extremities opposable; hallux with a flat nail or none; a well-defined caecum; *penis pendulous, testes scrotal;* always two pectoral mammary glands" (italics added).

usually scrotal, in the adults of some higher primates, e.g., *Macaca mulatta,* can be retractable into the lower portion of the inguinal canal because the lower ring of the canal does not fully close. Each testis is encapsulated in a tough white fibrous membrane, the tunica albuginea, with a large testicular artery coursing in a sinuous fashion along the anterior surface of the gonad. The parenchyma of the organ consists of many tortuous seminiferous tubules surrounded by intersitial tissue composed of Leydig cells, macrophages, nerves, blood vessels, and lymphatic vessels. In primates, the parenchyma is divided by fibrous tissue into lobules. Three types of germ cells, spermatogonia, spermatocytes, and spermatids, in addition to the somatic cells, named for Enrico Sertoli who identified their function 125 years ago *(14),* comprise the epithelium of the seminiferous tubules. The seminiferous epithelium is the site of spermatogenesis. Once spermatozoa are produced by the seminiferous epithelium they are released into the lumen of the tubule, and are transported through the tubulus rectus that forms when each seminiferous tubule loops around and rejoins itself to form this single straight tubule *(15).* The tubuli recti enter the anastomosing structure of the rete testis. The rete testis is embedded in dense connective tissue called the mediastinum, which, in most higher primates, runs through the long axis of the ovoid testis. The rete testis tubules join at the posterior surface of the testis into three to five ductuli efferentia that, in turn, form a single confluence that is the origin of the duct of the epididymis.

CYTOLOGY OF SPERMATOGENESIS

Spermatogenesis is a series of processes that produce a prodigious number of spermatozoa from a rather small finite population of stem spermatogonia. In addition to this quantitative aspect of spermatogenesis, meiosis results in an equally enormous number of haploid spermatozoa carrying different recombinations of the male's genes that contribute to the genetic diversity of the next generation. Moreover, spermatozoa are produced continuously throughout the life of the adult male primate, a time span that encompasses a few years in some nonhuman primates but 50 or more years in man. The cytology of spermatogenesis has been described for several Catarrhini *(16–22).* Because the types and arrangements of the germ cells are similar in these species, a general description is presented. Any differences are noted where appropriate.

Spermatogonia and Mitosis

Spermatogonia of mammals are always found adjacent to the basement membrane of the seminiferous tubule and are classified as either stem cells or differentiated spermatogonia *(19–26).* The first category, stem cells, are called type A spermatogonia, whereas differentiated spermatogonia are designated as type B spermatogonia. Type A spermatogonia in primates are further divided into dark type A, or Ad, spermatogonia, and pale type A, or Ap, spermatogonia *(17,19–26).* The Ap spermatogonia divide to produce either more Ap spermatogonia,[3] or the first generation of differentiated type B spermatogonia. Four generations of type B spermatogonia, designated B_1, B_2, B_3, and B_4, are present in the seminiferous epithelium of nonhuman primates of the Catarrhini. Humans are an exception in this regard, because only one generation of type B spermatogonia has been described in the seminiferous epithelia of men *(16–18,23,24,26).*

---

[3] The important topic of spermatogonial stem cells and the process of stem cell renewal is discussed in the section entitled Stem Cell Renewal.

The differentiated spermatogonia are committed to produce more type B spermatogonia. These germ cells are diploid and are destined to either proliferate or, if they fail to proliferate, die. The mitoses of the differentiated spermatogonia are symmetrical; the two daughter cells are identical to one another, but the nuclei have smaller diameters and contain more heterochromatin than those of the mother cell.

Spermatocytes and Meiosis

The last generation of type B spermatogonia divide and produce the primary spermatocytes. These are the last diploid germ cells in the production of spermatozoa. Historically, they were called resting spermatocytes, but this is a misnomer, because these cells are not quiescent *(13)*. The primary spermatocytes are the most mature germ cells to synthesize DNA in preparation for meiosis I and II. Moreover, these germ cells synthesize four times more DNA than is found in the haploid state. As the primary spermatocytes prepare for and enter the long prophase of meiosis I, they move from the basement membrane of the seminiferous tubule toward its lumen. At this point in the spermatogenesis process, germ cells bind to the Sertoli cells through specialized cellular junctions and remain so until the immature spermatozoa are released from the seminiferous epithelium. During this transition, the spermatocytes progress from leptonema, characterized by the formation of long, thin chromosomes, to zygonema, characterized by homologous chromosome pairing. As spermatocytes form the next cellular layer, the cytological event "crossing over" occurs. Because the chromosome pairs are thick, this phase of meiosis I is called pachynema. The duration of prophase of meiosis I is 2–3 wk, depending on the species. In rapid fashion after the completion of prophase I, the spermatocytes complete Meiosis I, forming haploid secondary spermatocytes that, in turn, complete meiosis II, resulting theoretically in four haploid spermatids.

Spermatids and Spermiogenesis

Spermiogenesis is the long phase of morphogenesis during which the haploid spermatids become highly motile cells ultimately capable of fertilizing ova. The major morphological changes occurring during this phase of spermatogenesis are the formation of the head of the spermatozoon, formation of the tail, and loss of cytoplasm *(13)*. The head of the mature spermatozoon in higher primates consists of the acrosome, a specialized lysosome containing enzymes needed at the time of fertilization, and the nucleus, which contains highly condensed chromatin. Several distinct steps in the formation of the acrosome during spermiogenesis, which are revealed by periodic acid-Schiff's staining of the putative organelle, are used to identify the temporal sequence of spermiogenesis.

The newly formed spermatid is distinguished from other germ cells by the presence of a small spherical nucleus in the cell cytoplasm. The Golgi region of the newly formed spermatid is pink under PAS-Schiff's staining and lies near the nuclear surface, producing a polarity in the spermatid. Spermatids with this morphology are identified as Step 1. Step 2 spermatids have two or more small red granules, usually between the Golgi region and the nucleus. Coalescence of the granules into a single large acrosomic granule indicates Step 3. Step 4 spermatids have a single red granule in a vesicle that contacts the nucleus of the cell. The formation of Step 4 spermatids marks the end of the first, or Golgi, phase of spermiogenesis. The vesicle and granule of the putative acrosome begin to spread along the nuclear surface. The next four steps of spermiogenesis, Steps 5, 6, 7, and 8, are distinguished by the extent of the cap-like formation, and these steps constitute the cap phase of acrosome formation. The next four steps of spermiogenesis, Steps 9–12, are characterized by formation of the final shape of the acrosome, condensation of the nuclear chromatin, and further growth of the spermatid tail. These steps form the acrosomic phase of spermiogenesis. The final phase of spermiogenesis, maturation phase, comprises Steps 13 and 14 in nonhuman primates. By Step 13, the spermatids have achieved the morphology of the spermatozoa, and little morphological change occurs during these steps, except for a further reduction of cytoplasm. Step 14 spermatids are often called testicular spermatozoa, and, with completion of this last step of spermiogenesis, the spermatozoa are released from the seminiferous epithelium.

KINETICS OF SPERMATOGENESIS AND CYCLE OF THE SEMINIFEROUS EPITHELIUM

The kinetics of spermatogenesis are the temporal relationships among the various germ cells within the seminiferous epithelium as they proceed through mitosis, meiosis, and spermiogenesis (13,16,17,20,21). The Sertoli cells, the only somatic cells found in the seminiferous epithelium, provide nourishment, growth factors, and organization to the germ cells (14). These somatic cells span the entire seminiferous epithelium, sitting on the basement membrane and stretching to the lumen of the seminiferous tubule. The seminiferous epithelium has, in addition to the Sertoli cells, one or two types of spermatogonia, spermatocytes, and spermatids. The spermatogonia lie on the basement membrane and, as described previously, are mitotically active. The spermatocytes, produced by the cell division of the last generation of differentiated spermatogonia, move toward the lumen of the tubule and, thus, constitute the next layer of the epithelium. The spermatocytes complete meiosis and produce the spermatids. The spermatids form the layers of the epithelium adjacent to the tubular lumen and proceed through the steps of spermiogenesis. The arrangement of the germ cells and the synchrony of the three processes of spermatogenesis, mitosis, meiosis, and spermiogenesis, result in a limited number of cell associations of fixed cellular composition (see Fig. 1). The steps of spermiogenesis define a finite number of cellular associations, usually 12 in nonhuman primates, and 6 in humans (16,17,20,21). The cellular associations are temporally related and form a sequence called the cycle of the seminiferous epithelium. Each cellular association is one stage of the cycle. The cycle of the seminiferous epithelium is defined as the occurrence of all stages in sequence in one area of a seminiferous tubule. In higher primates, the area of the seminiferous tubule in one stage of the cycle encompasses from 0.1 to 9 mm of the length of a seminiferous tubule, except in humans (20–21).

The duration of the cycle can be determined by administering a labeled nucleotide that is incorporated by all cells that are synthesizing DNA in preparation for mitosis. By precisely timing the interval between the administration of the labeled nucleotide and the removal of the testis, the duration of the cycle of the seminiferous epithelium can be studied. In addition, the frequency with which a stage is detected is directly related to the duration of that stage. Using the duration of the cycle and the individual stage frequencies, the duration of each stage can be determined. In turn, the duration of spermatogenesis can be estimated from the duration of each stage. The difficulty of determining the length of spermatogenesis results, in part, from the lack of consensus of when spermatogenesis precisely begins (see Stem Cell Renewal).

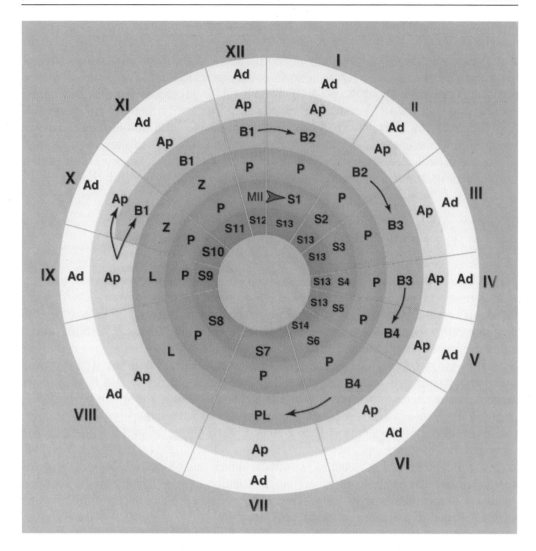

Fig. 1. The cycle of the seminiferous epithelium of the rhesus monkey depicted in a highly schematic manner to emphasize its recurring nature. The cellular associations that define the stages of the cycle are indicated with Roman numerals I–XII. The circumference represents time, and the width of each segment is proportional to the duration of each stage. The increasing darkness represents maturation of the cell types as the process of spermatogenesis unfolds. Spermatogenesis begins in stage IX, when half of the population of Ap spermatogonia divide and produce type B spermatogonia (B1). Coincidentally, the other half of the population of Ap spermatogonia also divide and produce Ap spermatogonia, thereby renewing the population of these stem cells. Spermatogenesis terminates in stage VI, when S14 spermatids are released into the lumen of the seminiferous epithelium. B1–B4, four generations of type B spermatogonia; PL, preleptotene spermatocytes; L, leptotene spermatocytes; Z, zygotene spermatocytes; P, pachytene spermatocytes; MII, completion of meiosis; S1–S14, spermatids at each of the 14 steps of spermiogenesis. The arrows or arrowheads indicate mitosis and the completion of meiosis, respectively. (From ref. *48.* Reprinted with permission of The Endocrine Society.)

In many higher primate species, a single cellular association forms the epithelium of a segment of the seminiferous tubule *(20,21)*. However, the seminiferous epithelium of man does not follow this orderly pattern *(16,17)*. In humans *(21)* and in two other primates, an Old-World monkey, the olive baboon, *P. anubis (27)*, and a New-World monkey, the common marmoset, *Callithrix jacchus (28)*, a cross-section of a tubule may contain more than one cellular association.

The duration of the cycle has been determined in several nonhuman primates to range from 9 to 12 d and is characteristic of each species *(13)*. To gain this information, the radionucleotide, tritiated thymidine, was administered to adult male primates. Testes were removed within 2–3 h after the injection. Other testes were removed at carefully timed intervals after radionucleotide administration. Using the most mature labeled cell at each interval, as well as stage frequencies, the duration of the cycle was determined. For example, tritiated thymidine was administered to several adult male stump-tailed macaques, *M. arctoides,* and the most mature labeled cells were determined in testes removed either 3 h or 12 d, 3 h later *(20)*. Using the stage frequencies that are directly related to the individual durations of each cycle stage, and the percentage of germ cells labeled at each time point, the duration of the stump-tailed macaque cycle was determined to be 11.5 d.

As stated previously, the seminiferous epithelium of man is less well organized than is that of other nonhuman primates. More than one cellular association may occur in a cross-section of the seminiferous tubule, and, frequently, some cellular associations are incomplete because one or more generations of germ cells may be absent. For these reasons, analysis of the kinetics of spermatogenesis in humans is problematic. Nonetheless, Heller and Clermont *(17)* were permitted in the early 1960s to inject tritiated thymidine into the testes of prisoner volunteers. Biopsies of the testes were performed 1 h, 16 d, and 32 d after the injection.

In the biopsies performed at 1 h, the most mature germ cells were preleptotene spermatocytes in Stage 3 of the six stages identified in man. At 16 d, pachytene spermatocytes in Stage 3 were the most mature germ cells labeled. At 32 d, after the administration of labeled nucleotide, Step 3 spermatids were the most mature germ cells labeled. From these results, the duration of the cycle in man was estimated to be 16 d. Spermatogenesis was defined to begin with the production of type B spermatogonia and extended for four cycles, or 64 d. Although this study will not be repeated for ethical reasons, it should be noted that biopsies are of limited value in a study of the kinetics of spermatogenesis. They are not representative of the entire testis, because too few seminiferous tubules are sampled to allow for a meaningful description of the cellular associations, their individual frequencies, and a sample that is sufficiently large to permit assessment of the percentage of each type of germ cell that incorporated the labeled nucleotide. All of these parameters are necessary to estimate the duration of the cycle of the seminiferous epithelium and, in turn, the duration of spermatogenesis. For these reasons, estimates of the kinetics of spermatogenesis of man that were reported in this early study must be considered preliminary *(17)*.

Wave of the Cycle

One final, but often misunderstood consequence of the organization of the seminiferous epithelium is the cycle wave *(13)*. The stages of the cycle occupy segments of the seminiferous tubule that are aligned more or less in sequence along the length of the tubule. This alignment of all stages of the cycle is the wave. Moreover, the length of a segment in a particular stage was assumed to be constant from one wave to another. Indeed, the wave was believed by many early investigators of spermatogenesis to represent in space what the cycle was in time, i.e., an orderly sequence that could be used to know precisely that the stage of the segments immediately adjacent were numerically one stage earlier or one later in the cycle.

A detailed study of the cycle wave in the rat indicated that the wave was not a spatial arrangement of stages that approached the orderly temporal sequence of the cycle *(29)*. The wave instead varied from an orderly spatial sequence in two ways. First, the segments of tubule in a particular stage were not consistently of similar length, and, in turn, the length of tubule containing the entire wave was also variable. Secondly, two types of modulations of the wave were observed. In the first type, the consecutive arrangement of the cycle stages along the tubule was interrupted, and the stages would be repeated. For example, if segments of tubule were in Stages 1, 2, and 3, then the next segment would not be Stage 4 as expected, but instead this segment would contain Stage 1 again, and subsequent segments would contain the remaining cycle stages. In the second variant, the sequence of stages would be reversed. For example, if the sequence was Stages 3, 4, and 5, then the next segments would be 4 and 3. The segments would then continue in sequence; that is, 4, 5, and 6.

STEM CELL RENEWAL

Stem cells are common to all epithelial systems because they have two fundamental properties *(30)*. First, stem cells have the ability to produce more stem cells (to maintain a constant number of these cells). Second, stem cells can produce differentiated progeny; this property of spermatogenetic stem cells was described in the Spermatogonia and Mitosis section. The former capability represents stem cell renewal.

Stem cell renewal is the mechanism that ensures that remarkably large numbers of spermatozoa are produced by a relatively small number of stem cells throughout the adult primate's life. Whether each stem cell produces one stem cell and one differentiated cell, asymmetrical mitosis, or one stem cell produces two stem cells while another adjacent stem cell produces two daughter cells, symmetrical mitosis, is not known for most epithelia *(31,32)*. As discussed later, evidence relating to this intriguing issue is presented that suggests that the renewing stem cells of some primates, if not all, divide symmetrically.

Historically, two fundamentally different models of stem cell renewal during mammalian spermatogenesis were postulated from the results of studies performed in rodents *(32)*. A review of the evidence supporting each model in rodents is necessary, because the original scheme of stem cell renewal has been generally accepted to occur in primates and the original scheme postulated from results in rodents has been replaced by the newer scheme. Moreover, the mechanism of stem cell renewal that is widely accepted in primates has recently been challenged by the notion that the newer model may be applicable to primates *(32)*.

Clermont and colleagues *(33)*, using mophometric analysis of histological sections and incorporation of tritiated thymidine during the DNA synthetic phase of the cell cycle, identified four morphologically distinct type A spermatogonia. These spermatogonia, called A_1–A_4, were distinguishable from each other by the increase of heterochromatin in the nuclei of spermatogonia of each succeeding generation. These workers determined that each type A_1 spermatogonium divided mitotically and theoretically produced two type A_2 spermatogonia. In turn, each type A_2 spermatogonium divided and potentially produced two type A_3 spermatogonia. Each type A_3 spermatogonium, in turn, divided, and produced two type A_4 spermatogonia. With the eventual appearance of type A_4 a departure from this straightforward system of spermatogonial proliferation was postulated. The type A_4 spermatogonia divided and produced either the differentiated intermediate type spermatogonia or the rather undifferentiated type A_1 spermatogonia. In other words, the most differentiated of the four generations of type A spermatogonia, A_4 cells, produced progeny that were either more differentiated or the least differentiated type A spermatogonia. Because of this potential to produce undifferentiated spermatogonia, all four generations of type A spermatogonia were considered renewing stem cells. This singular state of affairs was further complicated.

Indeed, another type A spermatogonia population was also described *(33)*. These type A spermatogonia were morphologically less differentiated than any of the other four type A spermatogonia and did not incorporate the labeled nucleotide that indicated a cell was preparing for mitosis. Furthermore, the number of these cells in the seminiferous epithelium did not change. Therefore, these rather undifferentiated type A spermatogonia were not mitotically active but were quiescent. These stem spermatogonia were designated type A_0 spermatogonia and postulated to represent stem cells held in reserve that would repopulate the seminiferous epithelium only when all more mature germ cells were destroyed by some catastrophe. The A_0 spermatogonia were postulated to divide mitotically and produce type A_1 spermatogonia until the seminiferous epithelium was reestablished. It was posited that one or all type A_{1-4} spermatogonia produced a factor, or factors, that normally held the A_0 stem cells in a quiescent state *(34)*. However, the search for this factor was not fruitful *(35–38)*.

The second scheme of stem cell renewal was posited by Huckins *(39,40)*, based on studies of rodent testes. A technique for isolating, fixing, and mounting long segments of seminiferous tubules for observation with the light microscope was developed. This technique permitted examination of the outer layer of the seminiferous tubule; that is, the layer containing the spermatogonia. The spermatogonia, both stem and differentiated, could be identified easily, and long strings of spermatogonial nuclei exhibiting the same morphology were readily apparent. Because the segments of seminiferous tubule were intact, the nuclei of each string were enumerated. In addition, the spacing of the nuclei was rather constant from one string to the other. Furthermore, when tritiated thymidine was administered to the rodent before removing the testes, all the nuclei in a string were labeled. The conclusion was that as the spermatogonial nuclei divided, cytokinesis was not completed and cytoplasmic bridges connected the spermatogonia. After the strings with identical morphology were examined, three kinds of nuclear strings were identified. Pairs of type A spermatogonia were identified but were too far from the next nuclei of similar morphology to expect that they were part of the same string. Longer strings, consisting of 4, 8, or 16 nuclei, were readily distinguished. The type A spermatogonia, with a nucleus that was clearly separated from the next nucleus with the same morphology, were called A isolated or A single (A_s). When two nuclei of similar morphology were adjacent to one another, they were called A paired (A_{pr}). The last class were strings of nuclei containing 4, 8, or 16 nuclei. These latter strings were called A aligned (A_{al}). These observations led to the conclusion that the type As were the renewing stem cells, whereas the remaining categories of nuclei strings were simply the result of mitosis without complete cytokinesis. Long strings of nuclei of type A_{1-4} were also recognized, but the results suggested that the Type A_{al} nuclei, whether strings of 4, 8, or 16, would, at the proper time in spermatogenesis, transform directly into type A_1 spermatogonia. This transformation of nuclei from strings of cells of different lengths is the greatest weakness of this model.

The latter scheme of stem cell renewal overcomes the problem of the former scheme, namely the dedifferentiation of type A_4 cells producing the undifferentiated type A_1 spermatogonia. This scheme, however, cannot explain easily how the transformation of nuclei strings with differing numbers can all transform simultaneously at the appropriate time to produce type A_1 spermatogonia. The greatest weakness of this model is that the cells can transform into A_1 whether they are in strings of 4, 8, or 16 nuclei. This poses a substantial problem, because the timing of the seminiferous epithelial cycle is clearly determined by the germ cells and not by external factors (41). It is difficult to conceive a mechanism whereby the chains of 4, 8, or 16 nuclei can detect the appropriate environment and directly transform.

In summary, the two schemes of stem cell renewal are distinctive in two respects. The first scheme has two types of stem cells, namely reserve stem cells and renewing stem cells. The reserve stem cells, type A_0 spermatogonia, are quiescent and only become active when the renewing stem cells, types A_{1-4} spermatogonia, are destroyed. The four generations of renewing stem cells require that a more differentiated cell, A_4 spermatogonium, produces less differentiated daughter cells, type A_1 spermatogonia. A mechanism that produces a pattern of differentiation immediately followed by dedifferentiation is difficult for the author to conceptualize. The second scheme of stem cell renewal is simpler than the first because no reserve stem cell is postulated, however, it has difficulty accounting for coordination of the strings of spermatogonial nuclei that have divided a different number of times, so that they all transform at the same time into the type A_1 spermatogonia. This coordination is required because, as described in the Wave of the Cycle section, the various types of germ cells and the processes of spermatoogonial proliferation, meiosis, and spermiogenesis are ordered and highly synchronized. Neither scheme is entirely satisfactory.

For stem cell renewal in higher primates, the mechanism is less complicated compared to that of rodents. Only two types of A spermatogonia are found in the seminiferous epithelia of these species, types Ad and Ap spermatogonia (see Spermatogonia and Mitosis section).

Type Ad spermatogonia are rather mitotically inactive.[4] This conclusion is based on two lines of evidence. First, the number of Ad spermatogonia in the higher primate testis is constant, and these cells rarely incorporate tritiated thyminidine, a marker of DNA synthesis preparatory to mitosis (18–20). Second, X-irradiation of the testes of adult rhesus monkeys destroyed all germ cells except the Ad spermatogonia (42). After documenting the decline and subsequent disappearance of all germ cells except Ad

---

[4] It should be noted that the initial descriptions of spermatogenesis in man (16) suggested that the Ad spermatogonia were the renewing stem cells. Later studies in monkey and man showed that few Ad spermatogonia incorporate radiolabeled nucleotides, suggesting that these cells were mitotically quiescent (20).

spermatogonia, all irradiation was stopped, and the seminiferous epithelia of the monkeys were allowed to recover. The type Ad spermatogonia transformed without mitosis directly into the type Ap spermatogonia. Once the population of Ap spermatogonia was reestablished, some of the Ap spermatogonia transformed back to Ad spermatogonia. These results unequivocally demonstrate that the Type Ad spermatogonia are reserve stem cells.

The case for Ap spermatogonia being the renewing stem cells is based on morphometric analyses and the pattern of incorporation of tritiated thymidine. Clermont and Antar *(20)* injected the testes of adult stump-tailed macaques *(M. arctoides)* with the radiolabeled nucleotide. Testes were removed either 3 h or 12 d and 3 h after the injection. In addition, the number of each cell type was enumerated. The number of Ad spermatogonia was unchanged at both 3 h and 12 d 3 h after injection. Few Ad spermatogonia were labeled with the tritiated thymidine, and 12 d later, none was identified. These results led to the notion that the Ad spermatogonia were reserve stem cells. By contrast, the Ap spermatogonia were increased in number, and incorporated the radiolabeled nucleotide at 3 h after injection. After the increase in Ap spermatogonia, the number of these cell types returned to the number before the increase. This transient increase in cell number was observed in the testes removed 14 d 3 h after the administration of tritiated thymidine. Moreover, Ap spermatogonia were labeled with tritiated thymidine in the testes removed 12 d 3 h after the single injection with labeled nucleotide.

Two schemata for the mechanism of stem cell renewal have been postulated *(20)*. The first scheme, which occurs in the rhesus monkey and African green monkey, and, perhaps, in man, is distinguished by a single peak of mitosis of the Ap spermatogonia. During that peak, all type Ap spermatogonia divide and yield either more Ap spermatogonia, thus renewing the population, or type B spermatogonia, beginning spermatogenesis. Whether this cell division is symmetrical or asymmetrical has not been determined, although cell counts and labeling patterns suggest that the mitosis of Ap spermatogonia mitosis is symmetrical; that is, half of the population of Ap spermatogonia divides and produces two daughter cells, both of which are Ap spermatogonia. The remaining half of the Ap spermatogonia divide, and produce two identical type B spermatogonia.

The other scheme, which occurs in the stump-tailed macaque and the crab-eating macaque, is distinguished by two peaks of Ap spermatogonia mitosis during every cycle of the seminiferous epithelium. The first peak results in a transitory doubling of the number of Ap spermatogonia and is followed in the same cycle by a second peak of mitosis. Only half of these newly formed type Ap spermatogonia divide during the second peak, resulting only in the production of the first generation of B spermatogonia. This scheme seems more likely to support the notion that the mitotic events are symmetrical.

HORMONAL REGULATION OF SPERMATOGENESIS

The central role of the pituitary to stimulate spermatogenesis[5] in adult primates was established nearly 60 yr ago *(5)*. Surgical removal of the pituitary gland in rhesus

---

[5] In the context of this discussion, spermatogenesis is defined as the production of testicular spermatozoa whether one or many.

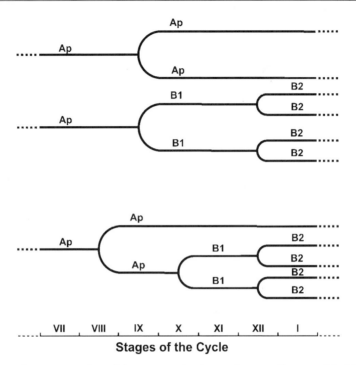

Stages of the Cycle

Fig. 2. A schematic representation of the two mechanisms of stem cell renewal in higher primates. The top two diagrams illustrate the scheme that is common to rhesus monkey *(Macaca mulatta),* African green monkey *(Cercopithecus atheops),* and, perhaps, man *(Homo sapiens).* All type Ap spermatogonia divide in stage IX; one half of the population produce more Ap spermatogonia and the other half divide and produce type B1 spermatogonia (B1). The B1 spermatogonia divide in stage XII and produce B2 spermatogonia (B2). The number of Ap spermatogonia remains constant throughout the cycle of the seminiferous epithelium of these primate species. The bottom diagram shows the scheme that is common to stump-tailed macaque *(M. arctoides)* and the crab-eating macaque *(M. fascicularis).* As in the first scheme, all Ap spermatogonia divide, but, in stage VIII and in contrast to the first scheme, only type Ap spermatogonia are produced, resulting in twice as many Ap spermatogonia stage IX. In stage X, half of the population of Ap spermatogonia divide and produce only type B1 spermatogonia. The remaining half of the Ap spermatogonia do not divide until stage VIII of the next cycle. As in the first scheme, the B1 spermatogonia divide in stage XII and produce B_2 spermatogonia (B2). This latter scheme of stem cell renewal suggests that the mitoses of Ap spermatogonia are symmetrical. (Drawn after ref. *20.)*

monkeys resulted in a precipitous decline in testicular size associated with the complete regression of the seminiferous epithelium to the extent that the tissue comprised only type A spermatogonia and Sertoli cells. More recent experiments using monkeys rendered hypogonadotropic, hypogonadal by either surgical or chemical hypophysectomy, have confirmed Smith's earlier observation and have extended it by demonstrating that replacement of testosterone stimulates testicular growth to approx 60% of the pretreatment size *(43–45).* The gonadal growth primarily resulted from stimulation of spermatogenesis by the androgen, but morphometric analysis of the seminiferous epithelium revealed that the smaller testicular size was accounted for by a deficit in the numbers of all type B spermatogonia. FSH replacement in testosterone-treated hypophysectomized adults resulted in a greater number of all four generations of type B spermatogonia (46). These results led to the conclusion that testosterone alone stimulates spermatogenesis but FSH is necessary to restore spermatogenesis completely. FSH was posited to accomplish this effect by rescuing type B spermatogonia from programmed cell death.

Unilateral orchidectomy in adult macaques results in the compensatory growth of the remaining testis (46,47). The number of Sertoli cells per testis was identical in the gonad removed at the time of unilateral orchidectomy and in the gonad that remained in the animal for 45 d. By contrast, the number of all germ cells more mature than type Ap spermatogonia was greater in the remaining testis than in the unilateral orchidectomy specimen. Moreover, the removal of one testis was occasioned by a transient decline in testosterone that, in turn, led to a transient increase in LH. By 4 d after surgery, the testosterone and LH concentrations returned to baseline values. The removal of one gonad in these primates was accompanied by a decline in inhibin B levels, which is secreted by Sertoli cells into the circulatory system. FSH concentrations in the circulation increased, confirming the important role of inhibin B in the negative feedback control of FSH secretion.

A model that describes the role and operation of the FSH-inhibin B feedback loop in the stimulation of spermatogenesis in the adult primate is shown in Fig. 3 (48). The circulating FSH concentration is postulated to set the level of sperm production above the basal rate induced by intratesticular testosterone. This FSH action on the germ cells is indirect and mediated by the Sertoli cells. The Sertoli cells stimulated by FSH produce a paracrine factor that rescues or prevents programmed cell death of the type B spermatogonia. The survival of these cells amplifies the basal level of germ cell production that is maintained by testosterone. FSH secretion is dependent on stimulation by pulsatile GnRH. The rate of FSH secretion is selectively dictated by the negative feedback action of testicular inhibin-B. The feedback arm of the loop (inhibin-B–FSH) must be more robust than the feedforward arm (FSH–inhibin-B) for a change in the testicular feedback signal (inhibin-B) to elicit a sustained perturbation to FSH secretion.

In contrast, other investigators have presented results that support the belief that the FSH action to increase the number of germ cells in the primate testis is indirect on type Ap spermatogonia, the renewing stem cells (49–51). For example, FSH administration to adult macaques resulted in an increase in the type Ap spermatogonia in the seminiferous epithelium; however, but an analysis using the kinetics of spermatogenesis does not support the theory that the increase in germ cell production results from an FSH action to increase the number of Ap spermatogonia (45,48).

In adult crab-eating macaques rendered hypogonadotropic for several weeks either by surgical ablation of the pituitary or by pharmacological suppression of gonadotropin secretion using GnRH-analogs or antagonists, a reduction in the total number of Ap spermatogonia was observed, in association with a profound depletion in all more mature germ cells (43,50–52). However, the population of Ap spermatogonia was not decreased in five normal men rendered hypogonadotropic during 19–24 wk of treatment with an androgen ester, testosterone enanthate, although a reduction of all germ cells more mature than type A spermatogonia was reported (53). That the loss of FSH action may have contributed to the reduction in the population of Ap spermatogonia during chemical hypophysectomy in the crab-eating macaque

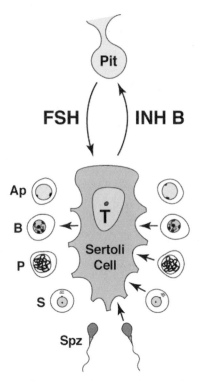

Fig. 3. A model of the negative feedback control system that regulates sperm production by the primate testis. According to this model, follicle-stimulating hormone (FSH) amplifies a basal level of spermatogenesis that is dependent on intratesticular testosterone (T). The degree of amplification is directly related to the circulating concentration of FSH, and the FSH drive is relayed to the seminiferous epithelium via the production of a paracrine factor by the Sertoli cell. This factor favors the survival of differentiated B spermatogonia (B), which leads to an increase in the number of subsequent generations of germ cells. The FSH concentration is regulated by the rate of secretion of inhibin-B (INH-B) by the Sertoli cell. Inhibin-B exerts a brake on FSH secretion by suppressing expression of FSHβ gene expression. The mechanism that controls the rate of inhibin-B secretion is controversial, but in the present model, a signal(s) from the differentiated germ cells is proposed to positively regulate inhibin-B production by the Sertoli cell. The intensity of the putative germ cell signal is posited to be related to the number of differentiated germ cells. P, primary spermatocyte; S, round spermatid; Spz, elongating spermatid and testicular spermatozoa; pit, pituitary gland. (From ref. *48*. Reprinted with permission of the Endocrine Society.)

was suggested by the finding that initiation of FSH treatment, coincident with the start of GnRH antagonist administration in another group of animals, prevented Ap spermatogonia depletion *(50)*. It should be noted that LH action may also maintain the population of Ap spermatogonia because the number of this cell type in the testis of testosterone-treated, hypophysectomized macaques was similar to that of intact animals *(43)*. This gonadotropin action on Ap spermatogonia may be permissive; that is, allowing these undifferentiated spermatogonia to divide each cycle and survive. In contrast, the regulatory action of FSH that determines the number of differentiated, or type B, spermatogonia that survive. Clearly, further study of the role of the gonadotropins in this regard is necessary.

PREPUBERTAL DEVELOPMENT
OF THE SEMINIFEROUS EPITHELIUM

Prepubertal Proliferation of Sertoli Cells

In humans and macaques, the ontogeny of Sertoli cell proliferation is different from that in rodents *(54–60)*. Cortes et al. *(56)*, using autopsy material from boys and men who had died in traumatic accidents, described two phases of Sertoli cell proliferation, one immediately after birth and one later at puberty. Each of these periods in higher primates is associated with elevated levels of gonadotropins *(61)*. In the rhesus monkey, the number of Sertoli cells per testis was increased fivefold from infancy to the juvenile phase of development, with a further sixfold increase from the juvenile to the adult phase. These increments in Sertoli cell number occurred during infancy and the pubertal period concomitant with the elevated gonadotropin levels that are characteristic of these developmental phases *(57)*. Moreover, GnRH administration to juvenile rhesus macaques that are naturally hypogonadotropic resulted in precocious LH and FSH secretion that, in turn, stimulated a premature increase in the number of Sertoli cells *(57)*. Finally, administration of synthetic human LH and FSH, either alone or in combination, to juvenile rhesus monkeys for 11 d resulted in an increase in the number of Sertoli cells *(59)*. Moreover, in contrast to the case in rodents, LH and FSH were equally effective in stimulating proliferation of Sertoli cells. The cellular and molecular actions of the two gonadotropins, LH and FSH, therefore, require further elucidation.

Prepubertal Proliferation of Spermatogonia

The ontogeny of the spermatogonia in primates has not been investigated as completely as that of the Sertoli cells *(57–60)*. Within the first days of life, the only germ cells observed in the rhesus monkey are type A spermatogonia, which are morphologically indistinguishable from the type A spermatogonia found in the adult testis *(57)*. The number of type Ad and Ap spermatogonia increases with age, and, as in the case of Sertoli cells, the major increases occur during puberty and may result from the increase in gonadotropins *(57)*.

SUMMARY

Spermatogenesis in higher primates have is characterized by distinct differences from the process in other genera. At birth, type Ad and Ap spermatogonia, indistinguishable from those cells in the adult testis, are the only germ cells present. Two distinct phases of Sertoli cell proliferation occur in higher primates: one during infancy and the second during puberty. In addition, LH and FSH are equally effective in stimulating Sertoli cell proliferation in the physioligically hypogonadotropic juvenile monkey. The mechanism of stem cell proliferation in primates is less complex than in rodents. The undifferentiated spermatogonia of primates have distinctively different roles. The Ad spermatogonia are usually mitotically quiescent and only become active when a depletion of all more mature cells occurs. These cells are the reserve stem cells of the seminiferous epithelium of the primate. The Ap spermatogonia are mitotically active in the adult seminiferous epithelium. They are the renewing stem cells that divide periodically and produce either Ap spermatogonia or differentiated, type B, spermatogonia. This period, or cell cycle time, of Ap cell division sets the duration of the cycle of the seminiferous epithelium.

REFERENCES

1. Romer AS. The vertebrate story. University of Chicago Press, Chicago, 1959.
2. Hill WCO. Primates Comparative Anatomy and Taxonomy, Vol 1. University Press, Edinburgh, 1953, Introduction, pp. 3–29.
3. Young JZ. The Life of Vertebrates, 2nd ed. New York, Oxford University Press, 1962, Primates, pp. 602–607.
4. Young JZ. The Life of Vertebrates, 2nd ed., New York, Oxford University Press, 1962, Rodents and Rabbits, pp. 654–660.
5. Smith PE. Comparative effects of hypophysectomy and therapy on the testes of monkeys and rats. In: Brouha L, ed. Hormones sexuelles. Paris, Comptes Rendus; 1938, pp. 201–209.
6. Clermont Y, Morgentaler H. Quantitative study of spermatogenesis in the hypophysectomized rat. Endocrinology 1955;57:369–382.
7. Huang HFS, Marshall GR, Rosenberg R, Nieschlag E. Restoration of spermatogenesis by high levels of testosterone in hypophysectomized rats after long-term regression. Acta Endocrinol (Copenh) 1987;116:433–444.
8. Smith PE. Maintenance and restoration of spermatogenesis in hypophysectomized rhesus monkeys by androgen administration. Yale J Biol Med 1944;17:281–287.
9. MacLeod J, Pazianos A, Ray B. The restoration of human spermatogenesis and of reproductive tract with urinary gonadotropins following hypophysectomy. Fertil Steril 1966;17:7–23.
10. Rea MA, Weinbauer GF, Marshall GR, Neischlag E. Testosterone stimulates pituitary and serum FSH in GnRH antagonistsuppressed rats. Acta Endocrinol (Copenh) 1986;113:487–492.
11. Rea MA, Marshall GR, Weinbauer GF, Nieschlag E. Testosterone maintains pituitary and serum FSH and spermatogenesis in gonadotropin-releasing hormone antagonist-suppressed rats. J Endocrinol 1986;108:101–107.
12. Sinha-Hikim AP, Swerdloff RS. Temporal and stage-specific changes in spermatogenesis of rat after gonadotropin deprivation by a potent gonadotropin-releasing hormone antagonist treatment. Endocrinology 1993;133:2161–2170.
13. Clermont Y. Kinetics of spermatogenesis in mammals: seminiferous epithelium cycle and spermatogonial renewal. Physiol Rev 1972;52:198–236.
14. Russell LD, Griswold MD, eds. The Sertoli Cell. Clearwater, FL, Cache River Press, 1993, pp. v–vi.
15. Setchell BP, Maddocks S, Brooks DE. Anatomy, vasculature, innevation, and fluids of the male reproductive tract. In: K Knobil, JD Neill, eds. The Physiology of Reproduction, 2nd ed., Vol. 1. Raven Press, New York, 1994, pp. 1063–1175.
16. Clermont Y. The cycle of the seminiferous epithelium in man. Am J Anat 1963:112:35–51.
17. Heller CG, Clermont Y. Kinetics of the germinal epithelium in man. Recent Prog Hormone Res 1964;20:545–575.
18. Clermont Y. Renewal of spermatogonia in man. Am J Anat 1966;118:509–524.
19. Clermont Y. Two classes of spermatogonial stem cells in the monkey (Cercopithecus aethiops). Am J Anat 1969;126:57–72.
20. Clermont Y, Antar M. Duration of the cycle of the seminiferous epithelium and the spermatogonial renewal in the monkey Macaca arctoides. Am J Anat 1973;136:153–165.
21. de Rooij DG, van Alphen MMA, van de Kant HJG. Duration of the cycle of the seminiferous epithelium and its stages in the rhesus monkey (Macaca mulatta). Biol Reprod 1986;35:587–591.
22. Cavicchia JC, Dym M. Ultrastructural characteristics of monkey spermatogonia and preleptotene spermatocytes. Biol Reprod 1978;18:219–228.
23. Schulze C. Morphological characteristics of the spermatogonial stem cells in man. Cell Tissue Res 1979;198:191–199.
24. Paniagua R, Nistal M, Amat P, Rodriguez MC, Alonso JR. Quantitative differences between variants of A spermatogonia in man. J Reprod Fertil 1986;77:669–673.
25. Fouquet JP, Dadoune JP. Renewal of spermatogonia in the monkey (Macaca fascicularis). Biol Reprod 1986;35:199–207.
26. Nistal M, Codesal J, Paniagua R, Santamarie L. Decrease in the number of human Ap and Ad spermatogonia and in the Ap/Ad ratio with advancing age: new data on spermatogonial stem cell. J Androl 1987;8:64–68.

27. Chowdhury AK, Marshall G, Steinberger E. Comparative aspects of spermatogenesis in man and baboon *(Papio anubis)*. In: Calaby JH, Tyndale-Biscoe CH, ed. *Reproduction and Evolution*. Australian Academy of Science, Melbourne, 1977, p. 143.
28. Millar MR, Sharpe RM, Weinbauer GF, Fraser H, Saunders PTK. Marmoset spermatogenesis: organizational similarities to the human. Int. J. Androl. 2000;23:266–277.
29. Perey B, Clermont Y, LeBlond CP. The wave of seminiferous epithelium in the rat. Am J Anat 1961;108:47–77.
30. Fuchs E, Segre JA. Stem cells: a new lease on life. Cell 2000;100:143–155.
31. Knoblich JA. Asymmetrical cell division during animal development. Nat Rev 2001;2:11–20.
32. de Rooij DG, Russell LD. All you wanted to know about spermatogonia but were afraid to ask. J Androl 2000;21:776–798.
33. Dym M, Clermont Y. Role of spermatogonia in the repair of the seminiferous epithelium following X-irradiation of the rat testis. Am J Anat 1970;128:265–282.
34. Irons MJ, Clermont Y. Spermatogonial chalone(s): effect on the phases of the cell cycle of type A spermatogonia in the rat. Cell Tissue Kinet 1979;12:425–433.
35. Clermont Y, Mauger A. Effect of a spermatogonial chalone on the growing rat testis. Cell Tissue Kinet 1976;9:99–104.
36. Thumann A, Bustos-Obregon E. An "in vitro" system for study of rat spermatogonial proliferative control. Andrologia 1978;10:22–25.
37. Cunningham GR, Huckins C. Failure to identify a spermatogonial chalone in adult irradiated testes. Cell Tissue Kinet 1979;12:81–89.
38. deRooij DG. Effects of testicular extracts on proliferation of spermatogonia in the mouse. Virchows Archiv B Cell Pathol 1980;33:67–75.
39. Huckins C. The spermatogonial stem cell population in adult rats. I. Their morphology, proliferation and maturation. Anat Rev 1971;169:533–557.
40. Huckins C. The spermatogonial stem cell population in adult rats. II. A radioautographic analysis of their cell cycle properties. Cell Tissue Kinet 1971;4:313–334.
41. Franca LR, Ogawa T, Avarbock MR, Brinster RL, Russell LD. Germ cell genotype controls cell cycle during spermatogenesis in the rat. Biol Reprod 1998;59:1371–1377.
42. van Alphen MM, van de Kant HJ, de Rooij DG. Repopulation of the seminiferous epithelium of the rhesus monkey after X irradiation. Radiation Res 1988;113(3):487–500.
43. Marshall GR, Wickings EJ, Ludecke DK, Nieschlag E. Stimulation of spermatogenesis in stalk-sectioned rhesus monkeys by testosterone alone. J Clin Endocrinol Metab 1983;57:152–159.
44. Marshall GR, Jockenhovel F, Ludecke D, Nieschlag E. Maintenance of complete but quantitatively reduced spermatogenesis in hypophysectomized monkeys by testosterone alone. Acta Endocrinol (Copenh) 1986;113:424–431.
45. Marshall GR, Zorub DS, Plant TM. Follicle-stimulating hormone amplifies the population of differentiated spermatogonia in the hypophysectomized testosterone-replaced adult rhesus monkey *(Macaca mulatta)*. Endocrinology 1995;136:3504–3511.
46. Ramaswamy S, Marshall GR, McNeilly AS, Plant TM. Dynamics of the follicle-stimulating hormone (FSH)-inhibin B feedback loop and its role in regulating spermatogenesis in the adult male rhesus monkey *(Macaca mulatta)* as revealed by unilateral orchidectomy. Endocrinology 2000;141:18–27.
47. Medhamurthy R, Aravindan GR, Moudgal NR. Hemiorchidectomy leads to dramatic and immediate alterations in pituitary follicle-stimulating hormone secretion and the functional activity of the remaining testis in the adult male bonnet monkey *(Macaca radiata)*. Biol Reprod 1993;49:743–749.
48. Plant TM, Marshall GR. The functional significance of FSH in spermatogenesis and the control of its secretion in male primates. Endocr Rev 2001;22:764–786.
49. van Alphen MMA, van de Kant HJG, de Rooij DG. Follicle-stimulating hormone stimulates spermatogenesis in the adult monkey. Endocrinology 1988;123:1449–1455.
50. Weinbauer GF, Behre HM, Fingscheidt U, Nieschlag B. Human follicle-stimulating hormone exerts a stimulatory effect on spermatogenesis, testicular size, and serum inhibin levels in the gonadotropin-releasing hormone antagonist-treated nonhuman primate *(Macaca fascicularis)*. Endocrinology 1991;129:1831–1839.
51. Zhengwei Y, Wreford NG, Schlatt S, Weinbauer GF, Nieschlag E, McLachlan RI. Acute and specific impairment of spermatogonial development by GnRH antagonist-induced gonadotrophin withdrawal in the adult macaque *(Macaca fascicularis)*. J Reprod Fertil 1998;112:139–147.

52. O'Donnell L, Narula A, Balourdos G, et al. Impairment of spermatogonial development and spermiation after testosterone-induced gonadotropin suppression in adult monkeys *(Macaca fascicularis).* J Clin Endocrinol Metab 2001;86:1814–1822.

53. Zhengwei Y, Wreford NG, Royce P, de Kretser DM, McLachlan RI. Stereological evaluation of human spermatogenesis after suppression by testosterone treatment: heterogeneous pattern of spermatogenic impairment. J Clin Endocrinol Metab 1998;83:1284–1291.

54. Orth JM. Proliferation of Sertoli cells in fetal and postnatal rats. Anat Rev 1982;203:485–492.

55. Kluin PM, Kramer MF, de Rooij DG. Testicular development in Macaca irus after birth. Int J Androl 1983;6:25–43.

56. Cortes D, Muller J, Skakkebaek NE. Proliferation of Sertoli cells during development of the human testis assessed by stereological methods. Int J Androl 1987;10:589–596.

57. Marshall GR, Plant TM. Puberty occurring either spontaneously or induced precociously in rhesus monkey *(Macaca mulatta)* is associated with a marked proliferation of Sertoli cells. Biol Reprod 1996;54:1192–1199.

58. Arslan M, Weinbauer GF, Schlatt S, Shahab M, Nieschlag E. FSH and testosterone, alone or in combination, initiate testicular growth and increase the number of spermatogonia and Sertoli cells in a juvenile non-human primate *(Macaca mulatta).* J Endocrinol 1993;136:235–243.

59. Ramaswamy S, Plant TM, Marshall GR. Pulsatile stimulation with recombinant single chain human luteinizing hormone elicits precocious Sertoli cell proliferation in the juvenile male rhesus monkey *(Macaca mulatta).* Biol Reprod 2000;63:82–88.

60. Schlatt S, Arslan M, Weinbauer GF, Behre HM, Nieschlag E. Endocrine control of testicular somatic and premeiotic germ cell development in the immature testis of the primate Macaca mulatta. Eur J Endocrinol 1995;133:235–247.

61. Plant TM. Puberty in primates. In: Knobil E, Neill JD, eds. The Physiology of Reproduction, Vol. 2. 2nd ed. Raven Press, New York, 1994, pp. 453–485.

4   Normal and Delayed Puberty

Leo Dunkel, MD

CONTENTS

DEFINITION

Approximately 99.6% of white boys have at least early signs of secondary sexual development by the age of 14, but the cutoff age for identifying boys who need to be evaluated for delayed puberty may vary in different ethnic groups. The most common reason for delayed puberty is constitutional (idiopathic), which is usually accompanied by a delay in height growth. Various endocrine disorders, causing hypogonadotropic or hypergonadotropic hypogonadism, must also be considered in boys with pubertal delay.

NORMAL PUBERTY

Physical Changes

Puberty is the maturational process of the reproductive endocrine system that results in final adult stature and adult body proportions, as well as final development of the genital organs and the capacity to reproduce. In this maturation of the hypothalamic–pituitary–gonadal axis, the levels of gonadotropins increase and the production of sex steroids rise, leading to gonadal development and the development of secondary sexual characteristics. In boys, the first physical signs of puberty are an increase in testis volume and penis size, at a mean age of approx 11.5 yr in most Western countries. Testis volume increases from prepubertal values of 1–2 mL to 3–8 mL even before pubic hair appears, and reaches 20–30 mL in adulthood *(1)*. Development of mature spermatogenesis is called spermarche (as opposed to menarche), at which time mature spermatozoa are found in the urine. This hallmark of gonadal maturation occurs at mean age of 13.5 years, when the mean testis volume reaches 11.5 mL *(2)*.

From: *Male Hypogonadism:*
Basic, Clinical, and Therapeutic Principles
Edited by: S. J. Winters © Humana Press Inc., Totowa, NJ

Secular Trends in Pubertal Development

Current trends in the timing of puberty have been reported recently in both sexes. In North American boys, recent data indicate earlier genital growth *(3)*. However, that study has elicited significant criticism, because the boys were not investigated thoroughly, although strong conclusions were drawn from the data. European studies do not support the American experience of strikingly earlier onset of puberty, e.g., in the Netherlands, a halt in the trend toward earlier puberty has been found during the last decades *(4)*. Therefore, further studies are needed to confirm the earlier onset of puberty in male and female American adolescents.

A subgroup of children having exceptionally early puberty are those adopted from developing countries. These children are often malnourished on arrival in their new home country. Early or even precocious puberty can result in a final height much lower than expected, but this height may not be much different from that of peers living in the country of origin. One speculation is that the intensive growth period after adaptation is "corrected" by an earlier onset of puberty, which results in a final height that is consistent with the original genetic growth potential.

Endocrine Changes During Puberty

GONADOTROPIN-RELEASING HORMONE AND GONADOTROPINS

The hypothalamus–pituitary–gonadal axis is already mature in the fetal period. Gonadotropin-releasing hormone (GnRH) is produced by hypothalamic neurons that originate from the medial olfactory placode of the nose. These neurons migrate during central nervous system (CNS) development and are finally located in the arcuate nucleus, in the preoptic area and in the medial basal hypothalamus. During gestation, there is an increase in GnRH content, which reaches its peak at 34–38 wk in the male fetus *(5)*. The secondary plexus of the portal capillary network is completed by weeks 19–21, coinciding with a striking rise of circulating gonadotropin levels at midgestation in both male and female fetuses. After midgestation, high circulating gonadotropin levels decrease to low levels at birth. This change in gonadotropin secretion results from the development of negative feedback system to sex steroids, as well as from the development of inhibiting influences from the CNS to the GnRH neurons (vide infra).

Luteinizing hormone (LH) and follicle-stimulating hormone secretion rise during the first month after birth, probably because the negative feedback effect of placental estrogens are withdrawn *(see* Figs. 1 and 2). LH is secreted in pulses during this postnatal period *(6)*. By the age of 6 to 12 mo, the GnRH pulse generator becomes quiescent, and gonadotropin levels decrease. However, LH pulses can be detected throughout childhood, with highly sensitive immunofluorometric methods *(7,8)*.

With the onset of puberty, LH secretion is augmented, first only during the night *(see* Fig. 2). In boys, this increase in LH is associated with an increase in plasma testosterone levels during the morning hours. With progression of puberty, LH secretion increases through an increase in both LH pulse frequency and amplitude. The day–night rhythm of gonadotropin secretion is evident during puberty, but it disappears in adulthood *(7,8)*.

SEX STEROIDS

LH controls sex steroid production by upregulating expression of the steroidogenic enzymes *(see* Chapter 2) and by controlling metabolic activity of the steroid-producing

LH/FSH concentration

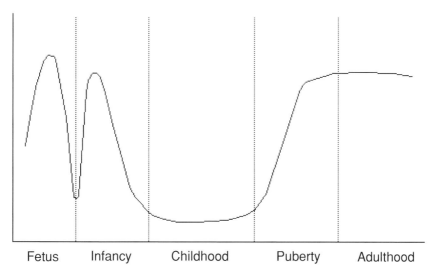

Fig. 1. Patterns of plasma gonadotropin secretion during sexual development.

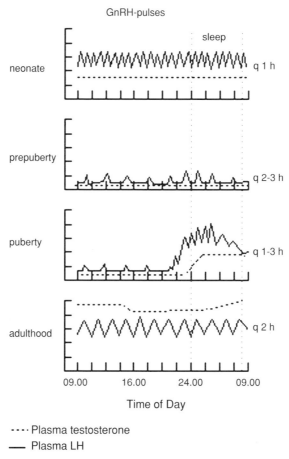

Fig. 2. Change in the patterns of pulsatile release of gonadotropin-releasing hormone (GnRH) and luteinizing hormone (LH) for 24 h during sexual maturation.

Table 1
Pubertal Stages (According to Tanner) With Respective
Testis Volumes and Plasma Testosterone Concentrations

Pubertal stage (Tanner)	Testicular volume (mL)	Plasma testosterone (ng/dL)
1	>4	<10
2	4–8	12–69
3	8–10	60–275
4	10–20	142–515
5	20–25	319–775

Note. Values adapted from ref. *1.*

Leydig cells. LH may also stimulate Leydig cell proliferation and differentiation *(9)*. During puberty, plasma testosterone levels increase dramatically. Table 1 summarizes the levels of testosterone at various developmental stages, with respective testis sizes. The pubertal increase in testis size results primarily from an increased number of proliferating and differentiating germ cells and, to a lesser extent, an increase in Sertoli cells *(10)*. The adult testes produce approx 6–7 mg of testosterone/d, with approx 5% synthesized in extratesticular tissues via peripheral conversion of adrenal steroids.

INHIBINS

Inhibin is a heterodimeric glycoprotein, which consists of an α-subunit linked either to a β_A subunit (inhibin-A) or to a β_B subunit (inhibin-B) *(see* Chapter 1). At least six different molecular weight isoforms of inhibin-B exist in the circulation *(11)*. The biological activity of these isoforms in not known, and they cannot be distinguished by current immunoassays. Several studies show that serum inhibin-B levels in children change in concert with the secretion of gonadotropins *(12–15)*. Between 1 wk and 7 mo of age, when the hypothalamic–pituitary–testicular axis is transiently activated *(16,17)*, serum inhibin-B levels increase to similar *(15,18)* or higher *(13)* levels than those observed in adolescent boys and adult men. This early inhibin-B secretion is sustained until the age of 18–24 mo; thereafter, serum concentrations decline to lower but readily measurable levels *(13)*. Early in puberty, between Tanner stages G1 and G2, serum inhibin-B concentrations again increase to reach peak levels at the Tanner stage G2, but then the levels plateau *(12,14)* *(see* Fig. 3). In contrast to inhibin-B, inhibin-A levels in human males are below the detection limit of the corresponding immunoassay *(18,19)*.

Hypotheses on Control of the Onset of Puberty

In 1931, Hohlweg presented a so-called "gonadostat" theory of puberty, which was based on the concept of a changing sensitivity of the gonadotropin-regulating system to the negative feedback effect of gonadal steroids *(20)*. This theory was further developed by Grumbach and colleagues *(21)*. Hohlweg and Junkmann observed that

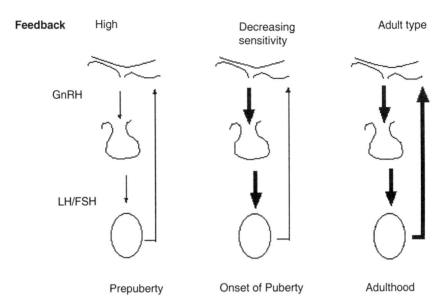

Fig. 3. The "gonadostat" hypothesis for puberty, i.e., a developmental change in the sensitivity of the gonadotropin-releasing hormone (GnRH) system in the regulation of gonadotropin secretion. During prepuberty, sensitivity to the negative feedback actions of gonadal steroids is highest, resulting in a low release of GnRH and gonadotropins. Initiation of puberty is secondary to a decrease in sensitivity to gonadal steroid feedback inhibition, resulting in increased GnRH and gonadotropin release, until a new equilibrium level is reached in adulthood. (Modified from ref. *21.*)

in castrated immature rats, small doses of steroid hormones prevented pituitary hypersecretion, whereas larger steroid doses were needed in adult rats *(22)*. Similarly in the human, pituitary gonadotropin secretion is sensitive to the suppressive effect of sex steroids, because small doses of estrogen are able to suppress gonadotropin levels *(21)*. Thus, according to this concept, the onset of puberty results from a decreasing sensitivity at the hypothalamic–pituitary level to the suppressive effect of sex steroids; consequently, gonadotropin secretion increases, and, in turn, there is an increase in gonadal steroid production (*see* Fig. 3). Testosterone infusion experiments in boys and men have shown a change in the mechanism of negative feedback with maturation. In boys, testosterone suppresses hypothalamic GnRH secretion, manifested by a decrease in LH pulse frequency but not amplitude, but the hypothalamus becomes resistant to testosterone negative feedback with puberty *(23–25)*. Thus, according to the gonadostat theory, at the time of puberty, gonadal steroid feedback inhibition of gonadotropin secretion reaches a new equilibrium at a higher setpoint.

In the 1980s, however, it was found, that agonadal subjects had a pattern of changes in gonadotropin concentrations that was similar to that of healthy subjects through infancy and childhood, a finding that contradicted the "gonadostat" hypothesis. Therefore, in the 1980s, an alternative theory, called the "intrinsic restraint concept," was

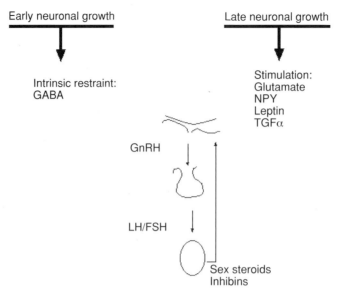

Fig. 4. Central nervous system (CNS) restraint hypothesis of puberty. Factors involved in the regulation of gonadotropin-releasing hormone (GnRH) secretion are listed. According to this idea, GnRH secretion is quiescent in childhood because of early neuronal growth, resulting in a restraint of GnRH release. Stimulating factors overcome this restraint and initiate GnRH release again at the onset of puberty.

proposed (*see* Fig. 4). According to this concept, in addition to sex steroid-mediated negative feedback, a central inhibitory system restrains GnRH release and maintains the prepubertal phase. At the onset of puberty, the intrinsic CNS restraint is inhibited or is dominated by a stimulatory system *(26)*. During the last decades, considerable evidence has been gathered to support this intrinsic restraint hypothesis (vide infra).

Yet a third hypothesis, called the "de-synchrony" theory, has been presented to explain the onset of puberty. This theory is based on a finding that GnRH concentrations in the hypothalamus of primates during prepuberty are comparable to those in the adult animals. Therefore, the lack of GnRH stimulation of the pituitary in prepuberty would result from the desynchronization of GnRH-secreting neurons *(27)*.

Factors Regulating GnRH secretion

The current view is that central inhibition of GnRH release results in a prepubertal "quiescence" of gonadotropin secretion, and the onset of puberty results from the removal of this central restraint *(28)*. Mechanisms related to the control of the onset of puberty have been extensively studied in various rodent models. However, in rodents, the interval between infancy and puberty is condensed, and these two developmental phases cannot be separated by a clearly demarcated juvenile phase of quiescence of the hypothalamic–pituitary–gonadal axis *(29,30)*. Therefore, some of the neurobiological mechanisms responsible for restraining the GnRH pulse generator in late infancy and for holding it in check during the prepubertal period, as well as those pathways that reaugment pulsatile GnRH release, all of which are aspects with significant relevance to human puberty, can be studied only in primate models.

γ-Aminobutyric acid (GABA) is the dominant inhibitory neurotransmitter in the hypothalamus, but in primates, direct innervation of GnRH neurons by GABA neurons has not been demonstrated. It is possible that the inhibition of GnRH neurons by GABA is mediated via glutamergic neurons, because a reciprocal innervation between GABA-ergic and glutamatergic neurons has been found *(31)*. During development, the GABA concentration and the number of GABA-ergic neurons increase from embryonic day 13 to the second postnatal week, which is then followed by a decline in the third postnatal week *(32)*. Before the onset of puberty, GABA release in the preoptic area decreases in female rats *(33)*, and in the rhesus monkey, GABA release in the median eminence decreases concomitant with the pubertal increase of GnRH secretion *(34)*.

The major excitatory amino acid neurotransmitter involved in the regulation of GnRH release is glutamate. Glutamatergic neurons provide axodendritic synaptic input to the hypothalamic GnRH neuronal network *(31)*. GnRH pulsatile release is regulated via two amino acid receptors: (1) inotropic receptors, which are coupled to ion channels (including receptor for *N*-methyl-D-aspartate, NMDA), and (2) metabotropic receptors, which are coupled to G proteins (for review see ref. *35*). The pubertal increase in GnRH secretion possibly results from increased glutaminase activity, the enzyme responsible for converting glutamine to glutamate. Furthermore, in male rats, an increase in NMDA receptor activity is seen before the onset of puberty, probably reflecting increased glutamate activity *(36)*. These peripubertal changes suggest that the neurotransmitter glutamate has a significant role in stimulation of GnRH release at the onset of puberty.

Neuropeptide Y (NPY) is involved in many CNS functions, including appetite control and reproduction. Infusion of NPY into the median eminence stimulates GnRH release in pubertal, but not in prepubertal, female monkeys, suggesting that NPY contributes to the pubertal process *(37)*. Furthermore, in male rhesus monkeys, the postnatal pattern of GnRH pulse generator activity is inversely related to that of NPY gene and protein expression in the mediobasal hypothalamus, and central administration of an NPY Y1 receptor antagonist to juvenile animals elicits precocious GnRH release *(38)*, suggesting a central role for NPY in the break restraining the onset of puberty in primates.

The peptide leptin exerts it effects in the CNS through NPY neurons by decreasing NPY-ergic signaling *(39,40)*. Absence of leptin signaling results in obesity and infertility, whereas leptin treatment decreases food intake and restores reproductive functions. Thus, in fasting, leptin levels decrease and gonadotropin secretion is suppressed. These findings imply that nutrition, especially fat tissue and leptin, could contribute to pubertal development. Clinical observations have further supported a role for leptin signaling in the onset of puberty, e.g., leptin or leptin receptor gene mutations result in the delay or absence of pubertal development on boys and girls *(41,42)* and, in a 12-yr-old girl with congenital leptin deficiency, treatment with recombinant leptin was followed by a pubertal pattern of LH release *(43)*. These observations have led to the speculation that leptin could serve as the somatic signal that inhibits hypothalamic NPY tone at the termination of prepuberty and, thereby, triggers the pubertal reaugmentation of the GnRH pulse generator activity. However, leptin is probably not an important metabolic trigger for the onset of puberty, because leptin levels remain constant in the prepubertal and postpubertal stages of development in primates *(44,45)* and, further, leptin gene expression in the hypothalamus is unchanged during development in the rat *(46,47)*. However, this conclusion does not detract from the hypothesis, derived from rat studies, that leptin serves as a permissive signal that allows a developmental program in GnRH pulse generator activity to unfold *(47)*.

Several growth factors secreted by glial cells regulate GnRH release, implying that the glial tissue may be involved in the regulation of GnRH release. However, the role of glia in triggering puberty remains uncertain. Of these growth factors, transforming growth factor-α (TGF-α) stimulates GnRH release and stimulates glial cells to produce bioactive substances, such as prostaglandin E_2 (PgE$_2$), which, in turn, stimulate the release of GnRH *(48)*. A role for TGF-α has also been postulated in the pathogenesis of precocious puberty associated with hypothalamic lesions: lesion-induced astrogliosis may be responsible for increased TGF-α in the hypothalamus.

The opioidergic system also plays a role in the control of GnRH secretion, because in humans, opioid peptides decrease gonadotropin levels *(49)*. Furthermore, the opiate receptor antagonist, naloxone, increases LH secretion after estradiol suppression in normal adult men and women, but it does not have this effect in prepubertal boys *(25)*. Thus, the opioidergic system becomes operative during pubertal development and possibly mediates, in part, the negative feedback action of sex steroids on GnRH.

DELAYED PUBERTY

Constitutional Delay of Puberty

The absence of a pathologic medical history, otherwise normal findings on physical examination, and a positive family history of delayed puberty in one or both parents suggest the diagnosis of constitutional delay. However, before making that diagnosis, important pathological conditions (e.g., CNS tumors) must be excluded. Boys with constitutional delay usually have delayed growth in childhood, and, consequently, they are short when compared with their peers. The bone age is retarded from the chronological age, but the developmental milestones are achieved at a normal bone age, i.e., onset of the first signs of pubertal development by a bone age of 14 yr. Gonadotropin and testosterone concentrations increase in concert with the advancement of the bone age. Thus, all stages of pubertal development occur at an age that is later than usual. However, boys with constitutional delay in growth and puberty do not reach their predicted adult height *(50)*. One explanation is that reduced estrogen concentrations for chronological age (but not for bone age), impair growth hormone (GH) secretion functionally and temporally. When this functional GH deficiency lasts for a sufficiently long time, it may also affect negatively on adult height. After the onset of puberty or the initiation of testosterone treatment, growth velocity and GH secretion normalize. Final height cannot be increased with GH or testosterone treatment, although these treatments temporarily increase growth velocity.

Finkelstein and colleagues reported decreased radial *(51)*, spinal *(51,52)*, and femoral *(52)* bone mineral density (BMD) in otherwise healthy adult men with history of delayed puberty, in comparison with controls (who had a normal onset of puberty). However, another study recently showed that young men with a history of delayed puberty have normal volumetric BMD, and the authors proposed that the reduced apparent BMD is likely the consequence of the influence of bone size on measured bone density *(53)*.

Hypogonadotropic Hypogonadism

GnRH and gonadotropin deficiency can be caused by various genetic or developmental defects of the hypothalamus or by destructive lesions, such as tumors, inflammatory processes, vascular lesion, or trauma. Patients with isolated gonadotropin deficiency are generally of normal height for age in the prepubertal period and contrast with boys with constitutional delay who are shorter. In patients with hypogonadotropic hypogonadism, gonadotropin responses to GnRH stimulation may be subnormal, but because of the functional hypogonadotropism in constitutional delay, the differential diagnosis between these two conditions may be difficult *(54,55)*.

TEMPORARY GONADOTROPIN DEFICIENCIES

Anorexia Nervosa. Anorexia nervosa, which results from a distorted body image, an obsessive fear of obesity, and avoidance of food, can be associated with severe, even fatal, weight loss. For unknown reasons, this disorder is much more common in girls than in boys. The boys' functional hypogonadotropic hypogonadism at least partly results from severe weight loss. The underlying pathophysiology of delayed puberty is GnRH deficiency, because the LH secretory pattern in adolescents with anorexia is similar to that of normal prepuberty: low or absent LH pulses and a blunted LH response to stimulation by exogenous GnRH *(56)*. Pulsatile administration of GnRH restores a pubertal pattern of LH secretion, confirming the hypothalamic location of the defect. The mechanism for GnRH deficiency may relate to the effects of stress *(57)*. Corticotropin-releasing factor (CRF) levels increase in stress, and CRF, in turn, stimulates β-endorphin levels, which then directly inhibit GnRH release. Recovery to normal weight will normalize most of the endocrine and metabolic disturbances, but in girls, amenorrhea may persist for years.

Athletic Training. Intensive exercise may inhibit GnRH secretion and arrest pubertal development. Although participation in sports in which weight control does not occur does not affect pubertal development, in some sports, such as long-distance running and weight lifting, the energy deficit may be sufficient to delay puberty *(58)*. Hypogonadotropic hypogonadism may occur even when the athletes are of normal weight but have less fat and more muscle mass than nonathletic boys *(57)*. The mechanism of delayed puberty is unclear, but interruption of intensive training advances puberty before any change in body composition or weight, suggesting a direct effect of physical activity on GnRH secretion, possibly through stress effects *(57)* (*see also* Chapter 16).

Malnutrition and Chronic Diseases. In malnutrition and chronic diseases, weight loss to below 80% of ideal body weight can delay or arrest pubertal development. Nutrition plays an important, but poorly understood, role in the control GnRH secretion, e.g., in regional enteritis gonadotropin secretion remains normal if nutrition is optimally balanced, whereas suboptimal nutrition will result in a hypogonadotropic state and arrested pubertal maturation. More than 50% of patients with regional enteritis have subnormal height velocity, and approx 25% will have short stature. The endocrine status is characterized by normal GH secretion and a slightly subnormal serum insulin-like growth factor (IGF)-1 levels, which is related to nutritional status *(59)*.

Chronic renal insufficiency delays pubertal development, but after successful renal transplantation, gonadotropin secretion is usually restored. GnRH secretion is disrupted in these patients as well.

CENTRAL NERVOUS SYSTEM TUMORS

Tumors causing delayed puberty most commonly interfere with GnRH synthesis or secretion. Deficiency of other anterior pituitary hormones, diabetes insipidus, and visual disturbance is common.

Craniopharyngioma. The most common neoplasm causing hypothalamic–pituitary dysfunction and hypogonadotropic hypogonadism is craniopharyngioma. It is a congenital tumor, which most commonly becomes symptomatic between the ages of 6 and 14 yr. At presentation, the most common symptoms are headache, visual disturbances, short stature, delayed puberty, polyuria, and polydipsia. Skull radiographs may show suprasellar or intrasellar calcification or an abnormality of the sella turcica. Computed tomography (CT) or magnetic resonance imaging (MRI) scans may reveal fine calcifications that are not apparent on routine skull radiographs. The structure of the tumor varies from solid to cystic. Treatment consists of surgery and radiotherapy, but the recurrence rate is high, even when complete surgical removal is attempted.

Langerhans Cell Histiocytosis. Langerhans cell histiocytosis, also called Hand-Schüller-Christian disease or Histiocytosis X, is characterized by infiltration of lipid-containing histiocytic cells in the skin, bone, and viscera. Cyst-like areas can be found by X-ray in the flat bones of the skull, pelvis, dorsolumbar spine, scapula, and long bones of the arms and legs. CNS involvement and, in particular, hypothalamic-pituitary involvement are well-described features of Langerhans cell histiocytosis. The precise incidence of CNS-Langerhans cell histiocytosis disease is unknown, and the natural history is poorly understood. Diabetes insipidus is reported to be the most common and well-described manifestation of hypothalamic–pituitary involvement (up to 50%). Anterior pituitary dysfunction occurs in up to 20% of patients with Langerhans cell histiocytosis and almost exclusively together with diabetes insipidus. Although histiocytosis is not a tumor, it can be treated with chemotherapeutic agents, especially vinblastine. The natural course of the disease fluctuates, which makes it difficult to evaluate treatment efficacy. Endocrine function does not improve after medical treatment of Langerhans cell histiocytosis with chemotherapy and glucocorticoids. All Langerhans cell histiocytosis with patients should undergo a thorough endocrine evaluation periodically.

Germinomas. Germinomas are uncommon extrasellar tumors that often cause delayed puberty. Polydipsia, polyuria, and visual disturbances are the most common presenting symptoms, followed by arrested growth and delayed puberty. Germinomas are located in the pituitary stalk, in the suprasellar region of the hypothalamus, or close to the pineal gland. Seeding of the tumor into the cerebrospinal fluid is common and can be used in diagnosis, i.e., examination of tumor markers (human chorionic gonadotropin [hCG]-β, or α-fetoprotein) or germ cells (with positive placental alkaline phosphatase staining). These laboratory findings, together with typical clinical features, and an excellent response to radiation therapy are so characteristic of this condition that surgery is rarely indicated, except for biopsy to establish a histological diagnosis *(60,61)*.

OTHER CENTRAL NERVOUS SYSTEM DISORDERS

Defects in Development. Various malformations affecting the development of the prosencephalon may cause hypogonadotropic hypogonadism together with deficiency of any, or all, other pituitary hormones. Midline malformations are often associated with optic dysplasia, and an absent septum pellucidum is often found by imaging techniques (septo-optic dysplasia). Other congenital midline defects, ranging from holoprosencephaly to cleft lip and palate, may also be associated with variable hypothalamic–pituitary dysfunction.

Genetic defects in the development of the anterior pituitary cause hypopituitarism, including hypogonadotropic hypogonadism. During fetal development of the anterior pituitary gland, several sequential processes occur that affect cell differentiation and proliferation. Recent advances in molecular biology have revealed several steps that are required for pituitary cell line specification, and several genes have been identified to play a role in the control of these steps. Mutations in *DAX1* gene cause X-linked adrenal hypoplasia congenita and mutations in the DAX1-related orphan nuclear receptor, steroidogenic factor-1; leptin and prohormone convertase-1 may influence GnRH release and processing of the GnRH receptor. The pituitary transcription factors, HESX-1, LHX3, and PROP-1, are important for gonadotroph development. Depending on the condition, different approaches for family counseling are needed. Despite recent advances, the pathophysiological basis of hypogonadotropic hypogonadism in the majority of individuals remains unclear.

Recently, compound heterozygous mutations in the GnRH receptor gene were described in males and females, and GnRH resistance was confirmed in vitro *(62,63)*. Because of various mutations, there is a wide spectrum of phenotypes, ranging from complete hypogonadotropic hypogonadism with lack of pubertal development to partial hypogonadism with pubertal arrest. In complete GnRH resistance, endogenous LH secretory patterns are abnormal: they are either apulsatile, or characterized by a low-normal pulse frequency with small pulses, or erratic pulses of low amplitude. In patients with partial resistance, basal LH plasma concentration are low, but FSH levels are in the normal range *(62)*.

Kallmann Syndrome. Kallmann syndrome is the most common form of isolated hypogonadotropic hypogonadism (*see* Chapter 5). Hypogonadism in these subjects results from GnRH deficiency. The other components of this syndrome include anosmia or hyposmia, resulting from hypoplasia of the olfactory lobes, and occasionally cleft lip and palate, unilateral renal agenesis, short metacarpals, sensory-neural hearing loss, and color blindness. Nearly 50% of Kallmann syndrome patients have mutations in the *KAL* gene on chromosome Xp22.3. This gene encodes an extracellular matrix protein that regulates axonal path-finding and cellular adhesion *(64)*. Defects in this gene cause failure of fetal GnRH neurons to migrate from the olfactory palacode to the mediobasal hypothalamus, resulting in hypoplasia of the olfactory sulci. Autosomal disorders (dominant or recessive) may also cause Kallmann syndrome, but those gene defects have not yet been characterized. Because approximately half of the patients have the X-linked disorder, the syndrome is more common in boys than in girls.

IATROGENIC GONADOTROPIN DEFICIENCIES

Treatment of CNS tumors, leukemia, or metastatic neoplasms with cranial irradiation may result in the gradual development of hypothalamic–pituitary failure. GH

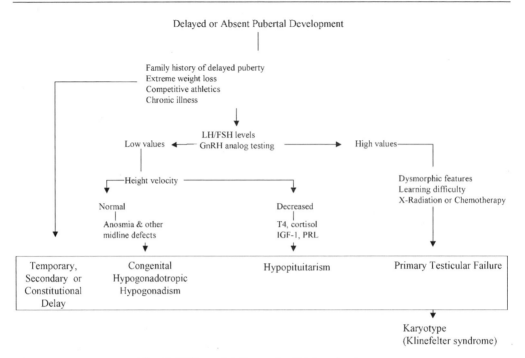

Fig. 5. Differential diagnosis of delayed puberty.

deficiency is the most common component of the radiation induced hormone disorder, but gonadotropin deficiency also occurs after sufficiently high radiation doses. Development of radiation-induced hypothalamic–pituitary failure usually develops over 1 to several years.

Hypergonadotropic Hypogonadism

Hypergonadotropic states (chromosomal alterations, syndromes, genetic disorders, and radiotherapy/chemotherapy) are covered elsewhere in this volume (*see* Chapters 9 and 13), and may present as pubertal delay. Testicular abnormalities are characterized by elevated gonadotropin and low inhibin-B concentrations, and patients with these abnormalities sometimes have specific physical features.

DIFFERENTIAL DIAGNOSIS OF DELAYED PUBERTY

The cutoff age for boys who need an evaluation for delayed puberty may vary in different ethnic groups, but in most populations, early signs of secondary sexual development should be present by age 14 yr.

A thorough medical history should note the symptoms and signs of anorexia nervosa, the intensity of athletic training, and the timing of puberty of both parents (*see* Fig. 5). In boys with constitutional delay of puberty, one parent often developed late as well. A history of chronic illness, such as celiac disease or inflammatory bowel disease, suggests a temporary or secondary delay of puberty. Stature and height velocity should be evaluated using appropriate growth charts. Height velocity is usually reduced in patients with constitutional delay but is normal in patients with isolated hypogonadotropic hypogonadism, but acquired hypogonadotropic hypogonadism is often associated with GH deficiency, short stature, and a slow growth rate. Likewise, bone age (X-ray film of left hand and wrist read according to standards such as Greulich and Pyle) delay provides useful information in the growth analysis but contributes little to the differential diagnosis.

Gonadotropin levels are generally increased in primary testicular failure or in Klinefelter syndrome, but single basal serum LH and FSH determinations are not useful in the differential diagnosis of constitutional delay vs hypogonadotropic hypogonadism. Dynamic testing, such as synthetic GnRH administration, may provide information for the differential diagnosis (54,55). Boys with constitutional delay who are destined to undergo spontaneous pubertal development within 6 to 12 mo may have a pubertal pattern of response to GnRH (post-GnRH maximum LH levels higher than maximum FSH levels), but a low prepubertal LH response to GnRH is usually found in boys with constitutional delay who will develop later than that, as well as in boys with hypogonadotropic hypogonadism. The LH response to a superactive GnRH agonist may be higher in a boy who will undergo spontaneous puberty than in one with permanent hypogonadotropic hypogonadism (65,66). Accurate differential diagnosis between constitutional delay and hypogonadotropic hypogonadism has been reported, using multiple overnight samples for LH analysis by a highly sensitive assay (67). Ultimately, third-generation supersensitive assays for LH and FSH may improve distinction between the two conditions (68). but patient follow-up is often necessary for definitive diagnosis.

MANAGEMENT OF DELAYED PUBERTY

For induction of puberty in boys with constitutional delay of puberty, the indication for treatment is usually psychosocial: boys with delayed puberty may suffer because of short stature and lack of pubertal progression. This distress may affect their school performance and their social relationships. Testosterone esters, given intramuscularly, remain the most commonly used treatment approach; therapy can be started with 50 mg of a mixture of testosterone propionate and testosterone enanthate every 4 wk. Often, a treatment course of 6 to 12 mo will accelerate growth and sexual maturation, and such a short treatment course is usually sufficient to alleviate psychosocial problems related to pubertal delay. Other treatment options are testosterone undecanoate by mouth, transdermal testosterone patches or gels, or oxandrolone. Compared with other treatment regimens, a short-course of low-dose depot testosterone intramuscularly is an effective, practical, safe, well-tolerated, and inexpensive regimen.

In boys with short parents, consideration should be given to delaying testosterone therapy to avoid compromising final height. On the other hand, a significant delay in pubertal development may also decrease final adult height, because in boys with delayed puberty, estrogen concentrations are low for chronological age (but not for bone age), and, consequently, GH secretion is functionally and temporally impaired for age. If this functional GH deficiency persists for a long time, adult height may be reduced.

In hypogonadal boys when testosterone therapy is required to induce pubertal development, the dosing and timing should be aimed at mimicking normal pubertal development, accounting for the individual's desire to begin puberty and also the family history of age at onset of puberty. Doses should be adjusted to the response of the individual

patient, which may be monitored in terms of the development of secondary sex characteristics and bone maturation. In boys with hypopituitarism, testosterone therapy should
be coordinated with the use of GH. This should be individualized for each patient to optimize growth and pubertal development.

For boys who are hypogonadal, testosterone substitution therapy should be initiated
at a low dose, because too large a dose may advance skeletal maturation disproportion-
ately and, thus, compromise final adult height. Furthermore, large doses may cause
acne, gynecomastia, or too-rapid change in libido. Doses are adjusted according to the
clinical response (Tanner stage and bone age). Most commonly, long-acting testosterone preparations, which are administered intramuscularly, are used for this purpose.
Esterification of testosterone with either propionic or enanthic acid at position 17 prolongs the metabolite's activity *(69)*. Testosterone propionate is not a suitable testosterone preparation for substitution therapy, because plasma concentration show wide
fluctuations, and the maximal between-injection interval is only 3 d with a 50 mg dose
(70). Testosterone enanthate at a dose of 250 mg intramuscularly has a half-life of 4.5
d. Based on multiple-dose pharmacokinetics, an injection interval of every 2 wk, with a
dose of 250 mg, leads to supraphysiological serum testosterone concentrations of up to
51 nmol/L and nadir level in the low normal range (12 nmol/L) before the next injection *(70)*. In male hypogonadism, a mixture of testosterone propionate and testosterone
enanthate is widely used for substitution therapy (*see* Chapter 18).

REFERENCES

1. Knorr D, Bidlingmaier F, Butenandt O. Plasma testosterone in male puberty. Acta Endocrinol
   1974;75:181–194.
2. Nielsen CT, Skakkebaek NE, Richardson DW, et al. Onset of the release of spermatozoa (spermarche)
   in boys in relation to age, testicular growth, pubic hair, and height. J Clin Endocrinol Metab
   1986;62:532–535.
3. Herman-Giddens ME, Wang L, Koch G. Secondary sexual characteristics in boys: estimates from the
   national health and nutrition examination survey III, 1988–1994. Arch Pediatr Adolesc Med
   2001;155:1022–1028.
4. de Muinich Keizer SM, Mul D. Trends in pubertal development in Europe. Hum Reprod Update
   2001;7:287–291.
5. Siler-Khodr TM, Khodr GS. Studies in human fetal endocrinology. Luteinizing hormone-releasing factor content of the hypothalamus. Am J Obstet Gynecol 1978;130:795–800.
6. Waldhauser F, Weissenbacher G, Frisch H, Pollak A. Pulsatile secretion of gonadotropins in early
   infancy. Eur J Pediatr 1981;137:71–74.
7. Dunkel L, Alfthan H, Stenman UH, Perheentupa J. Gonadal control of pulsatile secretion of luteinizing
   hormone and follicle-stimulating hormone in prepubertal boys evaluated by ultrasensitive time-
   resolved immunofluorometric assays. J Clin Endocrinol Metab 1990;70:107–114.
8. Dunkel L, Alfthan H, Stenman UH, Selstam G, Rosberg S, Albertsson-Wikland K. Developmental
   changes in 24-hour profiles of luteinizing hormone and follicle-stimulating hormone from prepuberty
   to midstages of puberty in boys. J Clin Endocrinol Metab 1992;74:890–897.
9. Chemes HE, Gottlieb SE, Pasqualini T, Domenichini E, Rivarola MA, Bergada C. Response to acute
   hCG stimulation and steroidogenic potential of Leydig cell fibroblastic precursors in humans. J Androl
   1985;6:102–112.
10. Rey RA, Campo SM, Bedecarras P, Nagle CA, Chemes HE. Is infancy a quiescent period of testicular
    development? Histological, morphometric, and functional study of the seminiferous tubules of the
    cebus monkey from birth to the end of puberty. J Clin Endocrinol Metab 1993;76:1325–1331.
11. Robertson DM, Cahir N, Findlay JK, Burger HG, Groome N. The biological and immunological char-
    acterization of inhibin A and B forms in human follicular fluid and plasma. J Clin Endocrinol Metab
    1997;82:889–896.

12. Andersson AM, Juul A, Petersen JH, Muller J, Groome NP, Skakkebaek NE. Serum inhibin B in healthy pubertal and adolescent boys: relation to age, stage of puberty, and follicle-stimulating hormone, luteinizing hormone, testosterone, and estradiol levels. J Clin Endocrinol Metab 1997;82:3976–3981.

13. Andersson AM, Toppari J, Haavisto AM, et al. Longitudinal reproductive hormone profiles in infants: peak of inhibin B levels in infant boys exceeds levels in adult men. J Clin Endocrinol Metab 1998;83:675–681.

14. Raivio T, Perheentupa A, McNeilly AS, et al. Biphasic increase in serum inhibin B during puberty: a longitudinal study of healthy Finnish boys. Pediatr Res 1998;44:552–556.

15. Byrd W, Bennett MJ, Carr BR, Dong Y, Wians F, Rainey W. Regulation of biologically active dimeric inhibin A and B from infancy to adulthood in the male. J Clin Endocrinol Metab 1998;83:2849–2854.

16. Forest MG, Sizonenko PC, Cathiard AM, Bertrand J. Hypophyso-gonadal function in humans during the first year of life. 1. Evidence for testicular activity in early infancy. J Clin Invest 1974;53:819–828.

17. Winter JS, Faiman C, Hobson WC, Prasad AV, Reyes FI. Pituitary-gonadal relations in infancy. I. Patterns of serum gonadotropin concentrations from birth to four years of age in man and chimpanzee. J Clin Endocrinol Metab 1975;40:545–551.

18. Bergada I, Rojas G, Ropelato G, Ayuso S, Bergada C, Campo S. Sexual dimorphism in circulating monomeric and dimeric inhibins in normal boys and girls from birth to puberty. Clin Endocrinol (Oxf) 1999;51:455–460.

19. Illingworth PJ, Groome NP, Byrd W, et al. Inhibin-B: a likely candidate for the physiologically important form of inhibin in men. J Clin Endocrinol Metab 1996;81:1321–1325.

20. Hohlweg W, Dohrn M. Beziehungen zwischen Hypophysenvorderlappen und Keimdrusen. Wiener Archivs Innere Medizin 1931;21:337–339.

21. Grumbach MM, Roth J, Kaplan SL, Kelch RO. Hypothalamic-pituitary regulation in man: evidence and concepts derived from clinical research. In: Grumbach MM, Grave GD, Mayer FE, eds. Control of the Onset of Puberty. Wiley & Sons, New York, 1974, pp.115–166.

22. Hohlweg W, Junkmann K. Hormonal-Nervöse Regulierung der Function des Hypophysenvorderlappens. Klinishe Wochenschrift 1932;8:321–324.

23. Hale PM, Khoury S, Foster CM, et al. Increased luteinizing hormone pulse frequency during sleep in early to midpubertal boys: effects of testosterone infusion. J Clin Endocrinol Metab 1988;66:785–791.

24. Foster CM, Hassing JM, Mendes TM, et al. Testosterone infusion reduces nocturnal luteinizing hormone pulse frequency in pubertal boys. J Clin Endocrinol Metab 1989;69:1213–1220.

25. Kletter GB, Padmanabhan V, Beitins IZ, Marshall JC, Kelch RP, Foster CM. Acute effects of estradiol infusion and naloxone on luteinizing hormone secretion in pubertal boys. J Clin Endocrinol Metab 1997;82:4010–4014.

26. Conte FA, Grumbach MM, Kaplan SL, Reiter EO. Correlation of luteinizing hormone-releasing factor-induced luteinizing hormone and follicle- stimulating hormone release from infancy to 19 years with the changing pattern of gonadotropin secretion in agonadal patients: relation to the restraint of puberty. J Clin Endocrinol Metab 1980;50:163–168.

27. Wetsel WC, Valenca MM, Merchenthaler I, et al. Intrinsic pulsatile secretory activity of immortalized luteinizing hormone-releasing hormone-secreting neurons. Proc Natl Acad Sci USA 1992;89:4149–4153.

28. Plant TM. Neurobiological bases underlying the control of the onset of puberty in the rhesus monkey: a representative higher primate. Front Neuroendocrinol 2001;22:107–139.

29. Fraser MO, Plant TM. Further studies on the role of the gonads in determining the ontogeny of gonadotropin secretion in the guinea pig (Cavia porcelus). Endocrinology 1989;125:906–911.

30. Ojeda SR, Urbanski HF. Puberty in the rat. In: Knobil E, Neill JD, eds. The Physiology of Reproduction. Vol. 2. Raven Press, New York, 1994, pp. 363–409.

31. Goldsmith PC, Thind KK, Perera AD, Plant TM. Glutamate-immunoreactive neurons and their gonadotropin-releasing hormone-neuronal interactions in the monkey hypothalamus. Endocrinology 1994;134:858–868.

32. Schaffner AE, Behar T, Nadi S, Smallwood V, Barker JL. Quantitative analysis of transient GABA expression in embryonic and early postnatal rat spinal cord neurons. Brain Res Dev 1993;72:265–276.

33. Goroll D, Arias P, Wuttke W. Preoptic release of amino acid neurotransmitters evaluated in peripubertal and young adult female rats by push-pull perfusion. Neuroendocrinology 1993;58:11–15.

34. Terasawa E, Luchansky LL, Kasuya E, Nyberg CL. An increase in glutamate release follows a decrease in gamma aminobutyric acid and the pubertal increase in luteinizing hormone releasing hormone release in the female rhesus monkeys. J Neuroendocrinol 1999;11:275–282.

35. Brann DD, Mahesh VB. Excitatory amino acids: evidence for a role in the control of reproduction and anterior pituitary hormone secretion. Endocr Rev 1994;15:3–49.
36. Bourguignon JP, Gerard A, Alvarex-Gonzalez ML, Fawe L, Franchimont P. Gonadal-independent developmental changes in activation of N-methy-D-aspartate receptors involved in gonadotropin-releasing hormone secretion. Neuroendocrinology 1992;55:634–641.
37. Terasawa E, Fernandez DL. Neurobiological mechanisms of the onset of puberty in primates. Endocr Rev 2001;22:111–151.
38. El Majdoubi M, Sahu A, Ramaswamy S, Plant TM. Neuropeptide Y: a hypothalamic brake restraining the onset of puberty in primates. Proc Natl Acad Sci USA 2000;97:6179–6184.
39. Kalra SP, Dube MG, Pu S, Xu B, Horvath TL, Kalra PS. Interacting appetite-regulating pathways in the hypothalamic regulation of body weight. Endocr Rev 1999;20:68–100.
40. Zhang Y, Proenca R, Maffei M, Barone M, Leopold L, Friedman JM. Positional cloning of the mouse obese gene and its human homologue. Nature 1994;372:425–432.
41. Clement K, Vaisse C, Lahlou N, et al. A mutation in the human leptin receptor gene causes obesity and pituitary dysfunction. Nature 1998;392:398–401.
42. Strobel A, Issad T, Camoin L, Ozata M, Strosberg AD. A leptin missense mutation associated with hypogonadism and morbid obesity. Nat Genet 1998;18:213–215.
43. Farooqi IS, Jebb SA, Langmack G, et al. Effects of recombinant leptin therapy in a child with congenital leptin deficiency. N Engl J Med 1999;341:879–884.
44. Mann DR, Akinbami MA, Gould KG, Castracane VD. A longitudinal study of leptin during development in the male rhesus monkey: the effect of body composition and season on circulating leptin levels. Biol Reprod 2000;62:285–291.
45. Plant TM, Durrant AR. Circulating leptin does not appear to provide a signal for triggering the initiation of puberty in the male rhesus monkey (Macaca mulatta). Endocrinology 1997;138:4505–4508.
46. Flier JS. Clinical review 94: What's in a name? In search of leptin's physiologic role. J Clin Endocrinol Metab 1998;83:1407–1413.
47. Cheung CC, Thornton JE, Nurani SD, Clifton DK, Steiner RA. A reassessment of leptin's role in triggering the onset of puberty in the rat and mouse. Neuroendocrinology 2001;74:12–21.
48. Ma YJ, Berg-von der Emde K, Rage F, Wetsel WC, Ojeda SR. Hypothalamic astrocytes respond to transforming growth factor-alpha with the secretion of neuroactive substances that stimulate the release of luteinizing hormone-releasing hormone. Endocrinology 1997;138:19–25.
49. Delitala G, Giusti M, Mazzocchi G, Granziera L, Tarditi W, Giordano G. Participation of endogenous opiates in regulation of the hypothalamic-pituitary-testicular axis in normal men. J Clin Endocrinol Metab 1983;57:1277–1281.
50. Albanese A, Stanhope R. Predictive factors in the determination of final height in boys with constitutional delay of growth and puberty. J Pediatr 1995;126:545–550.
51. Finkelstein JS, Neer RM, Biller BM, Crawford JD, Klibanski A. Osteopenia in men with a history of delayed puberty. N Engl J Med 1992;326:600–604.
52. Finkelstein JS, Klibanski A, Neer RM. A longitudinal evaluation of bone mineral density in adult men with histories of delayed puberty. J Clin Endocrinol Metab 1996;81:1152–1155.
53. Bertelloni S, Baroncelli GI, Ferdeghini M, Perri G, Saggese G. Normal volumetric bone mineral density and bone turnover in young men with histories of constitutional delay of puberty. J Clin Endocrinol Metab 1998;83:4280–4283.
54. Dunkel L, Perheentupa J, Sorva R. Single versus repeated dose human chorionic gonadotropin stimulation in the differential diagnosis of hypogonadotropic hypogonadism. J Clin Endocrinol Metab 1985;60:333–337.
55. Dunkel L, Perheentupa J, Virtanen M, Maenpaa J. GnRH and HCG tests are both necessary in differential diagnosis of male delayed puberty. Am J Dis Child 1985;139:494–498.
56. Mantzoros CS. Role of leptin in reproduction. Ann N Y Acad Sci 2000;900:174–183.
57. Opstad PK. Androgenic hormones during prolonged physical stress, sleep, and energy deficiency. J Clin Endocrinol Metab 1992;74:1176–1183.
58. Roemmich JN, Richmond RJ, Rogol AD. Consequences of sport training during puberty. J Endocrinol Invest 2001;24:708–715.
59. Savage MO, Beattie RM, Camacho-Hubner C, Walker-Smith JA, Sanderson IR. Growth in Crohn's disease. Acta Paediatr Suppl 1999;88:89–92.
60. Wara WM, Fellows CF, Sheline GE, Wilson CB, Townsend JJ. Radiation therapy for pineal tumors and suprasellar germinomas. Radiology 1977;124:221–223.

61. Mootha SL, Barkovich AJ, Grumbach MM, et al. Idiopathic hypothalamic diabetes insipidus, pituitary stalk thickening, and the occult intracranial germinoma in children and adolescents. J Clin Endocrinol Metab 1997;82:1362–1367.
62. de Roux N, Young J, Brailly-Tabard S, Misrahi M, Milgrom E, Schaison G. The same molecular defects of the gonadotropin-releasing hormone receptor determine a variable degree of hypogonadism in affected kindred. J Clin Endocrinol Metab 1999;84:567–572.
63. de Roux N, Young J, Misrahi M, et al. A family with hypogonadotropic hypogonadism and mutations in the gonadotropin-releasing hormone receptor. N Engl J Med 1997;337:1597–1602.
64. Rugarli EI. Kallmann syndrome and the link between olfactory and reproductive development. Am J Hum Genet 1999;65:943–948.
65. Ghai K, Cara JF, Rosenfield RL. Gonadotropin-releasing hormone agonist (nafarelin) test to differentiate gonadotropin deficiency from constitutionally delayed puberty in teen-age boys—a clinical research center study. J Clin Endocrinol Metab 1995;80:2980–2986.
66. Kletter GB, Rolfes-Curl A, Goodpasture JC, et al. Gonadotropin-releasing hormone agonist analog (nafarelin): a useful diagnostic agent for the distinction of constitutional growth delay from hypogonadotropic hypogonadism. J Pediatr Endocrinol Metab 1996;9:9–19.
67. Brown DC, Stirling HF, Butler GE, Kelnar CJ, Wu FC. Differentiation of normal male prepuberty and hypogonadotrophic hypogonadism using an ultrasensitive luteinizing hormone assay. Hormone Res 1996;46:83–87.
68. Haavisto AM, Dunkel L, Pettersson K, Huhtaniemi I. LH measurements by in vitro bioassay and a highly sensitive immunofluorometric assay improve the distinction between boys with constitutional delay of puberty and hypogonadotropic hypogonadism. Pediatr Res 1990;27:211–214.
69. Junkmann K. Long acting steroids in reproduction. Rec Prog Hormone Res 1957;13:389–419.
70. Behre HM, Oberpenning F, Nieshlag E. Comparative pharmacokinetics of androgen preparation: application of computer analysis and simulation. In: Behre HM, Nieschlag E, eds. Testosterone: Action, Deficiency and Substitution. Springer, Berlin, 1990, pp. 115–135.

5

Congenital Hypogonadotropic Hypogonadism

Clinical Features and Pathophysiology

William F. Crowley, MD
and Nelly Pitteloud, MD

NORMAL SEXUAL DEVELOPMENT IN THE HUMAN MALE

Ontogeny of Gonadotropin-Releasing Hormone Secretion

The pattern of gonadotropin-releasing hormone (GnRH) induced gonadotropin secretion in the human changes dynamically with sexual development (*see* Fig. 1). Therefore, understanding the ontogeny of GnRH secretion is essential for assessing normal sexual maturation and pathologic states, such as congenital hypogonadotropic hypogonadism.

GnRH neurons originate in the olfactory placode and migrate along the olfactory tract through the cribriform plate to the forebrain to reach their final destination, the arcuate nucleus of the hypothalamus. GnRH neurons have been observed in the human hypothalamus by the ninth week of gestation, and by 12–14 wk, gonadotropins are first detectable in the fetal circulation *(1)*. Their biosynthesis is at least partially dependent on GnRH, as evidenced by the ability of GnRH to induce luteinizing hormone (LH) synthesis and secretion in fetal human pituitary cell cultures *(2)*. Anencephalic fetuses, which lack a hypothalamus, secrete glycoprotein hormone α-subunit but do not produce LH-β or follicle-stimulating hormone (FSH)-β subunits, demonstrating the complete dependence of the dimeric gonadotropins on GnRH *(1)*.

During the neonatal period, increased pulsatile GnRH secretion induces a rise in gonadotropin secretion that, in turn, initiates gonadal hormone production *(3)*. During

From: *Male Hypogonadism:*
Basic, Clinical, and Therapeutic Principles
Edited by: S. J. Winters © Humana Press Inc., Totowa, NJ

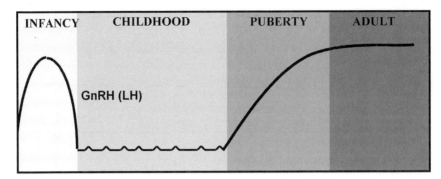

Fig. 1. Schematic drawing of the activity of the hypothalamic–pituitary–gonadal axis across the life cycle. During the neonatal window, pulsatile gonadotropin-releasing hormone (GnRH) stimulates luteinizing hormone (LH) and follicle-stimulating hormone (FSH) secretion, which induce adult levels of testosterone, estradiol, and inhibin B. Childhood is marked by a low-amplitude LH secretion and low testosterone levels. Pubertal reactivation of the hypothalamic–pituitary–gonadal axis subsequently triggers the onset of sexual maturation, initially in a sleep-entrained pattern.

childhood, the hypothalamic–pituitary axis is not completely quiescent, because the pulsatile release of gonadotropins has been shown in prepubertal boys using ultrasensitive LH assays *(4)*, as discussed more thoroughly in Chapter 4. The onset of puberty is marked by sleep-entrained reactivation of the reproductive axis, characterized by a striking increase in the amplitude of LH pulses, with less change in frequency, resulting in stimulation of the target gonad *(5,6)*. As puberty progresses, gonadotropin secretion occurs during both the day and the night, promoting the development of secondary sexual characteristics and the pubertal changes in body composition. During adulthood, gonadotropins are secreted in pulsatile fashion, with one pulse approximately every 2 h in adult men *(see* Fig. 2). There is considerable variability among individuals in both the frequency and the amplitude of LH pulses, as well as in the ensuing testosterone (T) levels. Indeed, in 15% of normal men, long interpulse intervals between LH secretory pulses were observed during a 12-h period of frequent blood sampling (every 10 min), resulting in a transient decrease in serum T levels to as low as 3.5 nmol/L *(see* Fig. 3) *(7)*.

Regulation of Gonadotropin Secretion

The regulation of gonadotropin secretion in the human male involves a complex interplay between stimulation by GnRH and inhibitory feedback by the sex steroids T and estradiol. In addition, FSH is negatively regulated by a feedback loop mediated by inhibin-B secretion from Sertoli cells *(8–11)*, as well as autocrine/paracrine regulation within the pituitary by activin and follistatin *(12)*. GnRH stimulation of gonadotropin secretion requires pulsatile release from the hypothalamus into the hypophysial portal circulation *(13)*. Although secretion pulses are clearly evident for LH in peripheral blood, FSH pulses are less evident because of their long-circulating half-life *(see* Chapter 1).

Normal Gonadal Development in the Male

Sexual maturation in males is heralded by increases in both sex steroid and inhibin-B secretion *(11,14)*. However, prior developmental changes in seminiferous tubule growth in the postnatal period and childhood are critical in setting the stage for these pubertal

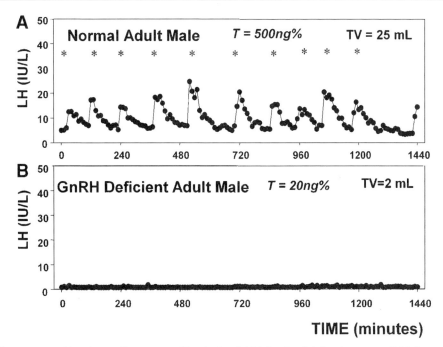

Fig. 2. Frequent blood sampling (every 10 min for 24 h) for luteinizing hormone (LH) in a normal man and a man with idiopathic hypogonadotropic hypogonadism (IHH). **(A)** Normal adult male pattern of gonadotropin-releasing hormone (GnRH) secretion with high amplitude LH pulsations (10 pulses in 24 h), normal serum testosterone levels, and normal testicular volume; **(B)** Apulsatile pattern of GnRH secretion in an IHH male as assessed by a complete absence of endogenous LH pulsations, low serum testosterone levels, and prepubertal sized testis.

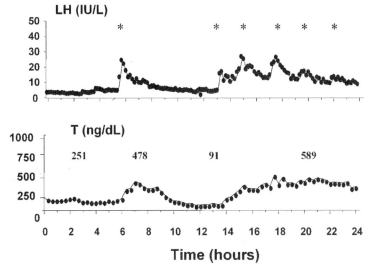

Fig. 3. Frequent blood sampling (every 10 min for 24 h) of serum testosterone and luteinizing hormone (LH), in a normal male revealing a nadir testosterone level of 91 ng/dL (to convert to nmol/L, multiply by 0.03467) after a long interpulse interval of LH secretion.

events. During the neonatal window, the initial activation of the hypothalamic–pituitary–gonadal axis triggers an elevation of T to levels close to those of adult men. These high T levels are believed to direct the completion of the inguinoscrotal phase of testicular descent and the further growth of the phallus (15). Before the onset of puberty, there is a gradual threefold increase in testis size, as evidenced by postmortem studies in monkeys and childhood trauma victims. This increase is caused by a lengthening of the seminiferous tubules, resulting mainly from intense proliferation of Sertoli cells and, to a lesser degree, of immature germ cells (16,17). These events occur before Sertoli cell maturation and the initiation of spermatogenesis. Two waves of postnatal Sertoli cell proliferation occur, the first during infancy and the second at early puberty (16). Both coincide with discrete developmental windows of neuroendocrine activity (16,18,19). The cessation of Sertoli cell proliferation and initiation of Sertoli cell maturation occur during early puberty and result in the establishment of the blood–testis barrier, formation of a lumen, high-protein synthesis capacity, and the initiation of spermatogenesis (20,21). Ultimately, this final complement of mature Sertoli cells is the major determinant of testes size, seminiferous tubular development, and sperm counts (22), because each Sertoli cell supports a finite number of germ cells (23,24).

Thereafter, a dramatic increase in meiotic germ cells promotes the most significant increase in testis size that occurs during puberty. Germ cell development is highly organized and precisely timed and involves the interaction of groups of germ cells with Sertoli cells. Finally, improvement of spermatogenic efficiency leads to complete maturation of the seminiferous tubules (20,25). Although intratesticular T plays a central role in stimulating spermatogenesis, both directly and in concert with FSH, the increase in systemic T levels also induces adult males' secondary sexual characteristics. The specific role of FSH in adult males is not yet well established. However, based on the phenotype of the males with mutations in either the FSH-β or FSH receptor (FSH-R) (see Chapter 6), FSH is necessary to maintain both qualitative and quantitative normal spermatogenesis.

CONGENITAL HYPOGONADOTROPIC HYPOGONADISM

Congenital abnormalities leading to hypogonadotropic hypogonadism are rare but are well described (Table 1). Congenital hypogonadotropic hypogonadism (CHH) is usually the consequence of deficient GnRH secretion or function. CHH can occur by itself (normosmic CHH) or can be associated with anosmia and other midline defects and is termed Kallmann syndrome. Mutations in both LH-β and FSH-β subunits have been reported to cause CHH. Recently, leptin and leptin-R gene mutations have also been demonstrated to cause hypogonadotropic hypogonadism. CHH may also be associated with impaired production of other pituitary hormones, often resulting from reduced or absent expression of transcription factors such as PROP-1 or HEXS-1. Finally, hypogonadotropic hypogonadism can be a component of complex syndromes with multiple somatic abnormalities, such as morbid obesity (Prader-Willi), cerebellar ataxia (26), cranial nerves palsies and peripheral neuropathy (27), congenital spherocytosis (28). CHH is differentiated from primary testicular disease by the demonstration of low/normal gonadotropin levels in the setting of low T levels and impaired spermatogenesis. The diagnosis also requires normal radiological imaging of the hypothalamic and pituitary region.

Table 1
Differential Diagnosis of Congenital Hypogonadotropic Hypogonadism

Congenital Idiopathic hypogonadotropic hypogonadism (CIHH)
   Anosmic (Kallmann syndrome)
   Nonansomic: normosmic IHH (nIHH)
   Fertile eunuch syndrome
   Adrenal hypoplasia congenita
Genetic defects of the gonadotropin subunits
   FSH-β mutations
   LH-β mutations
Genetic defects of leptin and leptin receptor genes
Hypogonadotropic hypogonadism associated with other pituitary hormone deficiencies
   Prop-1 mutations
   HERS1 mutations
Complex syndrome, including hypogonadotropic hypogonadism
   Prader-Willi syndrome
   Hypogonadotropic hypogonadism and congenital spherocytosis
   Hypogonadotropic hypogonadism and Moebius syndrome
   Hypogonadotropic hypogonadism and cerebral ataxia
   Hypogonadotropic hypogonadism and retinitis pigmentosa

Congenital Idiopathic Hypogonadotropic Hypogonadism (CIHH)

DEFINITION

CIHH is characterized by an isolated defect in GnRH secretion or function. Criteria for the diagnosis of CIHH include: (1) decreased T levels in the hypogonadal range (e.g., <3.5 nmol/L), (2) low/normal gonadotropin levels representing absent or reduced GnRH secretion, (3) otherwise normal hormonal testing of the anterior pituitary, (4) a normal ferritin level, and, (5) normal radiographic imaging of the hypothalamic–pituitary region.

Familial CIHH was reported in 1944, in association with anosmia and was termed Kallmann syndrome *(29,30)*. However, some hypogonadal patients do not present with an abnormal sense of smell but instead have the normosmic form of CIHH (nIHH). In our retrospective series of 78 men with CIHH, we found approx 60% with Kallmann syndrome and 40% with nIHH *(31)*. Several phenotypic abnormalities are described in CIHH, but it is not clear if they represent true associations. Synkinesia has been reported in patients with Kallmann syndrome *(29,32,33)*. Abnormal fast-conducting ipsilateral corticospinal tract projections were found in these patients *(34)*. Abnormalities in spatial perception have been found specifically in patients with Kallmann syndrome with synkinesia *(35)*. The association of renal agenesis is also reported in association with Kallmann syndrome *(32,36)*. Craniofacial and palate abnormalities have been described in Kallmann syndrome *(37)*. Finally, cardiovascular defects *(38,39)* have been associated with Kallmann syndrome. Because it is a rare disease, data on CIHH prevalence are limited and are estimated to be approx 1/10,000 to 1/86,000 *(40)*. Isolated GnRH deficiency is predominantly a male disease, with a 4:1 ratio based on analysis of more than 300 cases at the Massachusetts General Hospital.

CLINICAL FEATURES

Although the classification of CIHH based on the presence or absence of smell is frequently used in the literature, clinical phenotypic overlap is seen between Kallmann syndrome and nIHH *(31)*. Moreover, families have been documented with individuals having full Kallmann syndrome, nIHH, and isolated ansomia within a single sibship *(41)*. We have found recently that stratifying patients according to the time of onset and severity of GnRH deficiency provides greater insight into the clinical spectrum of CIHH *(31)*. In the absence of other congenital abnormalities, the clinical features of GnRH deficiency are first manifested at puberty; however, subjects may present at any age.

During the neonatal period, the presence of cryptorchidism or/and microphallus in a male fetus may indicate GnRH deficiency. Typically, gonadotropin, sex steroid, and inhibin levels are inappropriately low in such infants, because they are unable to normally activate the hypothalamic–pituitary–gonadal axis during the neonatal window *(42)*. Notably, these neonates have otherwise normal sexual differentiation. Indeed, the growth and differentiation of the male genitalia, which develop from the Wolffian ducts and the urogenital sinus, are stimulated by T production from fetal Leydig cells (*see* Chapter 2). After an initial gonadotropin-independent phase, steroidogenesis activation, as well as Leydig cell development and differentiation, are completely dependent on placental human chorionic gonadotropin (hCG) *(43)*. However, cryptorchidism and microphallus in patients with CHH indicates that in the late fetal/early neonatal period, endogenous GnRH secretion is necessary for inguinoscrotal descent of the testes and full growth of the external genitalia *(15)*.

Most often, however, the diagnosis of CIHH is delayed until adolescence. At that time, considerable clinical heterogeneity is observed with variable spontaneous pubertal development. The most common phenotype is represented by patients who fail to undergo puberty (*see* Fig. 4). Their clinical features include a lack of secondary sex characteristics, eunuchoidal body proportions (upper/lower body ratio <1 with an arm span >6 cm standing height) *(44,45)*, a high-pitched voice, slight anemia, delayed bone age, and prepubertal sized testes (1–3 mL). A large proportion of these subjects report a history of cryptorchidism (40%) or microphallus (20%) *(46)*. These latter two clinical signs provide evidence for the lack of activity of the hypothalamic–pituitary–gonadal axis during the feto-neonatal window and, thus, represent clinical surrogate markers of the failure to activate GnRH secretion at that stage of development. However, both of these markers lack sensitivity, because other factors may compensate for the lack of feto-neonatal T production. In addition, the incidence of microphallus in the men with CIHH with no prior puberty might be underestimated, given the reported successful induction of phallus growth with androgen therapy during childhood *(47)*. Although most men with CIHH (75%) fail to go through puberty, the remainder display some degree of spontaneous puberty as assessed by at least two of these criteria: (1) some testicular growth, (2) a growth spurt, (3) an increase in the number of erections, and (4) the initiation of shaving. At the milder end of the spectrum, lies the fertile eunuch variant (see following discussion). Gynecomastia is seen in approx 20–30% of men with CIHH and most often is not related to prior therapy with gonadotropins *(31,48)*.

Variant Forms of Congenital Hypogonadotropic Hypergonadism. *Fertile Eunuch Syndrome.* The first report of a man with the fertile eunuch variant of CIHH was in 1950 by McCullagh. These subjects harbor eunuchoidal proportions and

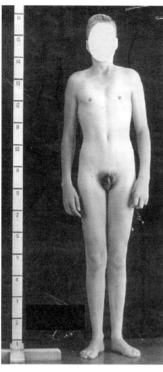

History
- **Good general health**
- **Absence of puberty**
- **Decreased/absent sense of smell**

Physical Exam
- **Arm span > height**
- **Little or/no axillary or pubic hair**
- **small testis**
- **Microphallus**
- **Cryptorchidism**

Fig. 4. Typical presentation of a man with idiopathic hypogonadotropic hypogonadism (IHH) with the most severe phenotype, including absence of puberty, eunuchoidal proportions, prepubertal testis, microphallus, and cryptorchidism.

undervirilization but have normal gonadal size and preserved spermatogenesis *(49)*. In this disorder, endogenous GnRH secretion, although decreased and insufficient to stimulate full virilization, produces adequate intragonadal T levels to support spermatogenesis and testicular growth. Indeed, these patients can be fertile either spontaneously or with T or human chorionic gonadotropin (hCG) therapy without the addition of FSH *(50,51)*. The clinical picture of the fertile eunuch thus resembles that of normal midpubertal boys; indeed, a nocturnal rise of LH and T secretion synchronous with sleep, as seen normally in midpuberty, was demonstrated in two men with the fertile eunuch syndrome *(52)*. These two cases of fertile eunuch syndrome may have resulted from defects in GnRH regulation. In contrast, we recently described a patient with the fertile eunuch variant who had detectable, but apulsatile, LH secretion associated with a partially inactivating mutation of the GnRH receptor (GnRH-R) *(53)*. These data underscore the clinical, genetic, and pathophysiological heterogeneity that exists in this syndrome.

Delayed Puberty. Delayed puberty is frequently reported in the family members of patients with CIHH *(41)*. In our series of 106 patients with CIHH, 12% had relatives with a history of delayed puberty *(41)*, as compared to 1% in the general population *(54)*. These data suggest that delayed puberty may represent the mildest end of the phenotypic spectrum of CIHH.

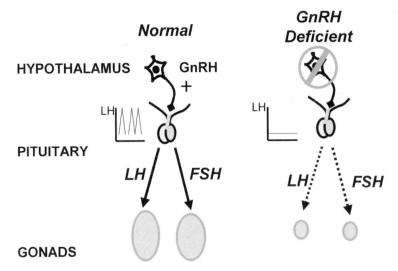

Fig. 5. Schematic drawing of the hypothalamic–pituitary–gonadal axis in a normal adult male and in congenital hypogonadotropic hypogonadism.

PATHOPHYSIOLOGY OF CIHH

Biochemical Studies. Despite variation in the clinical phenotype of CIHH men, their biochemical findings are similar. By definition, all patients have T levels in the hypogonadal range. Gonadotropins are low/normal in all subjects, which, in the setting of low T levels, indicate hypogonadotropic hypogonadism (*see* Figs. 5 and 6). Interestingly, mean LH and FSH levels are significantly higher in those patients with some degree of spontaneous puberty as compared with those men with no prior puberty *(31)*. This may explain partly the spontaneous testicular growth seen in those patients with partial puberty.

The Sertoli cell products inhibin-B and Müllerian inhibitory substance (MIS) can be measured in the serum and provide additional gonadal markers of the onset and extent of GnRH deficiency. In the normal ontogeny of inhibin-B secretion, levels rise during the neonatal activation of the hypothalamic–pituitary–gonadal axis *(55)* and then decline but remain readily measurable throughout childhood, despite low FSH levels. During the early stages of puberty, inhibin-B levels increase, plateau at stage II of puberty, and remain constant, unless spermatogenesis is disrupted *(56)*. In contrast to normal men, men with CIHH with absent pubertal development display low/undetectable inhibin-B levels *(11)*, which are well below those of normal children *(55)*. Therefore, prior gonadotropin exposure is required for normal inhibin-B production during childhood. Thus, inhibin-B levels represent a marker of reproductive axis activity during the fetal/neonatal period in patients with no sexual maturation. In men with IHH with partial puberty, baseline inhibin-B levels reach the normal range, despite low gonadotropins, presumably reflecting adequate Sertoli cell proliferation during the neonatal window and early puberty. MIS, the first detectable secretory product of fetal Sertoli cells *(57)*, is another biochemical marker of pubertal onset *(58,59)*. Indeed, MIS levels are high throughout fetal and postnatal life and decline thereafter with the onset of spermatogenesis and the activation of LH-Leydig cell function *(59)*. Accordingly,

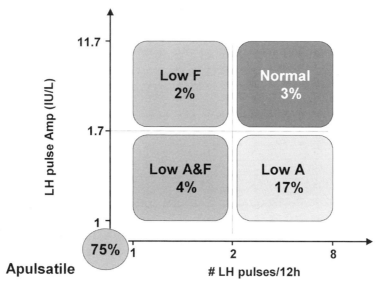

Fig. 6. Spectrum of gonadotropin-releasing hormone (GnRH) induced luteinizing hormone (LH) secretion abnormalities in men with idiopathic hypogonadotropic hypogonadism (IHH) based on our retrospective study on 78 men with CIHH (np). 75% of men with CIHH exhibit no detectable LH pulses. Seventeen percent had a normal LH frequency but a low LH amplitude. Three percent had a low LH amplitude and low frequency; 2% had a normal LH amplitude but low frequency. Finally, 2% had normal LH amplitude and frequency, deemed pathologic in the setting of hypogonadal testosterone levels.

MIS levels are high among men with CIHH with no pubertal development and are lower in those men with partial GnRH deficiency *(31)*.

Patterns of GnRH Secretion in Subjects With GnRH Deficiency. Because of low circulating levels and a short half-life (2–4 min), GnRH levels in the peripheral circulation do not accurately reflect its secretion *(60,61)*. Consequently, the study of GnRH secretion is limited to inferential approaches. Traditionally, LH is the most commonly used surrogate marker of the GnRH pulse generator *(62,63)*.

A spectrum of abnormalities in the neuroendocrine pattern of GnRH secretion is observed among men with CIHH. In our retrospective study of 78 men with CIHH, using every-10 min sampling for LH, 75% of patients failed to exhibit any detectable LH pulses, implying a lack of GnRH pulse generator activity *(see* Figs. 2 and 6) *(64,31)*. The remainder (25%) demonstrated abnormal but detectable LH pulses. Among the latter group, the majority of patients displayed a normal LH pulse frequency with a low LH pulse amplitude *(see* Fig. 6). Although a higher prevalence of apulsatile LH secretion (80%) is found among those who lack sexual development, detectable LH pulses were identified in up to 20% of subjects in this group *(31)*. Perhaps the initiation of puberty requires higher levels of GnRH stimulation than are required to maintain the neuroendocrine axis after puberty *(65)*. Also, 50% of patients with CIHH with some pubertal development did not exhibit any LH pulses *(31)*. This finding suggests that transient pubertal activation of the hypothalamic–pituitary–gonadal axis occurred, followed by a failure of the GnRH secretory program in these patients. Alternatively, we may have failed to detect a suppressed pulsatile pattern of GnRH, because the LH assay was not sufficiently sensitive. From these data, we conclude that neither mean gonadotropin levels nor the current LH secretion patterns are reliable surrogate markers for complete versus partial CHH.

GENETICS OF CIHH

Pattern of Inheritance. Considerable genetic heterogeneity underlies CIHH, which may be sporadic or familial *(41)*. Approximately 75% of cases are sporadic *(31,66)*. This may reflect a high rate of spontaneous mutations, or, alternatively, the syndrome may not be uniformly genetic. As more subjects are successfully treated to enhance fertility, the incidence of familial cases may increase. In the familial cases, CIHH can be inherited as an X-linked, autosomal-dominant, or autosomal-recessive trait *(41)*. Interestingly, in our cohort, the familial cases display a more severe phenotype, with 95% of the subjects presenting with absent pubertal development and a higher prevalence of cryptorchidism (71%) and microphallus (55%) *(31)*. To date, the genetic basis of both Kallmann syndrome and nIHH has been established in fewer than 20% of cases *(67–69)*. Interestingly, some subjects with Kallmann syndrome have family members with hypogonadism but normal olfaction, suggesting that the stratification between Kallmann syndrome and nIHH might be oversimplified *(54,70,71)*.

X-Linked Genes. *Kallmann Syndrome Gene (KAL).* In 1944, Kallmann described the clinical association of familial hypogonadotropic hypogonadism and ansomia *(29)* that has been classified as Kallmann syndrome. Both X-linked Kallmann syndrome (X-KS) and autosomal Kallmann syndrome pedigrees are well described *(72)*. Although the majority of familial cases of Kallmann syndrome are inherited autosomally *(73)*, much attention has focused on the X-linked form of Kallmann syndrome. Using contiguous gene strategy, X-KS and ichthyosis were found in patients with large Xp22.3 deletions *(69,74)*. In 1992, the first genetic defect in the KAL gene in Xp 22.3 was determined to underlie X-KS *(67)*. Since that report, several different KAL point mutations have been described *(73,75,76)*. Most KAL gene mutations are clustered in the four fibronectin type III repeat domains *(77–78)*. They cause alteration of splicing, frameshift, or stop codons and result in the synthesis of a truncated anosmin protein *(79)*. Missense mutations have rarely been described *(66,79)*. The X-linked form of Kallmann syndrome results from a disruption of the migration of GnRH neurons from the olfactory placode to their final destination in the hypothalamus. A study of a Kallmann syndrome fetus with a deletion from Xp22.31 to Xpter, i.e., including the entire KAL gene, confirmed the causative role of the KAL gene in the pathogenesis of X-KS. Histologic studies of the brain of a subsequent fetus revealed that the migration of GnRH and olfactory neurons was arrested at the cribriform plate *(80)*. This GnRH neuronal migration defect results in the failure to form normal axonal communication with the median eminence and to activate the hypothalamic–pituitary–gonadal axis in patients with X-KS, consistent with their severe phenotype. In our cohort, X-linked men with Kallmann syndrome display a complete absence of pubertal development, an apulsatile pattern of LH secretion, a high frequency of cryptorchidism and microphallus, low inhibin-B levels, and histologically immature testes *(31)*. There is some variability in the phenotypic expression of mutations, both within and between families *(75,81)*. Finally, no correlation has been demonstrated between phenotype and location of the mutation described *(79)*.

DAX-1 Gene. The DAX-1 gene (Xp21) encodes a nuclear hormone receptor with a novel DNA-binding domain *(82)*. Mutations of the DAX-1 gene cause X-linked adrenal hypoplasia congenita (AHC). Although most male subjects with a DAX-1 gene mutation display complete adrenal insufficiency in childhood and subsequent hypogonadotropism as teenagers *(83)*, clinical heterogeneity has also been reported, including men with IHH with normal adrenal function *(84)*. The response of patients with AHC to pulsatile GnRH therapy is variable, suggesting a hypothalamic and/or combined pituitary defect *(85)*. Finally, the failure of hCG to induce normal spermatogenesis implies an additional testicular defect *(85,86)*, a finding confirmed in the knockout mouse and our studies *(87)*.

Autosomal Genes. Based on the pattern of inheritance, autosomal genes account for the majority of familial cases of CHH. Of 36 familial cases with CIHH studied at Massachusetts General Hospital, only 21% could be attributed to X-linkage *(41)*. Moreover, when surrogate markers of IHH (isolated congenital anosmia and delayed puberty) were included in the analysis, the X-linked families comprised only 11%, autosomal recessive 25%, and autosomal dominant 64%. These data suggest that in familial cases, the X-linked form of GnRH deficiency is the least common. The genes responsible for most of these autosomal cases remain to be defined.

GnRH Gene. The GnRH gene itself, located at 8p21-8p11.2, is the most obvious autosomal candidate gene in CHH. Indeed, the hypogonadal *(hpg)* mouse, in which the GnRH gene has been deleted, presents with hypogonadotropic hypogonadism *(88)*. Surprisingly, however, no deletions, rearrangements, or point mutations in the GnRH gene have been described in humans to date *(89–91)*.

GnRH-Receptor Gene. A functional GnRH-R is crucial for both pubertal development and reproductive function. Indeed, hypothalamic GnRH secreted into the hypophysial portal blood interacts with high-affinity GnRH-R expressed in the cell membranes of gonadotrophs. Defects in the GnRH-R have recently emerged as the first autosomal cause of IHH *(68,85,92,93)*. GnRH-R is a G protein-coupled receptor (GPCR), with seven transmembrane segments, that activates phospholipase C, leading to the intracellular increase in inositol phosphate *(94,95)*. Although patients with a GnRH-R mutation were expected to present with complete hypogonadotropic hypogonadism and unresponsiveness to GnRH stimulation, milder variants have been described. De Roux et al. described the first family with a partially inactivating mutation in the GnRH-R *(68)*. The affected male had limited testicular growth (8-mL testes), detectable gonadotropins, and a normal response to a single pharmacologic dose of GnRH. Genetic analysis revealed a compound heterozygous mutation (Gln106Arg and Arg 262Gln substitutions). The parents were phenotypically normal, and each was heterozygous for one mutation. In CHO cells expressing Gln106Arg substitution localized in the first extracellular loop of the receptor, the level of GnRH binding and stimulation of IP$_3$ activity was markedly reduced. In contrast, in cells expressing the Arg262Gln substitution localized in the third intracellular loop of the receptor, hormone binding was normal, but IP$_3$ activation was impaired. Thereafter, several additional GnRH-R mutations (either homozygous or compound heterozygous) were found, which significantly impaired GnRH binding and/or signaling to varying degrees *(85,96,97)*. Interestingly, a spectrum of pubertal development has been observed in males with IHH with mutations in the GnRH-R, depending on the genotype, ranging from the fertile eunuch syndrome *(53)* to partial IHH *(68,92,98)* to the most severe form of GnRH deficiency characterized by cryptorchidism, microphallus, undetectable gonadotropins, and absent pubertal development *(85,96,97)*.

Congenital Hypogonadotropic Hypogonadism Caused by Genetic Defects of the Gonadotropin Subunit Genes

MUTATION IN THE GENE FOR LH-β SUBUNIT

A single case report from this institution described a male who had an inactivating mutation of the LH-β subunit *(99)*. The proband presented at the age of 17, with delayed puberty. He was from a family with several infertile male members. T levels were reduced in association with elevated LH and FSH levels. Testicular biopsy revealed spermatogenic arrest and absent Leydig cells. Long-term hCG therapy induced testicular growth and spermatogenesis. The mutant hormone had normal immunoreactivity but no biologic activity. These findings, together with the occurrence of infertility in three maternal uncles, suggested a genetic defect in the LH structure. A homozygous mutation of the LH-β subunit, A to G missense mutation, was found in codon 54, causing a Glu to Arg substitution. The proband's mother, sister, and uncles were heterozygous for the mutation. Coexpression of the mutated LH-β gene with the normal α-subunit gene in CHO cells resulted in the formation of immunoreactive LH α/β heterodimers, with no biological activity because of its inability to bind to the LH receptor. This rare case confirms that LH is not needed *in utero* for a normally masculinized fetus at birth; instead, placental hCG stimulates androgen production by the fetal testis. However, after birth, the endocrine function of the testis critically depends on LH, as demonstrated by the total absence of pubertal development in this case without bioactive LH.

MUTATIONS IN THE GENE FOR FSH-β SUBUNIT

Recently, two men with FSH-β subunit mutations have been described. The first subject, a 32-yr-old man, appeared normally virilized with normal LH and T levels but small testes, azoospermia, and undetectable FSH level *(100)*. Genetic analysis revealed a homozygous T to C mutation (Cys 82 to Arg). It was predicted that the lack of cysteine would result in the inability to form the proper disulfide bond of FSH-β with abnormal tertiary structure. The second reported case of an FSH-β gene mutation is an 18-yr-old man who presented with delayed puberty, small testes (1 and 2 mL), azoospermia, and undetectable FSH levels. The finding of a high LH and low T levels implies an additional unexplained defect in Leydig cell function *(101)*. Genetic analysis demonstrated a homozygous 2 bp deletion in codon 61. The mutation gives rise to an altered amino acid sequence, followed by a premature stop codon. Consequently, the translated FSH-β protein was truncated and unable to associate with the α-subunit, and serum FSH was undetectable.

Hypogonadotropic Hypogonadism Associated With Leptin and Leptin-R Mutations

The adipocyte-specific hormone, leptin, the product of the obese (ob) gene, acts on the hypothalamus to control appetite and energy expenditure *(102)*. Leptin acts through the leptin receptor (leptin-R), a single transmembrane-domain receptor of the cytokine-receptor family *(103)*. In 1997, Montague reported the first consanguineous family with two very obese prepubertal children who had congenital leptin deficiency *(104)*. The two cousins were homozygous for a frameshift mutation in the leptin gene. Leptin administration to one of these children led to a sustained reduction of weight mainly because of suppressed food intake. Moreover, the patient's basal and stimulated gonadotropin levels increased after 1 yr of leptin therapy and a nocturnal LH secretion pattern was observed, characteristic of midpuberty *(105)*. These findings might suggest a permissive role of leptin in the onset of puberty. In 1998, another consanguineous family with three affected obese individuals who had undetectable leptin levels was reported. Affected individuals were homozygous for a missense mutation (Arg105Try) in the leptin gene *(106)*. Among the sibship, a 24-yr-old man failed to undergo puberty. He had low T and low gonadotropin levels, but a normal response to exogenous hCG and GnRH. Similar to the ob/ob mice with leptin mutation, these patients had morbid obesity, hyperinsulinemia, and hypogonadotropic hypogonadism, but unlike the mice, these patients were not hyperglycemic, had normal glucocorticoid concentrations, and did not present with growth abnormalities. In 1998, three sisters with obesity, hypogonadotropic hypogonadism, and elevated serum leptin levels have a leptin-R mutation *(107)*. Genetic analysis revealed a homozygous mutation (G to A change) in the splice donor site of exon 16, resulting in skipping this exon during splicing. The resulted truncated receptor lacked the transmembrane and intracellular domains of the ob receptor. These results demonstrate the existence of hypothalamic hypogonadism in patients with leptin and leptin-R mutations and establish that leptin plays a key role in human reproduction *(108)*.

Hypogonadotropic Hypogonadism Associated With Other Pituitary Hormone Deficiencies

PROP-1 GENE MUTATIONS

Combined pituitary hormone deficiency has been associated with rare abnormalities in gene-encoding transcription factors that are necessary for pituitary development *(109)*. Prop-1 is required for the activation of genes involved in ventral differentiation and proliferation of the four ventral cell types (somatotropes, lactotropes, thyrotropes, and gonadotropes) *(110)*. Mutations in the gene Prop-1 (Prophet of Pit-1) are the most common cause of both familial and sporadic congenital combined pituitary hormone deficiency. Several different mutations in the Prop-1 gene have been identified and are inherited recessively. The hormonal phenotype includes deficiencies of growth hormone (GH), prolactin (PRL), and thyroid-stimulating hormone (TSH). Some subjects with Prop-1 mutations also present with LH and FSH deficiencies. However, there is variability in the clinical and hormonal expression of the cases reported thus far. Most affected patients fail to enter puberty and show consistently low LH and FSH responses to GnRH stimulation *(111)*. However, there is a report of two sibships with a homozygous mutation in PROP-1 (Arg120Cys), in which there was spontaneous initiation of puberty followed by pubertal arrest *(112)*. This finding suggests that Prop-1 is not needed for gonadotroph determination but may have a role in gonadotroph differentiation.

HESX1 GENE MUTATION

In contrast to the Prop-1 gene, HESX-1 gene is a transcriptional repressor and plays a broader role in the development of multiple placodally derived anterior structures *(110)*. A mutation in the homeobox gene HESX-1 was identified in one family of affected individuals presenting with septo-optic dysplasia, a disorder characterized by panhypopituitarism, optic nerve atrophy, and other midline CNS abnormalities, such as agenesis of the corpus callosum *(113)*. Two siblings were homozygous for an Arg53Cys missense mutation in the HESX-1 homeodomain, with a loss of ability to bind target DNA. During early mouse development, the mouse homolog of HESX- 1, Hesx1, is expressed in prospective forebrain tissue but is later restricted to Rathke's pouch, which becomes the anterior pituitary gland. Mice lacking Hesx1 exhibit variable anterior CNS defects and pituitary dysplasia. These data suggest an important role for Hesx1/HESX-1 in forebrain, midline, and pituitary development in mouse and human.

Prader-Willi Syndrome

Prader-Willi syndrome is a genetic disorder characterized by short stature, low lean body mass, hypotonia, mental retardation, behavioral abnormalities, dysmorphic features, excessive appetite, and progressive obesity. Most patients also present with reduced GH secretion and hypogonadism. The principal genetic mutation identified is a deletion of the paternally derived segment of chromosome 15 (15q11-15q13). Several other genetic abnormalities have been linked to the syndrome *(114,115)*. The majority of individuals with Prader-Willi syndrome present with delayed or partial pubertal development. There are no detailed studies of the neonatal or childhood period in children with Prader-Willi syndrome. Decreased gonadotropin levels, consistent with hypogonadotropic hypogonadism, have been found in some patients, whereas others have hypergonadotropic hypogonadism secondary to cryptorchidism *(116)*. In those with hypogonadotropic hypogonadism, the localization of the defect is unclear, because some affected individuals respond poorly to GnRH, whereas some individuals have a normal gonadotropin response to GnRH *(116–118)*. Finally, the contribution of morbid obesity to the changes in the hypothalamic–pituitary–gonadal axis has not yet been clarified in patients with Prader-Willi syndrome.

Other Causes of Hypogonadotropic Hypogonadism

STRUCTURAL DEFECT OF THE HYPOTHALAMIC–PITUITARY AREA

Structural lesions of the hypothalamus and pituitary can lead to an abnormal pattern of GnRH and/or gonadotropin secretion (*see* Chapter 8). Most patients with such tumors have multiple pituitary hormone deficiencies, whereas isolated hypogonadotropism is rare *(119,120)*. However, patients with mass lesions can present with hypogonadotropic hypogonadism without adrenal or thyroid hormone deficiency, but GH deficiency with or without hyperprolactimemia is almost always present. Indeed, a mass in the pituitary or hypothalamus is more likely to decrease the secretion of gonadotropins than that of adrenocorticotropic hormone (ACTH) or TSH. Craniopharyngioma is the most common tumor resulting in hypogonadotropic hypogonadism in childhood. It is often associated with growth retardation, diabetes insipidus, and visual field defects. Prolactinoma is the most frequent tumor causing hypogonadotropic hypogonadism in adult men *(121,122)*. Although rare, infiltrative hypothalamus or pituitary disorders, such as hemochromatosis *(123)*, sarcoidosis, lymphocytic hypophysitis *(124)*, and histiocytosis may also lead to hypogonadotropic hypogonadism. Irradiation therapy for CNS tumors or leukemia may lead to a progressive onset of hypothalamic–pituitary failure *(125–127)*. The degree of impairment depends on both the dose and the type of radiation and typically is the consequence of hypothalamic dysfunction, because the hypothalamus is significantly more radiosensitive than the pituitary gland. Sudden and severe hemorrhage into the pituitary can also result in permanent impairment of pituitary function, including hypogonadism *(128)*.

FUNCTIONAL HYPOGONADOTROPIC HYPOGONADISM

Functional forms of hypogonadotropic hypogonadism are characterized by a transient defect in GnRH secretion. This clinical presentation is well described in female hypogonadotropic subjects with hypothalamic amenorrhea (HA) but has received little study in men. In susceptible individuals, factors such as significant weight loss, exercise, or stress may precipitate HA *(129–131)*. However, in contrast to congenital hypogonadotropic hypogonadism, GnRH secretion in these subjects will resume after correcting the precipitating factor and menstruation will recur. In healthy men, moderate to severe dietary restriction is associated with mild decreased T levels, because GnRH secretion is impaired *(132,133)*. In addition, some *(134,135)*, but not all *(136,137)*, studies have shown that strenuous physical exercise may cause a transient decrease in T levels (*see* Chapter 16). However, to date, a clinical syndrome of functional GnRH deficiency in men, that is analogous to HA, has not been well characterized.

DRUG-INDUCED GnRH DEFICIENCY

The use of anabolic steroids may result in reversible hypogonadotropic hypogonadism (*see* Chapter 16) and is manifested by a decrease in T and dihydrotestosterone concentrations and suppressed spermatogenesis *(138,139)*. Suppression of the hypothalamic–pituitary–gonadal axis after androgen therapy may last more than 16 wk after discontinuation of the drug *(138)*. Chronic treatment with pharmacologic doses of glucocorticoids may also cause hypogonadism *(140)*. Chronic use of narcotic analgesics may also suppress LH secretion and result in reversible hypogonadotropic hypogonadism *(141)*.

CRITICAL ILLNESS

Any severe chronic *(142)* or acute illness, such as surgery *(143)*, myocardial infarction *(144)*, or burn injury *(145)* may result in decreased T levels *(146)*. Acute injury causes an immediate suppression of Leydig cell function *(147)*. Prolonged severe stress may inhibit pulsatile LH secretion, resulting in hypogonadotropic hypogonadism *(147)* (*see* Chapter 11).

Evaluation of Congenital Hypogonadotropic Hypogonadism

Hypogonadism is defined as a defect in one of the two major functions of the testes (i.e., production of T and spermatogenesis). Hypogonadism can reflect either a primary testicular defect (hypergonadotropic hypogonadism) or a disorder of the pituitary or hypothalamus (secondary or hypogonadotropic hypogonadism). Serum LH and FSH concentrations distinguish primary from secondary hypogonadotropic hypogonadism.

Primary hypogonadism is diagnosed in the presence of low serum T levels, oligospermia, or azoospermia, and elevated serum gonadotropin levels. In contrast, secondary hypogonadism is defined by a low T level and a reduced sperm count in the setting of low or inappropriately normal serum LH and FSH concentrations.

Given the diurnal rhythm of T secretion in normal men, T should be measured in a morning blood sample. If the initial level is low, repeat measurements should be performed. In secondary hypogonadism, the serum LH response to a single bolus of exogenous GnRH cannot determine if the defect is localized to the pituitary or hypothalamus, because a subnormal response may occur in both settings. Indeed, patients with complete GnRH deficiency are likely to have had no prior exposure to endogenous GnRH, and in this setting, repeated GnRH administration is needed to prime the gonadotropes and induce a gonadotropin response. Although not often used clinically, a pretreatment inhibin-B level may be a useful predictor of therapeutic outcome for men with CHH who desire to conceive *(31)*. Finally, although frequent blood sampling to characterize the pulsatile pattern of LH secretion may help refine the diagnosis in a research study, it is not practical in the clinical setting.

A semen analysis should be obtained in patients with congenital hypogonatropic hypogonadism who can produce an ejaculate and should include an assessment of the volume, sperm count, motility, and morphology. The World Health Organization (WHO) criteria for normal semen analysis parameters are a volume greater than 2 mL, a sperm count of ≥20 million/mL or more of ejaculate with motility 50% or greater, and normal morphology in 30% or greater. Because of the variability in sperm counts, it is worthwhile to obtain a second semen specimen if the first sample is abnormal.

Finally, in the case of secondary hypogonadism, it is critical to assess other pituitary functions (*see* Chapter 8), including a prolactin level, to ensure that the defect is isolated to the hypothalamic–pituitary–gonadal axis. A ferritin level should be measured to exclude hemochromatosis. Patients with hypogonadotropic hypogonadism typically undergo adrenarche at a normal age and should, therefore, have normal adult male dehydroepiandrosterone levels. Radiographic evaluation should include a bone age determination, MRI of the pituitary and hypothalamic area, and a DEXA scan to assess BMD.

ACKNOWLEDGMENT

This work was supported by Grants R01 HD15788 and M01-RR-01066, by NICHD/NIH through cooperative agreement (U54-HD-28138, U54 DK07028-24) as part of the Specialized Cooperative Centers Program in Reproduction Research.

REFERENCES

1. Kaplan SL, Grumbach MM. The ontogenesis of human foetal hormones. II. Luteinizing hormone (LH) and follicle stimulating hormone (FSH). Acta Endocrinol (Copenh) 1976;81:808–829.
2. Castillo RH, Matteri RL, Dumesic DA. Luteinizing hormone synthesis in cultured fetal human pituitary cells exposed to gonadotropin-releasing hormone. J Clin Endocrinol Metab 1992;75:318–322.
3. Sullivan KA, Silverman AJ. The ontogeny of gonadotropin-releasing hormone neurons in the chick. Neuroendocrinology 1993;58:597–608.
4. Apter D, Cacciatore B, Alfthan H, Stenman UH. Serum luteinizing hormone concentrations increase 100-fold in females from 7 years to adulthood, as measured by time-resolved immunofluorometric assay. J Clin Endocrinol Metab 1989;68:53–57.
5. Boyar RM, Rosenfeld RS, Kapen S, et al. Human puberty. Simultaneous augmented secretion of luteinizing hormone and testosterone during sleep. J Clin Invest 1974;54:609–618.
6. Ross JL, Loriaux DL, Cutler GB, Jr. Developmental changes in neuroendocrine regulation of gonadotropin secretion in gonadal dysgenesis. J Clin Endocrinol Metab 1983;57:288–293.
7. Spratt DI, O'Dea LS, Schoenfeld D, Butler J, Rao PN, Crowley WF, Jr. Neuroendocrine-gonadal axis in men: frequent sampling of LH, FSH, and testostcrone. Am J Physiol 1988;254:E658–E666.
8. Dubey AK, Zeleznik AJ, Plant TM. In the rhesus monkey *(Macaca mulatta),* the negative feedback regulation of follicle-stimulating hormone secretion by an action of testicular hormone directly at the level of the anterior pituitary gland cannot be accounted for by either testosterone or estradiol. Endocrinology 1987;121:2229–2237.
9. Illingworth PJ, Groome NP, Byrd W, et al. Inhibin-B: a likely candidate for the physiologically important form of inhibin in men. J Clin Endocrinol Metab 1996;81:1321–1325.

10. Anawalt BD, Bebb RA, Matsumoto AM, et al. Serum inhibin B levels reflect Sertoli cell function in normal men and men with testicular dysfunction. J Clin Endocrinol Metab 1996;81:3341–3345.

11. Nachtigall LB, Boepple PA, Seminara SB, et al. Inhibin B secretion in males with gonadotropin-releasing hormone (GnRH) deficiency before and during long-term GnRH replacement: relationship to spontaneous puberty, testicular volume, and prior treatment—a clinical research center study. J Clin Endocrinol Metab 1996;81:3520–3525.

12. Ying SY. Inhibins, activins, and follistatins: gonadal proteins modulating the secretion of follicle-stimulating hormone. Endocr Rev 1988;9:267–293.

13. Belchetz PE, Plant TM, Nakai Y, Keogh EJ, Knobil E. Hypophysial responses to continuous and intermittent delivery of hypothalamic gonadotropin-releasing hormone. Science 1978;202:631–633.

14. Seminara SB, Boepple PA, Nachtigall LB, et al. Inhibin B in males with gonadotropin-releasing hormone (GnRH) deficiency: changes in serum concentration after shortterm physiologic GnRH replacement—a clinical research center study. J Clin Endocrinol Metab 1996;81:3692–3696.

15. Hutson JM, Hasthorpe S, Heyns CF. Anatomical and functional aspects of testicular descent and cryptorchidism. Endocr Rev 1997;18:259–280.

16. Cortes D, Muller J, Skakkebaek NE. Proliferation of Sertoli cells during development of the human testis assessed by stereological methods. Int J Androl 1987;10:589–596.

17. Muller J, Skakkebaek NE. Quantification of germ cells and seminiferous tubules by stereological examination of testicles from 50 boys who suffered from sudden death. Int J Androl 1983;6:143–156.

18. Marshall GR, Plant TM. Puberty occurring either spontaneously or induced precociously in rhesus monkey (Macaca mulatta) is associated with a marked proliferation of Sertoli cells [published erratum appears in Biol Reprod 1996;55(3):728]. Biol Reprod 1996;54:1192–1199.

19. Rey R, Lordereau-Richard I, Carel JC, et al. Anti-mullerian hormone and testosterone serum levels are inversely during normal and precocious pubertal development. J Clin Endocrinol Metab 1993;77:1220–1226.

20. Russell LD, Bartke A, Goh JC. Postnatal development of the Sertoli cell barrier, tubular lumen, and cytoskeleton of Sertoli and myoid cells in the rat, and their relationship to tubular fluid secretion and flow. Am J Anat 1989;184:179–189.

21. Dym M, Cavicchia JC. Further observations on the blood-testis barrier in monkeys. Biol Reprod 1977;17:390–403.

22. Orth JM, Gunsalus GL, Lamperti AA. Evidence from Sertoli cell-depleted rats indicates that spermatid number in adults depends on numbers of Sertoli cells produced during perinatal development. Endocrinology 1988;122:787–794.

23. Russell LD, Peterson RN. Determination of the elongate spermatid-Sertoli cell ratio in various mammals. J Reprod Fertil 1984;70:635–641.

24. Russell LD, Ren HP, Sinha Hikim I, Schulze W, Sinha Hikim AP. A comparative study in twelve mammalian species of volume densities, volumes, and numerical densities of selected testis components, emphasizing those related to the Sertoli cell. Am J Anat 1990;188:21–30.

25. Orth JM. Proliferation of Sertoli cells in fetal and postnatal rats: a quantitative autoradiographic study. Anat Rev 1982;203:485–492.

26. Seminara SB, Acierno JS, Jr., Abdulwahid NA, Crowley WF, Jr., Margolin DH. Hypogonadotropic hypogonadism and cerebellar ataxia: detailed phenotypic characterization of a large, extended kindred. J Clin Endocrinol Metab 2002;87:1607–1612.

27. Kawai M, Momoi T, Fujii T, Nakano S, Itagaki Y, Mikawa H. The syndrome of Mobius sequence, peripheral neuropathy, and hypogonadotropic hypogonadism. Am J Med Genet 1990;37:578–582.

28. Vermeulen S, Messiaen L, Scheir P, De Bie S, Speleman F, De Paepe A. Kallmann syndrome in a patient with congenital spherocytosis and an interstitial 8p11.2 deletion. Am J Med Genet 2002;108:315–318.

29. Kallmann FJ, Schoenfeld WA. The genetic aspects of primary eunuchoidism. Am J Ment Defic 1944;158:203–236.

30. Zitzmann M, Nieschlag E. Hormone substitution in male hypogonadism. Mol Cell Endocrinol 2000;161:73–88.

31. Pitteloud N, Hayes FJ, Boepple PA, et al. The role of prior pubertal development, biochemical markers of testicular maturation, and genetics in elucidating the phenotypic heterogeneity of idiopathic hypogonadotropic hypogonadism. J Clin Endocrinol Metab 2002;87:152–160.

32. Quinton R, Duke VM, Robertson A, et al. Idiopathic gonadotrophin deficiency: genetic questions addressed through phenotypic characterization. Clin Endocrinol (Oxf) 2001;55:163–174.

33. Conrad B, Kriebel J, Hetzel WD. Hereditary bimanual synkinesis combined with hypogonadotropic hypogonadism and anosmia in four brothers. J Neurol 1978;218:263–274.

34. Krams M, Quinton R, Ashburner J, et al. Kallmann's syndrome: mirror movements associated with bilateral corticospinal tract hypertrophy. Neurology 1999;52:816–822.
35. Kertzman C, Robinson DL, Sherins RJ, Schwankhaus JD, McClurkin JW. Abnormalities in visual spatial attention in men with mirror movements associated with isolated hypogonadotropic hypogonadism. Neurology 1990;40:1057–1063.
36. Kirk JMW, Grant DB, Besser GM, et al. Unilateral renal aplasia in X-linked Kallmann's syndrome. Clin Genet 1994;46:260–262.
37. Molsted K, Kjaer I, Giwercman A, Vesterhauge S, Skakkebaek NE. Craniofacial morphology in patients with Kallmann's syndrome with and without cleft lip and palate. Cleft Palate Craniofac J 1997;34:417–424.
38. Moorman JR, Crain B, Osborne D. Kallman's syndrome with associated cardiovascular and intracranial anomalies. Am J Med 1984;77:369–372.
39. Cortez AB, Galindo A, Arensman FW, Van Dop C. Congenital heart disease associated with sporadic Kallmann syndrome. Am J Med Genet 1993;46:551–554.
40. Filippi G. Klinefelter's syndrome in Sardinia. Clinical report of 265 hypogonadic males detected at the time of military check-up. Clin Genet 1986;30:276–284.
41. Waldstreicher J, Seminara SB, Jameson JL, et al. The genetic and clinical heterogeneity of gonadotropin-releasing hormone deficiency in the human. J Clin Endocrinol Metab 1996;81:4388–4395.
42. Main KM, Schmidt IM, Skakkebaek NE. A possible role for reproductive hormones in newborn boys: progressive hypogonadism without the postnatal testosterone peak. J Clin Endocrinol Metab 2000;85:4905–4907.
43. Huhtaniemi IT, Korenbrot CC, Jaffe RB. HCG binding and stimulation of testosterone biosynthesis in the human fetal testis. J Clin Endocrinol Metab 1977;44:963–967.
44. Graner J, Buchanan B, Abraira C. Ratio of arm span to height not usually increased in Klinefelter's syndrome. N Engl J Med 1982;306:1490–1491.
45. Reeves SL, Varakamin C, Henry CJ. The relationship between arm-span measurement and height with special reference to gender and ethnicity. Eur J Clin Nutr 1996;50:398–400.
46. Bardin CW, Ross GT, Rifkind AB, Cargille CM, Lipsett MB. Studies of the pituitary-Leydig cell axis in young men with hypogodotropic hypogonadism and hyposmia: comparison with normal men, prepubertal boys, and hypopituitary patients. J Clin Invest 1969;48:2046–2056.
47. Bin-Abbas B, Conte FA, Grumbach MM, Kaplan SL. Congenital hypogonadotropic hypogonadism and micropenis: effect of testosterone treatment on adult penile size why sex reversal is not indicated. J Pediatr 1999;34:579–583.
48. Lieblich JM, Rogol AD, White BJ, Rosen SW. Syndrome of anosmia with hypogonadotropic hypogonadism (Kallmann syndrome). Am J Med 1982;73:506–519.
49. McCullagh EP, Beck JC, Schaffenburg CA. A syndrome of eunuchoidism with spermatogenesis, normal urinary FSH and low or normal ICSH: "Fertile." Eunuchs. J Clin Endocrinol Metab 1953;13:489–509.
50. Smals AG, Kloppenborg PW, van Haelst UJ, Lequin R, Benraad TJ. Fertile eunuch syndrome versus classic hypogonadotrophic hypogonadism. Acta Endocrinol (Copenh) 1978;87:389–399.
51. Rogol AD, Mittal KK, White BJ, McGinniss MH, Lieblich JM, Rosen SW. HLA-compatible paternity in two "fertile eunuchs" with congenital hypogonadotropic hypogonadism and anosmia (the Kallman syndrome). J Clin Endocrinol Metab 1980;51:275–279.
52. Boyar RM, Wu RH, Kapen S, Hellman L, Weitzman ED, Finkelstein JW. Clinical and laboratory heterogeneity in idiopathic hypogonadotropic hypogonadism. J Clin Endocrinol Metab 1976;43:1268–1275.
53. Pitteloud N, Boepple PA, DeCruz S, Valkenburgh SB, Crowley WF, Jr., Hayes FJ. The fertile eunuch variant of idiopathic hypogonadotropic hypogonadism: spontaneous reversal associated with a homozygous mutation in the gonadotropin-releasing hormone receptor. J Clin Endocrinol Metab 2001;86:2470–2475.
54. Styne DM. Puberty and its disorders in boys. Endocrinol Metab Clin North Am 1991;20:43–69.
55. Andersson AM, Muller J, Skakkebaek NE. Different roles of prepubertal and postpubertal germ cells and Sertoli cells in the regulation of serum inhibin B levels. J Clin Endocrinol Metab 1998;83:4451–4458.
56. Andersson AM, Juul A, Petersen JH, Muller J, Groome NP, Skakkebaek NE. Serum inhibin B in healthy pubertal and adolescent boys: relation to age, stage of puberty, and follicle-stimulating hormone, luteinizing hormone, testosterone, and estradiol levels. J Clin Endocrinol Metab 1997;82:3976–3981.

57. Tran D, Muesy-Dessole N, Josso N. Anti-Mullerian hormone is a functional marker of foetal Sertoli cells. Nature 1977;269:411–412.
58. Young J, Rey R, Couzinet B, Chanson P, Josso N, Schaison G. Antimullerian hormone in patients with hypogonadotropic hypogonadism. J Clin Endocrinol Metab 1999;84:2696–2699.
59. Lee MM, Donahoe PK, Hasegawa T, et al. Mullerian inhibiting substance in humans: normal levels from infancy to adulthood. J Clin Endocrinol Metab 1996;81:571–576.
60. Arimura A, Kastin AJ, Gonzales-Barcena D, Siller J, Weaver RE, Schally AV. Disappearance of LH-releasing hormone in man as determined by radioimmunoassay. 1974;3:421–425.
61. Pimstone B, Epstein S, Hamilton SM, LeRoith D, Hendricks S. Metabolic clearance and plasma half-disappearance time of exogenous gonadotropin-releasing hormone in normal subjects and in patients with liver disease and chronic renal failure. J Clin Endocrinol Metab 1977;44:356–360.
62. Clarke IJ, Cummins JT. The temporal relationship between gonadotropin-releasing hormone (GnRH) and luteinizing hormone (LH) secretion in ovariectomized ewes. Endocrinology 1982;111:1737–1739.
63. Levine JN, Pau KYF, Ramirez VD, Jackson GL. Simultaneous measurement of luteinizing hormone releasing hormone and luteinizing hormone release in unanesthetized, ovariectomized sheep. Endocrinology 1982;111:1449–1455.
64. Whitcomb RW, Crowley WF, Jr. Clinical review 4: diagnosis and treatment of isolated gonadotropin-releasing hormone deficiency in men. J Clin Endocrinol Metab 1990;70:3–7.
65. Spratt DI, Finkelstein JS, O'Dea LS, et al. Long-term administration of gonadotropin-releasing hormone in men with idiopathic hypogonadotropic hypogonadism. A model for studies of the hormone's physiologic effects. Ann Intern Med 1986;105:848–855.
66. Georgopoulos NA, Pralong FP, Seidman CE, Seidman JG, Crowley Jr WF, Vallejo M. Genetic heterogeneity evidenced by low incidence of KAL-1 gene mutations in sporadic cases of gonadotropin-releasing hormone deficiency. J Clin Endocrinol Metab 1997;82:213–217.
67. Bick D, Franco B, Sherins RJ, et al. Brief report: intragenic deletion of the KALIG-1 gene in Kallmann's syndrome [see comments]. N Engl J Med 1992;326:1752–1755.
68. de Roux N, Young J, Misrahi M, et al. A family with hypogonadotropic hypogonadism and mutations in the gonadotropin-releasing hormone receptor. N Engl J Med 1997;337:1597–1602.
69. Legouis R, Hardelin JP, Levilliers J, et al. The candidate gene for the X-linked Kallmann syndrome encodes a protein related to adhesion molecules. Cell 1991;67:423–435.
70. Jakacki RI, Kelch RP, Sauder SE, Lloyd JS, Hopwood NJ, Marshall JC. Pulsatile secretion of luteinizing hormone in children. J Clin Endocrinol Metab 1982;55:453–458.
71. Rugarli EI, Lutz B, Kuratani SC, et al. Expression pattern of the Kallmann syndrome gene in the olfactory system suggests a role in neuronal targeting. Nat Genet 1993;4:19–26.
72. Seminara SB, Hayes FJ, Crowley WF, Jr. Gonadotropin-releasing hormone deficiency in the human (idiopathic hypogonadotropic hypogonadism and Kallmann's syndrome): pathophysiological and genetic considerations. Endocr Rev 1998;19:521–539.
73. Oliveira LM, Seminara SB, Beranova M, et al. The importance of autosomal genes in Kallmann syndrome: genotype-phenotype correlations and neuroendocrine characteristics. J Clin Endocrinol Metab 2001;86:1532–1538.
74. Franco B, Guioli S, Pragliola A, et al. A gene deleted in Kallmann's syndrome shares homology with neural cell adhesion and axonal path-finding molecules. Nature 1991;353:529–536.
75. Quinton R, Duke VM, de Zoysa PA, et al. The neuroradiology of Kallmann's syndrome: a genotypic and phenotypic analysis. J Clin Endocrinol Metab 1996;81:3010–3017.
76. Hardelin JP, Levilliers J, Blanchard S, et al. Heterogeneity in the mutations responsible for X chromosome-linked Kallmann syndrome. Hum Mol Genet 1993;2:373–377.
77. Ballabio A, Carrozzo R, Parenti G, et al. Molecular heterogeneity of steroid sulfatase deficiency: a multicenter study on 57 unrelated patients, at DNA and protein levels. Genomics 1989;4:36–40.
78. Cohen-Salmon M, Tronche F, del Castillo I, Petit C. Characterization of the promoter of the human KAL gene, responsible for the X-chromosome-linked Kallmann syndrome. Gene 1995;164:235–242.
79. Hardelin JP, Levilliers J, Young J, et al. Xp22.3 deletions in isolated familial Kallmann's syndrome. J Clin Endocrinol Metab 1993;76:827–831.
80. Schwanzel-Fukuda M, Bick D, Pfaff DW. Luteinizing hormone-releasing hormone (LHRH)-expressing cells do not migrate normally in an inherited hypogonadal (Kallmann) syndrome. Mol Brain Res 1989;6:311–326.
81. Parenti G, Rizzolo MG, Ghezzi M, et al. Variable penetrance of hypogonadism in a sibship with Kallmann syndrome due to a deletion of the KAL gene. Am J Med Genet 1995;57:476–478.

82. Zanaria E, Muscatelli F, Bardoni B, et al. An unusual member of the nuclear hormone receptor super-family responsible for X-linked adrenal hypoplasia congenita. Nature 1994;372:635–641.

83. Habiby RL, Boepple P, Nachtigall L, Sluss PM, Crowley WF, Jr., Jameson JL. Adrenal hypoplasia congenita with hypogonadotropic hypogonadism: evidence that DAX-1 mutations lead to combined hypothalmic and pituitary defects in gonadotropin production [see comments]. J Clin Invest 1996;98:1055–1062.

84. Merke DP, Tajima T, Baron J, Cutler GB, Jr. Hypogonadotropic hypogonadism in a female caused by an X-linked recessive mutation in the DAX1 gene. N Engl J Med 1999;340:1248–1252.

85. Caron P, Chauvin S, Christin-Maitre S, et al. Resistance of hypogonadic patients with mutated GnRH receptor genes to pulsatile GnRH administration. J Clin Endocrinol Metab 1999;84:990–996.

86. Tabarin A, Achermann JC, Recan D, et al. A novel mutation in DAX1 causes delayed-onset adrenal insufficiency and incomplete hypogonadotropic hypogonadism. J Clin Invest 2000;105:321–328.

87. Seminara SB, Achermann JC, Genel M, Jameson JL, Crowley WF, Jr. X-linked adrenal hypoplasia congenita: a mutation in DAX1 expands the phenotypic spectrum in males and females. J Clin Endocrinol Metab 1999;84:4501–4509.

88. Mason AJ, Pitts SL, Nikolics K, et al. The hypogonadal mouse: reproductive functions restored by gene therapy. Science 1986;234:1372–1378.

89. Layman LC, Wilson JT, Huey LO, Lanclos LD, Plouffe Jr L, McDonough PG. Gonadotropin-releasing hormone, follicle-stimulating hormone beta, luteinizing hormone beta gene structure in idiopathic hypogonadotropic hypogonadism. Fertil Steril 1992;57:42–49.

90. Nakayama Y, Wondisford FE, Lash RW, et al. Analysis of gonadotropin-releasing hormone gene structure in families with familial central precocious puberty and idiopathic hypogondotropic hypogonadism. J Clini Endocrinol Metab 1990;70:1233–1238.

91. Weiss J, Crowley WF, Jr., Jameson JL. Normal structure of the gonadotropin-releasing hormone (GnRH) gene in patients with GnRH deficiency and idiopathic hypogonadotropic hypogonadism. J Clin Endocrinol Metab 1989;69:299–303.

92. de Roux N, Young J, Brailly-Tabard S, Misrahi M, Milgrom E, Schaison G. The same molecular defects of the gonadotropin-releasing hormone receptor determine a variable degree of hypogonadism in affected kindred. J Clin Endocrinol Metab 1999;84:567–572.

6

Male Hypogonadism Resulting From Mutations in the Genes for the Gonadotropin Subunits and Their Receptors

Ilpo T. Huhtaniemi, MD, PhD

CONTENTS

INTRODUCTION

The unraveling of the structure of the human genome has allowed for major advances in the diagnostics of inherited diseases. Besides clear disease-causing mutations, the emerging knowledge about single nucleotide and microsatellite polymorphisms in the human genome is adding a new level of complexity to genomic function, providing the structural basis for individual variability of the genome and its phenotypic expression. All mutations can, in principle, be classified as inactivating, activating, or neutral, i.e., with no effect on function of the encoded protein. The hormone ligand mutations that are known today are almost invariably inactivating. The polymorphisms, by definition, are neutral, or they have only minor effects at the functional level. In some cases, they may even offer a functional advantage to their carriers. In the case of hormone receptors, the inactivating mutations block receptor function through a variety of mechanisms, whereas with activating mutations, the receptor becomes constitutively activated in the absence of hormone, or it acquires novel functions not present in the wild-type (WT) receptor.

Reproductive functions, like all functions on the human body that are under genetic control, are affected by specific mutations and polymorphisms of key genes. The focus

From: *Male Hypogonadism:*
Basic, Clinical, and Therapeutic Principles
Edited by: S. J. Winters © Humana Press Inc., Totowa, NJ

of this chapter is to review the currently known mutations in the three gonadotropins, the pituitary luteinizing hormone (LH), its placental analog, human chorionic gonadotropin (hCG), and the pituitary follicle-stimulating hormone (FSH), as well as their cognate receptors (R), the LH-R and FSH-R. Specific forms of male gonadal dysfunction are caused by these mutations. Common polymorphisms exist in the gonadotropins and their receptor genes, and they may be responsible for borderline alterations of gonadal function. This review emphasizes the role of gonadotropin and gonadotropin receptor mutations in male gonadal dysfunction. The polymorphisms of these genes with phenotypic effects are also described, as well as the relevant genetically-modified animal models when they enhance the molecular pathogenesis of the mutations.

STRUCTURE OF THE GONADOTROPIN SUBUNIT AND GONADOTROPIN RECEPTOR GENES AND PROTEINS

Gonadotropin Subunits

FSH, LH, and hCG, together with thyroid-stimulating hormone (TSH), comprise the family of glycoprotein hormones. Each hormone is composed of two subunits that are coupled by noncovalent interactions: the common α-subunit of 92 amino acids (aa) and the β-subunit; 110 aa in FSH, 121 aa in LHβ, and 145 aa in hCGβ (see Fig. 1). The different β-subunits of the glycoprotein hormones are responsible for their functional specificity. hCG is structurally similar to LH, and both hormones have similar actions. Gonadotropins are glycosylated through N-linked bonds (see Fig. 1), and the carbohydrate content of LH is approx 15%, of FSH is 20%, and of hCG is 30% (1,2). Most conspicuously, the carbohydrate moieties increase the circulatory half-lives of the gonadotropins, which are approx 20 min for LH, approx 2 h for FSH, and 12–24 h for hCG. The long half-life of hCG is primarily explained by the 24-aa C-terminal extension of its β-subunit, in comparison to LHβ, which is heavily glycosylated through O-linked glycosylation sites (see Fig. 1). The short half-life of LH is a function of the high proportion of terminal sulphate groups in its carbohydrates; a specific hepatic receptor accelerates the elimination of this type of glycoprotein from the circulation (3).

The *common α-subunit* gene is located on chromosome 6q12.21, *FSHβ* is found on chromosome 11p13, and the cluster of *LHβ/hCGβ* genes, consisting of one *LHβ* and six *hCGβ* genes and pseudogenes, is located on chromosome 19q13.32 (4,5). The *common α-subunit* gene consists of four exons, and the β-subunits are composed of three exons. The crystal structures of deglycosylated hCG (6) and FSH (7) are similar and reveal that both subunits contain so-called "cysteine knot structures" that are similar to some remotely related growth factor-type signaling molecules. Each subunit has an elongated shape, with two β-hairpin loops on one side of the central cysteine knot and a long loop on the other side. The noncovalent interaction between the two subunits is stabilized by a segment of the β-subunit that extends like a "seatbelt" around the α-subunit and is "locked" by a disulfide bridge.

Gonadotropin Receptors

Like their ligands, the gonadotropin receptors are structurally related glycoproteins, belonging to the large family of G protein-coupled receptors (GPCRs) (see Figs. 2 and 3) (8–10). They each have a transmembrane domain that traverses the plasma membrane

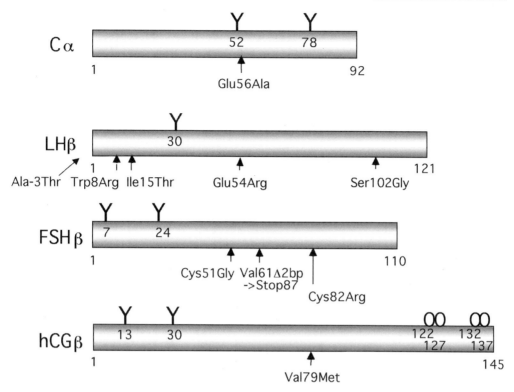

Fig. 1. Schematic presentation of sizes, locations of the carbohydrate side chains, and currently known mutations and polymorphisms in the gonadotropin subunits, i.e., common α-subunit (Cα), LHβ, FSHβ, and hCGβ. The numbers below the right ends of the bars indicate the numbers of amino acids in the mature subunit proteins. Symbols "Y" and "O" indicate the locations of *N*-linked and *O*-linked carbohydrate side chains, respectively. The arrows below the bars indicate the locations of point mutations and polymorphisms.

as seven α-helices connected by three extracellular and three intracellular loops. The glycoprotein hormone receptors form a subgroup within this gene family with a distinct long *N*-terminal extracellular domain, comprising approximately half the size of the receptor. The C-termini of the receptor proteins form short intracellular tails. Whereas the FSH-R binds only FSH, LH and hCG are so structurally similar that they bind to the same LH-R. Both gonadotropin receptor genes are localized on chromosome 2p21 *(11,12)*, and they carry considerable structural similarity, especially in their transmembrane domains. The clearest difference is that the first 10 exons encode the extracellular domain of LH-R, whereas this domain is encoded by 9 exons in the FSH-R. The last long eleventh exon in *LH-R* (tenth in *FSH-R*) encodes the transmembrane and intracellular domains.

Gonadotropins bind to the extracellular domain of their receptors. This domain contains several leucine-rich repeats that are found in various proteins responsible for protein-protein interactions. The domain is glycosylated in an *N*-linked fashion, but the role of these structures in receptor function is not clear. The extracellular and transmembrane domains are connected by a short hinge region that may influence ligand specificity, as shown with a human mutation of *LH-R* lacking this region *(13)*. The

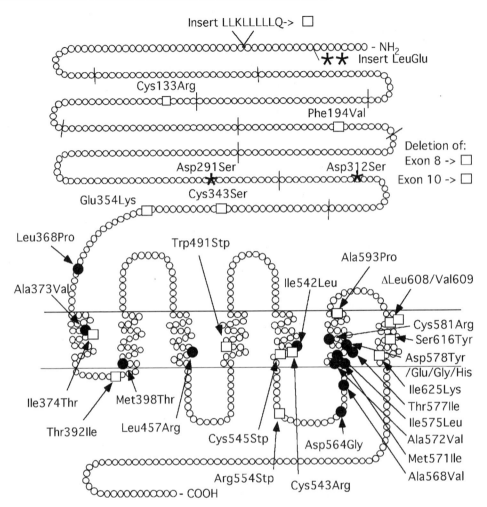

Fig. 2. Locations of the currently known mutations of the human luteinizing hormone receptor (LHR). □ inactivating mutation; ●, activating mutation; ⋆, polymorphism. The short lines across the peptide chain depict the exon boundaries.

transmembrane domain, with its seven membrane-spanning α-helices and intracellular and extracellular loops, resembles other GPCRs and is crucial for signal transduction. In particular, the third intracellular loop, the sixth transmembrane domain, and the cytoplasmic tail are closely involved in G protein coupling and signal transduction. The crystal structure of the gonadotropin receptors is not yet known.

The gonadotropin receptors are primarily coupled to a G protein that activates adenylyl cyclase and elevates intracellular cyclic adenosine monophosphate (cAMP) levels *(8,10)*. These receptors also activate other signaling pathways, including phosphatidylinositide turnover, intracellular Ca^{2+}, mitogen-activated protein kinases, and activation of the G_i protein *(8,10,14)*. The alternate signaling pathways are often activated at higher hormone concentrations, and their functions may be limited to special conditions in which gonadotropin levels are elevated, e.g., pregnancy or constitutively activating receptor mutations (see section on activating mutations).

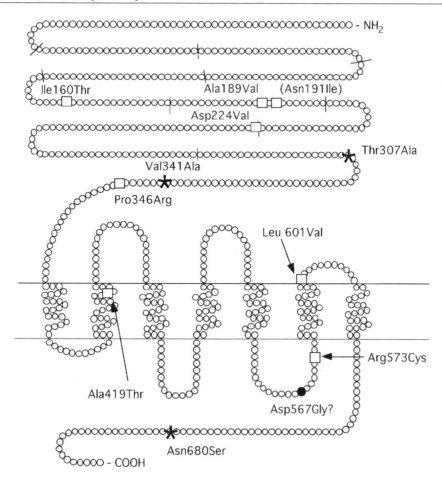

Fig. 3. Locations of the currently known mutations of the human follicle-stimulating hormone receptor (FSH-R). □, inactivating mutation; ●, activating mutation; ∗, polymorphism. The short lines across the peptide chain depict the exon boundaries. The Asn191Ile FSHR mutation has been found only in a heterozygous form in a normal subject. The activating Asp567Gly mutation has marginal constitutive activity in vitro.

The transcription of the gonadotropin receptors is characterized by a complex phenomenon of alternative splicing and several mRNA species; messages that are both shorter and longer than the one deduced from the expected translation product are observed *(8,10).* Both inhibitory and stimulatory interactions with the full-length receptors have been proposed for these putative receptor variants. However, no clear physiological or pathophysiological role for them has yet been demonstrated.

GONADOTROPIN SECRETION AND ACTIONS THROUGHOUT THE MALE LIFE SPAN

Physiological studies have clarified in great detail the role of gonadotropins in the development and mature functions of male reproduction. In the fetal period, placental hCG, a superagonist of pituitary LH, is responsible for the stimulation of testosterone production by fetal Leydig cells, which is essential for masculinization of the male reproductive organs (15). This occurs in collaboration with the Sertoli cell product, anti-Müllerian hormone (or Müllerian-inhibiting substance), and another Leydig cell product, insulin-like factor-3 (INSL-3) that regulate the transabdominal phase of testicular descent (16,17). Although FSH secretion begins in the fetus and fetal testes express FSH-R (18), FSH's role in the fetal period is uncertain. Data from animal models indicate that its first role is the stimulation of Sertoli cell proliferation in the prepubertal testis (19). Fetal pituitary gonadotropin secretion begins at the end of the first trimester, with high levels in midpregnancy, followed by a decline toward the end of gestation, apparently resulting from development of feedback regulation (20). A secondary increase occurs during the first 4–6 mo of postnatal life, which is accompanied by a similar peak in testosterone production (21). No function has been demonstrated for this period of activation, and it may represent an adaptation to extrauterine life and the hormonal milieu in the absence of placental hormones.

The prepubertal phase of male development is typified by low circulating gonadotropin levels, but they are not absent, and ultrasensitive assays can detect pulsatile LH secretion especially during the night (22). Prepubertal testes also have receptors for both gonadotropins, as shown indirectly by their functional responses to stimulation by hCG or FSH (23).

Puberty is the period of reawakening of gonadotropin secretion (see Chapter 4). At this time, both hormones reach adult levels and the pulsatile pattern of secretion. LH activates Leydig cell growth, proliferation, and steroid production, and FSH stimulates Sertoli cell proliferation and the metabolic functions that are needed for the maintenance of spermatogenesis. Whether FSH is mandatory for the pubertal initiation and adult maintenance of spermatogenesis is controversial, but it is clear that qualitatively and quantitatively normal spermatogenesis is possible only in the presence of all endocrine and paracrine factors, including FSH, that are functioning in the pituitary–gonadal axis (24).

Human testicular function is maintained through old age. However, mean testosterone levels and spermatogenesis decline with aging (25). This phenomenon of "andropause" and the effect of testosterone replacement therapy, have recently received a great deal of attention (see Chapter 14).

When considering the influence of gonadotropin or gonadotropin receptor mutations on male reproductive functions, specific phenotypic effects can be identified during all stages of the male life span.

GONADOTROPIN SUBUNIT MUTATIONS

Common α-Subunit and hCGβ-Subunit

Mutations in the gonadotropin subunit genes appear to be extremely rare, perhaps because of their deleterious effects on reproduction (see Table 1; 26–39). Probably for the same reason, not a single patient with a germline mutation in the common α-subunit gene has been noted. Such mutations would lead to defective hCG, LH, FSH, and TSH function, a condition that would probably be lethal, particularly because of lack of hCG. Nevertheless, α-subunit Knockout mice are viable, though hypogondal and hypothyroid (26), but because this species does not produce chorionic gonadotropin, the gestation regulation may be under differential hormonal control. Only one somatic α-subunit point mutation (Glu56Ala) in the ectopically produced hCG of a carcinoma has been described in the literature (*see* Fig. 1) *(26).* Likewise, no hCGβ mutations have been described. Besides several silent polymorphism in this gene, only one relatively common (4.5% allelic frequency) amino acid-altering point mutation, Val79Met, has been detected in heterozygous form (*see* Fig. 1) *(33).* This mutation hampers α/β dimer formation in vitro and, if present in homozygous form, could block sufficient bioactive hCG synthesis and be lethal. Milder forms of hCG mutations could, if they exist, cause intrauterine undermasculinization of male fetuses because of hCG's crucial role in the stimulation of fetal testicular testosterone synthesis.

Inactivating LHβ *Subunit Mutation*

Only one totally inactivating mutation of the *LHβ* gene has so far been detected *(27)* (Table 1). The proband was a male who presented with delayed puberty at the age of 17 yr and had a family history of male infertility on the father's side, but none on the mother's side. His serum testosterone level was low and immunoreactive LH was high. A normal serum testosterone response was found on challenge with exogenous hCG, but in vitro bioassay of serum LH revealed no activity. These findings, together with a family history of consanguinity, suggested an inherited defect in the LH structure, maintaining its immunoreactivity but abolishing bioactivity. After 2 yr of testosterone treatment, there was no evidence for spontaneous puberty after treatment was withdrawn. Testicular biopsy revealed arrested spermatogenesis and absent Leydig cells. Long-term hCG treatment resulted in testicular enlargement, normal virilization, and spermatogenesis.

Sequencing of the patient's *LHβ subunit* gene revealed a homozygous A-to-G missense mutation in codon 54, causing a glutamine (Gl) to arginine (Arg) substitution. The proband's mother, sister, and three uncles were heterozygotes for the same mutation. A gene conversion within the *CGβ/LHβ* gene cluster was excluded, which indicated that the alteration in *LHβ* structure represented a spontaneous germ line mutation. When the mutated *LHβ* was coexpressed with normal α-*subunit* in CHO cells, immunoreactive LH α/β heterodimers were formed, but they displayed no activity in a radioreceptor assay, i.e., the mutated hormone was devoid of biological activity because of its inability to bind to LH-R. The heterozygous family members, as expected, had reduced ratio of bioactivity/immunoreactivity of their serum LH, because half of this protein was encoded by the mutated gene.

This rare case clarifies some points about pituitary LH's developmental role. Because the affected man was apparently normally masculinized at birth and had descended testes, pituitary LH is not needed for the stimulation of testicular testosterone or INSL-3 production *in utero.* Indeed, fetal testicular testosterone production is initiated seemingly autonomously but becomes subsequently dependent on placental hCG *(15,41),* and fetal pituitary LH plays a minimal role *in utero.* However, the endocrine function of the postnatal testes is critically dependent on pituitary LH, as was demonstrated by the total absence of mature Leydig cells and spontaneous puberty in this patient who was lacking bioactive LH. It is intriguing that the prevalence of infertility was increased in heterozygous male family members, despite normal pubertal masculinization. Inasmuch as the proband's father was an obligate heterozygote, however, the importance of the heterozygosity for testicular function remains uncertain.

The heterozygous women, including the proband's mother, were asymptomatic. It is curious that no other human subjects homozygous for this type of mutation have been subsequently detected, and, although the phenotype of the single patient is in harmony with our knowledge of the ontogeny of LH action, some caution must be exercised when drawing conclusions on the basis of a single patient. The female phenotype would probably resemble those with inactivating *LH-R* mutation (see section on LH-R mutations). Comparison of these two conditions would elucidate the role of intrauterine LH/hCG action, if any, in ovarian development and function.

LHβ *Polymorphisms*

Several polymorphisms have been detected in the *LHβ* gene (*see* Table 1), and their occurrence has been studied in relation to various phenotypic signs of male and female gonadal dysfunction, including hypogonadism and infertility *(9,42)*. We review here the findings that are suggestive of the influence of these polymorphisms on testicular function.

Of particular interest is the Trp8Arg/Ile15Asn polymorphism resulting from two point mutations that are in linkage disequilibrium *(28–30)*. It is common in all populations, with considerable ethnic variability in carrier frequency, from 0% in the south of India to 53.5% in aboriginal Australians *(43)*. It was originally detected as an immunologically anomalous form of LH in a woman with normal reproductive function but undetectable LH, using a specific combination of monoclonal antibodies for detection of immunoreactive LH *(44)*. This variant (V) form of LH displays increased bioactivity in vitro but has a shortened circulating half-life *(45,46)*, and most of the studies on its clinical correlations indicate that it is a functionally less active form of LH when compared to the WT hormone. Besides the two point mutations in the coding region, there are eight additional point mutations in the promoter region of the *V-LHβ* allele, and they increase the transcriptional activity of the variant promoter by approx 50%, which may be a compensatory alteration to counteract the decreased half-life of the variant hormone *(47)*.

V-LH has been correlated with several clinical conditions related to LH action (reviewed in *9,42*). In women, it has mild, although statistically significant, effects on fertility, ovarian steroidogenesis, occurrence of certain types of polycystic ovarian syndrome, and breast cancer occurrence. In the male, three findings in particular are worthy of comment. When pubertal progression was compared in WT boys and heterozygotes for *V-LHβ*, there was no difference in the age of onset of puberty, which is mainly determined by the reawakening of hypothalamic gonadotropin-releasing hormone (GnRH) secretion. Instead, the tempo of pubertal progression was significantly slower in boys who were heterozygous for the V-LHβ allele *(48)*. When its occurrence was studied in cryptorchidism, the allele frequency in cryptorchid and healthy boys was similar, but when the frequency in cryptorchid boys was correlated with gestation duration, it increased significantly with increasing gestation duration, from 6% in boys born before week 30 to 45% in boys born beyond week 42 of pregnancy *(49)*. The final phase of testicular descent, from the inguinal region to the scrotum, depends on the testicular testosterone production in late gestation. The tropic stimulus for this activity is provided by the combined action of hCG and pituitary LH, and when the duration of pregnancy is prolonged, the pituitary LH role becomes more important. If this hormone is less active, as V-LH is then testosterone production may be compromised, predisposing to cryptorchidism in boys carrying the *V-LHβ* allele who are the products of post-term pregnancy. Finally, V-LH is more prevalent in older men who are obese and have low testosterone levels *(50)*. These findings, together with those in women, indicate that V-LH represents a clinically meaningful genetic variant of the hormone with milder overall gonadotropic action in vivo. Finally, the clinician must be aware of its occurrence, because some immunoassay kits for LH are unable to detect V-LH, which may explain unexpectedly low LH levels.

FSHβ *Subunit*

Only four women and three men with a total of four different inactivating mutations of the *FSHβ* gene have so far been described in the literature *(34–38,51)* (Table 1). All four women had similar phenotypes, with slightly variable severity, including sexual infantilism, lack of follicular development, and infertility, which are readily explained by the lack of FSH action on granulosa cell estrogen production and progression of follicular maturation beyond the early stages. The phenotypes of the three men with *FSHβ* mutation *(35,37,38,52)*, are discussed in the section on FSH-R mutations in more detail because they present a conundrum when compared with all other findings concerning the phenotypic effects of inactivation of FSH action in men and male experimental animals.

Of the reports of the three men with inactivating *FSHβ* Mutations, the one from Sweden described a 32-yr-old man of Serbian origin who presented with azoospermia, normal puberty and male physical characteristics, and a selective FSH absence *(37,52)*. His serum testosterone level was low normal (11 nmol/L) and LH was slightly elevated (12 IU/L). These findings may result from the small size of his testes (3mL/6mL) and the missing FSH effect on their growth at puberty.

Genetic analysis demonstrated a homozygous T to C mutation, predicting a Cys82Arg substitution in the FSHβ protein. It was postulated that the elimination of a cysteine would impair formation of the proper intramolecular disulphide bond of FSHβ. This would result in abnormal tertiary structure during FSHβ synthesis, with extensive intracellular degradation, inability to dimerize with the α-subunit, defective glycosylation, and, finally, inability to form biologically active hormone.

The second male, reported from Israel *(35)*, was an 18-yr-old with slight delay of puberty, small testes, azoospermia, and a plasma FSH concentration below 0.5 IU/L. Total testosterone was low (4.5 nmol/L), and LH was increased (24.5 IU/L), indicating a defect in testosterone biosysthesis. DNA sequencing revealed the same homozygous 2 bp deletion in codon 61 that was found previously in the female patients *(34,36,38)*. The mutation gave rise to a completely altered amino acid sequence between codons 61 and 86 of the FSHβ chain, which was followed by a premature stop codon, and lack of translation of amino acids 87 to 111. Consequently, the translated FSHβ protein was truncated and unable to associate with common β-subunit to form bioactive or immunoreactive α/β dimers.

The third man with inactivating FSHβ mutation, described from Brazil *(45)*, had had normal puberty but presented with infertility resulting from azoospermia. His serum testosterone at the age of 30 yr was normal (26 nmol/L), FSH was low, and LH was elevated. His testes were small (12 mL), and testicular biopsy revealed Leydig cell hyperplasia (LCH) and sparse, small seminiferous tubules with germinal cell aplasia, peritubular fibrosis, and few Sertoli cells. The C to A mutation in codon 76 of his *FSHβ* gene brought about a premature stop codon (TAA). Because the phenotype of the female patient reported with this mutation was less severe than those of women with the other *FSHβ* mutations *(41,43)*, it was hypothesized that the missing amino acids 76–110 of FSHβ may not bring about complete inactivation of FSH action *(45)*.

Table 1
List of Currently Known Mutations and Polymorphisms in Human Glycoprotein Hormone Subunit Genes

Gene	Location	Type	Nucleotide change	Amino acid change	Symptoms inpatient(s)*	Functional effect	Reference
Common α	Exon 3	Missense	$CA^{239}G \rightarrow CCG$	$Glu^{56} \rightarrow Ala$	Carcinoma	No association with β-subunit	26
LHβ	Exon 3	Missense	$CA^{221}G \rightarrow CGG$	$Gln^{54} \rightarrow Arg$	*Infertility, delayed puberty*	No binding to receptor	27
LHβ	Exon 2	2 missense mutations }	$T^{82}GG \rightarrow CGG$ $AT^{104}C \rightarrow ACC$	$Trp^{8} \rightarrow Arg$ $Ile^{15} \rightarrow Th$ }	Slightly supressed fertility Association with PCOS? *Delayed tempo of puberty*	Increased in vitro bioactivity Short half	28–30
LHβ	Exon 3	Missense	$A^{1502}GT \rightarrow GGT$	$Ser^{102} \rightarrow Gly$	Infertility	Not detected	31
LHβ	Exon 3	Missense	$G^{52}CA \rightarrow ACA$	$Ala^{-3} \rightarrow Thr$	Not studied	Slight decrease in signal transduction activity	32
hCGβ	Exon 3	Missense	$G^{295}TG \rightarrow ATG$	$Val^{79}Met$	Not studied	Insufficient assembly with α-subunit	33
FSHβ	Exon 3	2-bp deletion	$GTG \rightarrow GX^{236,237}$	$Val^{61} \rightarrow STOP^{87}$	Prim. amenorrhea, infertility *Azoospermia*	Truncated protein	34, 35
FSHβ	Exon 3	Missense	$T^{206}GT \rightarrow GGT$	$Cys^{51} \rightarrow Gly$	Prim. amenorrhea, infertility	Faulty tertiary structure of protein	36
FSHβ	Exon 3	Missense	$T^{298}GT \rightarrow CGT$	$Cys^{82} \rightarrow Arg$	*Azoospermia*	Faulty tertiary structure of protein	37
FSHβ	Exon 3	Nonsense	$TAC^{282} \rightarrow TAA$	$Tyr^{76} \rightarrow STOP^{87}$	Prim. amenorrhea, infertility *Azoospermia*	Loss of bioactivity	38
FSHβ	Exon 3	Silent	$TAT^{228} \rightarrow TAC$	No change (Tyr)	High FSH, association with PCOS?	Not detected	39

The nucleotide number was counted according to the translation start site (40), the intronic sequences are excluded.

*Findings on male subjects in *italic*.

Conspicuously, all three men with the *FSHβ* mutation were azoospermic. As elaborated in the section on FSH-R mutations, this is not the case with the five men reported to carry homozygous inactivating mutations in the *FSH-R* gene *(53)*. They each displayed variable suppression of spermatogenesis but were not azoospermic. Neither were the KO mice for *FSHβ (54)* or *FSH-R (55,56)* azoospermic, and, moreover, the phenotypes of women with inactivating *FSHβ* and *FSH-R* mutation were practically identical *(34,36,38,57)*. The more severe phenotype of the ligand mutation in men is curious also for the reason that animal data show the opposite *(58)*, most likely because of the slight constitutive activity of FSHR in the absence of ligand. Why then are the three men with *FSHβ* mutation azoospermic? This is discussed next in more detail in connection with *FSH-R* mutations.

GONADOTROPIN RECEPTOR MUTATIONS

Gonadotropin receptor mutations are also quite rare. There are both activating and inactivating mutations in these genes, with widely varying phenotypic effects. Activating receptor mutations can be classified into four categories: (1) receptor activation in the absence of ligand hormone; (2) increased sensitivity of the receptor to its normal ligand; (3) relaxed specificity of the receptor to ligands; and (4) acquired novel functions of the mutated receptor. All activating gonadotropin receptor mutations detected have been missense point mutations that are localized to the transmembrane region or its vicinity (*see* Figs. 2 and 3). These mutations produce a structural alteration, activating constitutively the signal transduction machinery of the transmembrane region. Most clearly, receptor activation without ligand explains the altered function of these mutations. Abnormal phenotypes occur in heterozygous individuals because activation of the translation product of a single allele is sufficient to initiate the altered functional response.

Several mechanisms can also underlie receptor inactivation: (1) decreased synthesis of receptor protein; (2) aberrant intracellular processing; (3) reduced or absent ligand-binding activity; (4) impaired or absent signal transduction; (5) inability to anchor to the plasma membrane; (6) inability to dimerize, if needed, for signal transduction; or (7) increased degradation. Unlike the activating mutations, the types of inactivating mutations vary from point nonsense and missense mutations to various size insertions and deletions. In this case, only homozygotes or compound heterozygotes for two different inactivating mutations produce a clear phenotype because the normal function of a single receptor allele supplies a sufficient number of functional receptors to sustain normal gonadotropin action.

LH-R Mutations

INACTIVATING MUTATIONS

In the human male, LH-R function is essential at all ages for testicular androgen production. Therefore, these mutations influence male sexual differentiation, development, and mature functions from the fetal period through adulthood. The inactivating *LH-R* mutations vary in completeness, and the phenotype of affected males depends on the extent of receptor inactivation *(9,59,60)*. In the mildest forms, the phenotype is hypospadias and/or micropenis, and in the completely inactivating form, the male phenotype is complete sex reversal, i.e., pseudohermaphroditism *(9)*. The latter group presents with total lack of male type sexual differentiation *in utero* or postnatal development. The phenotype resembles the complete form of androgen insensitivity syndrome but notably differs by the lack of pubertal breast development, which, in androgen insensitivity, is explained by the increased conversion of testosterone to estradiol. On histological examination, the testes of the individuals with complete LH-R inactivation are totally devoid of Leydig cells, which explains the lack of testosterone production and absent masculinization. However, it is apparent that even on complete LH-R inactivation, some testicular steroidogenesis is possible, because epididymides and vasa deferentia are present *(9)*. The explanation for these structures may be low, but functionally sufficient, constitutive steroidogenesis in precursor Leydig cells. This has also been shown with LH-R knockout mice that have a low, but detectable, basal level of steroidogenesis in their testes *(61)*.

In women, LH-R inactivation causes a milder phenotype with normal intrauterine female sex differentiation and a seemingly normal FSH-dependent component of ovarian function *(9)*. Affected women present with primary amenorrhea and normal primary and secondary sex characteristics, increased gonadotropin levels, and a lack of ovarian response to hCG treatment. Histological study of ovarian tissue revealed all stages of follicular development, with the exception of preovulatory follicles and corpora lutea *(62)*. These observations emphasize the importance of LH for ovulation and formation of corpora lutea. LH may also be needed for the maturation of antral to preovulatory follicles *(61)*.

ACTIVATING MUTATIONS

The first gonadotropin receptor mutations detected were those activating constitutively the *LH-R (63,64)*, perhaps because of their striking phenotype. The syndrome caused by this mutation, i.e., familial male-limited precocious puberty (FMPP), is a gonadotropin-independent form of precocious puberty, also called testotoxicosis. Boys with FMPP begin to exhibit signs and symptoms of puberty between 1 and 3 yr of age. If they remain untreated, puberty progresses rapidly, resulting in premature epiphysial closure and compromised adult height. The syndrome has been know for a long time and was originally assumed to result from a circulating nongonadotropic factor that induces premature LH-independent activation of Leydig cell function. However, the subsequent detection of point mutations in the *LH-R* gene, which, in transfection studies, caused constitutive activation of the LH signaling pathway in the absence of ligand, provided a logical molecular pathogenesis of FMPP. Today, more than 10 activating mutations of the *LH-R* gene are known (*see* Fig. 2), and they all are localized in or near the transmembrane region of the LHR, which is pivotal for LH signal transduction. The mutations change the conformation of the transmembrane region of the receptor so that it assumes, at least partially, an activated conformation in ligand absence. The consequence is premature activation of Leydig cell testosterone production before the pubertal onset of LH secretion. In cell transfections, the mutated receptor protein usually displays an approx 10-fold increase in basal cAMP production, whereas maximal stimulation is often suppressed. The latter alteration has no physiological importance, because at the circulating levels of LH, receptor occupancy remains relatively low. Whether other signalling pathways that are initiated by LH-R activation are activated to a similar extent has not been systematically studied.

Despite the distinct phenotype in males, no phenotype is known for females with activating LH-R mutation. One explanation is that the LH action initiation in the ovary requires FSH priming, and FSH-dependent paracrine factors may be needed to induce theca cell LH-R responsiveness. Because there is little FSH secretion in these women before the normal age of puberty, the constitutively activated LH-R would not be expected to be prematurely functional. The lack of LH-R in prepubertal granulosa cells is evident, because this receptor is acquired during the later stages of follicular maturation. Therefore, the presence of an activating mutation in the *LH-R* is functionally unimportant if the gene is not expressed before the age of normal puberty.

A novel phenotype of activating *LH-R* mutations associated with Leydig cell tumors (LCTs) was described recently in three unrelated boys with isosexual precocious puberty without a family history of this condition *(65)*. Besides the symptoms and findings of FMPP, unilateral testicular mass was found by ultrasonography in all boys. In each case, well-circumscribed tumors were removed that were composed of nested polygonal cells with abundant eosinophilic cytoplasm and round ovoid nuclei. Mitotic activity was low and Reincke's crystals were absent. Genomic DNA was extracted from the tumor tissues and peripheral blood leucocytes, and the sequence-encoding exon 11 of the LH-R was amplified. The tumor tissues, but not leucocytes, contained a heterozygous somatic mutation encoding an Asp578His replacement in LHR *(65)*. When the mutated receptor was transfected into COS-7 cells, it was found to initiate constitutive activation of cAMP production in ligand absence (*see* Fig. 4). In addition, inositol phosphate production was constitutively activated, a response that has not been made with other activating *LH-R* mutations. Besides the tumor phenotype, these subjects differ from FMPP because their *LH-R* mutations were somatic. This particular mutation has not been detected in the germ-line. Two further reports with similar phenotype and causative *LH-R* mutation have also been published *(66,67)*. It remains to be determined whether this mutation is the only one that causes Leydig cell tumorigenesis.

Another report described nodular LCH in a boy with FMPP, which is not a typical finding in this syndrome *(68)*. The genomic heterozygous Asp564Gly mutation detected in this boy caused only partial activation of cAMP production, and similar Leydig cell alterations were not found in other patients affected with the same mutation. Therefore, the mechanism of the nodular hyperplasia appears to differ from that in the three cases presented here.

A third type of testicular tumor that has occurred in one 36-yr-old patient with FMPP due to a germ-line Asp578Gly mutation is testicular seminoma *(69)*. Although no causative relationship was established for the *LH-R* mutation and seminoma, the possibility remains that a prolonged high intratesticular testosterone concentration resulting from LH-R stimulation could be oncogenic. However, transgenic (TG) mice that overexpressed hCG and produced high intratesticular testosterone levels showed no signs of testicular tumors beyond mild LCH (S. Rulli, M. Poutanen, & I. Huhtaniemi, unpublished data).

The situation with activating LH-R mutations and testicular tumors is somewhat analogous to familial nonimmunogenic hyperthyroidism and sporadic thyroid adenomas caused by germ-line and somatic mutations of the *TSH-R* gene, respectively *(70,71)*. As in these thyroid disorders, the somatic LH-R mutations brought about greater constitutive activity of the receptor than do germ-line mutations. The severe forms would probably be eliminated from the genetic pool because of their strong deleterious effects. The mutation detected occurred in a position where three other amino acid-substituting mutations have been detected in Asp578 to Tyr/Glu/Gly (9)

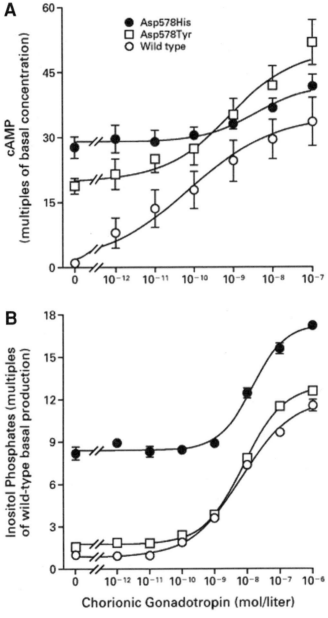

Fig. 4. Comparison of luteinizing hormone receptor (LH-R) cell signaling by the activating Asp578His or Asp578Tyr mutations and the wild-type (WT) LH-R. Mean basal and human chorionic gonadotropin (hCG)-stimulated accumulation of cAMP (panel A) and inositol phosphates (panel B) is shown in COS-7 cells transfected with DNA for the WT LH-R or receptors with the Asp578Tyr or Asp578His mutation. Basal activity of the WT receptor is the same as that of the pSG5 expression vector alone. (From *65*, with permission.)

(*see* Fig. 2). The other forms cause milder receptor activation and, at most, patchy LCH but no tumors. Hence, the high level of basal stimulation of the receptor is important for adenoma formation. Whether high cAMP production alone or additive or synergistic effect of the concomitantly stimulated phospholipase C pathway are involved in tumorigenesis remains to be established. In fact, the analogous mutation in the TSH-R, Asp633His, has been found in a patient presenting with insular thyroid carcinoma with metastases *(72)*.

These data emphasize that the same phenotype may be caused by both benign FMPP and by LCTs. Therefore long-term follow-up with testicular ultrasonography is advised for boys with FMPP to exclude Leydig cell adenoma. Genetic analysis of the *LH-R* mutation is also advisable if testicular biopsy material is available. Finally, another genetic cause for LCTs is activating mutation in the stimulatory G protein *(73)*.

FSH-R Mutations

INACTIVATING MUTATIONS

Several inactivating mutations have been detected in the *FSH-R* gene, most of them in women with hypergonadotropic hypogonadism (9) (*see* Fig. 3). The complete form of *FSH-R* mutation in women causes the total arrest of follicular development *(57)*, a process which is dependent on FSH action. The incomplete forms cause a partial phenotype that is responsive to high-dose gonadotropin treatment *(74,75)*. In addition to the Finnish-type FSHR inactivation (C → T transition, causing Ala189Val mutation), which has been found in multiple families *(57)*, all other FSH-R mutations detected have been sporadic *(9,74–77)*.

Five men with totally inactivating mutation of *FSH-R* have been described from Finland *(53)*. These men were identified because they were homozygous brothers of women with hypergonadotropic hypogonadism caused by *FSH-R* mutation. The men were normally masculinized, with normal puberty and virilization. Their testes were mildly or severely reduced in size, and all had pathological semen samples, although, conspicuously, none was azoospermic (Table 2). Moreover, two of the men each had fathered two children. As expected, the men had high FSH levels, low inhibin-B, normal or slightly elevated LH, but normal testosterone concentrations *(53)*. Both testicular sizes and the endocrine parameters of the five men displayed considerable variability. Besides the large age range of the subjects (29–55 yr), this may reflect the individual variability in the importance of FSH in maintaining testicular function. More detailed conclusions are limited by the small sample size. These findings were rather surprising because of the concept of a fundamental role for FSH in spermatogenesis, particularly the pubertal initiation of this process. Findings in these men demonstrated that FSH action *per se* is not necessary for qualitatively complete spermatogenesis. However, FSH is needed for qualitatively and quantitatively normal spermatogenesis but not necessarily for fertility. Subsequent experiments in mice in which *FSH-R* or *FSHβ* gene expression was disrupted produced similar results *(54–56);* the animals were fertile, but their testes were reduced in size and their spermatogenesis was qualitatively and quantitatively suppressed. The mild phenotype of the men with *FSH-R* mutation indicated that they cannot be readily distinguished phenotypically from other men with idiopathic oligozoospermia. In fact, when this was studied in a region with high allelic frequency (1%, northern Finland) for the

Table 2
Semen Analyses and Some Hormone Levels on Men Homozygous for the Inactivatin Ala189Val FSHR Mutation

Subject	Age (Yr)	Fertility	Testis size ml (right/left)	Sperm analysis sperm count/mL	vol. mL	(at age)	FSH (IU/L)	LH (IU/L)	Testosterone (nmol/L)	Inhibin B (ng/L)
1	47	Two children	16.5/ 16.5	5 x 10⁶	3.0	(47)	12.5	5.6	8.8	<15
2	55	Two children	13.5 / 15.8	< 0.1 x 10⁶	3.3	(55)	15.1	4.2	15.8	33
3	45	infertile	4.0 / 4.0	< 0.1 x 10⁶	4.8	(30)	23.5	16.3	14.5	62
4	29	unknown	8.6 / 6.0	42 x 10⁶	1.5	(29)	39.6	11.1	14.7	54
5	42	unknown	8.0 / 8.0	< 1.0 x 10⁶	2.5	(42)	20.6	16.2	26.2	53
Reference range				> 20 x 10⁶			1–10.5	1–8.4	8.2–34.6	76–447

From ref. 53.

inactivating *FSH-R* mutation, the frequency of the mutation was the same in a cohort of men with idiopathic oligozoospermia and in normal controls *(53)*. There was no apparent disturbance in pubertal development in these individuals. The sperm quality in the five men was highest in the youngest individual suggesting that the spermatogenic capacity in the absence of FSH action may be compromised—these men may be fertile only as young adults.

The discrepancy between the azoospermia of the three men with *FSHβ* mutation (see above) and the oligoasthenozoospermia, but not azoospermia, in the men with *FSH-R* mutation is puzzling. One explanation is that azoospermia is the real phenotype of total elimination of FSH action, and the receptor mutation described is only partial, with partial inactivation of FSH action that does not totally impede spermatogenesis. All evidence collected thus for about the inactivating Ala189Val *FSH-R* mutation shows, however, that it is near-totally inactivating because of the sequestration of the mutant receptor inside the cell *(78)*. A minute fraction of the mutated receptor may reach the cell surface but is unable to mediate the signal properly even at high FSH levels. Cells transfected with the mutated *FSH-R* gene are devoid of the basal constitutive adenylyl cyclase activity that can be displayed in cells transfected with WT *FSH-R (53)*. Likewise, women with this mutation are totally resistant to FSH treatment *(79)*. A second explanation is that oligozoospermia is the true phenotype of FSH deficiency, and the two subjects with inactivating *FSHβ* mutation have a second disturbance in the regulation of spermatogenesis predisposing to azoospermia. This is quite likely because spermatogenesis is a process that is regulated by a complex network of endocrine, paracrine, and autocrine mechanisms. Two key players in this process with paramount importance are testosterone and FSH. The importance of FSH may be relative; if all other factors function properly, FSH is not vital, and, therefore, men with *FSH-R* mutation have complete spermatogenesis. If, on the other hand, there is a failure in some other mechanism, then the function of FSH becomes critical. The Israeli patient *(35)* with *FSHβ* mutation had an additional failure in testosterone production that might explain the critical role of loss of FSH function. The Swedish patient was treated for extended periods of time with FSH, but there was no spermatogenic response *(52)*. It is possible in his case that key paracrine mechanisms had failed and FSH replacement could not compensate for those deficiencies. Furthermore, these two patients were studied because of azoospermia, whereas the *FSH-R* mutation patients were detected because they were the brothers of women homozygous for this mutation. Hence, the outcome of genotype/phenotype correlations partly depends on which end of the cascade the search is initiated.

In conclusion, the majority of information available implies that FSH action *per se* is not mandatory for the pubertal initiation of spermatogenesis or for male fertility. However, FSH improves spermatogenesis both qualitatively and quantitatively. The phenotype of men with defective FSH-R function varies from severe to mild impairment of spermatogenesis, in the face of apparently normal Leydig cell androgen production. The azoospermia of men with *FSHβ* mutation may result from additional contributing factors and not solely to FSH deficiency. However, it is apparent that additional cases of genetically proven FSH deficiency are needed before the existing discrepancy between the phenotypes of the ligand and receptor deficiency can be reconciled. At the moment, it may be useful to state that treatment of men with FSH, who have idiopathic oligozoospermia and normal to elevated FSH concentrations, has no scientific basis and that prospects for developing a male contraceptive method based on inhibition of FSH secretion or action are not promising.

ACTIVATING MUTATION

There is one somewhat controversial report of a man with an activating mutation of the *FSH-R* gene *(80)*. The patient previously underwent hypophysectomy and radiotherapy because of a pituitary tumor, and, despite panhypopituitarism and unmeasurable serum gonadotropin levels, he displayed persistent spermatogenesis during testosterone treatment. Detailed studies of this patient were undertaken because androgen treatment is usually not sufficient to maintain spermatogenesis in the absence of gonadotropins. A heterozygous Asp567Gly mutation was found in the third intracellular domain of exon 10 of his *FSH-R* gene *(see* Fig. 3), and it was shown in vitro to have marginal constitutive activity. Because the WT FSH-R has a considerable constitutive activity without ligand in such cell line transfection studies *(53)*, the marginal elevation of cAMP production in the presence of the *FSH-R* mutation must be interpreted with caution. Moreover, the patient's serum testosterone level was 5 nmol/L 3–4 mo after discontinuing testosterone replacement, a value fivefold to eightfold higher than in bilaterally orchidectomized men. Thus, his phenotype may not represent solely the effect of FSH alone on spermatogenesis or androgen synthesis in the absence of LH stimulation. In my view, a fair conclusion at this point is that undisputed information about the phenotype of an activating *FSH-R* mutation in man is not yet available. Such mutations are possible, however, as has been shown with site-directed mutagenesis *(81)*, but whether they cause a phenotype in vivo has not yet been resolved. A search for *FSH-R* mutations in candidate diseases, such as premature ovarian failure, ovarian tumors, megalotestes, precocious puberty, and twin pregnancies, has yielded negative results *(82–86)*. It also remains possible that activating *FSH-R* mutation has no abnormal phenotype, or that it differs totally from our educated guesses. An animal model would be seminal in resolving this intriguing question.

Gonadotropin Receptor Polymorphisms

Several polymorphisms have been detected in the gonadotropin receptor genes *(see* Figs. 2 and 3), but relatively little is known thus far about their functional correlates. The polymorphisms Thr307/Asn680 and Ala307/Ser680 in the FSHR gene are in linkage disequilibrium in some populations, and the frequency of both alleles is nearly equal, at least in whites *(87)*. It was recently reported from Germany that in women undergoing ovulation induction, the basal FSH concentration of the Asn/Asn genotype (6.4 ± 0.4 IU/L) was significantly lower than that of the Ser/Ser genotype (8.3 ± 0.6 U/L), and that the latter group required approx 50% more exogenous FSH to stimulate follicular growth *(87)*. However, this finding was recently disputed by the same authors when a larger group of anovulatory women from Germany and the Netherlands was studied, although the Ser/Ser patients again displayed higher basal FSH levels than did the Asn/Asn or Asn/Ser variants *(88)*. Likewise, no correlation was found between the *FSH-R* genotype and spermatogenesis in the original publication. Hence, the role of this polymorphism in gonadal function, if any, remains uncertain.

A recent study examined the relationship of known LH-R polymorphisms with male undermasculinization *(89)*. It was found that the polymorphism-encoding insertion of leucine and glutamine between codons 8 and 9 of the LH-R protein was significantly associated with those undermasculinized individuals that had a long polymorphic polyglutamine repeat (>26) in their androgen receptor, which is associated with suppressed androgen receptor activity *(90)*. Also, two single nucleotide polymorphisms of the *LH-R,* both altering the amino acid sequence (Asp291er and Asp312Ser), were found both alone and in combination to be associated with undermasculization.

Inconsistent findings on the phenotypic effects of polymorphisms are not unusual. For example, inconsistencies were observed when the frequency of the common LH polymorphism (see the section on LHβ Polymorphisms) was studied in women with polycystic ovary syndrome; the frequency and correlation with the syndrome varied according to ethnicity of the patient cohorts *(91)*. This is understandable because the phenotypic effects of mild alterations of function of gene products, such as the polymorphisms depend on the genetic background and combined effects of other genes, and, therefore, the phenotypic expression may differ between populations. Overall, the studies on phenotypic effects of the polymorphisms in gonadotropin and gonadotropin receptor genes are still in their infancy and more information about their potential effects on the individual variability in pituitary–gonadal function will undoubtedly be obtained in the future.

CONCLUDING REMARKS

No germ-line mutations of the glycoprotein hormone *common α-subunit* have been reported, apparently because of the dramatic phenotypic effects they would have (possibly embryo lethality). One inactivating *LHβ* mutation has been described in a man with normal prenatal masculinization but arrested pubertal development. Additional cases are needed before final conclusions about the phenotypic effect of missing LH action can be drawn. A common polymorphism exists in the *LHβ* subunit. It affects bioactivity of the hormone and has multiple mild phenotypic effects, including slow tempo of puberty in boys. It may be a contributing factor to the heterogeneous pace of pubertal development. It is also enriched in postterm boys with cryptorchidism. The three men so far described with *FSHβ* mutation were azoospermic, but additional patients are needed to confirm the phenotype, particularly because this phenotype conflicts with the findings in FSH-R inactivation.

Constitutively activating mutations of the *LH-R* gene give rise to FMPP. Inactivating *LH-R* mutation results in an array of male phenotypes ranging from micropenis and hypospadias to complete sex reversal (XY, pseudohermaphroditism), depending on the completeness of inactivation of the receptor. Inactivating *FSHR* mutations in men cause a decrease of testicular size and suppressed quality and quantity of spermatogenesis but not azoospermia. Some affected men may be fertile. FSH inactivation is unlikely to affect pubertal maturation. No unequivocally activating mutations of the *FSHR* have yet been described in either sex. Studies on candidate syndromes (e.g., precocious puberty and macro-orchia) have yielded negative results.

The discrepancy between the phenotypes of men with inactivating *FSH β-subunit* (azoospermia) and *FSH-R* (no azoospermia) mutations must be clarified with additional subjects. The male and female phenotypes of activating *FSH-R* mutation must be established. In addition, the phenotypic effects, if any, of the number of common polymorphisms detected in genes of the gonadotropin subunits and their receptors must be explored in more detail.

REFERENCES

1. Morgan FJ, Kammerman S, Canfield RE. Chemistry of human chorionic gonadotropin. In: Greep RO, Astwood EA, eds. Handbook of Physiology, Vol. II, Female Reproductive System, Part 2. American Physiology Society Edition, Washington, DC, 1973, pp. 311–322.
2. Sairam MR, Parkoff H. Chemistry of pituitary gonadotropins. In: Greep RO, Astwood EA, eds. Handbook of Physiology, Vol. IV. The Pituitary Gland and Its Neuroendocrine Control, Part 2. American Physiology Society Edition, Washington, DC, 1973, pp. 111–131.
3. Fiete D, Srivastava V, Hindsgaul O, Baenziger JU. A hepatic reticuloendothelial cell receptor specific for SO4-4GalNAc beta 1,4GlcNAc beta 1,2Man alpha that mediates rapid clearance of lutropin. Cell 1991;67:1103–1110.
4. Bo M, Boime I. Identification of the transcriptionally active genes of the chorionic gonadotropin beta gene cluster in vivo. J Biol Chem 1992;267:3179–3184.
5. Bousfield GR, Perry WM, Ward DN. Gonadotropins. Chemistry and biosynthesis. In: Knobil E, Neill JD, eds. The Physiology of Reproduction, 2nd ed. New York Raven Press, 1994, pp. 1749–1792.
6. Lapthorn AJ, Harris DC, Littlejohn A, et al. Crystal structure of human chorionic gonadotropin. Nature 1994;369:455–461.
7. Fox KM, Dias JA, Van Royen P. Three-dimensional structure of human follicle-stimulating hormone. Mol Endocrinol 2001;5:378–389.
8. Simoni M, Gromoll J, Nieschlag E. The follicle-stimulating hormone receptor: biochemistry, molecular biology, physiology, and pathophysiology. Endocr Rev 1997;18:739–773.
9. Themmen APN, Huhtaniemi IT. Mutations of gonadotropins and gonadotropin receptors: elucidating the physiology and pathophysiology of pituitary-gonadal function. Endocr Rev 2000;21:551–583.
10. Ascoli M, Fanelli F, Segaloff DL. The lutropin/choriogonadotropin receptor, a 2002 perspective. Endocr Rev 2002;23:141–174.
11. Rousseau-Merck MF, Misrahi M, Atger M, Loosfelt H, Milgrom E, Berger R. Localization of the human luteinizing hormone/choriogonadotropin receptor gene (LHCGR) to chromosome 2p21. Cytogenet Cell Genet 1990;54:77–79.
12. Rousseau-Merck MF, Atger M, Loosfelt H, Milgrom E, Berger R. The chromosomal localization of the human follicle-stimulating hormone receptor gene (FSHR) on 2p21-p16 is similar to that of the luteinizing hormone receptor gene. Genomics 1993;15:222–224.
13. Gromoll J, Eiholzer U, Nieschlag E, Simoni M. Male hypogonadism caused by homozygous deletion of exon 10 of the luteinizing hormone (LH) receptor: differential action between human chorionic gonadotropin and LH. J Clin Endocrinol Metab 2000;85:2281–2286.
14. Herrlich A, Kuhn B, Grosse R, Schmid A, Schultz G, Gudermann T. Involvement of Gs and Gi proteins in dual coupling of the luteinizing hormone receptor to adenylyl cyclase and phospholipase C. J Biol Chem 1996;271:16764–16772.
15. Huhtaniemi I. Fetal testis—a very special endocrine organ. Eur J Endocrinol 1994;130:25–31.
16. Teixeira J, Maheswaran S, Donahoe PK. Mullerian inhibiting substance: an instructive developmental hormone with diagnostic and possible therapeutic applications. Endocr Rev 2001;22:657–674.
17. Adham IM, Emmen JM, Engel W. The role of the testicular factor INSL3 in establishing the gonadal position. Mol Cell Endocrinol 2000;160:11–16.
18. Huhtaniemi IT, Yamamoto M, Ranta T, Jalkanen J, Jaffe RB. Follicle-stimulating hormone receptors appear earlier in the primate fetal testis than in the ovary. J Clin Endocrinol Metab 1987;65:1210–1214.
19. Orth JM. The role of follicle-stimulating hormone in controlling Sertoli cell proliferation in testes of fetal rats. Endocrinology 1984;115:1248–1255.
20. Kaplan SL, Grumbach MM, Aubert ML. The ontogenesis of pituitary hormones and hypothalamic factors in the human fetus: maturation of central nervous system regulation of anterior pituitary function. Recent Prog Horm Res 1976;32:161–243.
21. Forest MG, De Peretti E, Bertrand J. Hypothalamic-pituitary-gonadal relationships in man from birth to puberty. Clin Endocr (Oxf) 1976;5:551–569.
22. Wu FCW, Butler GE, Kelnar CJH, Stirling HF, Huhtaniemi I. Patterns of pulsatile luteinizing hormone and follicle-stimulating hormone secretion in prepubertal (midchildhood) boys and girls and patients with idiopathic hypogonadotropic hypogonadism (Kallmann's syndrome): a study using an ultrasensitive time-resolved immunofluorometric assay. J Clin Endocrinol Metab 1991;72:1229–1237.
23. Raivio T, Toppari J, Perheentupa A, McNeilly AS, Dunkel L. Treatment of prepubertal gonadotrophin-deficient boys with recombinant human follicle-stimulating hormone. Lancet 1997;350:263–264.

24. Plant TM, Marshall GR. The functional significance of FSH in spermatogenesis and the control of its secretion in male primates. Endocr Rev 2001;22:764–786.
25. Vermeulen A. Andropause. Maturitas 2000;34:5–15.
26. Nishimura R, Shin J, Ji I, et al. A single amino acid substitution in an ectopic alpha subunit of a human carcinoma choriogonadotropin. J Biol Chem 1986;261:10475–10477.
27. Weiss J, Axelrod L, Whitcomb RW, Harris PE, Crowley WF, Jameson JL. Hypogonadism caused by a single amino acid substitution in the beta subunit of luteinizing hormone. N Engl J Med 1992;326:179–183.
28. Pettersson K, Mäkelä MM, Dahlén P, Lamminen T, Huoponen K, Huhtaniemi I. Genetic polymorphism found in the LH beta gene of an immunologically anomalous variant of human luteinizing hormone. Eur J Endocrinol 1994;130 (suppl 2):65.
29. Furui K, Suganuma N, Tsukahara S, et al. Identification of two point mutations in the gene coding luteinizing hormone (LH) beta-subunit, associated with immunologically anomalous LH variants. J Clin Endocrinol Metab 1994;78:107–113.
30. Okuda K, Yamada T, Imoto H, Komatsubara H, Sugimoto O. Antigenic alteration of an anomalous human luteinizing hormone caused by two chorionic gonadotropin-type amino-acid substitutions. Biochem Biophys Res Comm 1994;200:584–590.
31. Liao WX, Roy AC, Chan C, Arulkumaran S, Ratnam SS. A new molecular variant of luteinizing hormone associated with female infertility. Fertil Steril 1998;69:102–106.
32. Jiang M, Lamminen T, Pakarinen P, et al. A novel Ala^{-3} Thr mutation in signal peptide of human luteinizing hormone beta-subunit: potentiation of the inositol phosphate signalling pathway and attenuation of the adenylate cyclase pathway by recombinant variant hormone. Mol Hum Reprod 2002;8:201–212.
33. Miller-Lindholm AK, Bedows E, Bartels CF, Ramey J, Maclin V, Ruddon RW. A naturally occurring genetic variant in the human chorionic gonadotropin-beta gene 5 is assembly inefficient. Endocrinology 1999;140:3496–3506.
34. Matthews CH, Borgato S, Beck-Peccoz P, et al. Primary amenorrhea and infertility due to a mutation in the beta-subunit of follicle-stimulating hormone. Nat Genet 1993;5:83–86.
35. Phillip M, Arbelle JE, Segev Y, Parvari R. Male hypogonadism due to a mutation in the gene for the beta-subunit of follicle-stimulating hormone. N Engl J Med 1998;338:1729–1732.
36. Layman LC, Lee EJ, Peak DB, et al. Delayed puberty and hypogonadism caused by mutations in the follicle-stimulating hormone beta-subunit gene. N Engl J Med 1997;337:607–611.
37. Lindstedt G, Nyström E, Matthews C, Ernest I, Janson PO, Chatterjee K. Follitropin (FSH) deficiency in an infertile male due to FSH-beta gene mutation. A syndrome of normal puberty and virilization but underdeveloped testicles with azoospermia, low FSH but high lutropin and normal serum testosterone concentrations. Clin Chem Lab Med 1998;36:663–665.
38. Layman LC, Porto ALA, Xie J, et al. FSHβ gene mutations in a female with partial breast development and male sibling with normal puberty and azoospermia. J Clin Endocrinol Metab 2002;87:3702–3707.
39. Liao WX, Tong Y, Roy AC, Ng SC. New AccI polymorphism in the follicle-stimulating hormone beta-subunit gene and its prevalence in three Southeast Asian populations. Hum Hered 1999;49:181–182.
40. Kendall SK, Samuelson LC, Saunders TL, Wood RI, Camper SA. Targeted disruption of the pituitary glycoprotein hormone alpha-subunit produces hypogonadal and hypothyroid mice. Genet Dev 1995;9:2007–2019.
41. Huhtaniemi IT, Korenbrot CC, Jaffe RB. hCG binding and stimulation of testosterone biosynthesis in the human fetal testis. J Clin Endocrinol Metab 1977;44:963–967.
42. Lamminen T, Huhtaniemi I. A common genetic variant of luteinizing hormone; relation to normal and aberrant pituitary-gonadal function. Eur J Pharmacol 2001;414:1–7.
43. Nilsson C, Jiang M, Pettersson K, et al. Determination of a common genetic variant of luteinizing hormone using DNA hybridization and immunoassay. Clin Endocr (Oxf) 1998;49:369–376.
44. Pettersson K, Ding YQ, Huhtaniemi I. An immunologically anomalous luteinizing hormone variant in a healthy woman. J Clin Endocrinol Metab 1992;74:164–171.
45. Haavisto A-M, Pettersson K, Bergendahl M, Virkamäki A, Huhtaniemi I. Occurrence and biological properties of a common genetic variant of luteinizing hormone. J Clin Endocrinol Metab 1995;80;1257–1263.
46. Manna PR, Joshi L, Reinhold VN, et al. Synthesis, purification, and structural and functional characterization of recombinant form of a common genetic variant of human luteinizing hormone. Hum Mol Genet 2002;11:301–315.

47. Jiang M, Pakarinen P, Zhang F-P, et al. A common polymorphic allele of the human luteinizing hormone beta-subunit gene: additional mutations and differential function of the promoter sequence. Hum Mol Genet 1999;8:2037–2046.

48. Raivio T, Huhtaniemi I, Anttila R, et al. The role of luteinizing hormone-beta gene polymorphism in the onset and progression of puberty in healthy boys. J Clin Endocrinol Metab 1996;81:3278–3282.

49. Kaleva M, Virtanen H, Haavisto A-M, et al. The prevalence of variant luteinizing hormone among cryptorchid boys increases with gestational age, submitted.

50. van den Beld AW, Huhtaniemi IT, Pettersson K, et al. Luteinizing hormone and different genetic variants, as indicators of frailty in healthy elderly men. J Clin Endocrinol Metab 1999;84:1334–1339.

51. Matthews C, Chatterjee VK. Isolated deficiency of follicle-stimulating hormone re-revisited. N Engl J Med 1997;337:642.

52. Lindstedt G, Ernest I, Nyström E, Janson PO. Fall av manlig infertilitet. Klinisk Kemi I Norden 1977;3:81–87 (In Swedish).

53. Tapanainen JS, Aittomäki K, Jiang M, Vaskivuo T, Huhtaniemi IT. Men homozygous for an inactivating mutation of the follicle-stimulating hormone (FSH) receptor gene present variable suppression of spermatogenesis and fertility. Nat Genet 1997;15:205–206.

54. Kumar TR, Wang Y, Lu N, Matzuk MM. Follicle stimulating hormone is required for ovarian follicle maturation but not male fertility. Nat Genet 1997;15:201–204.

55. Dierich A, Sairam MR, Monaco L, et al. Impairing follicle-stimulating hormone (FSH) signaling in vivo: targeted disruption of the FSH receptor leads to aberrant gametogenesis and hormonal imbalance. Proc Natl Acad Sci USA 1998;95:13612–13617.

56. Abel MH, Wootton AN, Wilkins V, Huhtaniemi I, Knight P, Charlton HM. The effect of a null mutation in the follicle-stimulating hormone receptor gene on mouse reproduction. Endocrinology 2000;141:1795–1803.

57. Aittomäki K, Dieguez Lucena JL, Pakarinen P, et al. Mutation in the follicle-stimulating hormone receptor gene causes hereditary hypergonadotropic ovarian failure. Cell 1995;82:959–968.

58. Baker PJ, Abel MH, Charlton HM, Huhtaniemi IT, O'Shaughnessy PJ. Failure of normal Leydig cell development in FSH receptor deficient mice but not in FSHβ-deficient mice. Endocrinology 200;144:138–145.

59. Kremer H, Kraaij R, Toledo SP, et al. Male pseudohermaphroditism due to a homozygous missense mutation of the luteinizing hormone receptor gene. Nat Genet 1995;9:160–164.

60. Misrahi M, Meduri G, Pissard S, et al. Comparison of immunocytochemical and molecular features with the phenotype in a case of incomplete male pseudohermaphroditism associated with a mutation of the luteinizing hormone receptor. J Clin Endocrinol Metab 1997;82:2159–2165.

61. Zhang F-P, Poutanen M, Wilbertz J, Huhtaniemi I. Normal prenatal but arrested postnatal sexual development of luteinizing hormone receptor knockout (LuRKO) mice. Mol Endocrinol 2001;15:182–193.

62. Toledo SP, Brunner HG, Kraaij R, et al. An inactivating mutation of the luteinizing hormone receptor causes amenorrhea in a 46,XX female. J Clin Endocrinol Metab 1996;81:3850–3854.

63. Kremer H, Mariman E, Otten BJ, et al. Co-segregation of missense mutations of the luteinizing hormone receptor gene with familial male-limited precocious puberty. Hum Mol Genet 1993;2:1779–1783.

64. Shenker A, Laue L, Kosugi S, Merendino JJ, Jr., Minegishi T, Cutler GBJr. A constitutively activating mutation of the luteinizing hormone receptor in familial male precocious puberty. Nature 1993;365:652–654.

65. Liu G, Duranteau L, Carel J-C, Monroe J, Doyle DA, Shenker A. Leydig-cell tumors caused by an activating mutation of the gene encoding the luteinizing hormone receptor. N Engl J Med 1999;341:1731–1736.

66. Canto P, Söderlund D, Ramón G, Nishimura E, Méndez JP. Mutational analysis of the luteinizing hormone receptor gene in two individuals with Leydig cell tumors. Am J Med Genet 2002;108:148–152.

67. Richter-Unruh A, Wessels HT, Menken U, et al. Male LH-independent sexual precocity in a 3.5-year-old boy caused by somatic activating mutation of the LH receptor in a Leydig cell tumor. J Clin Endocrinol Metab 2002;87:1052–1056.

68. Leschek EW, Chan WY, Diamond DA, et al. Nodular Leydig cell hyperplasia in a boy with male-limited precocious puberty. J Pediatr 2001;138:949–951.

69. Martin MM, Wu S-M, Martin ALA, Rennert OM, Chan W-Y. Testicular seminoma in a patient with a constitutively activating mutation of the luteinzing hormone/chorionic gonadotropin receptor. Eur J Endocrinol 1998;139:101–106.

70. Paschke R, Ludgate M. The thyrotropin receptor in thyroid diseases. N Engl J Med 1997;337:1675–1681.
71. Parma J, Duprez L, Van Sande J, et al. Diversity and prevalence of somatic mutations in the thyrotropin receptor and Gsa genes as a cause of toxic thyroid adenomas. J Clin Endocrinol Metab 1997;82:2695–2701.
72. Russo D, Tumino S, Arturi F, et al. Detection of an activating mutation of the thyrotropin receptor in a case of an autonomously hyperfunctioning thyroid insular carcinoma. J Clin Endocrinol Metab 1997;82:735–738.
73. Fragoso MC, Latronico AC, Carvalho FM, et al. Activating mutation of the stimulatory G protein (gsp) as a putative cause of ovarian and testicular human stromal Leydig cell tumors. J Clin Endocrinol Metab 1998;83:2074–2078.
74. Beau I, Touraine P, Meduri G, et al. A novel phenotype related to partial loss of function mutations of the follicle stimulating hormone receptor. J Clin Invest 1998;102:1352–1359.
75. Touraine P, Beau I, Gougeon A, et al. New natural inactivating mutations of the follicle-stimulating hormone receptor: correlations between receptor function and phenotype. Mol Endocrinol 1999;13:1844–1854.
76. Doherty E, Pakarinen P, Tiitinen A, et al. A novel mutation in the follicle-stimulating hormone receptor inhibiting signal transduction and resulting in primary ovarian failure. J Clin Endocrinol Metab 2002;57:1151–1155.
77. Allen LA, Achermann JC, Pakarinen P, et al. A novel loss of function mutation in exon 10 of the FSH receptor gene causing hypergonadotropic hypogonadism: clinical and molecular characteristics. Hum Reprod 2003;18:251–256.
78. Rannikko A, Pakarinen P, Manna P, et al. Functional characterization of the human FSH receptor with an inactivating Ala189Val mutation. Mol Hum Reprod 2002;8:311–317.
79. Vaskivuo TE, Aittomäki K, Anttonen M, et al. Effects of follicle-stimulating hormone (FSH) and human chorionic gonadotropin in individuals with inactivating mutation of the FSH receptor. Fertil Steril 2002;78:108–113.
80. Gromoll J, Simoni M, Nieschlag E. An activating mutation of the follicle-stimulating hormone receptor autonomously sustains spermatogenesis in a hypophysectomized man. J Clin Endocrinol Metab 1996;81:1367–1370.
81. Tao YX, Mizrachi D, Segaloff DL. Chimeras of the rat and human FSH receptors (FSHRs) identify residues that permit or suppress transmembrane 6 mutation-induced constitutive activation of the FSHR via rearrangements of hydrophobic interactions between helices 6 and 7. Mol Endocrinol 2002;16:1881–1892.
82. Gicalglia LR, da Fonte Kohek MB, Carvalho FM, Villares Fragaso MCB, Mendonca BB, Latronico AC. No evidence of somatic activating mutations on gonadotropin receptor genes in sex cord stromal tumors. Fertil Steril 2000;64:992–995.
83. Takakura K, Takebayashi K, Wang H-Q, Kimura F, Kasahara K, Noda Y. Follicle-stimulating hormone receptor gene mutations are rare in Japanese women with premature ovarian failure and polycystic ovary syndrome. Fertil Steril 2001;75:207–209.
84. Tong Y, Liao WX, Roy AC, Ng SC. Absence of mutations in the coding regions of follicle-stimulating hormone receptor gene in Singapore Chinese women with premature ovary failure and polycystic ovary syndrome. Hormone Metab Res 2001;33:221–226.
85. de la Chesnaye E, Canto P, Ulloa-Aguirre A, Mendez JP. No evidence of mutations in the follicle-stimulating hormone receptor gene in Mexican women wit 46,XX pure gonadal dysgenesis. Am J Med Genet 2001;98:129–135.
86. Montgomery GW, Duffy DL, Hall J, Kudo M, Martin NG, Hsueh AJ. Mutations in the follicle-stimulating hormone receptor and familial dizygotic twinning. Lancet 2001;357:773–774.
87. Perez Mayorga M, Gromoll J, Behre HM, Gassner C, Nieschlag E, Simoni M. Ovarian response to follicle-stimulating hormone (FSH) stimulation depends on the FSH receptor genotype. J Clin Endocrinol Metab 2000;85:3365–3369.
88. Laven JS, Mulders AG, Simoni M, Gromoll J, Fauser BC. Follicle-stimulating hormone (FSH) receptor genotype in normogonadotropic anovulatory infertile (WHO II) patients and normo-ovulatory controls. The Endocrine Society, Annual Meeting, June 2002, abstract OR60-1.
89. Mongan NP, Hughes IA, Lim HN. Evidence that luteinising hormone receptor polymorphisms may contribute to male undermasculinisation. Eur J Endocrinol 2002;147:103–107.

90. Ahmed SF, Hughes IA. The genetics of male undermasculinsation. Clin Endocrinol (Oxf) 2002;56:1–18.
91. Tapanainen JS, Koivunen R, Fauser BC, et al. A new contributing factor to polycystic ovary syndrome: the genetic variant of luteinizing hormone. J Clin Endocrinol Metab 1999;84:1711–1715.

7

Hypogonadism in Males With Congenital Adrenal Hyperplasia

Barto J. Otten, PhD, MD,
Nike M.M.L. Stikkelbroeck, PhD, MD,
and Ad R.M.M. Hermus, PhD, MD

CONTENTS

INTRODUCTION

Congenital Adrenal Hyperplasia: Impaired Steroid Synthesis in the Adrenal Gland

In congenital adrenal hyperplasia (CAH), the synthesis of cortisol by the adrenal gland is impaired as a result of an enzyme deficiency. Consequently, the secretion of adrenocorticotropin hormone (ACTH) by the pituitary gland is increased, resulting in hyperplasia of the adrenal cortex and excess production of steroids that do not require the specific deficient enzyme for their synthesis *(1)*. Figure 1 depicts the pathway for normal adrenal steroid synthesis. Mutations in the genes encoding for the enzymes 21-hydroxylase, 17-hydroxylase/17,20-lyase, 11-hydroxylase, 3β-hydroxysteroid dehydrogenase, or the protein StAR (intracellular cholesterol transport protein) lead to CAH. The most frequent cause of CAH (more than 90% of all cases) is 21-hydroxylase deficiency. This deficiency results in cortisol and aldosterone deficiency and an overproduction of 17-hydroxyprogesterone and androstenedione, leading to androgen excess.

From: *Male Hypogonadism:*
Basic, Clinical, and Therapeutic Principles
Edited by: S. J. Winters © Humana Press Inc., Totowa, NJ

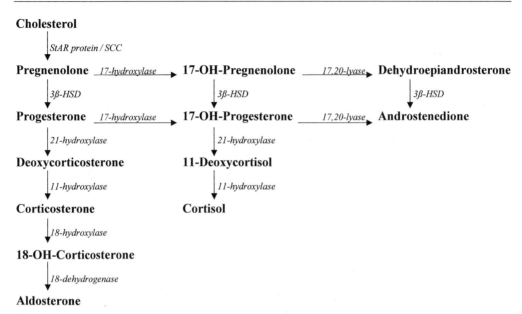

Fig. 1. Adrenal steroid synthesis. StAR, steroidogenic acute response protein; SCC, (cholesterol) side chain cleavage enzyme; 3β-HSD, 3β-hydroxysteroid dehydrogenase.

Prevalence

Most enzyme deficiencies that cause CAH are extremely rare, except for 21-hydroxylase deficiency and 11-hydroxylase deficiency. The prevalence of classic 21-hydroxylase deficiency worldwide is 1/10.000 to 1/18.000, as derived from results of neonatal screening. Nonclassic 21-hydroxylase deficiency is estimated to be more prevalent (1/600), but this diagnosis can easily be missed in men because signs of androgen excess may go unrecognized. The estimated prevalence of 11-hydroxylase deficiency is 1/100.000 *(1)*.

Presentation and Diagnosis

The symptoms and signs of CAH depend on the degree of enzyme deficiency. For 21-hydroxylase deficiency, this results in a broad clinical picture: complete 21-hydroxylase deficiency leads to cortisol and aldosterone absence and salt-wasting crisis in the newborn period. The androgen excess results in prenatal virilization of the external genitalia in women (classic salt-wasting form). Less severe 21-hydroxylase deficiency results in milder cortisol deficiency and milder prenatal androgen excess, with prenatal virilization in women, but no aldosterone deficiency (classic simple virilizing form). Patients with the mildest forms present with symptoms caused by androgen excess only: pseudo precocious puberty, hirsutism, menstrual irregularities and infertility, all of which are most readily detected in women (nonclassic form) *(1)*.

Genetics

All CAH forms are characterized by an autosomal recessive inheritance. The genes that encode the different enzymes have all been elucidated *(1)*. 21-Hydroxylase is encoded by the *CYP21* gene. *CYP21* and the homologous pseudogene *CYP21P* are located in the human leukocyte antigens (HLA) major histocompatibility complex on chromosome 6. *CYP21* and *CYP21P* are 98% identical, which explains the high mutation rate of the *CYP21* gene. One-third of the described mutations are deletions and large gene conversions that were caused by recombinations between the two homologous loci. The other mutations are small defects that are transferred from the *CYP21P* pseudogene to the active *CYP21* gene, resulting from nonhomologous pairing. The genotype–phenotype correlation is reported to be 80–90%, with the best predictions in the most severe and the mildest deficiencies *(1)*.

Of all types of congenital adrenal hyperplasia, 21-hydroxylase deficiency is the most frequent and the most extensively studied. Therefore, this chapter on male hypogonadism in CAH predominantly focuses on 21-hydroxylase deficiency.

FERTILITY IN MEN WITH 21-HYDROXYLASE DEFICIENCY

Reported Fertility in Men With 21-Hydroxylase Deficiency

Fertility can be documented by studying child rate or by indirect methods, such as the semen analysis or measurement of serum follicle-stimulating hormone (FSH) and luteinizing hormone (LH) levels.

Reports on child rate in males with CAH are rare. Jääskeläinen et al. *(2)* found a child rate of 0.07 in the complete Finnish male CAH population, compared to 0.34 in age-matched Finnish males. Other authors reported parenthood only as additional information in smaller and selected patient populations. Urban et al. *(3)* described 14 fathers in 20 male patients (aged 18 to 37 yr), Wüsthof et al. *(4)* reported paternity in 6 of 53 adult patients; Cabrera et al. *(5)* in 2 of 30 patients (aged 17 to 43 yr).

The results from the semen analysis are more frequently reported but usually only in a subgroup of the study population, because not all patients are willing to provide a semen sample for analysis. The semen analysis was normal in 8 of 10 patients studied by Urban et al. *(3)* (total patient group 20) but in only 8 of 53 patients reported by Wüsthof et al. *(4)* (total patient group 53), 7 of 16 patients from Cabrera et al. *(5)* (total patient group 30), and 4 of 11 patients reported by Stikkelbroeck et al. *(6)* (total patient group 17). Taking the results of these last three studies, 80 of the 100 patients agreed to provide semen for analysis. Of these 80 patients, only 19 (24%) had normal semen quality. Most reports on semen analysis, however, are results of single samples. This represents a limited assessment of semen quality, because the (daily) variability in semen quality is substantial based on data from healthy men *(7)*. In addition, fertility in CAH males may change throughout the years. This is illustrated by two men in the study by Cabrera et al. *(5)*, who had previously fathered a child but were later judged to be infertile based on semen analysis.

Measurements of serum FSH and LH levels are also used to assess fertility. A decreased FSH level may indicate hypogonadotropism (especially when associated with decreased LH levels), whereas a strongly elevated FSH level implies severe Sertoli cell damage. Jääkeläinen et al. *(2)* found no differences in the LH, FSH, and inhibin levels in 16 male patients with CAH and controls. In three other studies with 55 patients, abnormal FSH values were found in 13 men (24%): decreased levels in 4 (with LH decrease in 2 of them) and increased FSH levels in 9 patients (with LH increase in 2 of them) *(3,5,6)*.

In summary, there is substantial evidence that fertility can be impaired in male patients with CAH. This finding raises the question to what extent male subfertility in the general population is caused by undiagnosed CAH. Ojeifo et al. *(8)* investigated basal and ACTH-stimulated serum 17-hydroxyprogesterone levels in a population of 50 males with idiopathic infertility and compared the results with those of 25 controls. No differences in basal or stimulated levels were found, and they concluded that 21-hydroxylase deficiency is a rare cause of idiopathic male infertility.

Causes of Subfertility in Males With CAH

The most frequently reported cause of subfertility in males with CAH is the presence of adrenal rest tumors in the testes *(5,6,9)*. These tumors may interfere directly (mechanically or paracrine) or indirectly (endocrine) with testicular function *(10,11)*. Subfertility can also be caused by gonadotropin deficiency resulting from suppression of the hypothalamic–pituitary–gonadal axis by adrenal androgens (both directly and after conversion to estrogens) *(12–14)*. Other testicular abnormalities and psychological problems may also be important *(2)*. The next sections focus on these topics separately, although in practice, these factors may not be separated easily.

TESTICULAR TUMORS

Prevalence

The presence of testicular tumors in male patients with CAH resulting from 21-hydroxylase deficiency was first described in 1940 by Wilkins et al. *(15)*. Since then, the reported prevalence has varied between 0 and 94% *(2,3,5,6,9)*. The reported prevalence is strongly dependent on patient selection (prepubertal, adolescent, or adult), and on the method of tumor detection (physical examination or imaging techniques). Urban et al. *(3)* found no testicular tumors by physical examination in 30 adult patients. Using ultrasonography, adrenal rest tumors were reported in 2 of 14 adult patients *(2)*, 9 of 18 adult patients *(5)*, and 16 of 17 postpubertal patients *(6)*. Tumors have also been reported in prepuberty: of the 8 patients with testicular tumors described by Avila et al. in a population of 38 patients, 7 were younger than 16 yr old *(9)*. Shanklin et al. reviewed the autopsy material of patients with CAH and noted testicular nodules in 3 of 7 patients younger than 8 wk old and in all 14 patients older than 14 mo *(16)*.

Diagnostics

The physical examination reveals only a small proportion of all testicular tumors in CAH, depending on their size. For more accurate detection of these tumors, imaging techniques, such as ultrasound and magnetic resonance imaging (MRI), are required *(3,5,6,9,17,18)*. A comparative study in males with CAH concluded that ultrasound is the method of choice, because it is as sensitive as MRI and more accessible *(19)*. Reports of ultrasound features show a similar picture of hypoechoic lesions adjacent to the mediastinum testis, often lobulated and mostly bilateral *(see* Fig. 2) *(9,18–25)*. In larger tumors, we have observed hyperechoic reflections *(25a)*. Tumor margins may be blurred on ultrasound but are always well defined on MRI *(19,26)*. On MRI, most of the masses are isointense on T1-weighted images and hypointense on T2-weighted images, as are adrenal glands *(19)*.

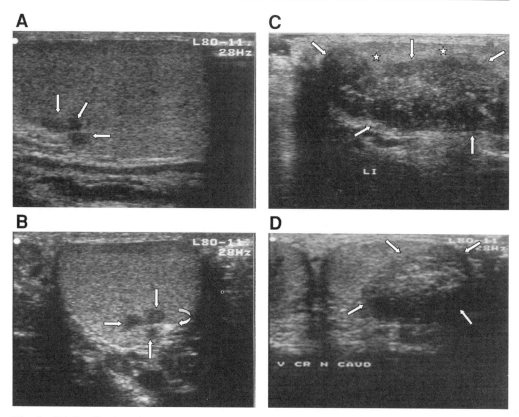

Fig. 2. (A) Small adrenal rest tumors in a 17.9-yr-old male patient with 21-hydroxylase deficiency. **(A)** Longitudinal ultrasonographic image of the left testis in the plane of the mediastinum showing three small well-delineated conflating tumors (arrows). The tumors are hypoechoic compared to the normal testicular tissue. Their maximal lengths were 0.4, 0.3, and 0.2 cm, respectively. **(B)** Ultrasonographic image obtained in the transverse plane. Note that the tumors are located around the mediastinum, which is visible as a small white line (curved arrow). **(C)** Large palpable adrenal rest tumor in a 17.3-yr-old male patient with 21-hydroxylase deficiency. Longitudinal ultrasonographic image of the left testis showing a well-delineated mass with marked irregular echo texture (arrows). Note that only a small rim of normal testicular tissue is visible (asterisks). **(D)** Ultrasonographic image obtained in the transverse plane. The tumor measured 3.8 × 3.8 × 2.0 cm. (Reproduced with permission from ref. 6.)

Testicular tumors in CAH may resemble malignant testicular tumors on ultrasonography and MRI (24,27). However, characteristics such as the bilateral presence of lesions and the location of the lesions adjacent to the mediastinum are helpful in differentiating between a testicular tumor in CAH and a malignant testicular lesion (21,26,28). On the other hand, the ultrasound characteristics of a testicular tumor can suggest the diagnosis CAH in males with previously undiagnosed CAH who present with a testicular mass (28). In that case, elevated 17-hydroxyprogesterone levels may indicate 21-hydroxylase deficiency. However, 17-hydroxyprogesterone production by a Leydig cell tumor (LCT) in a patient without CAH has also been reported once (29).

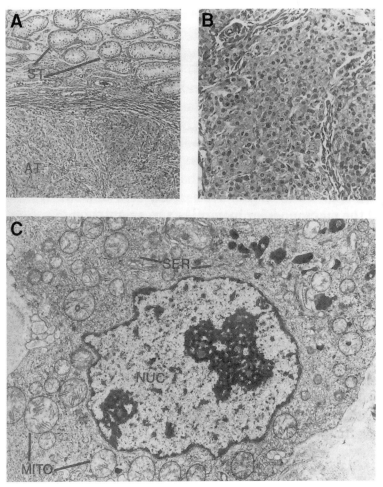

Fig. 3. (A) Light micrograph (original magnification ×130) showing hyperplastic nodular adrenal rest tissue (AT) and the adjacent area with few atrophic seminiferous tubules (ST) that contains Sertoli cells and a few spermatogonia and early spermatocytes. **(B)** Light micrograph (original magnification ×350) showing confluent polygonal eosinophilic cells of uniform appearance, with interspersed bands of connective tissue stroma. **(C)** Electron micrograph (original magnification ×6000) showing ultrastructural detail of representative cell from the adenomatous adrenal rest demonstrating abundant smooth endoplasmic reticulum (SER), mitochondria with tubular cristae (MITO), and nucleus (NUC) with dense heterochromatin and prominent nucleolus. (Reproduced with permission from ref. *38.*)

Histopathology

Histologically, the testicular tumors in patients with CAH resemble LCTs, and differentiation can be difficult (*see* Fig. 3) *(30)*. However, some differences may exist; testicular tumors associated with CAH are bilateral in 83% of the cases and LCTs are bilateral in only 3% of cases. Malignant degeneration has not been reported in testicular tumors associated with CAH, but it occurs in 10% of LCTs in adults *(30)*. In addition, the tumors are located in the mediastinum testis and often decrease in size when ACTH levels are suppressed by increasing the glucocorticoid dose *(11,28,31–34)*. Rich et al. *(30)* found that both the testicular tumors of CAH and LCTs are circumscribed, lobulated, nodular lesions. CAH tumors are typically encapsulated nodules that are dark brown (resulting from a greater concentration of lipochrome pigmentation), whereas LCTs are usually yellow intratesticular masses. The color distinction is not always reliable, however, because some LCTs are occasionally darker. Reinke's crystals, which can be found in 25–40% of LCTs, have never been observed in CAH tumors. In the surrounding parenchyma, seminiferous tubules show atrophic sclerosis in CAH tumors, whereas in LCTs seminiferous tubules are rarely found because they are replaced by the tumor *(31)*.

Steroid Production

Steroid production by testicular tumors has been investigated both in vitro and in vivo.

Cortisol production by the testicular tumor was demonstrated in vivo by testicular venous sampling after stimulation with ACTH in a patient with nonclassic CAH *(35)* and, surprisingly, also in a patient with salt-wasting *(36)*.

17-Hydroxyprogesterone production by a testicular tumor was demonstrated in vivo by testicular vein sampling after ACTH stimulation *(37)*.

11-Hydroxylated steroids, like 21-deoxycortisol (21-DF), 21-deoxycorticosterone (21-DB), and 11β-hydroxy-Δ⁴-androstenedione (11β-OHA), have been demonstrated in vitro *(37,38)*, as well as in vivo *(37,39,40)*. 11-Hydroxylase activity is usually restricted to the adrenal gland. Clark et al. demonstrated 11-hydroxylase activity in vitro in a testicular tumor from a patient with salt-wasting CAH *(38)*. That study identified abundant angiotensin II receptors but no gonadotropin receptors in tumor membranes. In vivo, 11-hydroxylase activity was demonstrated by testicular vein sampling by Blumberg-Tick et al. *(40)*. Combes-Moukhovsky et al. showed that stimulation with human chorionic gonadotropin (hCG) increased secretion of 11-hydroxylated steroids *(39)*. In humans, LH/hCG receptors have been found not only in the testes but also in the normal adrenal cortex *(41)*.

Testosterone production was shown in vitro by Franco Saenz et al. *(36)* but only after stimulation with ACTH or hCG. Interestingly, testosterone production was more responsive to ACTH stimulation than to hCG stimulation. The authors hypothesized the presence of specific receptors for ACTH and hCG in the same cells, a defective receptor with loss of specificity or the presence of two different cell lines. In vivo, Kirkland et al. showed increased testosterone production after ACTH infusion into the testicular artery *(42)*.

Benvenga et al. hypothesized from longitudinal observations in a single patient that at least three distinct types of testicular tumors in CAH can be discriminated, based on their response to dexamethasone-induced ACTH suppression *(43)*. The first type was ACTH dependent, in both growth and steroidogenesis. The second type was only partially responsive to ACTH, because growth suppression lagged behind the prompt suppression of steroidogenesis. In addition, this type was responsive to LH/hCG. In the third type, growth is unresponsive to dexamethasone-induced ACTH suppression, unresponsive to gonadotropins, and has lost the property to synthesize cortisol.

The Origin of the Testicular Tumors

Based on histopathology, steroid-producing properties, and ACTH responsiveness, these testicular tumors are believed to consist of adrenal tissue. Aberrant adrenal tissue has been identified in 7.5% of normal testes by Dahl et al. *(44)*. In the embryological phase, the adrenal glands develop in the immediate vicinity of the gonads. Aberrant adrenal tissue may descend with the testis or ovary along the course of their supplying arteries and end up in the testes, celiac plexus, broad ligament, or ovary *(44–48)*. The aberrant adrenal cells are believed to retain their potential for glucocorticoid production and to respond with hyperplasia to increased ACTH stimulation. The testicular tumors in males with CAH are, therefore, often called adrenal rest tumors.

Relationship Between the Presence of Testicular Tumors and Therapeutic Control

Early reports of testicular tumors in CAH were predominantly in poorly controlled patients *(10,11,14,28,38–40,49)*. Those observations led to the hypothesis that poor hormonal control and inadequate ACTH secretion suppression is a dominant etiological factor in the development of the testicular tumors in CAH. This hypothesis is supported by the development of tumors in other patients who have elevated ACTH levels, such as in Nelson's syndrome *(50,51)* and in Addison's disease *(52)*.

However, in more recent studies, no correlation was found between the presence of testicular tumors and the degree of hormonal control *(5,6,17,18,20)*. Nevertheless, other associations were found, such as a higher incidence of these tumors in patients with salt-wasting CAH *(5)* or larger tumors in patients with at least one deletion/conversion of the *CYP21* gene *(6)*.

Effect of Testicular Adrenal Rest Tumors on Fertility

Adrenal rest tumors may interfere directly (mechanically or paracrine) or indirectly (endocrine) with testicular function. The mechanical effect of the tumors can be considerable because of their central location adjacent to the mediastinum testis. It can lead to obstruction of the vascular supply and compression and atrophy of the seminiferous tubules. Pathological examination revealed that in cases of large tumors, the residual testicular parenchyma was abnormal and showed atrophy, sclerosis, or immaturity and decreased or absent spermatogenesis *(28)*. However, around small nodules, the testicular parenchyma was generally normal *(28)*. Murphy et al. showed in one patient that germ cells close to the mediastinum and the tumor were reduced and spermatogenesis was impaired. However, testicular aspiration in other areas showed normal spermatogenesis *(53)*.

In addition to direct mechanical effects (obstruction or destruction), tumors may have a paracrine effect on the surrounding tissue, i.e., steroids produced by the tumors could be toxic to Sertoli cells or germ cells *(53)*.

Indirect (endocrine) effects of testicular tumors in CAH on fertility could result from steroid secretion by the tumor, with suppression of the hypothalamic–pituitary–gonadal axis. The association between infertility, testicular adrenal rest tumors, and depressed serum LH and FSH levels in males with CAH has been described *(5,6,39,43,54)*. However, the effect of steroid secretion by the tumor cannot be readily separated from the effect of excess steroids secreted by the adrenal glands.

Therapy of Adrenal Rest Tumors

Intensified glucocorticoid–mineralocorticoid therapy is the preferred treatment for testicular tumors in CAH. By increasing the glucocorticoid dose, ACTH secretion is suppressed and the adrenal rest tissue is no longer stimulated. The need for tumor shrinkage and the side effects of increasing glucocorticoid therapy must be carefully balanced, especially in asymptomatic cases *(55)*. In 1988, Rutgers et al. reported tumor shrinkage in 75% of 16 patients after increasing the glucocorticoid dose *(28)*. In 1997, Walker et al. reviewed 75 cases of testicular tumors in CAH and stated that the majority of the masses regressed with an increase in glucocorticoid dose *(26)*. Increasing the glucocorticoid dose can also lead to improved semen quality.

If tumor size does not decrease with increasing glucocorticoid therapy, surgical intervention may be considered. Walker et al. reviewed the surgical management of these tumors and showed that the predominant intervention was orchiectomy in 19 of 28 patients (68%) *(26)*. In these patients, the tumors were steroid resistant or (initially) misdiagnosed as LCTs. Walker performed a testis-sparing enucleation in three boys with CAH with steroid-unresponsive testicular tumors. Postoperative MRI and ultrasound of the testis in two of the three patients showed good vascular flow in the remaining tissue and no evidence of recurrent tumor. No semen analysis could be performed.

Because fertility prognosis in CAH males is uncertain, cryopreservation of the semen can be proposed to young male patients. In the case of unwanted infertility, assisted reproduction can be considered. When there is obstructive azoospermia, testicular aspiration and intracytoplasmatic sperm injection may offer a solution, as reported by Murphy et al. *(53)*.

Other Testicular Tumors in CAH Males

There are a few reports of other types of testicular tumors in CAH males. Adesokan et al. presented a case of a testicular adrenal rest tumor in a patient with CAH in combination with a testicular myelolipoma (a tumor of adrenal origin) and a seminoma in a cryptorchid testis *(56)*. Davis described an LCT with metastases in a patient with CAH *(57)*.

SECONDARY HYPOGONADOTROPISM

In male patients with 21-hydroxylase deficiency, as in affected females, adrenal androgens may suppress the hypothalamic–pituitary–gonadal axis, both directly and after conversion to estrogens, thereby leading to hypogonadotropic hypogonadism *(12–14)*.

Augarten et al. described a patient who was referred for secondary infertility and was diagnosed with nonclassic 21-hydroxylase deficiency, as was his daughter *(58)*. Serum FSH and LH levels were decreased and unresponsive to GnRH stimulation. Treatment with prednisone resulted in a decrease in the serum levels of 17-hydroxyprogesterone and of androgens and restored a normal response to GnRH. After 4 mo of treatment, successful conception occurred *(58)*.

Wischusen et al. described a patient with partial 21-hydroxylase deficiency, azoospermia, small testes, normal to high serum testosterone levels, and suppressed serum levels of gonadotropins. After treatment with glucocorticoids for several months, the semen quality improved, and he fathered a child *(59)*.

Bonaccorsi et al. presented three cases of male infertility resulting from 21-hydroxylase deficiency with low serum gonadotropin levels that were unresponsive to GnRH stimulation in two patients *(12)*. Unresponsiveness to GnRH was proposed to result from increased hypothalamic estrogen production from local aromatization of androstenedione, leading to GnRH suppression.

Cabrera et al. described 5 patients (out of a group of 30 patients) with poor adrenal control and suppressed gonadotropin levels; azoospermia was documented in 3 of the patients *(5)*.

The cases described illustrate that hypogonadotropic hypogonadism may occur in males with undiagnosed 21-hydroxylase deficiency or as a result of poor adrenal control. Most reports show reversible hypogonadotropism and improved fertility after increasing glucocorticoid therapy.

Small testes are incidentally reported in males with CAH, especially in poorly controlled patients, who had low FSH levels *(12,14,59)*. In 101 patients, described in four recent studies, 6 patients had small testes, as measured by ultrasonography *(2,5,6,9)*. Plasma FSH levels in these 6 patients were normal in 2 *(5)*, decreased in 2 *(5)*, just above the normal range in 1 *(6)*, and not documented in 1 *(9)*. Therefore, small testes have been observed in patients with CAH, but not frequently, and they are generally found in men with low FSH levels (hypogonadotropism). Testicular volume is relevant with respect to fertility, because it is positively correlated with semen quality *(60,61)*.

OTHER CAUSES OF SUBFERTILITY IN CAH MEN

Other Testicular Abnormalities

Varicoceles and hydroceles also interfere with testicular function and have been documented by ultrasonography in 4 and 3 patients, respectively, in a group of 18 patients with CAH *(5)*. However, semen quality was normal, in three of the four men with varicoceles *(5)*.

Psychological Factors

Suboptimal psychosocial adaptation to chronic disease has been suggested as a cause for impaired fertility by Jääskeläinen et al., who found a lower child rate in males with CAH compared to the healthy male population, despite normal gonadal and pituitary function *(2)*.

FERTILITY IN MEN WITH OTHER ENZYMATIC DEFICIENCIES IN STEROID SYNTHESIS

CAH can also be caused by enzyme deficiencies other than 21-hydroxylase deficiency (*see* Fig. 1).

The first two enzymes in steroid synthesis (3β-hydroxysteroid dehydrogenase and 17α-hydroxylase/17,20-lyase) and the intracellular cholesterol transport protein (StAR), are present in both adrenals and gonads. A deficiency of these enzymes or in the StAR protein leads to cortisol and aldosterone deficiency and insufficient gonadal production of sex steroids. In the male patient, this results in prenatal hypovirilization, depending on the degree of the enzyme deficiency, varying from hypospadias to intersex conditions.

11-Hydroxylase deficiency leads to cortisol deficiency and to aldosterone deficiency. Characteristically, patients have hypertension as a result of desoxycorticosterone (DOC) overproduction, which acts as mineralocorticoid. Because androgen production is increased and the clinical picture resembles 21-hydroxylase deficiency in some reports on male fertility in CAH, patients who are both 21-hydroxylase and 11-hydroxylase deficient have been included.

CONCLUSION

Fertility in men with congenital adrenal hyperplasia can be impaired. Testicular tumors are the most frequent cause of impaired fertility. They arise from aberrant adrenal cells in the testes that are stimulated by ACTH. Their location adjacent to the mediastinum and their steroid-producing properties may interfere with spermatogenesis and Leydig cell function. Secondary hypogonadotropism is a second cause of impaired fertility, resulting from suppression of the hypothalamic–pituitary–gonadal axis by adrenal androgen excess or by production of steroids by testicular tumors. Other testicular abnormalities and psychological factors may also contribute to impaired fertility.

REFERENCES

1. White PC, Speiser PW. Congenital adrenal hyperplasia due to 21-hydroxylase deficiency. Endocr Rev 2000;21:245–291.
2. Jaaskelainen J, Kiekara O, Hippelainen M, Voutilainen R. Pituitary gonadal axis and child rate in males with classical 21-hydroxylase deficiency. J Endocrinol Invest 2000;23:23–27.
3. Urban MD, Lee PA, Migeon CJ. Adult height and fertility in men with congenital virilizing adrenal hyperplasia. N Engl J Med 1978;299:1392–1396.
4. Wuesthof AR, Willig RP, Schulze W, Hoepffner W, Knorr D, Schwarz HP. Spermatogenesis is impaired in men with congenital adrenal hyperplasia. Hormone Res 1998;50:104–104.
5. Cabrera MS, Vogiatzi MG, New MI. Long-term outcome in adult males with classic congenital adrenal hyperplasia. J Clin Endocrinol Metab 2001;86:3070–3078.
6. Stikkelbroeck NMML, Otten BJ, Pasic A, et al. High prevalence of testicular adrenal rest tumors, impaired spermatogenesis, and Leydig cell failure in adolescent and adult males with congenital adrenal hyperplasia. J Clin Endocrinol Metab 2001;86:5721–5728.
7. World Health Organization. WHO Laboratory Manual for the examination of human semen and sperm-cervical mucus interaction, 4th ed. Cambridge: Cambridge University Press, 1999.
8. Ojeifo JO, Winters SJ, Troen P. Basal and adrenocorticotropic hormone-stimulated serum 17 alpha-hydroxyprogesterone in men with idiopathic infertility. Fertil Steril 1984;42:97–101.
9. Avila NA, Premkumar A, Shawker TH, Jones JV, Laue L, Cutler GB. Testicular adrenal rest tissue in congenital adrenal hyperplasia: findings at gray-scale and color Doppler US. Radiology 1996;198:99–104.
10. Cutfield RG, Bateman JM, Odell WD. Infertility caused by bilateral testicular masses secondary to congenital adrenal hyperplasia (21-hydroxylase deficiency). Fertil Steril 1983;40:809–814.
11. Cunnah D, Perry L, Dacie JA, et al. Bilateral testicular tumours in congenital adrenal hyperplasia: a continuing diagnostic and therapeutic dilemma. Clin Endocrinol (Oxf) 1989;30:141–147.
12. Bonaccorsi AC, Adler I, Figueiredo JG. Male infertility due to congenital adrenal hyperplasia: testicular biopsy findings, hormonal evaluation, and therapeutic results in three patients. Fertil Steril 1987;47:664–670.
13. Molitor JT, Chertow BS, Fariss BL. Long-term follow-up of a patient with congenital adrenal hyperplasia and failure of testicular development. Fertil Steril 1973;24:319–323.
14. Moore GW, Lacroix A, Rabin D, McKenna TJ. Gonadal dysfunction in adult men with congenital adrenal hyperplasia. Acta Endocrinol (Copenh) 1980;95:185–193.
15. Wilkins L, Fleishmann W, Howard JE. Macrogenitosomia precox associated with hyperplasia of the androgenic tissue of the adrenal and death from corticoadrenal insufficiency. Endocrinology 1940;26:385–395.
16. Shanklin DR, Richardson AP Jr, Rothstein G. Testicular hilar nodules in adrenogenital syndrome. Am J Dis Child 1963;106:243–250.
17. Willi U, Atares M, Prader A, Zachmann M. Testicular adrenal-like tissue (TALT) in congenital adrenal hyperplasia: detection by ultrasonography. Pediatr Radiol 1991;21:284–287.

18. Vanzulli A, DelMaschio A, Paesano P, et al. Testicular masses in association with adrenogenital syndrome: US findings. Radiology 1992;183:425–429.
19. Avila NA, Premkumar A, Merke DP. Testicular adrenal rest tissue in congenital adrenal hyperplasia: comparison of MR imaging and sonographic findings. Am J Roentgenol 1999;172:1003–1006.
20. Avila NA, Shawker TS, Jones JV, Cutler-GB J, Merke DP. Testicular adrenal rest tissue in congenital adrenal hyperplasia: serial sonographic and clinical findings. Am J Roentgenol 1999;172:1235–1238.
21. Shawker TH, Doppman JL, Choyke PL, Feuerstein IM, Nieman LK. Intratesticular masses associated with abnormally functioning adrenal glands. J Clin Ultrasound 1992;20:51–58.
22. Keely EJ, Matwijiw I, Thliveris JA, Faiman C. Congenital adrenal hyperplasia with testicular tumors, aggression, and gonadal failure. Urology 1993;41:346–349.
23. Dieckmann K, Lecomte P, Despert F, Maurage C, Sirinelli D, Rolland JC. Bilateral testicular tumors in congenital adrenal hyperplasia. Arch Pediatr 1995;2:1167–1172.
24. Coakley FV, Hricak H, Presti JC. Imaging and management of atypical testicular masses. Urolog Clin North Am 1998;25:375.
25. Proto G, Di-Donna A, Grimaldi F, Mazzolini A, Purinan A, Bertolissi F. Bilateral testicular adrenal rest tissue in congenital adrenal hyperplasia: US and MR features. J Endocrinol Invest 2001;24:529–531.
25a. Stikkelbroeck NM, Suliman HM, Otten BJ, Hermus AR, Blickman JG, Jager GJ. Testicular adrenal rest tumors in postpubertal males with congenital adrenal hyperplasia: sonographic and MR features. Eur Radiol 2003;13:1597–1603.
26. Walker BR, Skoog SJ, Winslow BH, Canning DA, Tank ES. Testis sparing surgery for steroid unresponsive testicular tumors of the adrenogenital syndrome. J Urol 1997;157:1460–1463.
27. Strauss S, Gottlieb P, Kessler A, Graif M, Heyman Z, Manor H. Non-neoplastic intratesticular lesions mimicking tumour on ultrasound. Eur Radiol 2000;10:1628–1635.
28. Rutgers JL, Young RH, Scully RE. The testicular tumor of the adrenogenital syndrome: A report of six cases and review of the literature on testicular masses in patients with adrenocortical disorders. Am J Surg Pathol 1988;12:503–513.
29. Solish SB, Goldsmith MA, Voutilainen R, Miller WL. Molecular characterization of a Leydig cell tumor presenting as congenital adrenal hyperplasia. J Clin Endocrinol Metab 1989;69:1148–1152.
30. Rich MA, Keating MA. Leydig cell tumors and tumors associated with congenital adrenal hyperplasia. Urol Clin North Am 2000;27:519–528.
31. Knudsen JL, Savage A, Mobb GE. The testicular 'tumour' of adrenogenital syndrome—a persistent diagnostic pitfall. Histopathology 1991;19:468–470.
32. Newell ME, Lippe BM, Ehrlich RM. Testis tumors associated with congenital adrenal hyperplasia: a continuing diagnostic and therapeutic dilemma. J Urol 1977;117:256–258.
33. Kim I, Young RH, Scully RE. Leydig cell tumors of the testis. A clinicopathological analysis of 40 cases and review of the literature. Am J Surg Pathol 1985;9:177–192.
34. Burke EF, Gilbert E, Uehling DT. Adrenal rest tumors of the testes. J Urol 1973;109:649–652.
35. Fore WW, Bledsoe T, Weber DM, Akers R, Brooks RTJ. Cortisol production by testicular tumors in adrenogenital syndrome. Arch Intern Med 1972;130:59–63.
36. Franco-Saenz R, Antonipillai I, Tan SY, McCorquodale M, Kropp K, Mulrow PJ. Cortisol production by testicular tumors in a patient with congenital adrenal hyperplasia (21-hydroxylase deficiency). J Clin Endocrinol Metab 1981, 53:85–90.
37. Dominguez OV. Biosynthesis of steroids by testicular tumors complicating congenital adrenocortical hyperplasia. J Clin Endocrinol Metab 1961;21:663–674.
38. Clark RV, Albertson BD, Munabi A, et al. Steroidogenic enzyme activities, morphology, and receptor studies of a testicular adrenal rest in a patient with congenital adrenal hyperplasia. J Clin Endocrinol Metab 1990;70:1408–1413.
39. Combes-Moukhovsky ME, Kottler ML, Valensi P, Boudou P, Sibony M, Attali JR. Gonadal and adrenal catheterization during adrenal suppression and gonadal stimulation in a patient with bilateral testicular tumors and congenital adrenal hyperplasia. J Clin Endocrinol Metab 1994;79:1390–1394.
40. Blumberg-Tick J, Boudou P, Nahoul K, Schaison G. Testicular tumors in congenital adrenal hyperplasia: steroid measurements from adrenal and spermatic veins. J Clin Endocrinol Metab 1991;73:1129–1133.
41. Pabon JE, Li X, Lei ZM, Sanfilippo JS, Yussman MA, Rao CV. Novel presence of luteinizing hormone/chorionic gonadotropin receptors in human adrenal glands. J Clin Endocrinol Metab 1996;81:2397–2400.
42. Kirkland RT, Kirkland JL, Keenan BS, Bongiovanni AM, Rosenberg HS, Clayton GW. Bilateral testicular tumors in congenital adrenal hyperplasia. J Clin Endocrinol Metab 1977;44:369–378.

43. Benvenga S, Smedile G, Lo GF, Trimarchi F. Testicular adrenal rests: evidence for luteinizing hormone receptors and for distinct types of testicular nodules differing for their autonomization. Eur J Endocrinol 1999;141:231–237.
44. Dahl EV, Bahn RC. Aberrant adrenal cortical tissue near the testis in human infants. Am J Pathol 1962;40:587–598.
45. Graham LS. Celiac accessory adrenal glands. Cancer 1953;6:149–152.
46. Falls JL. Accessory adrenal cortex in the broad ligament. Incidence and functional significance. Cancer 1955;8:143–150.
47. Symonds DA, Driscoll SG. An adrenal cortical rest within the fetal ovary: report of a case. Am J Clin Pathol 1973;60:562–564.
48. Wilson BE, Netzloff ML. Primary testicular abnormalities causing precocious puberty Leydig cell tumor, Leydig cell hyperplasia, and adrenal rest tumor. Ann Clin Lab Sci 1983;13:315–320.
49. Srikanth MS, West BR, Ishitani M, Isaacs H, Applebaum H, Costin G. Benign testicular tumors in children with congenital adrenal hyperplasia. J Pediatr Surg 1992;27:639–641.
50. Hamwi GJ, Gwinup G, Mostow JH, Besch PK. Activation of testicular adrenal rest tissue by prolonged excessive ACTH production. J Clin Endocrinol Metab 1963;23:861–869.
51. Johnson RE, Scheithauer B. Massive hyperplasia of testicular adrenal rests in a patient with Nelson's syndrome. Am J Clin Pathol 1982;77:501–507.
52. Seidenwurm D, Smathers RL, Kan P, Hoffman A. Intratesticular adrenal rests diagnosed by ultrasound. Radiology 1985;155:479–481.
53. Murphy H, George C, de Kretser DD, Judd S. Successful treatment with ICSI of infertility caused by azoospermia associated with adrenal rests in the testes: case report. Hum Reprod 2001;16:263–267.
54. Radfar N, Bartter FC, Easley R, Kolins J, Javadpour N, Sherins RJ. Evidence for endogenous LH suppression in a man with bilateral testicular tumors and congenital adrenal hyperplasia. J Clin Endocrinol Metab 1977;45:1194–1204.
55. Merke DP, Bornstein SR, Avila NA, Chrousos GP. NIH conference. Future directions in the study and management of congenital adrenal hyperplasia due to 21-hydroxylase deficiency. Ann Intern Med 2002;136:320–334.
56. Adesokan A, Adegboyega PA, Cowan DF, Kocurek J, Neal DE. Testicular "tumor" of the adrenogenital syndrome: a case report of an unusual association with myelolipoma and seminoma in cryptorchidism. Cancer 1997;80:2120–2127.
57. Davis JM, Woodroof J, Sadasivan R, Stephens R. Case report: congenital adrenal hyperplasia and malignant Leydig cell tumor. Am J Med Sci 1995;309:63–65.
58. Augarten A, Weissenberg R, Pariente C, Sack J. Reversible male infertility in late onset congenital adrenal hyperplasia. J Endocrinol Invest 1991;14:237–240.
59. Wischusen J, Baker HW, Hudson B. Reversible male infertility due to congenital adrenal hyperplasia. Clin Endocrinol (Oxf) 1981;14:571–577.
60. Lenz S, Giwercman A, Elsborg A, et al. Ultrasonic testicular texture and size in 444 men from the general population: correlation to semen quality. Eur Urol 1993;24:231–238.
61. Arai T, Kitahara S, Horiuchi S, Sumi S, Yoshida K. Relationship of testicular volume to semen profiles and serum hormone concentrations in infertile Japanese males. Int J Fertil Womens Med 1998;43:40–47.

8

Male Hypogonadism Resulting From Disorders of the Pituitary and Suprasellar Region

Annamaria Colao, MD, PhD,
Giovanni Vitale, MD, *Michele De Rosa*, MD,
and Gaetano Lombardi, MD

CONTENTS

INTRODUCTION

The primary regulator of testicular function is gonadotropin-releasing hormone (GnRH) that is secreted episodically by hypothalamic neurons into the portal vascular system. GnRH stimulates the synthesis and secretion of luteinizing hormone (LH) and follicle-stimulating hormone (FSH), which are produced by gonadotrophs of the anterior pituitary. LH stimulates testosterone synthesis after binding to specific receptors on Leydig cells, whereas Sertoli cells in the seminiferous tubules are the primary target of FSH *(1,2)*. Accordingly, mass lesions and other disorders of the suprasellar region or pituitary that disrupt GnRH or LH/FSH production result in impaired testicular function that is designated hypogonadotropic hypogonadism because of the deficiency of LH and FSH. These disorders are the subject of this chapter.

From: *Male Hypogonadism:*
Basic, Clinical, and Therapeutic Principles
Edited by: S. J. Winters © Humana Press Inc., Totowa, NJ

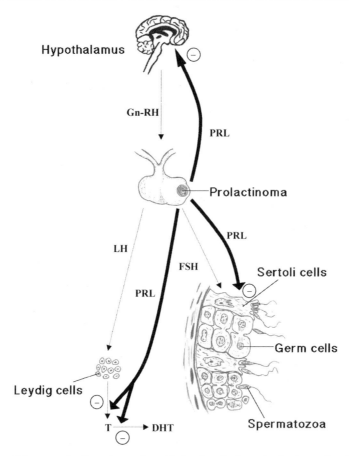

Fig. 1. Effects of hyperprolactinemia on hypothalamic–pituitary–testicular axis. ABP, androgen-binding globulin; AEC, aromatase enzyme complex; T, testosterone; DHT: dihydrotestosterone; E, estradiol; 5αR, 5α-reductase.

PROLACTINOMAS

Physiopathology of Hypogonadism

Prolactinomas are the most common functional adenomas of the anterior pituitary (representing 60% of hormone-secreting pituitary tumors). Men with prolactinomas usually present with macroadenomas (tumors ≥10 mm in diameter) and with high prolactin (PRL) levels, erectile dysfunction, loss of libido and/or infertility. These symptoms are related to the hypogonadism that occurs secondary to hyperprolactinemia *(3)*.

PRL affects the testis directly. PRL receptors are present in all stages of the cycle of the seminiferous epithelium, the surface of Sertoli and Leydig cells, and all phases of spermatogonia and spermatocytes in male rats *(4)*. PRL modulates testosterone production by regulating precursor steroid levels for bioconversion under LH influence. These findings imply that PRL plays a role in the process of spermatogenesis, and normal serum PRL levels are required for normal testicular function.

Hyperprolactinemia disrupts male gonadal function at several levels (*see* Fig. 1).

Table 1
Clinical Manifestations Secondary to Hypogonadism
in Men With Prolactinoma

Infertility
Decreased libido
Impotence
Gynecomastia
Galactorrhea
Loss of pubic hair
Osteoporosis
Apathy
Loss of muscle mass
Decreased sense of well-being

High levels of PRL suppress GnRH secretion and, consequently, decrease gonadotropin and testosterone production *(5,6)*. In some cases, hyperprolactinemia induces clinical hypogonadism notwithstanding normal serum FSH, LH, and testosterone levels. There is an exaggerated diurnal variation in testosterone in men with PRL-producing tumors, so that normal morning values do not guarantee normal values throughout the day *(7)*. Others have suggested a reduced conversion of testosterone to dihydrotestosterone (DHT) *(8,9)*. If so, the hypogonadism associated with hyperprolactinemia may not solely result from the decrease in serum testosterone. In fact, testosterone replacement therapy may not reverse the loss of libido that is typical of men with prolactinoma until the PRL level is normalized by the administration of a dopamine agonist *(10)*. Furthermore, human chorionic gonadotropin (hCG) administration did not increase DHT levels in men with hyperprolactinemia induced by sulpiride treatment, although testosterone levels were significantly increased *(11)*. Another mechanism to explain the suppression of gonadal function in men with prolactinoma is a direct tumor mass effect on gonadotrophs. Large adenomas often cause deficiency of anterior pituitary hormones, including the gonadotropins. However, a tumor mass effect is less important than hyperprolactinemia in the development of hypogonadism in prolactinomas. In fact, there is no significant difference in the prevalence of testosterone deficiency between microprolactinomas and macroprolactinomas, either before or after medical treatment *(12)*. Therefore, hyperprolactinemia produces sexual dysfunction and affects seminal fluid through several mechanisms, causing spermiogenic arrest and impairing sperm motility and/or quality. The development of a mouse line knockout for the PRL receptor could be used to better evaluate the multiple functions of PRL and the effects on testicular function *(13)*.

Diagnosis

Prolactinoma is readily detected in menstruating women because of galactorrhea and irregular menses, but in men, this tumor can be difficult to recognize. Symptoms and signs of hypogonadism (*see* Table 1) may not become obvious, unless the tumor becomes large, or hyperprolactinemia and gonadotropin deficiency become severe. Therefore, in men, the diagnosis of prolactinoma is often delayed until a visual field defect or other symptoms secondary to tumor pressure on surrounding structures occur (e.g., headaches, seizures, altered personality, cranial nerve palsies, symptoms related to the deficiencies of other pituitary hormones, and hydrocephalus). With long-standing hypogonadism, the testes are usually soft but of normal size and the semen analysis frequently reveals low semen volume, oligospermia, or azoospermia *(14–16)*. Most men with hyperprolactinemia have low-normal serum levels of LH, testosterone, and DHT, and low-frequency and low-amplitude spontaneous LH secretory episodes *(17)*, together with a normal increase in serum LH levels after GnRH administration *(10)*. The identification of high PRL levels is the beginning of the diagnostic process; however, hyperprolactinemia should be correctly identified and other causes should be excluded. PRL levels in patients with PRL-secreting adenomas are usually higher than 100 ng/ml and are proportional to the size of the tumor. Lower values may be associated with drugs, pituitary stalk compression, renal failure, cirrhosis, hypothyroidism, and polycystic ovary disease *(14)*. Macroprolactinemia is a molecular weight variant increasing the serum PRL levels because of reduced hormone clearance; it is usually unassociated with clinical problems. Computed tomography (CT) and magnetic resonance imaging (MRI) allow for detailed noninvasive imaging of the pituitary gland. Both methods are effective in identifying large pituitary tumours; CT is better for defining bone erosions and calcified structures, but MRI with gadolinium enhancement provides superior anatomical detail to detect prolactinomas and their relationship to neighboring structures. MRI is more efficacious than CT to identify microadenoma *(18–20)*.

Therapy

As noted earlier, testosterone replacement therapy does not cure sexual dysfunction, and does not normalize high serum PRL levels *(10)*. The therapeutic management of prolactinomas is primarily accomplished with dopamine agonists for the patient with a microadenoma or a macroadenoma *(21)*. Dopamine agonist therapy was developed based on the finding that the synthesis and secretion of PRL are regulated by the tonic inhibitory effects of hypothalamic dopamine, which acts on dopamine D2 receptors on the surface of lactotrophs *(16)*. Bromocriptine mesylate is a semisynthetic ergot alkaloid and long-acting dopamine receptor agonist. It normalizes PRL levels in 80–90% and 60–75% of patients with microprolactinomas and macroprolactinomas, respectively *(14,22)*. Treatment should be started with a dose of 1.25 mg administered at night consumed with a snack. After 1 wk, 1.25 mg is added in the morning. An additional dose of 1.25 mg/d may be added to the treatment regimen as tolerated every 7 d until an optimal response is achieved to a total dose of 2.5–15 mg/d. In resistant patients, however, doses higher than 15 mg/d may be necessary, although the basis for resistance is not completely known *(22)*. Headache, nasal congestion, nausea, vomiting, and dizziness are common side effects. Quinagolide is a more selective D2 agonist with only mild antagonistic effects at α_1-adrenoceptors. It is better tolerated, 100 times more potent than bromocriptine, and readily crosses the blood–brain barrier *(15,21)*. This drug induces an excellent response in both normalizing PRL levels and restoring gonadal function, with normalization of libido and improvement in the ejaculate. Usual doses are 0.15–0.6 mg/d. However, at least 6–12 mo of treatment is needed to obtain a significant improvement in seminal fluid parameters and circulating testosterone levels *(23)*. At present, the most commonly used dopamine agonist is cabergoline because of its prolonged duration of action and lower incidence of side effects. Tumor shrinkage and/or disappearance was observed in 60–88% of cases *(21,24)*. Cabergoline is more efficacious than bromocriptine in normalizing PRL levels and restoring gonadal function *(24)*. Normalization of serum PRL levels was followed by restoration of gonadal function in all patients with microprolactinomas, and in most patients with macroadenomas *(25,26)*. Moreover, the beneficial effects occurred more rapidly than with bromocriptine or quinagolide *(27)*. In patients treated with cabergoline, the percentage of immature germ cells was lowered and sperm viability, swollen tails, and penetration into bovine cervical mucus was increased significantly during the first 3 mo of treatment *(28)*. The recommended dosage of cabergoline for beginning therapy is 0.25 mg twice a week. The dosage may be increased up to 1–3 mg twice weekly in relation to the change in serum prolactin values. Dosage increases should occur every 4 wk. In addition, cabergoline may be effective in patients who are resistant to bromocriptine and quinagolide treatment *(27,29)*.

Surgery may be necessary in men who have not tolerated or have not responded to medical therapy, with invasive macroadenomas and visual field impairment with no immediate response to dopamine agonists, or in patients with complications, such as intratumoral hemorrhage or cerebrospinal fluid fistula *(16,22,28)*. A transsphenoidal approach is the preferred technique for microadenomas and most macroadenomas, whereas craniotomy is rarely necessary. Surgical success rates are highly dependent on the size of the tumor and the surgeon's experience and skill *(30)*. Pituitary adenomas are benign tumors, and the preservation or restoration of anterior pituitary function, including gonadal function, is an important goal of surgery *(31)*.

Because of the excellent therapeutic responses to medical therapy and surgery, radiotherapy is generally not considered as a primary treatment for prolactinomas, but is used for patients refractory to medical and surgical therapy. Hypopituitarism, including hypogonadism, is a frequent side effect after radiotherapy *(30)*.

In the uncommon case of hyperprolactinemia and hypogonadism induced by prolactinoma that is resistant or intolerant to medical therapy and with contraindications to surgery, gonadotropin therapy can be used to induce virilization and advance spermatogenesis sufficiently to achieve fertility *(32)*.

ACROMEGALY

Physiopathology of Hypogonadism

Acromegaly is a disease characterized by the excessive production of growth hormone (GH). More than 99% of cases of acromegaly result from a tumor of the pituitary gland secreting either GH or both GH and PRL. Gangliocytomas of the hypothalamus or pituitary and ectopic neuroendocrine tumors secreting GH-releasing hormone (GHRH) account for less than 1% *(33)*.

Hypogonadism has been reported in 49% to 70% of patients with acromegaly *(31,34)*. Secretion of PRL by the tumor, together with GH or stalk disruption by suprasellar growth, have been implicated in hypogonadism development *(35)*. However, Katznelson et al. *(35)* described low testosterone levels in 39% of men with somatotroph microadenomas, most of whom had normal PRL levels. Therefore, other factors may contribute to the pathogenesis of hypogonadism in acromegaly. GH lowers the level of sex hormone-binding globulin (SHBG), so that free testosterone levels should be measured. Hypogonadism occurs more often in patients with macroadenomas than in those with microadenomas *(34,35)* because of the tumor mass effect on surrounding normal tissue.

The primary factor mediating gonadal damage in acromegaly is GH excess. GH regulates testicular function, by stimulating the local production of insulin-like growth factor (IGF)-1, which modulates steroidogenesis and spermatogenesis. In fact, GH administration increases Leydig and Sertoli cell responses to FSH and LH *(36,37)*. However, high GH and IGF-1 levels induce severe testicular alterations and disrupt the hypothalamic–pituitary–testicular axis. Repeated administration of high doses of GH in dogs reduced testicular weight with germ cell degeneration and epithelial atrophy *(38)*. The extent of testicular damage is related to the severity of acromegaly. In fact, serum GH and IGF-1 levels correlate negatively with serum DHT levels *(see* Fig. 2). Several mechanisms have been proposed to explain these findings, including a change in androgen metabolism *(39)*, FSH and LH suppression by increased somatostatin tone, a decrease in the serum concentration of SHBG, and lactogenic effects of GH separate from those of PRL *(40–43)*. In addition, prostatic dysfunction leading to alterations of the seminal fluid may occur in acromegaly. In fact, GH/IGF-1 excess causes prostate enlargement with a high prevalence of prostatic abnormalities *(44,45)*.

Diagnosis

The symptoms of hypogonadism in men with acromegaly are similar to those of men with prolactinomas, including oligospermia and reduced sperm motility. These manifestations, like the specific acromegalic clinical features *(see* Table 2), progress slowly. Therefore, the diagnosis of acromegaly is often delayed for as many as 5 to 15 yr *(22)*.

The specific clinical manifestations of acromegaly are caused by excessive GH/IGF-1 secretion. In addition, pituitary tumor mass effects (headaches, hypopituitarism, and visual disturbances) are common, because of the high prevalence of macroadenomas (approx 75% of somatotroph adenomas) *(22,46)*.

An elevated random serum GH level is not absolutely necessary for the diagnosis of acromegaly. On the contrary, serum IGF-1 levels are invariably high in acromegaly. If IGF-1 is increased and the random GH level is normal, an oral glucose tolerance test (75 g) is used to establish the diagnosis. A normal response is a decrease in the serum GH level to less than 1 µg/L, but patients with acromegaly do not suppress normally, and 20% of patients have a paradoxical GH rise *(14,47)*.

After the clinical and endocrine diagnosis of acromegaly is made, radiological evaluation of the pituitary gland should be performed, preferably by MRI with gadolinium enhancement to localize and delineate the tumor from the surrounding tissues. GH-secreting tumors are larger than prolactinomas at the time of the radiographic evaluation, perhaps because of a later clinical presentation *(19)*.

Therapy

The treatment goals for men with hypogonadism secondary to acromegaly are the normalization of serum GH, IGF-1, and PRL levels when hyperprolactinemia is present, and the preservation and restoration of gonadotropin secretion and testicular function.

Trans-sphenoidal adenomectomy is the preferred treatment for GH-secreting tumors, inducing an endocrine remission in 80% of patients with microadenomas and 50% of macroadenomas in experienced centers *(22,48,49)*. It is likely that many cen-

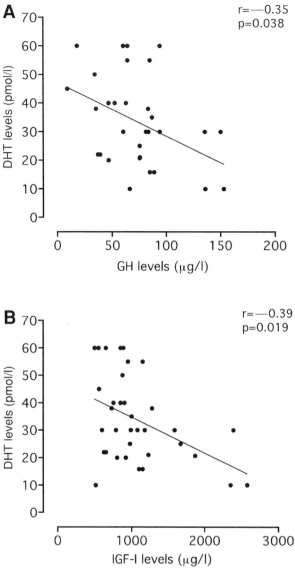

Fig. 2. Relationship of serum growth hormone (**A**) and insulin-like growth factor-1 (**B**) levels to serum dihydrotestosterone. (From ref. *53.*)

ters do not achieve these success rates, and this is a matter of concern. Surgery relieves the compression of adjacent structures, including the pituitary stalk and surrounding pituitary cells. If gonadotropin secretion is normal before surgery, gonadal function can be restored with a decrease in the serum GH concentration. Tominaga et al. *(31)* reported serum testosterone concentrations of less than 300 ng/dL in 14 of 20 patients (70%) with active acromegaly. Postoperatively, the serum GH level was normalized in 14 patients, whereas testosterone concentration normalized in 11 patients (79%), restoring gonadal function *(31).*

Table 2
Specific Clinical Features of Acromegaly

Recent acral growth
Prognathism and malocclusion
Frontal bossing
Widened spaces between the teeth
Increased breadth of the nose
Generalized visceromegaly
Cardiomyopathy
Hypertension
Osteoarthrosis
Kyphosis
Carpal tunnel syndrome
Proximal muscle weakness
Fatigue
Deep and resonant voice
Hyperhidrosis
Psychological disorders

Somatostatin analogs normalize IGF-1 levels in 60% to 70% of patients and achieve tumor shrinkage in approx 40% of patients. At present, long-acting analogs of somatostatin are available and improve compliance. Octreotide-LAR consists of octreotide incorporated into microspheres of a biodegradable polymer. It is injected intramuscularly at a dose of 10, 20, or 30 mg (every 4 wk). Slow-release lanreotide is a similar preparation, and is administered intramuscularly at a dose of 30 mg (every 1–2 wk) or 60 mg (every 4 wk). A new aqueous preparation of lanreotide (lanreotide autogel) was recently introduced. This preparation achieves the same results as slow-release lanreotide, but is longer acting. It is administered by deep subcutaneous injection at a dose of 120 mg (every 6–8 wk). Important side effects of somatostatin analogs are gallstone formation, which is generally silent; abdominal cramps, and decreased glucose tolerance *(50–52)*. It is interesting that short-term suppression of GH and IGF-1 levels after surgery or somatostatin analog therapy for 6 mo produces a significant increase in testosterone and DHT levels in most hypogonadal patients, with associated improvement in sperm number and motility *(53)*.

Dopamine agonists are less effective than are somatostatin analogs in normalizing IGF-1 levels (10–30% of patients) and reducing the tumor mass (<20% of cases). However, dopamine agonists are effective in GH-secreting tumors that also secrete prolactin or immunostain positive for prolactin. In addition, combined treatment with somatostatin analogs and dopamine agonists induces a greater suppression of IGF-1 compared with either drug alone and improves testicular function *(22,54)*.

Whereas somatostatin analogs and dopamine agonists bind to specific tumor receptors and inhibit GH secretion, a new drug, pegvisomant, blocks the ability of GH to stimulate IGF-1 production, the main mediator of the somatotropic actions of GH. Pegvisomant is a genetically manipulated analog of human GH that functions as a highly selective GH receptor antagonist, normalizing IGF-1 levels in approx 90% of patients with acromegaly *(55–57)*. However, there are no studies reporting the effects of GH antagonists on hypogonadism secondary to acromegaly at this time.

Radiation therapy should be considered for patients with contraindications to pituitary surgery or whose operation and/or medical treatment has failed. Radiotherapy induces a slow response and may damage normal pituitary tissues, leading to hypopituitarism and worsening hypogonadism in 50% of patients 10 yr after irradiation. It must be administered during over an extended period of approx 6 wk, and in multiple fractions to minimize radiation damage to surrounding structures (49).

CUSHING'S DISEASE

Physiopathology of Hypogonadism

Cushing's disease is characterized by chronic glucocorticoid excess secondary to hypersecretion of adrenocorticotropic hormone (ACTH) and other proopiomelanocortin peptides. It is commonly caused by a pituitary corticotroph adenoma. Hypogonadism is common in Cushing's disease. High levels of glucocorticoids decrease serum testosterone levels in men through several mechanisms (see Fig. 3). Excessive production of glucocorticoids may produce gonadotropin deficiency by acting at the pituitary and hypothalamic levels (58). Two regions of the mouse GnRH promoter (distal and proximal negative glucocorticoid response elements) regulate transcriptional repression by glucocorticoids. Glucocorticoid receptors induce glucocorticoid repression of GnRH gene transcription by their association within a multiprotein complex at the negative glucocorticoid response element (59). In addition, elevated glucocorticoid levels directly suppress testicular function, inducing apoptosis in Leydig cells (60), inhibiting LH receptor signal transduction, decreasing the oxidative activity of 11β-hydroxysteroid dehydrogenase, and impairing Leydig cell steroidogenesis (61).

Diagnosis

Since the description by Cushing at the beginning of the 20th century, it is well known that hypogonadism is common in active Cushing's disease (62).

Men have loss of libido, impotence, oligospermia, and histological damage to the testes. Basal LH and FSH levels are commonly decreased, the response to GnRH is impaired, and testosterone levels are low. However, hypogonadism occurs with other clinical features (see Table 3) secondary to chronically elevated cortisol production (47,63).

When Cushing's syndrome is suspected, initial laboratory testing to detect hypercortisolism includes measurement of 24-h urinary-free cortisol (UFC) excretion, and/or the 1-mg overnight dexamethasone suppression test (64). The sensitivity and specificity of the first test in detecting cortisol excess are 95% and 98%, respectively. Because of the difficulty in obtaining 24-h urine collection in many outpatients, some physicians use the 1-mg overnight dexamethasone suppression test (sensitivity 98% and specificity 80%). A newer diagnostic approach is the late-night (11 PM) salivary cortisol determination (65). In fact, cortisol in the saliva is highly stable and correlated with free serum or plasma cortisol levels and is independent of the rate of the saliva flow (65).

Once the diagnosis of Cushing's syndrome is established, the source of the excess cortisol production must be determined. The ACTH plasma level in the late afternoon is useful in identifying the ACTH-dependent pathologic state in almost half of cases. At this time of day, plasma ACTH levels exceed 10 ng/L in Cushing's disease, whereas

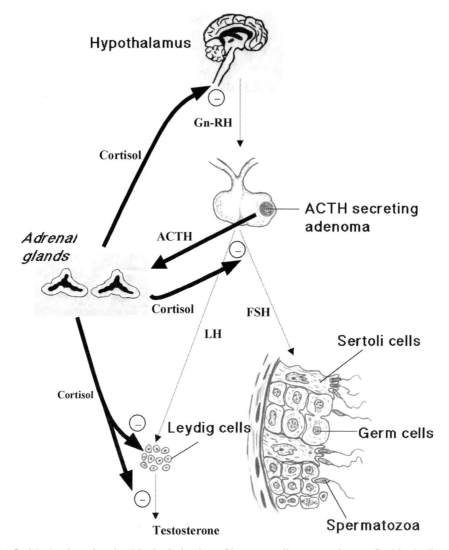

Fig. 3. Mechanisms involved in the induction of hypogonadism secondary to Cushing's disease.

plasma ACTH levels are generally suppressed in Cushing's syndrome secondary to adrenal disease *(66)*. The standard high-dose dexamethasone test (8 mg) and the corticotropin-releasing hormone (CRH) test are performed to obtain a clearer differential diagnosis. In Cushing's disease, serum cortisol levels and 24-h UFC excretion are suppressed after the 8-mg dexamethasone test and ACTH levels respond to CRH stimulation. The combination of these two tests may identify 60–80% of patients with Cushing's disease *(66)*.

Pituitary ACTH-secreting adenomas are most often microadenomas with a diameter less than 5 mm in 45% of cases, and only 10–20% of patients with Cushing's disease have a macroadenoma *(67)*. Therefore, pituitary MRI is often normal in patients with corticotropinomas. However, MRI of the pituitary is required in all patients with ACTH-dependent Cushing's syndrome. MRI should be performed with thin overlap-

Table 3
Clinical Features of Cushing's Syndrome

Centripetal obesity
Buffalo hump
Moon face
Facial plethora
Purple striae
Skin thinning
Easy bruising
Acne, oily skin
Skin infections
Proximal myopathy
Lethargy
Psychiatric disturbances
Hypertension
Backache, vertebral collapse, and fracture
Polydipsia and polyuria
Renal calculi
Hyperpigmentation
Abdominal pain

ping sections and high field strength (1.5 tesla) magnets *(68)*. In the absence of a detectable pituitary tumor, bilateral inferior petrosal venous sinus and peripheral vein catheterization with simultaneous collection of samples for measurement of ACTH should be performed to establish the diagnosis of Cushing's disease, as well as identify the location of ACTH production *(69,70)*. Stimulation with CRH, together with bilateral and simultaneous sampling, increases the sensitivity of this procedure *(65,71)*.

Therapy

The hypogonadotropic hypogonadism that is characteristic of male Cushing's disease is a reversible phenomenon. In fact, cure of hypercortisolism restores the decreased plasma testosterone and FSH and LH levels to normal and improves sexual and gonadal disturbances *(58,72,73)*.

Selective trans-sphenoidal adenomectomy after accurate preoperative localization of the corticotroph adenoma represents the treatment of choice for Cushing's disease. In experienced hands, a cure rate of 80–90% may be expected in microadenomas. However, the cure rate decreases to 50% with macroadenomas *(63,67)*. A trans-sphenoidal approach was also successfully used in ACTH-producing adenomas located in the pituitary stalk *(74)*.

Patients who are unresponsive to surgical treatment or those in whom surgery is deemed inappropriate (large invasive tumors or high surgical risk) are referred for pituitary irradiation with adjunctive medical therapy, and/or bilateral adrenalectomy. Conventional radiotherapy is given in 25 fractional doses throughout 35 d, for a total dose of 4500 cGy (rad) using a three-field technique. This strategy may cure up to 15% of patients after several years, but it can lead to hypopituitarism and worsening hypogonadism *(14,68)*.

Medical therapy is adjunctive in Cushing's disease. It is suitable for patients who are undergoing surgery, in those treated with radiotherapy to achieve early biochemical remission, and whenever definitive treatment must be delayed *(75)*. Current medical therapies include drugs to decrease ACTH secretion, inhibit corticosteroid synthesis, or block their peripheral actions. The first class of drugs (serotonin antagonists, dopamine agonists, γ-aminobutyric acid [GABA]-agonists and somatostatin analogs) inhibit ACTH release. However, few cases so treated have achieved permanent remission *(75)*. The second group of drugs includes inhibitors of steroidogenesis (mitotane, metyrapone, aminoglutethimide, and ketoconazole). These drugs have the advantage of being rapidly effective in most cases. However, the mechanism(s) of action has little selectivity, and extra-adrenal effects are likely to occur. Ketoconazole inhibits various cytochrome P450 enzymes, including C17–20 lyase involved in the synthesis of sex steroids. Thus, the drug not only lowers cortisol levels but also decreases testosterone levels such that gynecomastia, impotence, loss of libido, and oligospermia could occur *(71)*. The third class of drugs is represented by the glucocorticoid antagonist (mifepristone). Although a potentially important therapy, mifepristone has been used to treat only a few patients, and further clinical studies are needed to assess its long-term effectiveness and safety *(75)*. A few studies reported the efficacy of cabergoline treatment in patients with Cushing's disease and Nelson's syndrome. However, only a limited number of case reports have been published *(76,77)*.

Finally, bilateral adrenalectomy is reserved for cases in which other treatment modalities have failed. However, the risk for Nelson's syndrome is high with this approach *(14)*.

NONFUNCTIONING PITUITARY ADENOMAS

Physiopathology of Hypogonadism

Clinically nonfunctioning pituitary adenomas (NFPAs) represent approx 25–30% of pituitary tumors and are the most commonly encountered macroadenomas *(78–80)*. Hypogonadism is present in approximately half of the patients with NFPA, 50% of whom have mild hyperprolactinemia *(31)*, reflecting stalk compression that might contribute to impaired gonadal function.

The majority of nonfunctional tumors are inefficiently secreting rather than nonsecreting. They usually synthesize and immunostain for FSH and/or LH and/or free α-subunits and β-subunits. The gonadal dysfunction in males with NFPA is primarily related to intrasellar expansion of the tumor with compression of residual glandular tissue *(31)*. In fact, NFPAs usually are macroadenomas, causing hypopituitarism by both direct compression of the portal vessels that limits delivery of hypothalamic releasing factors and focal ischemic necrosis of the normal pituitary tissue. LH secretion is impaired in approx 53% of NFPAs *(78,81,82)*. However, disruption of ACTH, thyroid-stimulating hormone (TSH), and GH secretion may further inhibit gonadal function. In fact, corticotropin releasing factor (CRF)/ACTH/cortisol, thyroid hormones, and GH/IGF-1 modulate spermatogenesis and steroidogenesis.

Diagnosis

The majority of NFPAs are diagnosed incidentally or as a result of the mass effect (headache, visual disturbances, and neurological symptoms). Less often, deficient pitu-

itary hormone secretion, including gonadotropin deficiency, bring the patient to medical attention. These tumors can attain considerable size before manifesting clinically.
A mild or moderate increase in the PRL level is common, but this increase is disproportionate to the tumor dimensions. A complete endocrine evaluation, including measurement of FSH, LH, testosterone, TSH, Free Thyroxine (FT)4, ACTH, cortisol, GH,
and IGF-1, as well as prolactin, should be performed to exclude hypopituitarism. MRI
with gadolinium enhancement and CT with intravenous contrast represent the best way
to detect a pituitary tumor *(78–80)*.

Therapy

Trans-sphenoidal resection of the adenoma is the preferred and most effective treatment for symptomatic NFPA, because it may improve visual field defects and permits
recovery of pituitary function *(83)*. A two-stage procedure, craniotomy followed by
trans-sphenoidal resection, is often used in patients with extremely large tumors. More
than 80% of patients with microadenomas are cured by surgery. On the other hand,
only 15–30% of macroadenomas are completely cured. In hypogonadism, patients with
NFPAs less than 40 mm in size may experience a restoration of gonadal function *(31)*.
In these patients, the normal pituitary gland is often not destroyed, and its ability to
secrete gonadotropin is regained after decompression. In NFPAs larger than 40 mm,
surgery may further impair hypogonadism. In fact, with these tumors, it is common to
observe a decrease in testosterone levels after surgery. This reflects the difficulty in preserving or restoring anterior pituitary function in patients with large tumors *(31)*.

However, because of their large size, surgery alone is often not curative, and pituitary
irradiation is recommended for patients who have residual tumor after surgery *(80)*.

Somatostatin and dopamine receptors have been identified in some NFPAs. This
suggests that somatostatin analogs or dopamine agonists can be useful to treat refractory NFPA. However, these drugs benefit only a minority of patients, and additional
studies are needed to investigate whether subgroups of patients with NFPA will
respond to medical therapy *(84,85)*.

Gonadotropin or GnRH therapy is indicated if the patient desires spermatogenesis
and fertility (*see* Chapter 19). If fertility is not the requested outcome, testosterone is
administered to stimulate virilization, improve sexual function, and maintain bone and
muscle mass (*see* Chapter 18). In patients with multiple pituitary hormone deficiencies,
replacement therapy of all deficient hormones is required for complete improvement of
gonadal function. It is worth noting that cortisol therapy (10–20 mg hydrocortisone in
the early morning and 5–10 mg in the afternoon or 25–37.5 mg cortisone acetate in the
early morning and 12.5–25 mg in the afternoon) should be replaced first, followed by
thyroxine (1–2 µg/kg/d) and sex steroids once the patient's condition has stabilized.
This is important, because thyroxine therapy can exacerbate the features of glucocorticoid deficiency. If indicated, GH (5–10 µg/kg/d) can be administered as well *(86)*.

NONPITUITARY SELLAR AND PARASELLAR TUMORS

Physiopathology of Hypogonadism

Nonpituitary intrasellar and parasellar tumors include craniopharyngioma, Rathke's
cleft cyst, epidermoid, infundibuloma, chordoma, lipoma, colloid cyst, germinoma,
dermoid, teratoma, dysgerminoma, ectopic pinealoma, glioma, oligodendroglioma,

ependymoma, astrocytoma, meningioma, enchondroma, metastatic tumors, and lymphoma. These masses interfere with GnRH synthesis and secretion or directly impair FSH and LH production, inducing hypogonadotropic hypogonadism. In addition, the modest hyperprolactinemia that occurs secondary to hypothalamic stalk compression could impair gonadal function *(87,88)*.

Diagnosis

Many patients with nonpituitary sellar and suprasellar tumors have symptoms of anterior pituitary hormone failure. The most common hormone insufficiency is gonadotropin deficiency. Hypogonadism is diagnosed by a decrease in serum FSH, LH, and testosterone levels. Hyperprolactinemia is often detected, particularly in patients with craniopharyngiomas, meningiomas, or cystic lesions *(87)*.

Visual field impairment and decreased visual acuity are frequent events, because of the proximity of the optic nerves, chiasm, and optic tracts to the sella turcica. The tendency of these tumors to infiltrate parasellar structures causes cranial neuropathy. Tumors that are obstructing cerebrospinal fluid (CSF) flow (craniopharyngioma, meningioma, and germinoma) increase intracranial pressure. This event is characterized by visual impairment and headaches. Masses compressing the deep subfrontal region of the brain may induce personality changes and dementia. In addition, these lesions may impair hypothalamic function and disrupt appetite control, causing polyphagia and massive obesity or starvation *(87–89)*.

Although it is difficult to reach a specific preoperative diagnosis on MRI, many lesions have characteristic findings that are useful in the differential diagnosis. For example, calcifications are suggestive of craniopharyngiomas, meningiomas, chordomas, teratomas, and gliomas. Erosion of the sella floor is frequently observed in meningiomas of the middle fossa and Rathke's cleft cyst *(87)*.

Therapy

Gonadal impairment secondary to nonpituitary intrasellar and parasellar masses may recover after treatment of the lesion. The choice of treatment depends on the nature of the disease. However, surgery represents the first option in most cases. Surgical treatment generally involves trans-sphenoidal decompression of the mass, when possible, attempting to limit damage and restore normal function of the pituitary gland. Contraindications to the trans-sphenoidal approach include dumb-bell tumors and inaccessible extrasellar extension *(18)*.

Radiotherapy is recommended for residual tumor after surgery and for brain metastases. Medical therapy is not generally performed with dysgerminomas or metastatic lesions that require radiotherapy and chemotherapy, respectively, and hamartomas producing GnRH that respond to treatment with GnRH analogs. Long-acting GnRH analogs suppress gonadotropin secretion but do not affect the tumor. However, GnRH analogs may be the logical therapeutic option if the hamartoma does not cause other complications related to mass effects, because surgery may not be curative or may result in extensive complications, including fatality *(89)*.

When hypogonadism persists after surgical treatment or remains after conventional treatment, androgen replacement therapy is used to restore physiologic serum concentrations of testosterone. If fertility is desired, Leydig cell function is stimulated by the

Table 4
Nontumorous Causes of Acquired
Hypogonadotropic Hypogonadism

Pituitary apoplexy
Empty sella syndrome
Aneurysm
Pituitary abscess
Tuberculosis
Sarcoidosis
Giant cell granuloma
Lymphocitic hypophysitis
Histiocytosis X
Hemochromatosis
Arachnoid cyst
Mucocele
Postsurgery/irradiation
Head trauma

administration of hCG. Spermatogenesis may be restored; however, human follicle-stimulating hormone (hFSH) is sometimes necessary as well *(19)*. In patients with hypopituitarism, adequate replacement therapy further improves gonadal function.

NONTUMOROUS CAUSES OF ACQUIRED HYPOGONADOTROPIC HYPOGONADISM

Physiopathology of Hypogonadism

Several nonneoplastic diseases (*see* Table 4) may induce hypogonadotropic hypogonadism *(19)*. In these disorders, hypogonadism primarily results from gonadotropin deficiency secondary to hypothalamic–pituitary damage. In addition, GH/IGF-1, thyroid hormone, and CRF/ACTH/cortisol play a permissive role in the spermatogenesis and testosterone production regulation. In fact, these hormones regulate the gonadotrophin responsiveness of Leydig and Sertoli cells. Therefore, deficiency of all or some anterior pituitary hormones, together with the increase in PRL, may induce hypogonadism.

Pituitary apoplexy results in anterior pituitary failure secondary to hemorrhagic or ischemic infarction. In men, hemorrhage usually occurs into a pituitary tumor, whereas ischemia may involve a normal pituitary gland in the setting of increased intracranial pressure or during anticoagulation therapy. Hormone deficiencies after apoplexy include GH (88%), gonadotropins (58–76%), ACTH (66%), TSH (42–53%), and PRL (67–100%) *(90)*.

Empty sella is defined as a sella that is completely or partially filled by CSF, owing to arachnoid herniation into the pituitary fossa. This herniation remodels and enlarges the bony sella and flattens the pituitary gland against the sella floor. Empty sella is usually an incidental anatomical finding, and functional pituitary damage is infrequent, particularly in primary empty sella. That patients are usually asymptomatic derives from the large functional reserve of the adenohypophysis. However, hypogonadism is not rare, and hyperprolactinemia occurs in approx 15% of cases *(90)*.

Aneurysms of the cavernous sinus, as well as infectious (bacterial or fungal abscesses, tuberculosis, and toxoplasmosis) and inflammatory processes (sarcoidosis, giant cell granuloma, lymphocytic hypophysitis, and histiocytosis X) can mimic a pituitary adenoma, causing mass effect and hypothalamic-hypophyseal endocrine dysfunction secondary to infiltration of normal tissue (91).

Arachnoid cyst is a diverticulum of the arachnoidal membrane of Liliequist. Of these cysts, 15% occur in the sellar and parasellar regions. This mass may compress the hypothalamic–pituitary unit, inducing endocrine disorders, including hypogonadism-producing impotence or low libido (88).

Mucoceles are slowly expanding, mucous-filled cystic lesions that arise in the paranasal sinuses. These cysts result from the accumulation and retention of mucous secretions in a sinus secondary to the occlusion of the ostium draining the sinus. Sphenoid mucocele with suprasellar extension can also increase prolactin levels by compressing the pituitary stalk (92).

Radiation of the head for treatment of primary central nervous system (CNS) tumors or brain metastases may cause the gradual onset of hypothalamic-pituitary failure. The most frequent endocrine abnormalities after cranial radiotherapy are hypothyroidism (65%), hypogonadism (61%), and mild hyperprolactinemia (50%). Although the mechanism of radiation damage to the hypothalamus and pituitary gland is not known, it must involve a direct injury to the secreting cells or to the stroma or its microvasculature or damage the vascular channels that transfer the hypothalamic hormones to the pituitary (93).

Head trauma may induce hypogonadism. This is a common event. Lee et al. observed hypotestosteronemia in 67% of patients within 1 wk of severe traumatic brain injury (94). The gonadotropins are the most fragile hormones (95), with deficiency occurring in almost 100% of cases with post-head trauma hypopituarism. ACTH, TSH, and GH deficiency occur in 53%, 44%, and 24% of cases, respectively. In addition, stalk lesions may increase PRL levels in approx 50% of the cases, further worsening gonadal function (96).

Diagnosis

These diseases are characterized by extensive damage to pituitary function. Therefore, hypogonadism is rarely reported as an isolated manifestation but, instead, is frequently associated with hypopituarism and diabetes insipidus. In addition, headache, vomiting, ophthalmoplegia, and visual loss occur with acute onset in pituitary apoplexy or head trauma and occur progressively in the empty sella syndrome, infectious and inflammatory processes, mucocele, arachnoid cyst, giant cell granuloma, and echinococcal cystis (90).

Considering the importance of hypopituitarism in hypogonadism induction, anterior pituitary function testing (GnRH stimulation to assess gonadotroph function by measuring FSH and LH, insulin tolerance testing to assess corticotroph and somatotroph secretion by measuring serum cortisol and GH levels, and TRH stimulation test to assess TSH levels), blood PRL profile, as well as measurement of the serum testosterone level and the semen analyses, are mandatory in this group of patients (90).

Currently, MRI is an essential tool in the differential diagnosis of sellar masses and in the evaluation of head trauma. However, biopsy and histology are often necessary to confirm the diagnosis (19).

Therapy

The treatment goals in this group of patients with hypogonadism are as follow: (1) reduce or eliminate the mass effects of the lesion; (2) correct hormonal deficiencies, including those that impair gonadal function; and (3) preserve residual pituitary function. The specific treatments for the various diseases discussed are beyond the scope of this chapter. However, most lesions are initially treated surgically to eliminate the mass effects. Androgen replacement therapy is used to correct hypogonadism. When fertility is desired, treatment with exogenous gonadotropins (hCG ± hFSH) is generally successful. Finally, when panhypopituarism is present, hormonal replacement therapy is mandatory.

REFERENCES

1. Griffin JE, Wilson JD. Disorders of the testes and the male reproductive tract. In: Wilsom JD, Foster DW, Kronenberg HM, Larsen PD eds. Williams Textbook of Endocrinology, 9th ed. WB Saunders Company, Philadelphia, 1998, pp. 819–875.
2. Lin T, Clark R. Disorders of male reproductive function. In: Moore WT, Eastman RC, eds. Diagnostic Endocrinology, 2nd ed., St. Louis: Mosby, 1996, pp. 339–371.
3. Shimon I, Melmed S. Management of pituitary tumors. Ann Intern Med 1998;129:472–483.
4. Cheung CY. Prolactin suppresses luteinizing hormone secretion and pituitary responsiveness to luteinizing hormone-releasing hormone by a direct action at the anterior pituitary. Endocrinology 1983;113:632–638.
5. Bouchard P, Lagoguey M, Brailly S, Schaison G. Gonadotropin-releasing hormone pulsatile administration restores luteinizing hormone pulsatility and normal testosterone levels in males with hyperprolactinemia. J Clin Endocrinol Metab 1985;60:258–262.
6. Hondo E, Kurohmaru M, Sakai S, Ogawa K, Hayashi Y. Prolactin receptor expression in rat spermatogenic cells. Biol Reprod 1995;52:1284–1290.
7. Winters SJ. Diurnal rhythm of testosterone and luteinizing hormone in hypogonadal men. J Androl 1991;12:185–190.
8. Manandhar MS, Thomas JA. Effect of prolactin on the metabolism of androgens by the rat ventral prostate gland in vitro. Invest Urol 1976;14:20–22.
9. Waeber C, Reymond O, Reymond M, Lemarchand-Beraud T. Effects of hyper- and hypoprolactinemia on gonadotropin secretion, rat testicular luteinizing hormone/human chorionic gonadotropin receptors and testosterone production by isolated Leydig cells. Biol Reprod 1983;28:167–177.
10. Franks S, Jacobs HS, Martin N, Nabarro JD. Hyperprolactinemia and impotence. Clin Endocrinol 1978;8:277–287.
11. Magrini B, Ebiner JR, Burckhardt P, Felber JP. Study on the relationship between plasma prolactin and androgen metabolism in man. J Clin Endocrinol Metab 1976;43:944–947.
12. Pinzone JJ, Katznelson L, Danila DC, Pauler DK, Miller CS, Klibanski A. Primary medical therapy of micro- and macroprolactinomas in men. J Clin Endocrinol Metab 2000;85:3053–3057.
13. Kelly PA, Binart N, Lucas B, Bouchard B, Goffin V. Implications of multiple phenotypes observed in prolactin receptor knockout mice. Front Neuroendocrinol 2001;22:140–145.
14. Shimon I, Melmed S. Diagnosis and treatment of pituitary disease. Psycother Psychosom 1998;67:119–124.
15. Conner P, Fried G. Hyperprolactinemia: etiology, diagnosis and treatment alternatives. Acta Obstet Gynecol Scand 1998;77:249–262.
16. Biller BMK, Luciano A. Guideliness for the diagnosis and treatment of hyperprolactinemia. J Reprod Med 1999;44(suppl):1075–1084.
17. Winters SJ, Troen P. Altered pulsatile secretion of luteinizing hormone in hyponadal men with hyperprolactinemia. Clin Endocrinol 1984;21:257–263.
18. Anderson JR, Antoun N, Burnet N, et al. Neurology of the pituitary gland. J Neurol Neurosurg Psychiatry 1999;66:703–721.
19. FitzPatrick M, Tarataglino L, Hollander MD, Zimmerman RA, Flanders AE. Imaging of sellar and parasellar pathology. Radiol Clin North Am 1999;37:101–121.

20. Naidich MJ, Russel EJ. Current approach to imaging of the sellar region and pituitary. Endocrinol Metab Clin North Am 1999;28:45–79.
21. Colao A, di Sarno A, Pivonello R, di Somma C, Lombardi G. Dopamine receptor agonists for treating prolactinomas. Expert Opin Investig Drugs 2002;11:787–800.
22. Colao A, Lombardi G. Growth hormone and prolactin excess. Lancet 1998;352:1455–1461.
23. Colao A, De Rosa M, Sarnacchiaro F, et al. Chronic treatment with CV 205–502 restores the gonadal function in hyperprolactinemic males. Eur J Endocrinol 1996;135:548–552.
24. Verhelst J, Abs R, Maiter D, et al. Cabergoline in the treatment of hyperprolactinemia: a study in 455 patients. J Clin Endocrinol Metab 1999;84:2518–2522.
25. Ferrari CI, Abs R, Bevan JS, et al. Treatment of macroprolactinomas with cabergoline: a study of 85 patients. Clin Endocrinol 1997;46:409–412.
26. Cannavò S, Curtò L, Squadrito S, Almoto B, Vieni A, Trimarchi F. Cabergoline: a first-choice treatment in patients with previously untreated prolactin-secreting pituitary adenoma. J Endocrinol Invest 1999;22:354–359.
27. De Rosa M, Colao A, Di Sarno A, et al. Cabergoline treatment rapidly improves gonadal function in hyperprolactinemic males: a comparison with bromocriptine. Eur J Endocrinol 1998;138:286–293.
28. Colao A, Annunziato L, Lombardi G. Treatment of prolactinomas. Ann Med 1998;30:452–459.
29. Colao A, Di Sarno AM, Sarnacchiaro F, et al. Prolactinomas resistant to standard dopamine agonists respond to chronic cabergoline treatment. J Clin Endocrinol Metab 1997;82:876–883.
30. Molitch ME. Medical treatment of prolactinomas. Endocrinol Metab Clin North Am 1999;28:143–169.
31. Tominaga A, Uozumi T, Arita K, et al. Effects of surgery on testosterone secretion in male patients with pituitary adenomas. Endocr J 1996;43:307–312.
32. Isurugi K, Kajiwara T, Hosaka Y, Minowada S. Successful gonadotrophin treatment of hypogonadism in postoperative patients with macroprolactinoma and persistent hyperprolactinaemia. Int J Androl 1993;16:306–310.
33. Wass JA, Sheppard MC. New treatments for acromegaly. J Royal Coll Physic London 1998;32:113–117.
34. Molitch ME. Pathologic hyperprolactinemia. Endocrinol Metab Clin North Am 1992;21:877–901.
35. Katznelson L, Kleinberg D, Vance ML, et al. Hypogonadism in patients with acromegaly: data from the multi-centre acromegaly registry pilot study. Clin Endocrinol 2001;54:183–188.
36. Bartlett JMS, Charlton HM, Robinson IC, Nieschlag E. Pubertal development and testicular function in the male GH-deficient rat. J Endocrinol 1990;126:193–201.
37. Spiteri-Grech J, Barlett JMS, Nieschlag E. Regulation of testicular insulin-like growth factor-I in pubertal growth hormone-deficient male rats. J Endocrinol 1991;131:279–285.
38. Sjogren I, Joussou M, Madej A, Johansson HE, Ploen L. Effects of very high doses of human growth hormone (hGH) on the male reproductive system in the dog. Andrologia 1998;30:37–42.
39. Roellsema F, Moblenaar AJ, Frolich M. The influence of bromocriptine and transsphenoidal surgery on urinary androgen metabolic excretion in acromegaly. Acta Endocrinol 1984;107:302–311.
40. Zweirska-Korczala K, Ostrowska Z, Zych F, Buntner B. The levels of pituitary-testicular axis hormones and SHBG in active acromegaly following bromocriptine treatment. Endocr Regul 1991;25:211–216.
41. Schwander J, Hauri C, Zapf J, Froesch E. Synthesis and secretion of insulin-like growth factor and its binding protein by the perfused rat liver; dependence on growth hormone status. Endocrinology 1983;113:297–305.
42. Lindstedt G, Lindberg P, Hammond G, Vihko R. Sex hormone binding globulin-still many questions. Scand J Clin Lab Invest 1985;45:1–6.
43. Kleinberg DL, Todd J. Evidence that human growth hormone is a potent lactogen in primates. J Clin Endocrinol Metab 1980;51:1009–1013.
44. Colao A, Marzullo P, Spiezia S, et al. Effect of growth hormone (GH) and insulin-like growth factor-1 on prostate disease: an ultrasonographic and endocrine study in acromegaly, GH deficiency and healthy subjects. J Clin Endocrinol Metab 1999;84:1986–1991.
45. Colao A, Marzullo P, Ferone D, et al. Prostate hyperplasia: an unknown feature of acromegaly. J Clin Endocrinol Metab 1998;83:775–779.
46. Duncan E, Wass AH. Investigation protocol: acromegaly and its investigation. Clin Endocrinol 1999;50:285–293.
47. Veznedaroglu E, Armonda RA, Andrews DW. Diagnosis and therapy for pituitary tumors. Curr Opin Oncol 1999;11:27–31.
48. Newman CB. Medical therapy for acromegaly. Endocrinol Metab Clin North Am 1999;28:171–190.

49. Ben-Shlomo A, Melmed A. Acromegaly. Endocrinol Metab Clin North Am 2001;30:565–583.
50. Caron P, Morange-Ramos I, Cogne M, Jaquet P. Three year follow-up of acromegalic patients treated with intramuscular slow-release lanreotide. J Clin Endocrinol Metab 1997;82:18–22.
51. Newman CB, Melmed S, Snyder PJ, et al. Safety and efficacy of long-term octreotide therapy of acromegaly: results of a multicenter trial in 103 patients—a clinical research center study. J Clin Endocrinol Metab 1995;80:2768–2775.
52. Flogstad AK, Halse J, Bakke S, Lancranjan I, Bruns C, Jervell J. Sandostatin LAR in acromegalic patients: long-term treatment. J Clin Endocrinol Metab 1997;82:23–28.
53. Colao A, De Rosa M, Pivonello R, et al. Short-term suppression of GH and IGF-1 levels improves gonadal function and sperm parameters in men with acromegaly. J Clin Endocrinol Metab 2002;87:4193–4197.
54. Colao A, Ferone D, Marzullo P, et al. Effect of different dopaminergic agents in the treatment of acromegaly. J Clin Endocrinol Metab 1997;82:518–523.
55. Van der Lely AJ, Hutson RK, Trainer PJ, et al. Long-term treatment of acromegaly with pegvisomant, a growth hormone receptor antagonist. Lancet 2001;358:1754–1759.
56. Trainer P, Drake W, Katznelson L, et al. Treatment of acromegaly with growth hormone-receptor antagonist pegvisomant. N Engl J Med 2000;342:1171–1177.
57. Herman-Bonert VS, Zib K, Scarlett JA, Melmed S. Growth hormone receptor antagonist therapy in acromegalic patients resistant to somatostatin analogs. J Clin Endocrinol Metab 2000;85:2958–2961.
58. Luton JP, Thieblot P, Valcke JC, Mahoudeau JA, Bricaire H. Reversible gonadotropin deficiency in male Cushing's disease. J Clin Endocrinol Metab 1977;45:488–495.
59. Chandran UR, Attardi B, Friedman R, Zheng ZW, Roberts JL, Defranco DB. Glucocorticoid repression of the mouse gonadotropin-releasing hormone gene is mediated by promoter elements that are recognized by heteromeric complexes containing glucocorticoid receptor. J Biol Chem 1996;271:20412–20420.
60. Gao HB, Tong MH, Hu YQ, Guo QS, Ge R, Hardy MP. Glucocorticoid induces apoptosis in rat Leydig cells. Endocrinology 2002;143:130–138.
61. Sankar BR, Maran RR, Sudha S, Govindarajulu P, Balasubramanian K. Chronic corticosterone treatment impairs Leydig cell 11β-hydroxysteroid dehydrogenase activity and LH-stimulated testosterone production. Horm Metab Res 2000;32:142–146.
62. Cushing H. The basophil adenomas of the pituitary body and their clinical manifestations. Bull Johns Hopkins Hosp 1932;137:50–54.
63. Katz J, Bouloux PMG. Cushing's: how to make the diagnosis. Practitioner 1999;243:118–123.
64. Contreras LN, Hane S, Tyrrell JB. Urinary cortisol in the assessment of pituitary-adrenal function: utility of 24-hour and spot determination. J Clin Endocrinol Metab 1986;62:965–969.
65. Findling JW, Raff H. Newer diagnostic techniques and problems in Cushing's disease. Endocrinol Metab Clin North Am 1999;28:191–210.
66. Findling JW. Diagnosis and differential diagnosis of Cushing's syndrome. Meet The Professor—Endo 2002. San Francisco, June 19–22, 2002, pp. 87–94.
67. Invitti C, Pecori Giraldi F, De Martin M, Cavagnini F, The Study Group of the Italian Society of Endocrinology on the Pathophysiology of the Hypothalamic-Pituitary-Adrenal axis. Diagnosis and management of Cushing's syndrome results of an Italian multicentre study. J Clin Endocrinol Metab 1999;84:440–448.
68. Tsigos C, Kamilaris TC, Chrousos GP. Adrenal disease. In: Moore WT, Eastman RC, eds. Diagnostic Endocrinology, 2nd ed., St. Louis: Mosby, 1996, pp. 125–156.
69. Colao A, Faggiano A, Pivonello R, Giraldi FP, Cavagnini F, Lombardi G. Study Group of the Italian Endocrinology Society on the Pathophysiology of the Hypothalamic-Pituitary-Adrenal Axis. Inferior petrosal sinus sampling in the differential diagnosis of Cushing's syndrome: results of an Italian multicenter study. Eur J Endocrinol 2001;144:499–507.
70. Colao A, Merola B, Tripodi FS, et al. Simultaneous and bilateral inferior petrosal sinus sampling for the diagnosis of Cushing's syndrome: comparison of multihormonal assay, baseline multiple sampling and ACTH-releasing hormone test. Horm Res 1993;40:209–216.
71. Zarrilli L, Colao A, Merola B, et al. Corticotropin-releasing hormone test: improvement of the diagnostic accuracy of simultaneous and bilateral inferior petrosal sinus sampling in patients with Cushing syndrome. World J Surg 1995;19:150–153.
72. McKenna TJ, Lorber D, Lacroix A, Rabin D. Testicular activity in Cushing's disease. Acta Endocrinol (Copenh) 1979;91:501–510.

73. Smals AG, Kloppenborg PW, Benraad TJ. Plasma testosterone profiles in Cushing's syndrome. J Clin Endocrinol Metab 1977;45:240–245.

74. Mason RB, Nieman LK, Doppman JL, Oldfield EH. Selective excision of adenomas originating in or extending into the pituitary stalk with preservation of pituitary function. J Neurosurg 1997;87:343–351.

75. Sonino N, Boscaro M. Medical therapy for Cushing's disease. Endocrinol Metab Clin North Am 1999;28:211–222.

76. Colao A, Lombardi G, Annunziato L. Cabergoline. Expert Opin Pharmacother 2000;1:555–574.

77. Pivonello R, Faggiano A, Di Salle F, Filippella M, Lombardi G, Colao A. Complete remission of Nelson's syndrome after 1 year treatment with cabergoline. J Endocrinol Invest 1999;22:860–865.

78. Klibanski A. Nonsecreting pituitary tumors. Endocrinol Metab Clin North Am 1987;16:793–804.

79. Katznelson L, Alexander JM, Klibanski A. Clinical review 45. Clinically nonfunctioning pituitary adenomas. J Clin Endocrinol Metab 1993;76:1089–1094.

80. Snyder PJ. Clinically nonfunctioning pituitary adenomas. Endocrinol Metab Clin North Am 1993;22:163–175.

81. Arafah BM. Reversible hypopituarism in patients with large nonfunctioning pituitary adenomas. J Clin Endocrinol Metab 1986;62:1173–1179.

82. Arafah BM, Kailani SH, Nekl KE, Gold RS, Selman WR. Immediate recovery of pituitary function after transphenoidal resection of pituitary macroadenomas. J Clin Endocrinol Metab 1994;79:348–354.

83. Ebersold MJ, Quast LM, Laws ERjr, Scheithauer B, Randall RV. Long-term results in transsphenoidal removal of nonfunctioning pituitary adenomas. J Neurosurg 1986;334:246–254.

84. Nobels FRE, de Herder WW, van den Brink WM, et al. Long-term treatment with the dopamine agonist quinagolide of patients with clinically non-functioning pituitary adenoma. Eur J Endocrinol 2000;143:615–621.

85. Colao A, Ferone D, Lastoria S, et al. Hormone levels and tumor size response to quinagolide and cabergoline in patients with prolactin-secreting and clinically non-functioning pituitary adenomas: predictive value of pituitary scintigraphy with ^{123}I-methoxybenzamide. Clin Endocrinol 2000;52:437–445.

86. Lamberts SWJ, de Herder WW, van der Lely AJ. Pituitary insufficiency. Lancet 1998;352:127–134.

87. Freda PU, Post KD. Differential diagnosis of sellar masses. Endocrinol Metab Clin North Am 1999;28:81–117.

88. Shin JL, Asa SL, Woodhouse LJ, Smyth HS, Ezzat S. Cystic lesions of the pituitary: clinicopathological features distinguishing craniopharyngioma, Rathke's cleft cyst, and arachnoid cyst. J Clin Endocrinol Metab 1999;84:3972–3982.

89. Molitch ME. Sellar masses. Meet the Professor—Endo 2002. San Francisco, June 19–22, 2002, pp. 272–277.

90. Thorner MO, Lee Vance M, Laws ER, Howath E, Kovacs K. The anterior pituitary. In: Wilsom JD, Foster DW, Kronenberg HM, Larsen PD, eds. Williams Textbook of Endocrinology, 9th ed. WB Saunders Company, Philadelphia, 1998, pp. 249–340.

91. Bloom DL. Mucocle of the maxillary and sphenoidal sinuses. Radiology 1965;85:1103–1110.

92. Herzog KM, Tubbs RR. Langherans cell histiocytosis. Adv Anat Pathol 1998;5:347–358.

93. Constine LS, Woolf PD, Cann D, et al. Hypothalamic-pituitary dysfunction after radiation for brain tumors. N Engl J Med 1993;328:87–94.

94. Lee SC, Zasler ND, Kreutzer JS. Male pituitary-gonadal dysfunction following severe traumatic brain injury. Brain Inj 1994;8:571–577.

95. Benvenga S, Campenni A, Ruggeri RM, Trimarchi F. Hypopituarism secondary to head trauma. J Clin Endocrinol Metab 2000;85:1353–1361.

96. Valenta LJ, De Feo DR. Post-traumatic hypopituarism due to a hypothalamic lesion. Am J Med 1980;68:614–617.

9

Klinefelter's Syndrome

John K. Amory, MD
and William J. Bremner, MD, PhD

Contents

INTRODUCTION
HISTORICAL DESCRIPTION OF KLINEFELTER'S SYNDROME
PATHOPHYSIOLOGY OF KLINEFELTER'S SYNDROME
CLINICAL FEATURES OF KLINEFELTER'S SYNDROME
MORBIDITY ASSOCIATED WITH KLINEFELTER'S SYNDROME
DIAGNOSIS OF KLINEFELTER'S SYNDROME
ANDROGEN REPLACEMENT THERAPY
KLINEFELTER'S SYNDROME AND INFERTILITY
REFERENCES

INTRODUCTION

Klinefelter's syndrome (KS) is the most common sex chromosome disorder in men, affecting roughly 1 in 400–600 men throughout all ethnic groups *(1,2)*. It is also the most common cause of primary testicular failure, resulting in impairments in both spermatogenesis and testosterone production. The hypogonadism associated with KS can range from mild to severe, leading to a marked variation in clinical presentation. Men with KS possess at least one additional or "supernumerary" X chromosome, resulting in a 47, XXY genotype. The clinical phenotype in the adult is that of severely impaired spermatogenesis (usually azoospermia) and varying degrees of hypogonadism, manifested by a tall body habitus with sparse body and facial hair, gynecomastia, diminished libido, and small testes. In childhood, common presenting features can include delayed speech development, learning difficulties at school, unusually rapid growth in mid-childhood, and truncal obesity. Laboratory analysis reveals low or low-normal serum testosterone and elevated serum gonadotropin levels, with follicle-stimulating hormone (FSH) elevated to a greater degree than luteinizing hormone (LH). The clinical diagnosis is confirmed using chromosomal analysis (karyotyping) of either peripheral blood leukocytes or tissue, which usually reveals a 47, XXY genotype, although, infrequently, additional X chromosomes may be present or an individual may be mosaic (47, XXY/46, XY). Treatment consists of testosterone therapy for

From: *Male Hypogonadism:*
Basic, Clinical, and Therapeutic Principles
Edited by: S. J. Winters © Humana Press Inc., Totowa, NJ

improved virilization, sexual function, bone density, and quality of life. Gynecomastia is treated with cosmetic surgery after androgen replacement has begun. New approaches to the treatment of infertility, including intracytoplasmic injection of sperm aspirated from the testes, have been recently reported for KS patients and may be successful in the subset of patients in whom sperm are present on testicular biopsy. However, for most men with KS, artificial insemination with donor sperm or adoption remain the only options for fertility. This chapter summarizes the initial historical description of KS, as well as the current understanding of the pathophysiology, clinical manifestations, associated conditions, and treatment of individuals with KS. In addition, the effect of newly described assisted reproductive techniques on the potential for fertility in men with KS is discussed.

HISTORICAL DESCRIPTION OF KLINEFELTER'S SYNDROME

In 1940, Harry F. Klinefelter, Jr., a native of Baltimore and a graduate of the Johns Hopkins Medical School, spent a year working as a "traveling fellow" with Dr. Fuller Albright in the Metabolic Ward of the Massachusetts General Hospital in Boston (3). At that time, Dr. Albright was at the height of his formidable academic career and, among many other subjects, was interested in the endocrinology of sexual development and the therapeutic applications of the recently available steroid hormones. Dr. Albright had identified a group of adult men with a previously uncharacterized syndrome typified by gynecomastia, small testes, and varying degrees of eunuchoidism. Dr. Albright assigned Dr. Klinefelter the task of further describing this syndrome for publication.

Klinefelter, Albright, and their colleague Dr. Edward Reifenstein, Jr. published their description of the syndrome in a classic article in *The Journal of Clinical Endocrinology* in 1942 (4). In this article, they described a cohort of nine men "characterized by gynecomastia, aspermatogenesis without a-Leydigism, and increased excretion of follicle-stimulating hormone." The authors noted the presence of testosterone-producing Leydig cells in testicular biopsy specimens, as well as a marked increase in FSH production, comparable to that seen in castrated men. The authors suggested that the markedly elevated FSH levels were secondary to the absence of a testicular hormone other than testosterone. This postulated hormone, called inhibin by prior researchers, is, in fact, lacking in individuals with KS, but its identity and role in endocrine feedback in the male would not be fully elucidated for more than 50 yr (5).

Klinefelter and his colleagues were uncertain of the cause of the syndrome. They excluded testicular inflammation, infection, or obstruction of the vas deferens and noted on testicular biopsy specimens that the lesion involved the seminiferous tubules without dramatically affecting the histology of the Leydig cells, testicular interstitium, or epididymis. They recommended testosterone therapy (available since the late 1930s) for those men with signs or symptoms of hypogonadism but noted that this therapy did not improve the gynecomastia or infertility.

Although Klinefelter, Reifenstein, and Albright first described the clinical and endocrine manifestation of KS in 1942, it wasn't until 1956, after the ascertainment of DNA as the main instrument of heredity, that the additional X chromosomes, or "Barr bodies," were identified in tissue from patients with KS (6,7). Three years later, Jacobs and Strong confirmed the association between the extra X chromosome and KS by

Table 1
Mechanism of Origin of Additional X Chromosome in 47, XXY Males (10)

Sex chromosomes	Responsible cell division	X-Chromosome pattern	Frequency (%)
$X^M X^P Y$	Paternal meiosis	Identical to father	53
$X^{M1} X^{M2} Y$	Maternal meiosis-I	Identical to mother	34
$X^{M1} X^{M1} Y$	Maternal meiosis-II	Single maternal chromosome with heterozygosity	9
$X^{M1} X^{M1} Y$	Mitotic (postzygotic)	Single homozygous maternal chromosome	3

cytogenetic analysis of metaphase chromosomes, establishing KS as a sex chromosome disorder with a 47, XXY karyotype (8). Further work has demonstrated that some individuals may be mosaic (47, XXY/46, XY) with the extra X chromosome detectable in only peripheral blood or the testes; rare individuals with 48, XXXY and 49, XXXXY karyotypes have also been described (9).

PATHOPHYSIOLOGY OF KLINEFELTER'S SYNDROME

Most cases of KS occur through sporadic chromosomal nondisjunction during parental gametogenesis in either the sperm or the egg. A seminal study using DNA probes to X chromosome restriction-site polymorphisms demonstrated that in one series of 32 individuals with KS the additional X chromosome was of paternal origin in 17 (53%) of cases and of maternal origin in 14 (44%) of cases and resulted from a postzygotic mitotic error in 1 (3%) case (see Table 1) (10). Because these are sporadic errors in gametogenesis, there is no evidence that KS is familial or is likely to recur within a given family after one child is born with KS. Recent chromosomal analysis of sperm has demonstrated that older men produce higher frequencies of XY sperm that could increase their chances of fathering a child with KS (11).

In an individual with KS, the extra X chromosome forms a dense chromatin mass, or "Barr body," within the nuclei of somatic cells; but exactly how the presence of this extra chromosome leads to testicular failure remains a mystery. Testicular biopsy specimens from infants with KS may reveal only a reduced number of germ cells (12). After puberty, fibrosis of the seminiferous tubules begins, eventually leading to small, firm testes and azoospermia (4). Testicular biopsy specimens from adults with KS reveal marked seminiferous tubule hyalinization, with focal areas of immature seminiferous tubule formation and fibrosis with a resulting increase in the amount of interstitium (see Fig. 1). An absence of functional Sertoli cells in the seminiferous tubules is accompanied by low levels of serum inhibin-B (5), the hormone whose existence Klinefelter and colleagues had hypothesized in their original article.

The hormonal axis in boys with KS can appear normal until puberty, with no apparent differences in the levels of testosterone LH, or FSH when compared to controls (13–15). In addition, gonadotropin production in response to gonadotropin-releasing hormone (GnRH) stimulation is normal. However, at the time of puberty, elevated basal FSH and LH levels and an exaggerated FSH and LH response to GnRH stimula-

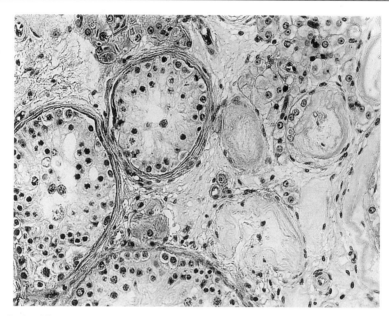

Fig. 1. Testicular biopsy specimen from a 21-yr-old with Klinefelter's syndrome. The peripheral blood karyotype and the karyotype of 100 cells grown from a testicular biopsy sample was 47, XXY. Note focal areas of immature seminiferous tubules interspersed with completely hyalinized tubules and an increase in intersitial tissues. (Photo courtesy of Dr. C. Alvin Paulsen.)

tion and low or low-normal testosterone levels are seen, presaging the hormonal abnormalities seen in adults with KS. Testosterone production in men with KS declines with aging in a fashion similar to normal men *(16)*.

The cause of the language difficulties often encountered by individuals with KS is not well understood; however, recently, high-resolution magnetic resonance imaging (MRI) scans of the brains of individuals with KS has demonstrated a relative reduction in left temporal lobe gray matter compared with control subjects *(17)*. Interestingly, individuals with KS who had been treated with testosterone had larger left temporal lobe volumes than individuals with KS who had not received testosterone therapy. Moreover, verbal fluency scores were significantly improved in the testosterone-treated KS patients compared with the individuals with KS who were never treated with testosterone. This finding implies that levels of testosterone, especially during development, may play a major role in the verbal and language problems related to KS.

The pathophysiology of KS-related gynecomastia is also not entirely clear. Individuals with KS do exhibit mildly elevated plasma levels of estradiol, probably from increases in peripheral aromatization and decreased clearance. However, histologic analysis of breast tissue from individuals with KS demonstrates *intra*ductal hyperplasia rather than the ductal hyperplasia seen in high estrogen states in the male, such as cirrhosis *(18)*.

CLINICAL FEATURES OF KLINEFELTER'S SYNDROME

The clinical manifestations of KS are those of prepubertal androgen deficiency and infertility. Because testicular failure occurs before puberty, the developmental changes

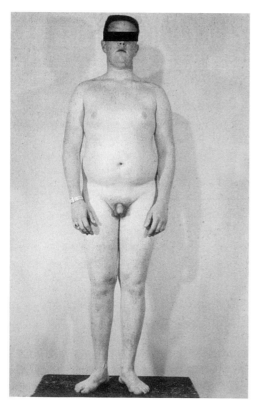
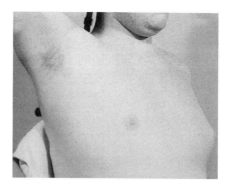
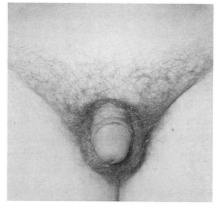

Fig. 2. An individual with Klinefelter's syndrome. Note tall body proportions, gynecomastia, relative paucity of facial and body hair, and small testis. (Photos courtesy of Dr. C. Alvin Paulsen.)

of puberty do not progress normally. This leads to the classic phenotype of KS: long legs, with an arm span frequently greater than height, gynecomastia, decreased muscle mass and increased abdominal adiposity, decreased facial and body hair, and small testes—which often measure less than 5 mL in volume (*see* Fig. 2). The penis may be decreased in size but is often of normal length. Gynecomastia is variable but is often prominent and may require surgical correction. Mosaicism may present more subtly, because affected individuals can appear anywhere along a phenotypic spectrum between classical KS and "normal." Infertility is almost universal; however, human leukocyte antigen (HLA)-confirmed children fathered by individuals with KS have been reported *(19)*. Moreover, assisted reproductive techniques may allow some men with KS to father children (see section on KS and infertility). The frequency of various symptoms and signs of KS is summarized in Table 2.

Hormonally, the majority of affected men have decreased total testosterone levels, and those with normal total testosterone levels may, in fact have decreased free testosterone, because serum sex hormone-binding globulin (SHBG) levels are elevated in KS *(18)*. More than 90% of men have increased levels of serum gonadotropins, particularly FSH, because inhibin-B levels are low in individuals with KS *(5)*. Because of low androgen levels, individuals with KS can have low bone mineral density and are at increased risk of developing osteoporosis, despite seemingly adequate androgen

Table 2
Clinical Characteristics of Men
With Klinefelter's Syndrome

Feature	%
Infertility	99–100
Small testes	99–100
Elevated gonadotropins	90–100
Low testosterone levels	65–85
Gynecomastia	50–75
Reduced facial and pubic hair	50–80
Reduced penis size	10–25

therapy *(20)*. This may result from the failure to achieve peak bone mass early in life, because testosterone replacement before the age of 20 can improve bone mass to normal levels, whereas testosterone therapy started later in life has a less potent effect *(21)*. As a result, calcium and vitamin D supplementation, as well as baseline densitometry, are probably prudent in individuals with KS, especially those who began androgen therapy later in life.

At one time, individuals with KS were believed to be frequently retarded and/or at increased risk of criminal behavior *(22,23)*. Those studies were often misleading, because they were based on preselected (usually committed or incarcerated) populations; however, such populations were not representative of the syndrome as a whole. Subsequent population-based studies have demonstrated a nonsignificant, but slightly increased, rate of incarceration among individuals with KS. The increased rate of imprisonment is most likely accounted for by a lower average score on IQ tests when compared to controls *(24)*.

When tested, groups of adult individuals with KS do exhibit significant deficits in language-processing skills, including reading and spelling, verbal processing speed, verbal and nonverbal executive abilities, and motor dexterity *(25,26)*. In general, this leads to lower average school performance and an increased frequency of psychological consultation. In addition, adolescent males with KS exhibit lowered sexual activity compared with their peers *(27)*. It is important to remember that individual variation in mental function is marked; some individuals with KS perform well above average on intelligence tests. Moreover, it seems likely that early developmental interventions and language tutoring in boys can assist in preventing disabling difficulties with language skills later in adult life *(28,29)*.

MORBIDITY ASSOCIATED WITH KLINEFELTER'S SYNDROME

Data from large population-based studies of chromosome abnormalities at birth have demonstrated that the KS occurs in approx 1 in 400–600 male births *(30–32)*. In adults, overall age-matched mortality is roughly doubled *(33,34)*. Most of this increase is from non-neoplastic diseases of the cardiovascular, respiratory, and digestive systems, and diabetes; however, the incidence of breast cancer and autoimmune disease is also increased *(35)*.

The risk of breast cancer is 20-fold higher in men with KS, who account for 4% of all breast cancer cases in men. Fortunately, breast cancer in men is rare, so the absolute risk of breast cancer in an individual with KS is well under 1%, and screening with mammography is not generally recommended *(36)*. There is also an increased risk of extragonadal germ cell tumors in individuals with KS *(37)*. Affected patients are young and frequently present with advanced disease, often of the mediastinum. It is believed that these neoplasms arise from primordial germ cells that failed to completely migrate to the fetal testes during embryogenesis. These germ cell precursors may then undergo malignant transformation, partly in response to the elevated gonadotropin levels seen in individuals with KS. Fortunately, these tumors are rare even in individuals with KS, and most of these tumors respond well to chemotherapy.

There may be an increased risk for autoimmune disease in individuals with KS. Systemic lupus erythematosis, rheumatoid arthritis, ankylosing spondylitis, and even rare vascular disorders, such as Takaysu's arteritis, have been reported in patients with KS, although the true relative increase in risk is difficult to calculate because of the small number of affected individuals *(38–40)*. It has been speculated that this possible increased risk of autoimmune disease results from an increase in the estrogen to testosterone ratio, because it is believed that elevated circulating estrogen levels may place premenopausal women at increased risk of autoimmune disease *(41)*. Alternative explanations for this increased risk of autoimmune disease in individuals with KS include abnormalities in the T-lymphocyte subsets, including a reduced number of T-suppressor cells (CD8+), because this is occasionally found in women with autoimmune disease. It is interesting to note that androgen therapy may both improve the clinical symptoms of autoimmune disease and correct some of the laboratory features of autoimmunity *(42)*.

Diabetes mellitus is more common in individuals with KS than in the general population *(43,44)*. Fortunately, the severity of illness is most frequently mild. The mechanism of diabetes in individuals with KS probably results from increased resistance to insulin action *(45)*.

Taurodontism (an enlargement of the pulp in molar teeth) is seen in almost half of individuals with KS *(46)*. Taurodontism is diagnosed by dental X-rays and predisposes to premature dental caries and tooth loss. Good dental hygiene and frequent cleaning may be protective.

Early varicose veins are a feature of KS, with 20% of men having severe varicosities at a relatively early age *(47)*. In addition to lower extremity venous ulcers, an increased risk of deep-vein thrombosis has been noted *(48,49)*. There is speculation that a defect in venous basement membrane connective tissue is present in some individuals with KS.

DIAGNOSIS OF KLINEFELTER'S SYNDROME

KS is unique because it can be diagnosed at almost any age: *in utero,* in a prepubertal boy, in an adolescent, or even in an adult male presenting to either a general practice or an infertility clinic. Chromosomal karyotyping of cells in amniotic fluid obtained from amniocentesis for an abnormal triple screen or for advanced maternal age will reveal KS with great accuracy. KS is suggested in prepubertal children by a testicular length of less than 2 cm after the age of 6 yr *(50)*. Additional clues to the diagnosis of

KS in a prepubertal boy are verbal learning disabilities and taurodontism, the unusual enlargement of the pulp of the tooth seen roughly half of men and boys with KS *(46)*. After puberty, individuals with KS will often exhibit tall stature (usually greater than 184 cm) with proportionally long legs and will frequently manifest an arm span that is greater than their height *(51)*. In adults, the diagnosis of KS should be considered in men with gynecomastia, primary hypogonadism, infertility, or osteoporosis. Because serum testosterone levels may be normal, serum gonadotropins should also be measured. Peripheral blood karyotyping can be used to confirm the diagnosis, although this test can be negative in mosaic individuals, and tissue karyotype may be necessary *(9)*.

ANDROGEN REPLACEMENT THERAPY

Testosterone therapy results in a more "male" phenotype, with increases in facial and pubic hair, muscle size and strength, libido, and bone mineral density, and improved mood *(21,47,52,53)*. We recommend testosterone therapy beginning at the time of puberty to allow boys with KS to experience pubertal changes in tandem with their peers. In addition, this approach may allow for optimal enhancement of bone mineral density. Even if testosterone therapy is delayed until adulthood, it is still associated with beneficial improvements in mood, behavior, and sense of well-being *(53)*. Testosterone therapy has no beneficial effect on infertility or gynecomastia, which is best treated with surgical resection if bothersome.

Testosterone therapy is safely and easily accomplished either by periodic intramuscular injection of testosterone esters or with newer (and more expensive) transdermal patches and gels described in detail elsewhere in this volume (*see* Chapter 18). Replacement doses for the intramuscular esters of testosterone are 100–200 mg intramuscularly every other week in adults, whereas adolescents are started at lower doses (e.g., 50–100 mg every 2–4 wk) and are gradually increased to adult doses over 2–3 mo *(13)*. Testosterone therapy side effects include weight gain, mostly owing to increases in lean body mass, and acne. In older men, erythrocytosis is seen with some frequency. Induction or a worsening of sleep apnea has also been reported *(52)*. In general, testosterone therapy is both beneficial and well-tolerated by individuals with KS, most of whom continue therapy long-term *(54)*. Twenty-year follow-ups of cohorts of men with KS treated with testosterone have demonstrated marked improvements in mental health, working capacity, social adjustment, and interpersonal relationships that are similar to improvements seen in hypogonadal control cohorts *(55)*. As a result, most health care providers believe that early diagnosis and treatment with testosterone is of great benefit to the long-term health and welfare of individuals with KS.

KLINEFELTER'S SYNDROME AND INFERTILITY

Previously, donated sperm or adoption were the only options for men with KS to have children, however, dramatic advances in infertility treatment for individuals with KS have recently occurred. Several reports of births resulting from intracytoplasmic sperm injection (ICSI) of sperm obtained from testicular biopsy specimens in patients with KS have been published *(56–58)*. Although most patients with nonmosaic KS do not have sperm on testicular biopsy *(59,60)*, this technique offers a chance at fertility for those who do. Unfortunately, analysis of spermatozoa obtained by testicular biopsy in individuals with KS has revealed an increased prevalence of sperm with an additional X chromosome *(61)*, higher rates of aneuploidy *(62)*, and trisomy 21 *(63)*, implying an increased risk of genetic abnormalities in offspring of individuals with KS born using ICSI. Additional selection of sperm from testicular biopsy specimens in individuals with KS may be required to prevent the transmission of genetic abnormalities.

Physicians and patients interested in obtaining further information about Klinefelter's syndrome, including support-group resources, can contact: Klinefelter's Syndrome and Associates, P.O. Box 119, Roseville, CA 95678–0119; e-mail: ksxxy@ix.netcom.com.

REFERENCES

1. Smyth CM, Bremner WJ. Klinefelter syndrome. Arch Intern Med 1998;158:1309–1314.
2. Amory JK, Anawalt BD, Paulsen CA, Bremner WJ. Klinefelter's syndrome. Lancet 2000;356:333–335.
3. Beighton P, Beighton G, Klinefelter, HF Jr. In: The Man Behind the Syndrome. Springer-Verlag, Berlin, 1986, p. 214.
4. Klinefelter HF Jr., Reifenstein EC Jr., Albright F. Syndrome characterized by gynecomastia, aspermatogenesis without a-Leydigism and increased excretion of follicle-stimulating hormone. J Clin Endocrinol 1942;2:615–627.
5. Anawalt BD, Bebb RA, Matsumoto AM, et al. Serum inhibin B levels reflect Sertoli cell function in normal men and men with testicular dysfunction. J Clin Endocrinol Metab 1996;81:3341–3345.
6. Bradbury IT, Bunge RG, Boccabella RA. Chromatin test in Klinefelter's syndrome. J Clin Endocrinol Metab 1956;16:689–690.
7. Plunkett ER, Barr ML. Testicular dysgenesis affecting the seminiferous tubules principally, with chromatin-positive nuclei. Lancet 1956;183:302–303.
8. Jacobs PA, Strong JA. A case of human intersexuality having a possible XXY sex-determining mechanism. Nature 1959;183:302–303.
9. Paulsen CA, Gordon DL, Carpenter RW, Gandy HM, Drucker WD. Klinefelter's syndrome and its variants: a hormonal and chromosomal study. Recent Prog Horm Res 1968;22:245–270.
10. Jacobs PA, Hassold TJ, Whittington E, et al. Klinefelter's syndrome: an analysis of the origin of the additional sex chromosome using molecular probes. Ann Hum Genet 1988;52:93–109.
11. Lowe X, Eskenazi B, Nelson DO, Kidd S, Alme A, Wyrobek AJ. Frequency of XY sperm increases with age in fathers of boys with Klinefelter syndrome. Am J Hum Genet 2001;69:1046–1054.
12. Mikamo K, Aguereif M, Hazeglin P, Martin-DU PR. Chromatin-positive Klinefelter's syndrome: a quantitative analysis of spermatogonadal deficiency at 3, 4 and 12 months of age. Fertil Steril 1968;19:731–739.
13. Winter JS. Androgen therapy in Klinefelter syndrome during adolescence. Birth Defects 1991;26:234–245.
14. Sorensen K, Nielson J, Wohlert M, Bennett P, Johnsen SG. Serum testosterone of boys with karyotype 47,XXY (Klinefelter's syndrome) at birth. Lancet 1981;2:1112–1113.
15. Salbenblatt JA, Bender BG, Puck MH, Robinson A, Faiman C, Winter JS. Pituitary-gonadal function in Klinefelter's syndrome before and during puberty. Pediatr Res 1985;19:82–86.
16. Gabrilove JL, Freiberg EK, Thornton JC, Nicolis GL. Effect of age on testicular function in patients with Klinefelfter's syndrome. Clin Endocrinol (Oxf) 1979;11:343–347.
17. Patwardhan AJ, Eliez S, Bender B, Linden MG, Reiss AL. Brain morphology in Klinefelter syndrome: extra X chromosome and testosterone supplementation. Neurology 2000;54:2218–2223.
18. Wang C, Baker HW, Burger HG, DeKretser DM, Hudson B. Hormonal studies in Klinefelter's syndrome. Clin Endocrinol (Oxf) 1975;4:399–411
19. Laron Z, Dickerman Z, Zamir R, Galatzer A. Paternity in Klinefelter's syndrome-a case report. Arch Androl 1982;8:149–151.
20. Van den Bergh JP, Hermus AR, Spruyt AI, Sweep CG, Corstens FH, Smals AG. Bone mineral density and quantitative ultrasound parameters in patients with Klinefelter's syndrome after long-term testosterone substitution. Osteoporos Int 2001;12:55–62.
21. Kubler A, Schulz G, Cordes U, Beyer J, Krause U. The influence of testosterone substitution on bone mineral density in patients with Klinefelter's syndrome. Exp Clin Endocrinol 1992;100:129–132.
22. Barr ML, Shaver EL, Carr DH, Plunkett ER. The chromatin-positive Klinefelter syndrome among patients in mental deficiency hospitals. Resident J Ment Defic 1960;4:89–107
23. Schroder J, de la Chapelle A, Hakola P, Virkkunen M. The frequency of XYY and XXY men among criminal offenders. Acta Psychiatr Scand 1981;63:272–276.

24. Witkin HS, Mednich SA, Schulsinger F, et al. Criminality in XYY and XXY men. Science 1976;193:547–555.
25. Boone KB, Swerdloff RS, Miller BL, et al. Neuropsychological profiles of adults with Klinefelter's syndrome. J Int Neuropsychol Soc 2001;7:446–456.
26. Sorensen K. Physical and mental development of adolescent males with Klinefelter syndrome. Horm Res 1992;37(Suppl 3):55–61.
27. Samango-Sprouse C. Mental development in polysomy X Klinefelter syndrome: effects of incomplete X inactivation. Sem Reprod Med 2001;19:193–202.
28. Visootsak J, Aylstock M, Graham JM Jr. Klinefelter syndrome and its variants: an update and review for the primary pediatrician. Clin Pediatr 2001;40:639–651.
29. Manning MA, Hoyme HE. Diagnosis of management of the adolescent boy with Klinefelter syndrome. Adolesc Med 2002;13:367–374.
30. Maclean N, Harnden DH, Court-Brown WM. Abnormalities of sex chromosome constitution in newborn babies. Lancet 1961;2:406–408.
31. Hamerton JL, Canning N, Ray M, Smith S. A cytogenetic survey of 14,069 newborn infants. Clin Genet 1975;8:223–243.
32. Neilsen J, Wohlert M. Sex chromosome abnormalities found among 34,910 newborn children: results from a 13-year incidence study in Arhus, Denmark. Hum Genetics 1991;87:81–83.
33. Price WH, Clayton JF, Wilson J, Collyer S, DeMey R. Causes of death in X-chromatin positive males (Klinefelter's syndrome). J Epidemiol Community Health 1985;39:330–336.
34. Swerdlow AJ, Hermon C, Jacobs PA, et al. Mortality and cancer incidence in persons with numerical sex chromosome abnormalities: a cohort study. Ann Hum Genetics 2001;65:177–188.
35. Sasco AJ, Lowefels AB, Pasker-DeJong. Epidemiology of male breast cancer: a meta-analysis of published case-controlled studies and discussion of epidemiologic factors. Int J Cancer 1993;53:538–549.
36. Hasle H, Mellemgaard A, Nielsen J, Hansen J. Cancer incidence in men with Klinefelter syndrome. Br J Cancer 1995;71:416–420.
37. Lee MW, Stephens RL. Klinefelter's syndrome and extragonadal germ cell tumors. Cancer 1987;60:1053–1055.
38. French MA, Hughes P. Systemic lupus erythematosis and Klinefelter's syndrome. Ann Rheum Dis 1983;42:471–473.
39. Berginer VM, Paran E, Hirsh M, Abelliovich D. Klinefelter's and Takayasu's syndromes in one patient—a pure coincidence? Angiology 1983;34:170–175.
40. Armstrong RD, Macfarlane DG, Panayi GS. Anklyosing spondylitis and Klinefelter's syndrome: does the X chromosome modify disease expression? Br J Rheumatol 1985;24:277–281.
41. Grossman CJ. Regulation of the immune system by sex steroids. Endocr Rev 1984;5:435–455.
42. Bizzarro A, Valentini G, DiMartino G, et al. Influences of testosterone therapy on clinical and immunological features of autoimmune disease associated with Klinefelter's syndrome. J Clin Endocrinol Metab 1987;63:32–36.
43. Hsueh WA, Hsu TH, Federman DD. Endocrine features of Klinefelter's syndrome. Medicine 1978;57:447–461.
44. Neilsen J. Diabetes mellitus in patients with aneuploid chromosome aberrations and the parents. Humagenetik 1972;16:171–176.
45. Pei D, Sheu WH, Jeng C, Liao W, Fuh M. Insulin resistance in patients with Klinefelter's syndrome and idiopathic gonadotropin deficiency. J Formos Med Assoc 1998;97:534–540.
46. Jorgenson RJ. The conditions manifesting taurodontism. Am J Med Genet 1982;11:435–442.
47. Becker KL. Clinical and therapeutic experiences with Klinefelter's syndrome. Fertil Steril 1972;23:568–578.
48. Campbell WA, Newton MS, Price WH. Hypostatic leg ulceration and Klinefelter's syndrome. J Ment Defic Res 1980;24:115–117.
49. Campell WA, Price WH. Venous thromboembolic disease in Klinefelter's syndrome. Clin Genet 1981;19:275–280.
50. Laron Z, Hochman H. Small testes in prepuberal boys with Klinefelter's syndrome. J Clin Endocrinol Metab 1971;32:671–672.
51. Leonard JM, Bremner WJ, Capell PT, Paulsen CA. Male hypogonadism: Klinefelter and Reifenstein syndromes. Birth Defects 1975;11:17–22.
52. Matsumoto AM. Hormonal therapy of male hypogonadism. Endocrinol Metab Clin North Am 1994;23:857–875.

53. Nielsen J, Pelson B, Sorensen K. Follow-up of 30 Klinefelter males treated with testosterone. Clin Genet 1988;33:262–269.

54. Mackey MA, Conway AJ, Handelsmen DJ. Tolerability of intramuscular injections of testosterone ester in an oil vehicle. Hum Reprod 1995;10:862–865.

55. Nielsen J, Pelsen B. Follow-up 20 years later of 34 Klinefelter males with karyotype 47,XXY and 16 hypogonadal males with karyotype 46,XY. Hum Genet 1987;77:188–192.

56. Palermo GP, Schlegel PN, Sills ES, et al. Births after intracytoplasmic injection of sperm obtained by testicular extraction from men with non-mosaic Klinefelter syndrome. N Eng J Med 1998;338:588–590.

57. Ron-El R, Friedler S, Strassburger D, Komarovsky D, Schachter M, Raziel A. Birth of a healthy neonate following the intracytoplasmic injection of testicular spermatozoa from a patient with Klinefelter's syndrome. Hum Reprod 1999;14:368–370.

58. Nodar F, De Vincentiis S, Olmedo SB, Papier S, Urrutia F, Acosta AA. Birth of twin males with normal karotype after intracytoplasmic sperm injection with use of testicular spermatozoa from a nonmosaic patient with Klinefelter's syndrome. Fertil Steril 1999;71:1149–1152.

59. Gordon DL, Krmpotic E, Thomas W, Gandy HM, Paulsen CA. Pathologic testicular findings in Klinefelter syndrome. Arch Intern Med 1972;130:726–729.

60. Okada H, Fujioka H, Tatsumi N, et al. Klinefelter's syndrome in the male infertility clinic. Hum Repro 1999;14:946–952.

61. Foresta C, Galeazzi C, Bettella A, et al. Analysis of meiosis in intratesticular germ cells from subjects affected by classic Klinefelter syndrome. J Clin Endocrinol Metab 1999;84:3807–3810.

62. Bergere M, Wainer R, Nataf V, et al. Biopsied testis cells of four 47,XXY patients: fluorescence in-situ hybridization and ICSI results. Hum Reprod 2002;17:32–37.

63. Hennebicq S, Pelletier R, Bergues U, Rousseaux S. Risk of trisomy 21 in offspring of patients with Klinefelter's syndrome. Lancet 2001;30:2104–2105.

10 Cryptorchidism

Peter A. Lee, MD, PhD, Barry A. Kogan, MD, and Michael T. Coughlin, MA

CONTENTS

INTRODUCTION

A requirement for a priesthood candidate in the Middle Ages was "Duo testes, bene pendulum." Although one could wonder why, considering the goals of celibacy and chastity, this rule attests to the recognition of the importance of descended testes. In John Hunter's early observations and considerations about cryptorchidism in *Observation on Certain Parts of the Animal Economy* in 1786, he not only noted that testes normally descend during the last 3 mo of gestation but also noted the conundrum that abnormal testes may fail to descend, whereas, conversely, failure to descend may result in abnormal testes.

Currently, the dilemma of whether a cryptorchid testis has an innate defect in addition to potential or actual acquired damage persists, making it difficult to determine ideal therapy. In this chapter, the definition, prevalence, etiologies, natural history, and consequences of testicular maldescent are discussed. Recent data suggest that the major consequences, infertility and malignancy, may not be as prevalent as reported previously, although data must be interpreted with caution, because different populations may have

From: *Male Hypogonadism:*
Basic, Clinical, and Therapeutic Principles
Edited by: S. J. Winters © Humana Press Inc., Totowa, NJ

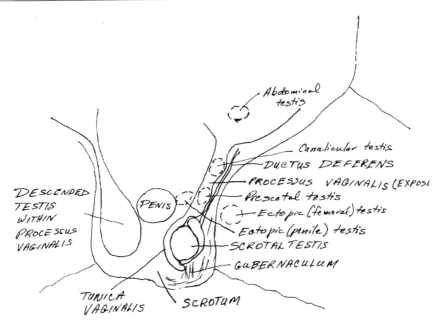

Fig. 1. Schematic drawing showing the pathway of normal testicular descent into the scrotum and ectopic locations.

been studied. Regarding testicular function, the primary traditional concern continues to relate to spermatogenesis and fertility, although recent data suggest that Leydig cell function may be compromised somewhat as well *(1)*.

DEFINITION

Cryptorchidism is the condition in which one (unilateral) or both (bilateral) testes are not fully descended into a scrotal position. In recent studies of a large cohort of men constituting the Children's Hospital of Pittsburgh cryptorchid group *(2,3)*, 86% had a history of unilateral and only 14% had bilateral cryptorchidism. Composite data from earlier reports *(4)* also revealed that 77% of patients had unilateral cryptorchidism (46% were right sided and 31% were on the left).

The etiology of the term derives from the Greek word *kryptos,* meaning hidden, and *orchis,* meaning testis. In fact, cryptorchid testes may or may not be completely hidden, because they may be visible or palpable. Undescended testes may be palpated at various locations along the usual path of descent or at ectopic locations that deviate from that path (*see* Fig. 1). The undescended testis is evidence for a developmental defect that may involve genetic, hormonal, or anatomic problems, resulting in failure of the testis(es) to descend into the scrotum. Cryptorchidism is a physical finding, and, although the control of testicular descent is not well understood, there are numerous proposed etiologies. Furthermore, the differentiation of the truly cryptorchid testis from the temporary but easy retraction of the descended testis may be difficult during childhood. On the other hand, although the term *cryptorchidism* implies that the testis is present but hidden, the nonpalpable testis may instead be absent.

Table 1
Prevalence of Cryptorchidism in Relation to Age
and Gestational Age

At birth	%
Overall	2.7–6.7
Bilateral	3.0
Unilateral	1.9
Related to birth and gestational age	
>2500 g	2.7–5.5
<2499 g	21.0–28.9
>37 wk	2.1
At 3 mo of age	
Overall	0.9–1.6
3 mo from estimated date of birth	1.3
Based on birth weight	
<2000 g	7.7
2000–2500 g	1.7–4.6
>2500 g	0.9–1.4

From refs. *9,10,12,14.*

In a prepubertal male, confirming that a testis is cryptorchid may require more than a single physical examination. It has been demonstrated that interobserver variation is a substantial bias in diagnosing undescended testes *(5)*. From 6 mo of age, the cremasteric reflex is active and the testes retract readily into the upper scrotum or even to the external inguinal ring if a boy is anxious, nervous, or cold, all of which are common occurrences during a medical examination. Because boys with normal testicular descent may have retractile testes, particularly during the mid-childhood years when the cremasteric reflex is most pronounced *(6)*, it is important to verify cryptorchidism and to exclude a retractile testis before considering treatment.

The major detrimental effects of the undescended testis are an increased risk of infertility and malignancy. Although concerns that detrimental psychological effects relating to body image may occur as a consequence of lack of testes in the scrotum have been raised *(7)*, a study that focused on gender identity development and sexual behavior identified no problems *(8)*. When given the choice, most young men choose to have two scrotal testes, even if one or both are synthetic, whereas older men often decline this option.

EPIDEMIOLOGY

Cryptorchidism is one of the most frequent developmental abnormalities of human men. However, there is considerable variation in the reported prevalence of cryptorchidism in newborns, ranging from 2% to 5% in full-term infants *(9–15)*. In premature infants, the prevalence is as high as 21%, with lower values as gestational age and birth weight increase. The prevalence of cryptorchidism changes considerably between birth and 3 mo of age *(see* Table 1); at 3 mo it is approx 1% *(14)*, with a slight decline to 0.8% at 9 mo *(12)*.

There is a greater chance of spontaneous testicular descent during early infancy among cryptorchid babies who weigh less than 2500 g at birth or who are born at less than 37 wk of gestation *(10)*. It is likely that such testes are normal, and the delayed descent represents a continuum of a normal process that may extend beyond 40 wk after conception. In addition, there is a greater likelihood of descent in the 3 mo after birth if the maldescent is bilateral, suggesting a delay of the usual process, and if the scrotum is large and well developed at birth, suggesting greater stimulation by testosterone *(11)*.

Although the estimated prevalence of undescended testes varies, the most consistent figures indicate that after 1 yr of age, 0.7% to 1% of males have one or two cryptorchid testes *(4,11,16,17)*. These prevalence figures are similar to the 0.82% found in Nigerian schoolboys aged 5 to 13 yr, none of whom had been treated *(18)*.

Although there have been reports suggesting a trend toward an increased incidence of cryptorchidism during recent decades *(9)*, such trends have not been verified in all populations, and the prevalence varies considerably from different sampling regions *(19,20)*. Taken together with evidence that cryptorchidism has increased in recent decades *(9,11)* are concerns that the incidence of other urogenital malformations, perhaps in association with cryptorchidism, is also rising and may result from chemicals, such as pesticides, with hormone-disrupting actions. For example, an increased risk (relative risk [RR] 1.67) of cryptorchidism was reported in the sons of women working in gardening but not in the sons of men working in farming or gardening *(21)*. Data to date are inconclusive, necessitating further studies to document the rising incidence of cryptorchidism and any association with environmental agents.

NORMAL DEVELOPMENT OF THE MALE REPRODUCTIVE SYSTEM: DESCENT OF THE TESTIS

Testicular development begins at conception under complicated genetic direction *(22)*. This involves a cascade of sequential steps under the control of numerous genes, most of which are yet to be identified. Key to testicular differentiation is the sex-determining region Y (SRY) gene. Genetic components upstream from SRY that are essential for gonadal development include splicing factor 1 (SF1), Wilm's tumor 1 gene (WT1), and Double sex and MAb-3-Related Transcription Factor 1 (DMRT1). Downstream from SRY are DAX1 (associated with dosage sensitive sex reversal), Wnt-4 (Wingless-type MnTV Integration Site Family, Member 4 (in which duplication is associated with XY sex reversal), and sex-related box (SOX9), in which mutations cause XY sex reversal and duplication with XX sex reversal. A scheme that may regulate downstream testicular differentiation is hypothesized to involve SRY suppression of Wnt-4, expression that, in turn, suppresses DAX1 expression, allowing for SOX9 expression, and leading to testicular differentiation. This would be normal sequence in the 46XY male, resulting in normal testicular development. Conversely, in the absence of SRY, Wnt-4 and DAX1 are expressed, inhibiting SOX9 expression and abolishing testicular differentiation, as in the 46XX female.

With the appropriate genetic direction and substrates, primitive sex cords become testicular cords to provide the framework for the developing testis. Primitive mesenchyme cells differentiate into Sertoli cells that can be seen in the testicular cords by 7 wk of gestation, with Leydig cells recognizable by 8 wk. Testosterone production also begins at this time. Concomitantly, primitive germ cells from the endoderm of the yolk sac first appear in the genital ridge. After this, Leydig cells proliferate and the testicular cords become canalized forming seminiferous tubules. Hence, the primordial gonad begins its differentiation into a testis in early fetal life and becomes functional by the middle of the first trimester with testosterone synthesis and release. Testosterone secretion is necessary for the subsequent development of the testis and the accessory male reproductive structures, as well as for the normal descent of the testes (23).

Concomitant with this early testicular differentiation is a series of other key developmental events that relate to testicular descent. Early in gestation, tissues begin to organize to form the associated ducts, the gubernaculum, and the tunica vaginalis (the serous membrane eventually covering a portion of the testes and epididymis). By 5 wk after conception, the initial concentrations of the mesenchyme begin to organize and develop into the ligamentous band of tissue that will develop into the gubernaculum. This structure eventually connects the lower end of the epididymis and the base of the scrotum. By 10 wk of fetal life, a small invagination that will become the processus vaginalis can be found next to the internal inguinal ring. This peritoneal outpocketing, adjacent to the gubernaculums, elongates progressively through the inguinal canal. The testicular ductal system develops under testosterone stimulation, beginning at week 7 to 8. The paired Wolffian ducts become rete testes, adjacent to the testes with the ejaculatory ducts at the distal end. Concomitantly, the testes secrete Müllerian-inhibiting hormone, precluding further differentiation of the paired Müllerian ducts. Externally, there is concomitant male differentiation of the genitalia under the control of dihydrotestosterone (DHT) that is essentially completed by 12 wk of fetal life.

Testicular descent in the developing male fetus is a complex process that is only understood partially. Descent has been described as consisting of either two or three phases (24,25), each with different regulatory mechanisms. Three phases are described: (1) repositioning of the testis, (2) transabdominal descent, and (3) transscrotal migration. The three-phase model includes an initial phase of morphologic reorientation that is the same in both sexes and involves repositioning of the testis caudally, concomitant with regression of the mesonephros as the metanephros migrates cranially. At this point early in gestation, the position of the testis is at the level of the lower pole of the metanephric kidney. It is unclear whether adjacent anatomic structures or hormonal factors are involved in the relative repositioning of the testis in phases 1 and 2 that occurs between the 8th and 26th wk to a posterior position at the level of the anterior iliac supine. Transabdominal migration culminates in the testis locating to a position that is clearly different from that of the ovary, the shift occurs from the posterior abdominal wall to the inguinal region. This movement is accomplished primarily between 10 and 15 wk of fetal life.

The cranial suspensory ligaments that are attached to the developing gonad anteriorly may play a role in testicular descent. Normally, these ligaments regress in males but persist in females. Regression allows both the relative intra-abdominal testicular repositioning and the transinguinal migration. Persistence of these ligaments in humans and mice with androgen insensitivity syndrome (24,26), failure of regression in male rats treated prenatally with anti-androgen (27), and regression of these ligaments and a more caudal ovarian location in newborn female rats treated in utero with androgens (28), together suggest that regression of these ligaments is under androgenic control. Because androgens play a role in the regression of these ligaments and such regression is important in both the abdominal and the transinguinal migration phases of testicular descent, androgens are crucial for both of these phases. Although Müllerian-inhibiting hormone has been hypothesized to participate in the transabdominal phase, this has not been verified.

The final phase of descent is called transinguinal migration, occurring after 26 wk of fetal life and lasting 4 to 6 wk. During this time, the testes pass through the inguinal canal (29) to the bottom of the scrotum. Thus, complete descent is generally accomplished by the 32nd wk of gestation but may not be fully complete until the first few months of postnatal life.

During this final phase, the testis carries the processus vaginalis (the peritoneal-lined outpocket into the inguinal canal) into a scrotal position. This phase has long been considered to be androgen dependent and to involve the gubernaculum, the cremaster muscle, the genitofemoral nerve, neurotransmitters, cytokines, intra-abdominal pressure, and epididymal maturation. The specific roles of the epididymis and the gubernaculum (the fetal ligament attached to the lower end of the epididymis and the bottom of the scrotum) are unclear. Epididymides with no attachment to the testes have been reported in some patients with maldescent (30). This defect may not only play a role in the lack of descent but also will cause infertility.

The anatomical changes and position of the gubernaculum led to the suggestion that this structure plays a role in the migration of the testis from the abdomen into the inguinal canal, although it is unclear whether an active or a passive process is involved (31,32). Before the transinguinal migration phase, the gubernaculum increases in size from the 15th to 24th wk of gestation. Gubernacular growth is characterized by mesenchymal cell hyperplasia and hypertrophy, with a marked increase of the extracellular matrix related to the hydrophilic properties of hyaluronic acid. The cremaster muscle is intertwined in the gubernaculum. Concomitant with the transinguinal migration phase is a phase of regression of the gubernaculum (29). During testicular migration, the gubernacular connective tissue changes into a fibrous structure containing considerable collagen and elastic fibers. These changes result in its decreased size (33). This regression may also cause a relative negative pressure, drawing the testis through the inguinal canal. An active process involving the cremaster muscle pulling the testis is unlikely. Most likely, the gubernaculum plays an important passive role by guiding the testis along the channel of descent. As shown in Fig. 1, testes may have an ectopic location. There are usually five points of attachment of the gubernaculum, with the primary one at the base of the scrotum. The mechanism for ectopic locations is likely to be an abnormal primary attachment of the gubernaculum to structures other than the base of the scrotum, such as laterally or medially in the femoral, penile, or perineal area.

Although transinguinal migration is clearly under androgenic control, such stimulation directs a cascade of metabolic responses involving paracrine factors and catabolic enzymes, such as acid phosphatase, which stimulate gubernacular regression (34). A role for the genitofemoral nerve is suggested from animal studies in which division of the nerve during early fetal life results in premature regression of the gubernaculum and prevents testicular descent (25,35). It has been hypothesized that this nerve secretes the neuropeptide, calcitonin gene-related peptide (CGRP) that has been found in its nucleus. The control of CGRP secretion by the genitofemoral nerve may reside in spinal cord nuclei, a hypothesis consistent with the increased prevalence of cryptorchidism in patients with spina bifida and in rats after spinal cord transection (36). Receptors for CGRP are found in the cremasteric muscle in the rat gubernaculum and are upregulated after denervation of the genitofemoral nerve (37,38). Exogenous

CGRP stimulates gubernacular development, whereas a synthetic CGRP antagonist (CGRP 8-37) delays testicular descent *(39,40)*. Also, in vivo administration of CGRP results in contraction in the gubernaculum in the rat *(41)*. Other factors may include an insulin-like peptide isolated from Leydig cells *(42)* and an insulin-like factor (INSL)-3/relaxin-like factor (RLF) gene that is expressed in Leydig cells *(43)*.

Even with the many potential genetic regulators of testicular descent, identifible genetic causes of cryptorchidism, or infertility in relation to cryptorchidism, are rare. Human studies have failed to find karyotypic abnormalities or an increased frequency of mutations in males with cryptorchidism *(44)*. There is evidence that INSL-3 (Leydig insulin-like or relaxin-like factor) plays a role in establishing gonadal position and in cryptorchidism in animals *(45,46)*. Although reports differ concerning the association of INSL-3 mutations and human cryptorchidism *(47–50)*, mutations in the coding region of the INSL-3 gene are an uncommon cause of human cryptorchdism *(61)*.

Given the complexity of the process, it is obvious that there may be multiple etiologies for failure of testicular descent. In particular, systemic factors are likely to be important in patients with bilateral cryptorchidism, whereas paracrine regulators may be disrupted when only one testis is undescended. Anatomic problems precluding descent could include a detached epididymis *(30)*, testicular-splenic, or testicular hepatic fusion *(52)*. Etiologies that result in a dysgenetic testis preclude normal function, even with correct scrotal positioning. However, if an anatomic problem has not compromised the vascular supply and can be corrected, the testis may develop normally, with the potential for normal function.

A concomitant inguinal hernia is a common finding with cryptorchidism. It is often unclear whether the hernia is related to the cause or is a result of the maldescent, although the latter has been presumed. If other malformations are present, the likelihood of a common etiology is increased. Almost one-half of cryptorchid fetuses and infants without inguinal hernias had associated diagnoses (e.g., dysplasia of the kidneys, ureters, or spinal column, suggesting a general insult or defect), whereas only approximately one-fifth of those with a hernia had such defects *(53)*.

ENDOCRINE ASPECTS OF TESTICULAR DESCENT

A role for hormones in testicular descent was demonstrated more than 70 yr ago when a urinary extract from pregnant monkeys (containing hCG) was used to treat monkeys with cryptorchidism *(54)*. It remains unclear whether that was a direct gonadotropin effect or an indirect effect from increased testosterone production. The factors controlling testicular descent are clearly more complicated than hormone insufficiency alone, because only a portion of hypogonadotropic patients with Kallmann syndrome have cryptorchidism. Furthermore, most patients with congenital primary hypogonadism (e.g., Klinefelter's syndrome) do not have cryptorchidism. Although the absence of cryptorchidism as a universal finding may be a consequence of the amount of gonadotropin or androgen present during differentiation, these examples are further evidence that many factors are involved in testicular descent, most of which are not yet understood.

There is a similar lack of understanding of the role of androgen action in testicular maldescent in 46XY patients with mutations in the LH receptor and those with androgen receptor defects producing complete androgen insensitivity syndrome. In these patients, the testes descend as far as is anatomically possible, because the absence of a scrotum precludes further descent. Thus, such examples fail to provide evidence for or against the role of androgens in testicular descent.

The available animal data are consistent with androgen stimulation of both the abdominal and the inguinal phases of descent (55,56). Although the androgenic effect is limited to a specific time period (56). Orchiectomy will halt gubernacular regression in the dog, a finding that is reversible with testosterone treatment (57,58). This property may be related to testosterone itself, rather than to DHT, because administration of a 5-α reductase inhibitor had little effect on testicular descent (59). Estrogen treatment prevents testicular descent in newborn rats (60,61). However, androgen and gonadotropin replacement were unable to reverse this effect in mice, raising the possibility of a direct estrogenic effect rather than via suppression of the hypothalamic–pituitary axis (62). Estrogen also been proposed to prevent testicular descent through downregulation of INSL-3 expression. In humans, a case-control study found no association between cryptorchidism and either exogenous estrogen exposure or pregnancy-related variables that are hypothesized to be indirect indicators of endogenous estrogens (63).

The hypothalamic–pituitary–testicular axis differentiates by midgestation. Testosterone, gonadotropins, and Müllerian-inhibiting hormone are present in the fetal circulation, and each could play a crucial role in testicular descent. During the first few months after birth, the hypothalamic–pituitary–testicular axis is active, with near-adult circulating levels of testosterone that peak between 1 to 3 mo of age. Thereafter, concentrations diminish gradually to low childhood levels by 6 mo of age (64). This neonatal testosterone rise is likely to be related to "imprinting" maleness and may be critical for normal differentiation of germ cells, as well as the spontaneous descent of undescended testes that occurs during the first 6 mo of life in males born with maldescent. These observations and the testosterone secretion pattern are also consistent with the finding that testes that fail to descend within the first 6 mo of life are unlikely to descend spontaneously thereafter.

Decreased testosterone levels have been reported in cryptorchid infants (65), consistent with diminished LH secretion (66,67), with lower levels in both the postnatal week and the second month of life in preterm infants with cryptorchidism, when compared to those without cryptorchidism (68). Although antipituitary antibodies have been found in mothers of cryptorchid infants, no correlation was found with postnatal testosterone levels (67).

Müllerian-inhibiting hormone, associated with regression of the Müllerian duct, is produced by Sertoli cells. Diminished levels in boys with cryptorchidism (69) led to the hypothesis that Müllerian-inhibiting hormone plays a role in testicular descent. Lower levels have also been reported in boys with bilateral than in unilateral cryptorchidism, and this difference has been interpreted to suggest that Müllerian-inhibiting hormone could be involved in the transabdominal phase of descent (70). Circumstantial evidence supporting this idea is that this phase occurs concurrent with the highest Müllerian-inhibiting hormone levels. However, animal data do not support this hypothesis insofar as male offspring of female rabbits immunized against Müllerian-inhibiting hormone had persistent Müllerian duct derivatives but descended testes (71).

During childhood, LH, FSH, and testosterone levels in boys with cryptorchidism are low and are similar to those of boys without cryptorchidism. Diminished LH responses to gonadotropin-releasing hormone (GnRH) stimulation have been reported in prepubertal boys with undescended testes (72). These and other data support the diagnosis of

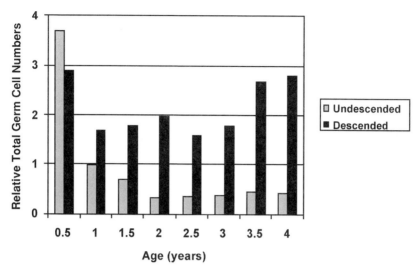

Fig. 2. Germ cell numbers vs age in young boys with unilateral cryptorchidism and in their contra-lateral descended testes.

mild hypogonadotropic hypogonadism in boys with cryptorchidism during childhood. However, hypergonadotropism, particularly involving FSH, is common in affected adults, whereas hypogonadotropism is rare in adults with a history of cryptorchidism *(73)*. Elevated FSH levels may become apparent as puberty approaches, suggesting at least partial gonadal failure *(74)*. On the other hand, inhibin-B levels are within the normal range in boys with either unilateral or bilateral cryptorchidism *(75)*.

GERM CELL DEVELOPMENT IN THE CRYPTORCHID TESTIS

Germ cell numbers and testicular and epididymal weights, but not body weights, were lower in stillborns with cryptorchidism than in those with full testicular descent *(53)*. Twenty-three percent of these fetuses had decreased numbers of germ cells per tubular cross-section. Furthermore, in contrast to the descended testis, germ cells in the cryptorchid testis were reduced in number with increasing fetal age.

Figure 2 shows that germ cells in cryptorchid testes at birth do not differ in number from those in descended testes *(53,76)*. Although not verified, it is generally assumed that such a testis has a normal potential for spermatogenesis. However, it is clear that testes that remain cryptorchid beyond infancy acquire a progressively more abnormal microscopic appearance. Although the histological appearance of the unilateral unde-scended testis cannot be distinguished from a normal testis based on germ cell number at birth *(77)*, changes are apparent by the second or third month, with defective trans-formation of gonocytes into adult dark spermatogonia *(78)*. Untransformed gonocytes persist until the second half of the first year of life; then secondary degeneration occurs, decreasing the total germ cell count. As illustrated in Fig. 2, germ cell number in the cryptorchid testes is reduced by age 1 yr and consistently so by 2 yr of age *(53,76,77,79–83)*, with a further decrease with increasing age *(84)*. Progression is apparent when the percentage of boys with abnormally low germ cell numbers is analyzed as a function of age; 22% of boys with cryptorchidism have values below the normal range during the first year of life, compared to 92% in the 1- to 3-yr-old group (53). During the first 5 yr of life, there is no difference in the number of germ cells between undescended testes that are intra-abdominal or canalicular (85), consistent with the lack of correlation between pretreatment testicular location and fertility in adulthood (86).

The number of germ cells in undescended testes from birth to 1 yr of age was statistically less among boys without an inguinal hernia than with a hernia, the latter being not different from normal (53). This difference was lost by 3 yr of age.

Key steps in the maturation of the descended testis include the disappearance of gonocytes (the fetal stem cell pool), with the subsequent appearance of adult dark spermatogonia (the adult stem cell pool) by 3 mo of age and the appearance of primary spermatocytes at the onset of meiosis by age 5 yr. Both of these steps are impaired in the undescended testis. Total and differential germ cell counts in testicular biopsies of cryptorchid testes in boys under 1 yr of age indicate that the adult stem cell pool is not yet fully established. This delay or defect is further reflected in the biopsies from boys 4 to 5 yr of age, which demonstrate a lack of primary spermatocytes; only approx 20% of contralateral testes contain these cell forms (87).

However, in the undescended testes of boys older than 5 yr of age, seminiferous tubules decrease progressively in size, with Sertoli cell hypoplasia, a marked reduction in spermatogonia number and peritubular hyalinization with thickening and fibrosis of the lamina propria (88). Biopsies of cryptorchid testes from boys aged 13 to 18 yr demonstrate changes that are similar to those of prepubertal boys, except for the development of Leydig cells and more Sertoli cell junctions. Cryptorchid testes from 19- to 27-yr-old men had changes ranging from complete spermatogenesis to isolated spermatogonia, mature to hyperplastic Sertoli cells, and normal to thickened lamina propria. A normal lamina propria was associated with mature Sertoli cells, whereas thickening involved peritubular cell alterations.

Reports conflict concerning the status of germ cells in the scrotal testis contralateral to an undescended testis. No differences in comparison with control descended testes have been reported (89). However, abnormal maturation and germ cell numbers have been reported in the scrotal testis that is contralateral to the unilaterally undescended testis. The contralateral testis has more germ cells than the undescended testis but fewer germ cells than in age-matched normal testes (90). There is variation between subjects, because in another report, 30% of contralateral testes had diminished numbers of germ cells, with a few testes demonstrating severe reduction (31). Histological changes have also been described in the contralateral testes of prepubertal boys who had unilateral torsion and atrophy, with decreased numbers and delay in maturation of germ cells, with variably diminished tubular diameter and Sertoli cell hyperplasia (91). As in unilateral cryptorchidism, contralateral changes could represent either an acquired immunological or congenital defect. Although it is unclear to what extent the altered testicular histology of the undescended testis is reversible and whether differences result from maturational lag or permanent damage, some postpubertal cryptorchid testes are devoid of germ cells.

The findings presented here are the basis for the current recommendation for treatment of cryptorchidism before 18 mo of age, even as young as age 6 mo. Based primarily on the findings of decreased germ cell numbers with age, the recommended age for treatment has declined progressively throughout the past 40 yr to the current young age. For decades, it was believed that orchiopexy should be performed at early puberty if spontaneous descent had not occurred. This reasoning was consequent to the inaccurate perception that the testes are inert during childhood. The recommended treatment age progressively declined as the risk of diminished testicular function, primarily reduced germ cell numbers with increasing age, was realized (92). The most recent recommendation is for treatment around 9 mo of age, because testes are not likely to descend spontaneously after the first 3 to 4 mo of life and germ cells are already declining by this age (80,86), with greater and earlier decreases with bilateral than with unilateral maldescent (80). Indeed, it was shown that orchiopexy was safe at age 1 yr (93). Although a study failed to find any improvement of germ cell numbers (30), more outcome data are needed to determine if fertility is improved by earlier treatment.

To determine if hormonal therapy will affect germ cell development, two studies suggested that orchiopexy followed by long-term gonadotropin stimulation improves germ cell numbers and subsequent fertility (94,95). Furthermore, a GnRH analog administered once daily in a nasal spray to stimulate rather than inhibit gonadotropins has also been reported to induce testicular descent and increase numbers of germ cells (96).

Evaluation based on numbers of germ cells alone may be insufficient. A study of young adult men who had undergone orchiopexy and testicular biopsy before 2 yr of age included semen for analysis. All men who had surgery before 6 mo of age had a normal number of germ cells on biopsy, whereas those older than 6 mo of age at the time of surgery had reduced germ cell numbers (94). Two thirds of the men provided semen for analysis as adults, but these findings did not correlate with the total number of germ cells at childhood biopsy. However, a diminished sperm count was found in men who did not have adult (dark) spermatogonia on biopsy 20 to 25 yr earlier. This finding implies irreparable damage rather than simply delayed maturation.

Another cohort of adult men who had a biopsy at orchiopexy at ages 10 to 12 yr has been studied (97). A positive correlation was found between the number of spermatogonia at biopsy and sperm count, volume of the operated testis, and total testicular volume. Negative correlations were found between FSH levels and testicular volume, sperm concentration, and total sperm count.

OTHER DEVELOPMENTAL ANATOMICAL ABNORMALITIES

Developmental abnormalities of the ductal system leading from the testes are frequently present in men with testicular maldescent and may contribute to infertility. For example, epididymal abnormalities have been noted in up to 40% of patients (30,98,99).

Retractile Testes

True cryptorchidism must be distinguished from the retractile testis. A retractile testis is usually descended and resides in the scrotum, but it readily and frequently temporarily enters the inguinal canal. If this occurs during a physical examination, cryptorchidism may be misdiagnosed. Most retractile testes are believed to function normally, whereas some may be abnormal but less so than cryptorchid testes (100).

Outcome data of fertility after cryptorchidism are compromised if study cohorts include men with retractile testes. Retractile testes may also bias assessments of hormonal treatment of testicular descent. In the cohort reported from the Children's Hospital of Pittsburgh Male Fertility study, men were included in the cryptorchid group only if they had undergone orchiopexy. All males with retractile testes were excluded, including those misdiagnosed as cryptorchid who had descended testes while under general anesthesia.

Ascending Testis

Ascent during childhood of a previously normally descended testis has been suggested for nearly two decades *(101)*. The ascending testis becomes tethered above the scrotum in an unacceptable position. This may occur consequent to shortening of the processus vaginalis because of inadequate elongation of the spermatic cord *(102)* or as a complication of inguinal hernia surgery *(103)*. The increased prevalence of cryptorchidism during late childhood than during late infancy and early childhood *(4)* could also be explained by missed diagnoses in younger boys or by a retractile testes being diagnosed as undescended in older boys. It is widely accepted that testes may ascend from the full scrotal position during mid-childhood years. There are documented cases of boys with undescended testes whose earlier medical records clearly noted descended or retractile testes *(104–106)*. Ascending testis may occur more frequently in boys born with undescended testes who undergo spontaneous descent in early infancy by 3 mo of age *(107)*. The age distribution of orchiopexy is bimodal, with an initial and larger peak within the first 5 yr of life and a second peak in surgical procedures between 8 and 11 yr of age. This distribution could be a consequence of acquired cryptorchidism or ascending testes *(108)*. Ascending testes are believed to be healthy and to have the potential for normal function, although they must be evaluated just like any undescended testis. It has been suggested that retractile testes may retract higher, perhaps becoming ascending testes, with abnormal development *(109)*. In general, ascending testes are viewed as a continuum between retractile testes and more severe forms of testicular maldescent.

PHYSICAL EXAMINATION

A careful physical examination is essential to determine whether a testis is cryptorchid or retractile *(110)*. If the scrotum is empty, it is fundamental to decide whether the testis is palpable. Repeated physical examinations may be necessary if it is unclear whether a testis is present or to determine the location of a palpable testis. Incompletely descended testes are not usually fixed in position. A testis may at one examination be just palpable at the internal inguinal ring and on another occasion be impalpable, or the location may be high scrotal on one occasion and in the inguinal canal on another. Also, the location on physical examination may differ from that when the patient is under general anesthesia in preparation for surgery.

If a testis is not palpable, laparoscopy may determine not only its presence but also its location *(111,112)*. As noted in the section on hormonal treatment, hormone stimulation (hCG, GnRH, or GnRH analog) may also be used to determine the presence of testicular tissue, because a rise in the serum testosterone level indicates the presence of functional Leydig cells. However, this test is only needed when neither testis is palpable.

TREATMENT

The rationale for treatment of cryptorchidism includes the increased risk of infertility and testicular cancer, the need to correct hernias, and decreasing the risk of torsion. It is considered, with the exceptions noted here, that bilateral cryptorchidism is associated with infertility if the testes remain undescended beyond puberty. However, it has not been shown clearly that treatment during childhood has any beneficial effect on fertility *(113)*. A meta-analysis revealed that in men with bilateral cryptorchidism treated during childhood, there were similar percentages of subjects with azoospermia and oligospermia (<20 million/mL) regardless of the type or age of treatment.

Furthermore, particularly for boys with unilateral cryptorchidism, it has been questioned whether treatment to bring the testis into a scrotal location influences fertility or modifies the risk of tumor development. The percentages of men with azoospermia or oligospermia have been reported to be similar for men who had surgical, hormonal, or both treatments or no treatment at all *(113)*. In one report, 42% of men who had received no treatment for unilateral undescent had sperm density greater than 20×10^6 (45% had oligospermia and 13% had azoospermia) *(114)*. Evaluations of semen in men with unilateral cryptorchidism suggest that treatment has not made a difference regarding fertility, although it must be realized that treatment in these studies was generally at ages considerably older than is recommended currently.

Although semen analysis may be abnormal, it was unclear until recently whether fertility was decreased for men with a history of unilateral cryptorchidism. As discussed in detail later, recent evidence suggests that when this population is compared to a control population, there is no significant difference in paternity rates *(2,115)*.

Surgical Treatment

Orchiopexy is one of the most frequent surgical procedures in males. Unpublished data from the National Hospital Discharge Survey by the National Center for Health Statistics indicate that there are approx 26,670 orchiopexies in the United States each year, with approx 75% (20,000) in males under 15 yr of age. Success after orchiopexy can be defined in various ways, such as a palpable testis in the scrotum, a normal-sized testis in the scrotum, normal testicular tissue on biopsy, normal semen analysis, or natural paternity. Success rates in achieving a palpable testis in the scrotum after surgery vary from 73 to 89% *(116)*, depending, in part, on the procedure used. The inguinal procedure has the highest success rate *(116,117)*, although the procedure is only appropriate for testes in this region. A meta-analysis has shown a relationship between anatomic location of the undescended testis and surgical success, with progressively better success rates, ranging from 74 to 92%, in association with a lower location of the testis *(116)*.

Surgical techniques have been refined and have changed markedly over the years, with some testes requiring staged surgery *(118)*. Recently, diagnostic laparoscopy has been used to determine the location of a nonpalpable testis *(111)*. The diagnostic laparoscopy is used to plan the surgical approach, and, when no evidence for a testis or associated vasculature is found, it will prevent unnecessary open surgical exploration *(112)*. Furthermore, the diagnostic laparoscopy can be converted to a laparoscopic orchiopexy when an intraabdominal testis is found *(118)*.

Hormonal Treatment

Human chorionic gonadotropin (hCG) and gonadotropin-releasing hormone (GnRH) are being used in patients with cryptorchidism for both diagnostic and therapeutic purposes. No uniform regimen for hCG is superior for either purpose, and it is likely that most regimens provide maximal stimulation. Treatment for 3 to 4 d is practical and provides a reliable assessment of testicular responsiveness *(119)*. The use of the diagnostic test is limited to the situation in which neither testis is palpated. In the boy with bilateral nonpalpable testes that may be either absent or abdominal, hCG stimulation is useful during the childhood years *(120)*. Testes may become palpable, or testosterone levels may rise. Because testes will respond to brief stimulation by hCG during childhood with increased testosterone secretion, this test is useful in determining the presence of testicular tissue containing responsive Leydig cells. This test does not differentiate between unilateral anorchia and a unilateral undescended testis, and an increase in testosterone does not ensure a normal testis. Because of the transient physiological increase in gonadotropin secretion, an infant male with absent testes will likely have markedly elevated LH levels consistent with primary hypogonadism. However, gonadotropin levels are low beyond infancy until the peripubertal period. It has also been reported that inhibin-B levels rise in young boys in response to hCG stimulation. This may prove to be a method by which Sertoli cell integrity can be assessed *(75);* however, false negative results may occur *(121)* from a lack of differentiated Leydig cells. During childhood, there is dedifferentiation or apoptosis of Leydig cells that were functional during infancy, with other Leydig cells becoming functional at puberty or after gonadotropin stimulation *(22)*.

Hormonal treatment with hCG or gonadotropin-releasing hormone (GnRH) analogs *(96)* or historically with FSH, human menopausal gonadotropin (hMG), and testosterone has been used for undescended testes. There are no data to indicate that the success rate in inducing permanent testicular descent differs between hCG and GnRH *(123,124)*. Overall, a meta-analysis showed that both treatments are more effective than placebo, but each was only approx 20% successful *(125)*. Earlier reports of 50–70% success rates likely resulted from the inadvertent inclusion of many patients with retractile testes.

Hormonal therapy with either hCG or GnRHa has become a secondary treatment modality, because only a small portion of patients respond with full descent *(126)*. An immediate response rate as high as 40% has been reported, although some studies found a higher response in the unilateral group *(126),* and others find no difference between those with unilateral or bilateral cryptorchidism *(124)*. A significant percentage of medically treated patients have subsequent re-ascent of the testis. The portion of boys with descent after hormonal stimulation is inversely related to age, with such a poor response in the first 2 yr of life that some authors recommend that medical therapy should not be used *(124)*.

The results of testicular biopsies at orchiopexy in boys treated unsuccessfully with GnRH showed a negative correlation between germ cell count and age at surgery *(127)*. This was interpreted as evidence to favor early surgery. Moreover, prolonged GnRH therapy has been reported to increase numbers of germ cells *(96)*. More recent data suggest, however, that hCG or GnRHa treatment may have a detrimental effect on germ cell numbers when given to boys younger than 4 yr of age *(128)*.

Successful hormonal treatment is precluded when an anatomic problem prevents descent (e.g., ectopic testes). In one series, 40% of patients with unsuccessful hormonal therapy subsequently had successful surgical treatment *(110)*. Hormonal therapy is generally reserved for special circumstances: (1) patients with nonpalpable testes, (2) patients in whom the testis is in the upper scrotum, (3) patients with a high likelihood of retractile testes that cannot be confirmed by routine physical examination, and (4) patients with a high anesthesia risk. It has been suggested that with hormonal therapy,

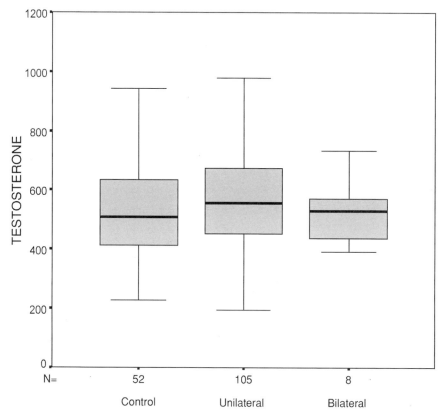

Fig. 3. Testosterone levels (ng/dL) in men who formerly had unilateral or bilateral cryptorchidism and control men. Solid line depicts the median, the shaded area the interquartile range, and the crosslines the minimum and maximum values.

the abdominal testis, its vascular supply, and its supporting structures may enlarge and descend partially, making the testis palpable and enhancing subsequent surgery. However, there are no data to support this contention. For the low-lying, but not fully descended, testis, the goal is to achieve full descent with hormone stimulation. It is noteworthy that boys with cryptorchidism with Klinefelter's syndrome have poorer hormonal and descent responses than other patients with cryptorchidism to hormonal therapy *(29)*. In cases in which the history is strongly suggestive of previously descended testes but the child is difficult to examine and has highly retractile testes, successful hormonal therapy might well be reassuring and obviate unnecessary orchiopexy.

CONSEQUENCES OF CRYPTORCHIDISM

Hormone Production, Sexual Development, and Activity

HORMONE PRODUCTION

Testosterone levels are generally normal in men with cryptorchidism, even those who were not treated *(73,130)*. Although testosterone levels are within the normal range in men who were formerly cryptorchid (*see* Fig. 3) without other problems, a

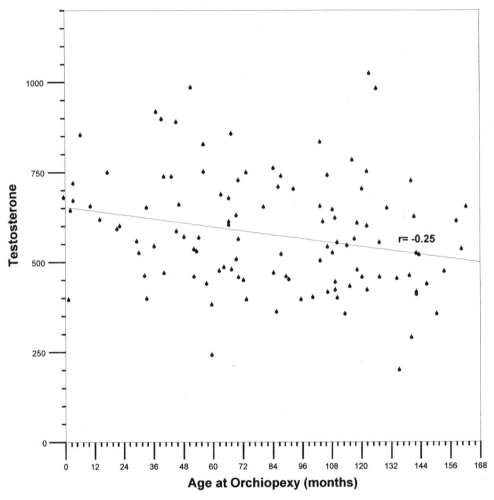

Fig. 4. Testosterone levels (ng/dL) in men who were formerly cryptorchid plotted against age of orchidopexy. These data suggest lower levels in men with orchiopexy at older ages *(1)*.

recent study found an inverse relationship between testosterone levels in adulthood and age at orchiopexy (*see* Fig. 4), suggesting a subtle progressive detrimental consequence of a nonscrotal testis during childhood *(1)*.

LH levels are generally within the broad normal adult male range, although GnRH stimulation testing may unmask subtle abnormalities. Elevated responses provide evidence for borderline diminished testicular function that likely involves Leydig cells. Results have ranged from an excessive rise in LH levels in more than 50% of men with unilateral and the majority of men with bilateral cryptorchidism in one study *(130)* to all responses within the broad normal adult male range *(131)*. Both studies also had a small subgroup of men who were formerly bilateral cryptorchid who had subnormal responses, suggesting partial gonadotropin deficiency *(130,131)*.

Although LH regulates Leydig cells, serum levels of inhibin-B and FSH relate more directly to seminiferous tubule function. Increased basal and GnRH-stimulated FSH

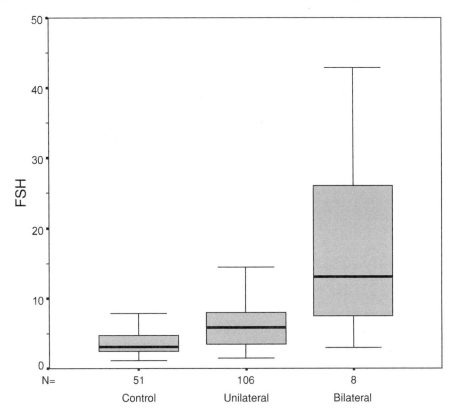

Fig. 5. Circulating follicle-stimulating hormone (FSH) levels in formerly cryptorchid men compared with control men. The majority of men in the unilateral group have FSH levels in the normal range, where almost half of men who had bilateral cryptorchidism had elevated FSH levels. Solid line depicts the median, the shaded area the interquartile range, and the cross-lines the minimum and maximum values.

levels are a common finding in men who were cryptorchid *(73)*. Basal FSH levels are frequently elevated (*see* Fig. 5) and are inversely related to sperm density (*see* Fig. 6) *(131,132)*. GnRH stimulation testing may identify an exaggerated abnormal response, which is more common and more severe in bilateral (88% in one series) than in unilateral (66%) cryptorchidism *(130)*. It is impossible to determine if this abnormality is a consequence of an abnormal cryptorchid testis, operative injury, or both.

Mean inhibin-B levels were lower in men who were formerly cryptorchid than control men (*see* Fig. 7) *(133)*. These levels correlated inversely with other hormonal markers, including FSH levels when controlled for LH, LH levels when controlled for FSH, GnRH-stimulated LH and FSH levels, testosterone, free testosterone, sperm density, sperm motility, and sperm morphology. In contrast, inhibin-B levels in control men correlated only with FSH and LH. Also, in cryptorchid but not control men, inhibin-B levels were significantly higher in men with normal sperm counts than men with low sperm counts (*see* Fig. 7). Likewise, men with cryptorchidism who were successful at paternity had higher inhibin-B levels than those who were unsuccessful. This difference was not observed in the control group. Inhibin-B is a sensitive marker of testicular dysfunction, implying diminished Sertoli cell number and/or function, and the findings suggest that a larger portion of the men

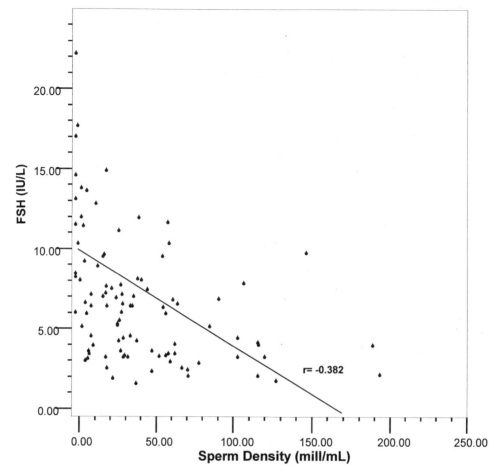

Fig. 6. An inverse relationship is apparent between follicle-stimulating hormone (FSH) levels and sperm density in men who were formerly cryptorchid.

who were formerly cryptorchid have compromised testicular function than indicated by paternity data. Elevated FSH and low inhibin-B levels and decreased sperm density are all indicative of a high risk of infertility.

As noted in the above figures, men with treated cryptorchidism have mean hormone levels that are similar to those of normal men *(86,131,133,134)*. Although a minority of unilateral men who formerly had cryptorchidism have elevated FSH and low inhibin-B levels, implying compromised seminiferous tubule function, the majority of men who had orchiopexy for bilateral cryptorchidism had elevated FSH and low inhibin-B levels *(139)*. In 45 men who were reported to have spontaneous bilateral descent after age 10 yr, 58% had elevated FSH levels, 62% had decreased testicular volume, and 53% had a sperm density less than 20 million/mL *(135)*. These data imply diminished function after a nonscrotal location of the testis during childhood years but also document that some men who were formerly cryptorchid have normal parameters.

The Children's Hospital of Pittsburgh study found that men who had orchidopexy for unilateral cryptorchidism had similar FSH, LH, testosterone, and inhibin-B levels

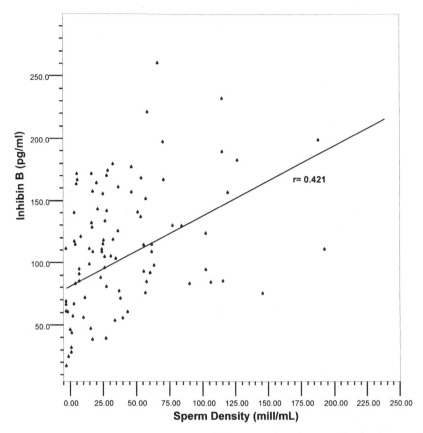

Fig. 7. A direct relationship is present between inhibin-B levels and sperm density in men who were formerly cryptorchid.

to controls *(131,133)*. When the men who had unilateral cryptorchidism were analyzed based on success or lack of success at attempted paternity, no differences were found in these hormone levels *(115)*. Men who had unilateral cryptorchidism have varying degrees of compromised seminiferous tubule function but may nevertheless be able to achieve paternity. Inhibin-B and FSH levels are only two of many markers of fertility and cannot be used to reliably predict infertility. Because numerous factors combine to cause reproductive success or failure, it is not surprising that no single finding short of azoospermia can predict infertility.

SEXUAL DEVELOPMENT

Normal testosterone production in patients with cryptorchidism, even those with unilateral anorchia or an atrophic testis, results in full stimulation of growth and maturation in androgen-responsive tissues. Hence, genital development and pubertal virilization are complete and normal, with the exception of diminished testicular volume in previously undescended testes *(130,142)*.

The cryptorchid testis varies considerably in size and may be small, even during the prepubertal years *(136)*. Catch-up growth is more likely after orchiopexy for the palpable than the nonpalpable testis *(137)* if it is brought to a scrotal location before 18 mo of age *(136)*. However, when adult testicular volume was evaluated in relation to previous germ cell counts at biopsy in prepubertal boys with cryptorchidism, prepubertal testicular size did not predict adult germ cell count *(138)*. There is also a lack of correlation between testicular volume at orchiopexy and paternity, hormone levels, sperm count, and testicular volume in adulthood when studied in both unilateral and bilateral men with cryptorchidism *(115,132,139)*.

Compensatory hypertrophy of the nonaffected testis in unilateral cryptorchidism or in the less affected testis in bilateral cryptorchidism, may occur before puberty, either before or after correction of the cryptorchidism. The mechanism for the hypertrophy is likely to involve decreased inhibin-B and, thereby, increased FSH production, even during the prepubertal years. Testicular volume differences become most significant at mid-puberty, approximately age 14 yr, when increases in testicular volume for the contralateral testis become greater than 15 mL *(140)*.

In infertile men overall, there is a significant correlation between testicular volume and indices of spermatogenesis (sperm density and motility and FSH levels) *(141)*. LH levels are related to testicular volume but not to testosterone levels. Adult previously undescended testes generally have diminished volume *(130,142)*. As a consequence of compensatory hypertrophy of the contralateral descended testis, mean testicular volume for men with corrected unilateral maldescent is usually within the normal adult range *(130)*. Occasionally, combined volume may be greater than expected, suggesting hypertrophy.

SEXUAL ACTIVITY

Although there is no reason to expect a disturbance in sexual activity because men who were formerly cryptorchid have normal development and testosterone levels and a normal interest and abilities for sexual functioning, an early report suggested that "sexual drive seemed to be diminished" *(130)*. Also, men who were formerly cryptorchid have been reported to be less sexually active as adults when judged by frequency of intercourse, although the mean age of onset of masturbation and coitus were not different than normal. It is of interest that a direct relationship was found between frequency of intercourse and both testicular volume and testosterone levels *(142)*. Also, unpublished data from the Children's Hospital of Pittsburgh cohort of formerly cryptorchid men indicate that frequency of intercourse is lower than in control men. These data are not well substantiated.

Infertility

Cryptorchidism may be a prominent cause of male infertility. Although there are no truly accurate indicators of male infertility, this number has been inferred from the portion of infertile couples whose infertility is believed to result from a male factor. It is estimated that 13 to 14% of couples in which the female partner is less than 45 yr of age are infertile (excluding those who are surgically sterile) *(143)*. In US studies, it is not possible to estimate what portion of these cases result from male factors, because all studies involve selected populations. However, a study from Great Britain evaluated a random sample of couples in a regional health district. In that study, 26% of the infertility was ascribed to problems with the man *(144)*. Applying this percentage to the 13 to 14% of couples in the United States who are infertile suggests that approx 3.5% of men are infertile *(143)*. Because the prevalence of cryptorchidism is estimated to be 0.7 to 2% of men after infancy *(11,17,42)*, this condition could account for a substantial portion of all infertile men.

There are multiple potential etiologies of cryptorchidism, and the different etiologies could result in varying potential for sperm production. Consequently, there may be considerable variation in the indices of fertility in different studies. Furthermore, it is not clear that treatment alters the potential for fertility. It has been considered an established fact that bilateral cryptorchidism is associated with infertility when the testes remain undescended beyond puberty. However, there are some interesting exceptions to this idea. Although testicular location is a potential key factor in relation to infertility, this may apply primarily to abdominal but not to lower positioned testes. Bilateral abdominal testes remaining in this location after puberty are universally associated with infertility.

Until recently, the prevalence of infertility after bilateral cryptorchidism has not been clearly documented, nor has it been shown that treatment during childhood has any beneficial effect *(113)*. A meta-analysis of 27 published studies *(113)* indicated that no men with untreated bilateral cryptorchidism had normal fertility potential based on sperm density, whereas 25% of those who were treated had normal sperm density. In patients with bilateral cryptorchidism who were treated during childhood, similar percentages of patients had azoospermia and oligospermia (density <20 million/mL), regardless of the type or age at treatment. This report, however, did not include men who were treated during infancy or early childhood.

Testicular sperm extraction (TESE) and testicular sperm aspiration (TESA) with intracytoplasmic sperm injection (ICSI) may be attempted in men who were formerly cryptorchid. Success with TESE and ICSI was reported in a man with prepubertal bilateral orchiopexy and azoospermia *(45)*. It is possible that these techniques may be successful, even for men with untreated bilateral intra-abdominal cryptorchidism.

RISK FACTORS

It has been hypothesized that disruption of the blood–testis barrier caused by testicular biopsy or by the placement of a suture through the testis to anchor it in the scrotum may have a detrimental effect on spermatogenesis, resulting from the development of antisperm antibodies. However, a study searching for antisperm antibodies in the semen of men who had had testicular biopsy at puberty failed to demonstrate antibodies *(146)*. An assessment of the Children's Hospital of Pittsburgh cohort of men who were formerly cryptorchid also found no increase in the prevalence of sperm antibodies in boys who were operated on during childhood (unpublished data). An earlier analysis seeking risk factors for infertility in this same cohort found evidence of an increased risk in association with the placement of a testicular suture (RR 7.56, 95% CI 1.66–34.39) *(147)*. However, subsequent analyses of the entire cohort failed to confirm this increased risk. Other risk factors for infertility were bilateral cryptorchidism (when compared within the entire cohort), the presence of a varicocele, hCG treatment for cryptoorchidism, and a partner with a fertility problem.

GERM CELL COUNTS (UNILATERAL AND BILATERAL)

Reports relating germ cell counts on biopsy at the time of orchiopexy to indices of fertility in adulthood are inconsistent, suggesting that germ cell number and maturation alone do not predict fertility potential or sperm density. Germ cell counts have correlated positively with sperm density and combined testicular volume and negatively with FSH levels in men who had bilateral orchiopexy between 10 and 16 yr of age

(148,149). The greatest sperm density was found in the men with testes in the superficial inguinal pouch. However, in another biopsy study, the percentage of the sections that contained spermatogonia (tubular fertility index) did not predict sperm density in adulthood *(150).*

A more recent assessment involved a group of men who had orchiopexy for either unilateral or bilateral cryptorchidism before 2 yr of age *(94,95),* of whom two-thirds had normal sperm density. In these men, testicular biopsy at the time of orchiopexy revealed that germ cells had undergone the second stage of maturation to adult dark (Ad) spermatogonia. Conversely, the remaining one-third of men who had low sperm densities had evidence for impaired germ cell maturation 20–25 yr earlier. Again, low sperm densities do not necessarily mean lack of paternity.

Most concerning are the prepubertal boys with cryptorchidism who have a complete lack of germ cells on biopsy. Although they are a minority of the total group, the absence of germ cells represents a significant independent risk of subsequent infertility *(97).* An age relationship is present with all patients who had a biopsy at orchiopexy before 2 yr of age having germ cells, but an increased risk for germ cell absence with orchiopexy at older ages *(151).* Overall, 30% of the bilateral cryptorchids and 20% of the unilateral group had no germ cells visualized. Conversely, 19% of the bilateral and 83% of the unilateral group had normal sperm densities.

AGE AT TREATMENT AND FERTILITY

It has been hypothesized that earlier treatment decreases the risk of infertility, but this has not been demonstrated convincingly. A 1975 report of 79 men found that fertility was greater when patients were younger at the time of orchiopexy *(152).* Another study of men with bilateral cryptorchidism also reported an inverse correlation between age at orchiopexy and sperm concentration *(148).* However, a meta-analysis *(113)* found no difference in the percentage of men with azoospermia or oligospermia with unilateral or bilateral cryptorchidism who were treated before vs. after 9 yr of age. Unfortunately, no patients in the meta-analysis were treated during the first few years of life. Efficacy of early therapy has been questioned, particularly for unilateral cryptorchidism. The percentage of men with azoospermia or oligospermia in the unilaterals was similar after surgical, hormonal, both treatments, or no treatment. A study of 329 men, including 66 married men, also failed to show a relationship between age of treatment and fertility, but, once again, the youngest age at therapy was 7 yr *(153).* Another study comparing patients who had surgery between 2 and 7 yr of age with those treated between 10 and 12 yr of age found no difference in fertility potential in adulthood based on testicular volume, LH, FSH and testosterone levels, and semen analyses *(97).* Finally, in the Pittsburgh study of men who had either unilateral or bilateral cryptorchidism corrected in childhood, sperm density did not correlate with age at surgery *(133).*

Successive analyses of the Children's Hospital of Pittsburgh Male Fertility Study seeking a relationship between age of orchiopexy and fertility parameters have also failed to show any such relationship *(115,139,154).* These analyses have involved men who had orchidopexy throughout childhood, including 23 men who had surgery before age 2 yr. No relationship was demonstrated between the age of orchiopexy and successful attempts at paternity, gonadotropin levels, or semen characteristics. Although the subjects in the unilateral group who had attempted paternity included 23 men who had had orchiopexy before 2 yr of age, paternity may not be a sufficiently sensitive or specific index for the relationship between age of orchiopexy and fertility *(115,155)* partly because of fertility issues in the partner. However, this study remains incomplete, because only a portion of the men have attempted paternity (359 of 609 in the unilateral cohort) and even fewer (105 of the 359) have been available for physical examination, hormone, and semen studies.

Interestingly, in the Pittsburgh cohort, a relationship is suggested between age at orchiopexy and testosterone levels in the unilateral group *(1)*. Although all men evaluated had circulating testosterone levels within the adult male range, there was an inverse relationship between testosterone and age at orchiopexy. This subtle finding is surprising and implies a risk of diminished Leydig cell function, with the retention of the testis after infancy. The finding is also consistent with the finding of Leydig cell atrophy in the cryptorchid testis *(156)*.

SPERMATOGENESIS

According to the World Health Organization (WHO) classification, sperm density greater than 20×10^6/mL is considered to be normal; oligospermia is defined as less than 20×10^6 sperm/mL, and azoospermia is 0 sperm/mL. Early reports of relatively small series suggested that sperm counts are higher in both unilateral and bilateral groups after hCG treatment than after surgery *(157)*, a large percentage of men who had unilateral cryptorchidism have subnormal sperm density *(158)*, and the fertility and potential for fertility are compromised more than suggested by recent studies. However, it is unclear whether patients with retractile testes accounted for a large portion of those treated with hCG, whether those in the hCG treatment group were less severely affected, or whether a large portion had surgical complications. Changes in surgery and surgical techniques were not considered.

Using semen analyses as an index of fertility, variable results in men who had cryptorchidism suggest considerable differences in fertility potential. In the Children's Hospital of Pittsburgh study, the sperm density was normal in only 4% of men with bilateral maldescent and in 23% with unilateral cryptorchidism *(133)*. Other studies have found normal sperm density in 0 to 20% of men who had bilateral cryptrochidism, with 23 to 36% demonstrating oligospermia, and 45 to 77% having azoospermia *(114,130)*. The outcome of patients with a history of unilateral cryptorchidism was better as a group than those with bilateral but was still largely abnormal *(60,113,159)*. Two-thirds of men with unilateral cryptorchidism have decreased sperm counts *(73,160)*, with normal density reported in only 35 to 72% *(114,130)*. Oligospermia was found in 21 to 27%, with 0 to 8% having azoospermia *(114,130)*. Sperm density results in the Children's Hospital of Pittsburgh Cryptorchid group are shown in Fig. 8.

In an attempt to determine the importance of age at orchiopexy, a study was conducted of patients who were operated on for unilateral or bilateral cryptorchidism at an older age of 7–13 yr *(153)*. That study found no improvement with earlier age at orchiopexy, although a relationship with pretreatment testicular position was present, with the lower testis resulting in better semen parameters. In the unilateral group, approximately two-thirds of the 40 men had normal semen volume, sperm density, morphology, and motility. In the bilateral group, 30% had normal sperm density.

An early assessment of sperm density in men with unilateral cryptrochidism from the Children's Hospital of Pittsburgh cohort revealed lower values than among control

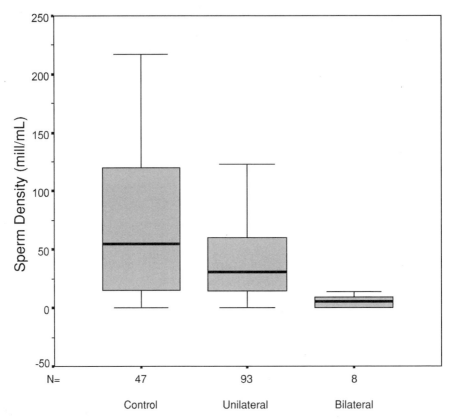

Fig. 8. Sperm density in men who were formerly cryptorchid shows diminished levels in all men who were formerly bilaterally cryptorchid, whereas the majority from the unilateral group are normal. Note that control men are men who did not have cryptorchidism but may have reproductive abnormalities. Solid line depicts the median, the shaded area the interquartile range, and the cross-lines the minimum and maximum values.

men *(131)*, as well as an inverse correlation with circulating FSH levels. However, subsequent analyses with an enlarged cohort (*see* Fig. 9) found no significant difference in sperm density between men who had or had not been successful at paternity. This is likely to result from the considerable variation in values in both the cryptorchid and the control group *(115)*. The successful fathers in the men who were formerly cryptorchid had a sperm density of $45.2 \pm 40.2 \times 10^6$/mL (M $\pm$ SD), whereas in those who were unsuccessful, the value was $27.0 \pm 30.1 \times 10^6$/mL. The control group of men in this study also had wide variation in sperm density ($82.3 \pm 82.8 \times 10^6$/mL), primarily because some men had high densities *(115)*. In addition to the wide ranges in both groups, the findings in the cryptorchid group attest to the fact that men with "subnormal" sperm counts can father children and that multiple other factors are involved in fertility. Only a limited number of men in this cohort had bilateral cryptorchidism; however, there were no men with normal sperm density, and counts ranged from azoospermia to 13.3×10^6/mL *(39)*.

It has been suggested that after unilateral cryptorchidism, the formerly undescended testis may have little sperm production, with most or all of the mature sperm arising from the contralateral testis. Two reports of men who had had unilateral cryptorchidism

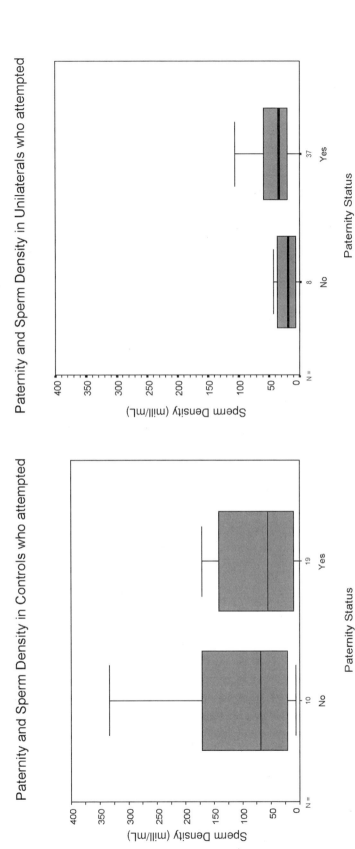

Fig. 9. Sperm density in fertile and infertile men in TE control group or with unilateral cryptorchidism. Solid line depicts the median, the shaded area the interquartile range, and the cross-lines the minimum and maximum values.

assessed semen samples after unilateral vasectomy of the contralateral testis *(161,162)*. These reports of men who had fathered children suggest that previously undescended testes produce relatively few sperm and that orchiopexy may, therefore, have little effect on sperm output. In one of these reports, 8 of 12 subjects had azoospermia after vasectomy of the contralateral testis, and the remainder had sperm densities of $2.2–9 \times 10^6$/mL *(162)*. These studies can be criticized, because surgery was done at a relatively old age. Nonetheless, the findings suggest that paternity derives primarily from the descended testis, with the previously undescended testis having poor function or severe abnormalities of the epididymis. Such an interpretation agrees with the finding that fertility is not different between men who have unilateral cryptorchidism and successful orchiopexy and men who had an absent or atrophic testis or who required orchioectomy during surgery for unilateral cryptorchidism *(114,163)*. It should also be considered that with current infertility treatments, orchiopexy may permit testicular sperm retrieval to be followed by ICSI.

PATERNITY

If accurately reported, paternity is the most valid index of fertility. A significant percentage of normal fertile men have sperm counts that are within the range considered as oligospermia ($<20 \times 10^6$/mL) *(164,165)*. In addition, sperm motility and morphology may be better indicators of paternity but are more difficult to accurately define than is the sperm count. For example, Vietnam veterans with agent-orange exposure were found to have decreased sperm counts but normal paternity rates *(166)*.

Older studies of paternity in men with a history of unilateral cryptorchidism indicated that 71 to 92% of married men reported fathering one or more children *(73,167–171)*. Overall, a composite assessment of these data indicates that 212 (80.9%) of the 262 married subjects reported children. Therefore, sperm density is not predictive of paternity.

In the recent studies of the cohort of men living in Allegheny County, Pennsylvania, during childhood (Children's Hospital of Pittsburgh male fertility study), men with unilateral cryptorchidism have paternity rates (*see* Fig. 10) that are not different from those of a control group *(2,115,154,172)*. The entire cohort included 609 men who had had orchiopexy for unilateral cryptorchidism. Each subject completed a detailed questionnaire concerning general health, marriages, cohabitation, use of birth control, frequency of intercourse, information on all children conceived in a committed relationship of 1 yr or longer, and several lifestyle factors, including alcohol, drug, and tobacco use and exposure to chemicals and irradiation. In this group, 359 men indicated that they had attempted paternity. Of these men, 89.7% had been successful in fathering one or more children, with this value not significantly different from the control group in which 93.7% were successful *(115)*. The control group consisted of men who did not have cryptorchidism or major illness. Of the 708 men, 443 completed the questionnaire, indicating that they either had fathered one or more children or had attempted paternity for more than 12 mo. A sensitive measure of fertility is time to conception; the median time was 3 mo for both the formerly unilateral and control groups, and the mean ($\pm$SD) was 7.1 ± 0.7 mo for the unilateral group and 6.9 ± 2.3 mo for the control group.

In exploring factors relevant to paternity in the men in the Pittsburgh cohort, no correlation was found between paternity and either age at orchiopexy or testicular size at

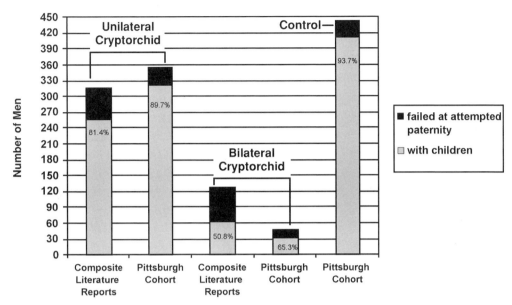

Fig. 10. Paternity data from a meta-analysis of reported cases and patients from the Pittsburgh cohort. The first two columns are from men who were formerly unilaterally cryptorchid, the next two from men who were formerly bilateral cryptorchid, and the final column the control group from the Pittsburgh study.

orchiopexy *(115,173)*. Although no statistically significant differences in paternity rates were found when analyzed by preoperative testicular location, men who had an abdominal testis had the lowest success rate (83.3%), and the lowest likelihood (60%) of achieving conception within 12 mo *(115)*. Increased risk of failure at attempted paternity was found for the presence of varicocele (7.1), major illness (3.6), and marijuana use (2.1), whereas no increased risk was found for history of mumps, prostate problems, sexually transmitted disease, or tobacco or alcohol use.

Paternity rates are significantly lower in men with a history of bilateral when compared to unilateral cryptorchidism or normal men (*see* Fig. 10). Paternity rates from various reports indicate that 33 to 62% of married men who were formerly bilaterally cryptorchid father children *(169,170,171,174)*. In the Pittsburgh cohort, we likewise found a markedly diminished paternity rate in this group *(3,154)*. In the bilateral group, only 65.3% of men were successful at paternity, compared with the 89.7% in the unilateral group and 93.2% in the control group *(140)*. In this group of men, no relationship was found between preoperative testis location and success at attempted paternity, except that the failure rate was high for bilateral but not unilateral men with an abdominal testis location. Also supportive is that time to conception was increased significantly, compared with control men and those with unilateral cryptorchidism *(175)*.

FERTILITY IN UNTREATED MALES

There are isolated case reports of fertility, based on paternity, in men with bilateral cryptorchidism not corrected until after puberty. One man who had palpable testes of normal volume located in the superficial inguinal ring until corrected at 23 yr of age subsequently fathered 4 children *(176)*. Although reported, this is clearly the exception rather than rule, and nearly all would agree that patients with untreated bilateral cryptorchidism are infertile.

Testicular Cancer

Together with infertility, increased testicular cancer risk is considered to be a major potential consequence of cryptorchidism. The origin of malignant cells is germ cells that remain in the early stages of differentiation. This may be a consequence of excessive proliferation of precursor germ cells, with associated loss of intercellular communications *(177)* or from a failure of maturation of these precursors. Testicular carcinoma-*in-situ* (CIS) precedes germ cell tumors *(178)*, although it is not clear that all CIS instances ultimately develop into tumors. Placenta-like alkaline phosphatase antibody positive cells (a marker of both undifferentiated germ cells and unclassified germ cell neoplasia) have been identified at biopsy during orchiopexy at young ages *(149)*. Thus far, no patient with these markers who was followed for two subsequent decades has developed testicular cancer.

Traditional reports suggested that patients with cryptorchidism had a 4- to 10-fold increased risk of tumors *(179)*. In all men who have cryptorchidism, the lifetime risk of a testicular cancer has been reported to be 2 to 3%, which is at least four times greater than the general population *(180,181)*. Based on the development of testicular tumors in men with a history of cryptorchidism, the risk was 4.7, compared with the general population *(179)*. The odds ratio was 9.3 in men with bilateral cryptorchidism and 2.4 in the unilateral group. Even the contralateral descended testis is at increased cancer risk. Furthermore, a much greater cancer risk is present in men with uncorrected cryptorchidism (RR 15.9 or 11/69) *(182)*. However, many of the rates reported may be falsely reduced by the inclusion of patients who had retractile testes.

The rate of development of testicular cancer has typically been assessed as the proportion of testicular cancer patients with a history of cryptorchidism, rather than the percentage of men who were formerly cryptorchid *(114)* who develop testicular tumors. In either situation, the risk may differ depending on the inclusion of patients with unilateral or bilateral cryptorchidism, age and mode of therapy, occurrence of spontaneous descent or ascent, location of the undescended testis, and the presence of other developmental anomalies.

A case-control study of men with testicular germ cell tumors found a significant association with cryptorchidism, with an odds ratio of 3.8 *(183)*. The odds ratio was 5.9 for bilateral and 2.7 for unilateral cryptorchidism. When the men in the unilateral group who had a tumor in the contralateral testis were assessed separately, the odds ratio for the ipsilateral testis was 4.0 and 1.4 for the contralateral testis. Positive associations with testicular cancer for the entire population, not just those who had cryptorchidism, were also noted for early onset of puberty (voice change and shaving), infertility, and a sedentary lifestyle. A protective effect of exercise was found, but no association with vasectomy was identified.

In addition to the generalized increased risk with cryptorchidism, certain factors stand out as adding to the cancer risk. In one study, testicular neoplasia, including CIS, was seen in 7 of 1249 biopsies of undescended testes *(184)*. This and previous reports *(178)* suggest an increased cancer risk in boys with intra-abdominal testes, an abnormal karyotype, or abnormal external genitalia. This reasoning has led to the proposal that testicular biopsy should be considered at the time of initial surgery. Inclusion of such patients may explain the high relative risk of testicular cancer in various study cohorts. Also, testicular biopsy itself may increase the cancer risk. In a cohort of 1124 men with cryptorchidism treated with surgery or hormones between 1951 and 1964 in which outcome data were obtained for 792 (70%) *(185)*, the risk was reported to be increased 8.5-fold for unilateral cryptorchidism, with a risk of 14.4-fold for the undescended testis and 2.1-fold for the scrotal testis. In that cohort, there was a substantial increase in risk in testes that were biopsied at orchiopexy, although this was done in only 9% of testes (120 of 1305 undescended testes from 1075 boys). The increase in cancer risk may relate to the reason the testes were biopsied, such as a dysgenetic appearance or the surgeon's view that the risk of neoplasia was increased.

TUMORS AND AGE AT ORCHIOPEXY

It is not known whether bringing the testis into a scrotal location reduces the risk of testicular cancer. Indeed, a relatively small study in which most surgery was done in late childhood found no effect of age of treatment on risk of cancer *(182)*. Conversely, when age at correction was considered for patients with previous unilateral cryptorchidism *(183)*, no increased risk of cancer was found for those who had successful surgery before the age of 10 yr (odds ratio 0.60), whereas the risk was increased with surgery at age 10 yr or older (odds ratio 6.75). It is noteworthy that the risk associated with undescended testes was eliminated in that study by orchiopexy before the age of 10 yr. In addition, there was a significant association between age at orchiopexy (age 3 to > 14 yr) and risk of cancer.

Although the benefits of orchiopexy in reducing the risk of neoplasia may be unclear, the general view is that bringing the testis into a scrotal or near-scrotal position is indicated. A scrotal position would allow for earlier detection of physical changes that might indicate malignancy. For this reason, orchiopexy has been recommended, even for postpubertal males who are healthy except for cryptorchidism, because the risk of malignancy is considered to exceed the perioperative morbidity and mortality *(186)*. Most also recommend biopsy of the testis at the time of orchiopexy in pubertal and postpubertal boys. In the past, some have argued for orchiectomy for the unilateral high testis, but this approach is less acceptable in the current era of assisted reproductive technology in which a single sperm may be sufficient to father a child.

SUMMARY

Cryptorchidism, the condition in which one or both testes are not descended fully into the scrotum, is one of the most frequent developmental anomalies of the human male. Although there is spontaneous descent in the first few months of life in many males born with this condition, the prevalence thereafter is about 1%. Genetic direction of testicular descent is only poorly understood. There are multiple etiologies of cryptorchidism, both anatomic and hormonal, with some testes having the potential for normal function.

Germ cells in the undescended testis fail to undergo normal differentiation from early infancy; hence, the recommendation for treatment by 1 yr of age. Frequently, men with undescended testes have impaired sperm production and decreased inhibin-B and elevated FSH levels during adulthood. Only a small portion of men who had unilateral cryptorchidism are infertile based on paternity, whereas nearly half of men with previous bilateral cryptorchidsm are infertile. The risk of developing testicular tumors, primarily of germ cell origin, is increased substantially particularly in the bilateral group and those not corrected before puberty.

REFERENCES

1. Lee PA, Coughlin MT. Leydig cell function after cryptrochidism: evidence of the beneficial result of early surgery. J Urol 2002;167:1824–1827.
2. Lee PA, O'Leary LA, Songer NJ, Coughlin MT, Bellinger MF, LaPorte RE. Paternity after unilateral cryptorchidism. Pediatrics 1996;98:676–679.
3. Lee PA, O'Leary LA, Songer NJ, Coughlin MT, Bellinger MF, LaPorte RE. Paternity after bilateral cryptorchidism: a controlled study. Arch Pediatr Adolesc Med 1997;151:260–263.
4. Thorup J, Cortes D. The incidence of maldescended testes in Denmark. Pediatr Surg Int 1990;5:2–5.
5. Olsen LH. Inter-observer variation in assessment of undescended testes. Brit J Urol 1989;64:644–648.
6. Caesar RE, Kaplan GW. The incidence of the cremasteric reflex in normal boys. J Urol 1994;152:779–780.
7. Cytryn L, Cytryn E, Rieger RE. Psychological implications of cryptorchidism. J Am Acad Child Psychiatr 1967;6:131–165.
8. Meyer-Bahlburg HFL, Aceto T, Pinch L. Cryptorchidism, development of gender identity, and sex behavior. In: Friedman RC, Richart RM, Vander Wiele RL, eds. Sex Differences in Behavior. Wiley and Company, New York, 1974, pp. 281–299.
9. John Radcliffe Hospital Cryptorchid Study Group. Cryptorchidism—an apparent substantial increase since 1960. Brit Med J 1986;293:401–1404.
10. John Radcliffe Hospital Cryptorchidism Study Group. Clinical diagnosis of cryptorchidism. Arch Dis Child 1988;63:587–591.
11. John Radcliffe Hospital Cryptorchidism Study Group. Cryptorchidism: a prospective study of 7500 consecutive male births, 1984–8. Arch Dis Child 1992;67:892–899.
12. Scorer CG. The descent of the testes. Arch Dis Child 1964;39:605–609.
13. Jackson MB, Chilvers C, Pike M, Ansell P, Bull D. Cryptorchidism: an apparent substantial increase since 1960. Brit Med J 1986;293:1401–1404.
14. Berkowitz GS, Lapinski RH, Dolgin SE, Gazella JG, Bodian CA, Holzman IR. Prevalence and natural history of cryptorchidism. Pediatrics. 1993;92:44–49.
15. Villumsen A, Zachau-Christiansen B. Spontaneous alteration in position of the testes. Arch Dis Child 1966;41:198–200.
16. Colodny AH. Undescended testes—is surgery necessary? N Engl J Med 1986;314:510–511.
17. Koyle MA, Rajfer J, Ehrlich RM. The undescended testis. Pediatr Ann 1988;17:39, 42–46.
18. Okeke AA, Osegbe DN. Prevalence and characteristics of cryptorchidism in a Nigerian district. Br J Urol Int 2001;88:941–945.
19. Toppari J, Kaleva M, Virtanen HE. Trends in the incidence of cryptorchidism and hypospadias, and methodological limitations of registry-based data. Hum Reprod Update 2001;7:282–286.
20. Kaleva M, Virtanen H, Haavisto AM, Main K, Skakkebaek NE, Toppari J. Incidence of cryptorchidism in Finnish Boys. Horm Res 2001;55:54.
21. Weidner IS, Moller H, Jenson TK, Skakkebaek NE. Cryptorchidism and hypospadias in sons of gardeners and farmers. Environmental Health Perspectives 1998;106:793–796.
22. Witchel SF, Lee PA. Ambiguous genitalia. In: Sperling MA, ed. Pediatric Endocrinology. Saunders, Philadelphia, 2002, pp. 111–133.
23. Grumbach MM, Hughes IA, Conte FA. Disorders of sex differentiation. In: Larsen PR, Kronenberg HM, Melmed S, Polonsky, eds. Willaims Textbook of Endocrinology, 10th ed. Saunders, Philadelphia, 2003, 842–1002.
24. Hutson JM, Donahoe PK. The hormonal control of testicular descent. Endocr Rev 1986;7:270–283.
25. Hutson JM, Baker M, Terada M, Zhou B, Paxton G. Hormonal control of testicular descent and the cause of cryptorchidism. Reprod Fertil Dev 1994;6:151–156.
26. Barthold JS, Kumasi-Rivers K, Upadhyay J, Shekarriz B, Imperato- Meginley J. Testicular position in the androgen insensitivity syndrome: implications for the role of androgens in testicular descent. J Urol 2000;164:497–501.

27. van der Schoot P, Elger W. Androgen-induced prevention of the outgrowth of cranial gonadal suspensory ligaments in fetal rats. J Androl 1992;13:534–542.

28. Lee SM, Hutson JM. Effect of androgens on the cranial suspensory ligament and ovarian position. Anat Rec 1999;255:306–315.

29. Heyns CF. The gubernaculums during testicular descent in the human fetus. J Anat 1987;153:93–112.

30. Schindler AM, Diaz P, Cuendet A, Sizonenko PC. Cryptorchidism: a morphological study of 670 biopsies. Helv Paediatr Acta 1987;42:145–158.

31. Heyns CF, Human HJ, DeKlerk DP. Hyperplasia and hypertrophy of the gubernaculums during testicular descent in the fetus. J Urol 1986;135:1043–1047.

32. Heyns CF, Human HJ, Werely CJ, DeKlerk DP. The glycosaminoglycans of the gubernaculums during testicular descent in the fetus. J Urol 1990;143:612–617.

33. Costa WS, Sampaio FJB, Favorito LA, Cardoso LEM. Testicular migration: remodeling of connective tissue and muscle cells in human gubernaculums testis. J Urol 2002;167:2171–2176.

34. Levy JB, Husmann DA. The hormonal control of testicular descent. J Androl 1995;16:459.

35. Beasley SW, Hutson JM. Effect of division of genitofemoral nerve on testicular descent in the rat. Aust N Z J Surg 1987;57:49–51.

36. Hutson JM, Beasley SW, Bryan AD. Cryptorchidism in spina bifida and spinal cord transection: a clue to the mechanism of transinguinal descent of the testis. J Pediatr Surg 1988;23:275–277.

37. Yamanaka J, Metcalfe MA, Hutson JM. Demonstration of calcitonin gene- related peptide receptors in the gubernaculum by computerized densitometry. J Pediatr Surg 1992;27:876–878.

38. Yamanaka J, Metcalfe SA, Hutson JM, Mendelsohn FA. Testicular descent. II. Ontogeny and response to denervation of calcitonin gene-related peptide receptors in neonatal rat gubernaculum. Endocrinology 1993;132:280–284.

39. Samarakkody UK, Hutson JM. Intrascrotal CGRP 8–37 causes a delay in testicular descent in mice. J Pediatr Surg 1992;27:874–875.

40. Griffiths AL, Middlesworth W, Goh DW, Hutson JM. Exogenous calcitonin gene-related peptide causes gubernacular development in neonatal (Tfm) mice with complete androgen resistance. J Pediatr Surg 1993;28:1028–1030.

41. Park WH, Hutson JM. The gubernaculum shows rhythmic contractility and active movement during testicular descent. J Pediatr Surg 1991;26:615–617.

42. Adham IM, Burkhardt E, Bonahmed M, Engel W. Cloning of a cDNA for a novel insulin-like peptide of the testicular Leydig cells. J Biol Chem 1993;268:26668–26672.

43. Zimmermann S, Steding G, Emmen JM, et al. Targeted disruption of the *Insl3* gene causes bilateral cryptorchidism. Mol Endocrinol 1999;13:681–691.

44. Cortes D, Thorup JM, Visfelt J, Schwartz M. Is fertility after surgery for cryptorchidism congenital or acquired? Pediatr Surg Int 1998;14:6–8.

45. Nef S, Shipman T, Parada LF. A molecular basis for estrogen-induced cryptorchidism. Dev Biol 2000;224:354–361.

46. Adham IM, Emmen JM, Engel W. The role of the testicular factor INSL3 in establishing the gonadal position. Mol Cell Endocrinol 2000;160:11–16.

47. Marin P, Ferlin A, Moro E, Garolla A, Foresta C. Different insulin-like 3 (InSL3) gene mutations not associated with human cryptorchidism. J Endocrinol Invest 2001;24:RC13–RC15.

48. Marin P, Ferlin A, Moro E, et al. Novel insulin-like 3(INSL3) gene mutation associated with human cryptorchidism. Am J Med Genet 2001;103:348–349.

49. Koskimies P, Virtanen H, Lindstrom M, et al. A common polymorphism in the human relaxin-like factor (RLF) gene: no relationship with cryptorchidism. Pediatr Res 2000;47:538–541.

50. Tomboc M, Lee PA, Mitwally MF, Schneck FX, Bellinger M, Witchel SF. Insulin-like 3/relaxin-like factor gene mutations are associated with cryptorchidism. J Clin Endocrinol Metab 2000;85:4013–4018.

51. Baker LA, Nef S, Nguyen MT, Stapleton R, Pohl H, Parada LF. The insulin-3 gene: lack of a genetic basis for human cryptorchidism. J Urol 2002;167:2534–2537.

52. Lund JM, Bouhadiba N, Sams V, Tsang T. Hepatotesticular fusion: an unusual case of undescended testes. Br J Urol Int 2001;88:439–440.

53. Cortes D, Thorup JM, Beck BL. Quantitative histology of germ cells in the undescended testes of human fetuses, neonates and infants. J Urol 1995;154:1188–1192.

54. Engle ET. Experimentally induced descent of the testis in the Macacus monkey by hormones from the anterior pituitary and pregnancy urine. Endocrinology 1932;16:513.

55. Husmann DA, McPhaul MJ. Time-specific androgen blockade with flutamide inhibits testicular descent in the rat. Endocrinology 1991;129:1409–1416.

56. Husmann DA, McPhaul MJ. Reversal of flutamide-induced cryptrochidism by prenatal time-specific androgens. Endocrinology 1992;131:1711–1715.

57. Baumans V, Dijkstra G, Wensing CJ. The effect of orchidectomy on gubernacular outgrowth and regression in the dog. Int J Androl 1982;5:387–400.

58. Baumans V, Dijkstra G, Wensing CJ. The role of a non-androgenic testicular factor in the process of testicular descent in the dog. Int J Androl 1983;6:541–552.

59. Spencer JR, Torrado T, Sanchez RS, Vaughan ED, Jr. Effects of flutamide and finasteride on rat testicular descent. Endocrinology 1991;129:741–748.

60. Kogan SJ. Fertility in cryptrochidism. Eur J Pediatr 1987;146(suppl 2):S21–S24.

61. Juenemann KP, Kogan BA, Abozcid MH. Fertility in cryptorchidism: an experimental model. J Urol 1986;136:214–216.

62. Hutson JM, Watts LM, Montalto J, Greco S. Both gonadotropin and testosterone fail to reverse estrogen-induced cryptorchidism in fetal mice: further evidence for nonandrogenic control of testicular descent in the fetus. Pediatr Surg Int 1990;5:13–18.

63. McBride ML, Van Den Steen N, Lamb CW, Gallagher RP. Maternal and gestational factors in cryptorchidism. Int J Epidemiol 1991;20:964–970.

64. Forest MG, Cathiard AM, Bertrand JA. Evidence of testicular activity in early infancy. J Clin Endocrinol Metab 1973;37:148–151.

65. Gendrel D, Job JC, Roger M. Reduced post-natal rise of testosterone in plasma of cryptorchid infants. Acta Endocrinol 1978;89:372–378.

66. Gendrel D, Roger M, Job JC. Plasma gonadotropin and testosterone values in infants with cryptorchidism. J Pediatr 1980;97:217–220.

67. Pouplard A, Job JC, Luxembourger I, Chaussain JL. Antigonadotropic cell antibodies in the serum of cryptorchid children and infants and of their mothers. J Pediatr 1985;107:26–30.

68. Baker BA, Morley R, Lucas A. Plasma testosterone in preterm infants with cryptorchidism. Arch Dis Child 1988;63:1198–1200.

69. Donahoe PK, Ito Y, Morikawa Y, Hendren WH. Mullerian inhibiting substance in human testes after birth. J Pediatr Surg 1977;12:323–330.

70. Yamanaka J, Baker M, Metcalfe S, Hutson SM. Serum levels of Mullerian inhibiting substance in boys with cryptorchidism. J Pediatr Surg 1991;26:621–623.

71. Tran D, Picard JY, Vigier B, Berger R, Josso N. Persistence of mullerian ducts in male rabbits passively immunized against bovine anti-mullerian hormone during fetal life. Dev Biol 1986;116:160–167.

72. Job J-C, Garnier PE, Chaussain J-L, Toublanc JE, Canlorbe P. Effect of synthetic luteinizing hormone-releasing hormone on the release of gonadotropins in hypophysogonadal disorders of children and adolescents. J Pediatr 1974;84:371–374.

73. Lipschulz LI, Caminos-Torees R, Greenspan CS, Snyder PJ. Testicular function after orchiopexy for unilateral undescended testis. New Eng J Med 1976;295:15–18.

74. Lee PA, Hoffman WH, White JJ, Engel RME, Blizzard RM. Serum gonadotropins in cryptorchidism. an indicator of functional testes. Am J Dis Child 1974;127:530–532.

75. Christiansen P, Andersson A-M, Skakkebaek NE, Julul A. Serum inhibin B, FSH, LH, and testosterone levels before and after human chorionic gonadotropin stimulation in prepubertal boys with cryptorchidism. Euro J Endocrinol 2002;147:95–101.

76. Hadziselimovic F, Herzog B, Buser M. Development of cryptorchid testes. Eur J Pediatr 1987;146(suppl 2):S8–S12.

77. Huff DS, Hadziselimovic F, Duckett JW, Elder JS, Snyder HM. Germ cell counts in semi-thin sections of biopsies of 115 unilateral cryptorchid testes: the experience from the Children's Hospital of Philadelphia. Eur J Pediatr 1987;146(suppl 2):S25–S27.

78. Huff DS, Hadziselimovic F, Snyder HM, Blyth B, Duckett JW. Early postnatal testicular maldevelopment in cryptorchidism. J Urol 1991;116:624–626.

79. Mengel W, Heinz HA, Sippe WG, Hecker WC. Studies on cryptorchidism: a comparison of histological findings in the germinative epithelium before and after the second year of life. J Pediatr Surg 1974;9:445–450.

80. Hedinger C. The histopathology of the cryptorchid testis. In: Bierich JR, Rager K, Ranke MB, eds. Maldescensus Tesis. Urban and Schwarzenberg, Munchen, 1977, pp. 29–37.

81. Hedinger C. Histological data in cryptorchidism. In: Job J-C, ed. Cryptorchidism, Diagnosis and Treatment. Pediatric and Adolescent Endocrinology, Vol 6. Karger, New York, 1979, pp. 3–13.

82. Hedinger CE. Histopathology of undescended testes. Eur J Pediatr 1982;139:266–270.

83. Hadziselimovic F. Histology and Ultrastructure of normal and cryptorchid testes. In: Hadziselimovic F, ed. Cryptorchidism, Management and Implications. Berlin, Springer-Verlag, 1983, pp. 35–58.

84. Mancini RE, Rosenberg E, Cullen M, et al. Cryptorchid and scrotal human testes. I. Cytological, cytochemical and quantitative studies. J Clin Endocr Metab 1965;25:927–942.

85. Wilkerson ML, Bartone FF, Fox L, Hadziselimovic F. Fertility potential: a comparison of intra-abdominal and intracanalicular testes by age groups in children. Horm Res 2001;55:18–20.

86. Lee PA, Coughlin MT, Bellinger MF. Paternity and hormone levels after unilateral cryptorchidism: relationship to pretreatment testicular location. J Urol 2000;164:1697–1700.

87. Huff DS, Fenig DM, Canning DA, Carr MG, Zderic SA, Snyder HM, 3rd. Abnormal germ cell development in cryptorchidism. Horm Res 2001;55:11–17.

88. Paniagua R, Martinez-Onsurbe P, Santamaria L, Saez FJ, Amat P, Nistal M. Quantitative and ultrastructural alterations in the lamina propria and Sertoli cells in human cryptorchid testes. Int J Androl 1990;13:470–487.

89. Kirby RS, Chapple CR, Ward SP, Williams C. Is the scrotal testis normal in unilateral cryptorchidism? Br J Urol 1985;57:187–189.

90. Hadziselimovic F. Cryptorchidism. In: Gillenwater JY, Grayhack JT, Howards SS, et al., eds. Adult and Pediatric Urology, Vol. 2. Mosby-Year Book, Chicago, 1991, pp. 2217–2228.

91. Dominguez C, Martinez Verduch M, Estornell F, Garcia F, Hernandez M, Garcia-Ibarra F. Histological study in contralateral testis of prepubertal children following unilateral testicular torsion. Eur Urol 1994;26:160–163.

92. Kogan SJ, Tennenbaum S, Gill B, Reda E, Levitt SB. Efficacy of orchiopexy by patient age 1 year for cryptorchidism. J Urol 1990;144:508–509.

93. Rezvani I. Cryptorchidism: a pediatrician's view. Pediatr Clin North Am 1987;34:735–746.

94. Hadziselimovic F, Herzog B. Importance of early postnatal germ cell maturation for fertility of cryptorchid males. Horm Res 2001;55:6–10.

95. Hadziselimovic F, Herzog B. The importance of both early orchidopexy and germ cell maturation for fertility. Lancet 2001;358:1156–1157.

96. Bica DT, Hadzisellimovic F. Buserelin treatment of cryptorchidism: a randomized, double-blind, placebo-controlled study. J Urol 1992;148:617–621.

97. Cortes D, Thorup JM, Lindenberg S. Fertility potential after unilateral orchiopexy: simultaneous testicular biopsy and orchiopexy in a cohort of 87 patients. J Urol 1996;155:1061–1065.

98. Koff WJ, Scaletscky R. Malformation of the epididymus in undescended testis. J Urol 1990;143:340–343.

99. Mollaeian M, Mehrabi V, Elahi B. Significance of epididymal and ductal anomalies associated with undescended testis: study in 652 cases. Urology 1994;43:857–860.

100. Puri P, Nixon MH. Bilateral retractile testes-subsequent effects on fertility. J Pediatr Surg 1977;12:563–566.

101. Atwell JD. Ascent of the testis: fact or fiction. Brit J Urol 1985;57:474–477.

102. Hutson JM, Goh DW. Can undescended testes by acquired? Lancet 1993;341:504.

103. Hadziselimovic F, Herzog B. Importance of early postnatal germ cell maturation for fertility of cryptorchid males. Horm Res 2001;55:6–10.

104. Lamah M, McCaughey ES, Finlay FO, Burge DM. The ascending testis: is late orchioipexy due to failue of screening or late ascent? Pediatr Surg Int 2001;17:421–423.

105. Mayr J, Rune GM, Holas A, Schimpl G, Schmidt B, Haberlik A. Ascent of the testis in children. Eur J Pediatr 1995;154:893–895.

106. Garcia J, Navarro E, Guirado F, Pueyo C, Ferrandez A. Spontaneous ascent of the testis. Br J Urol 1997;79:113–115.

107. John Radcliffe Hospital Cryptorchidism Study Group. Boys with late descending testes: the source of patients with "retractile" testes undergoing orchiopexy? Br Med J 1986;293:789–790.

108. Fenton EJ, Woodward AA, Hudson IL, Marschner I. The ascending testis. Pediatr Surg Int 1990;5:6–9.

109. Wyllie GG. The retractile testis. Med J Aust 1984;140:403–405.

110. Giannopoulos MF, Vlachakis IG, Charissis GC. 13 years' experience with the combined hormonal therapy of cryptorchidism. Horm Res 2001;55:33–37.

111. Tsujihata M, Miyake O, Yoshimura K, et al. Laparoscopic diagnosis and treatment of nonpalpable testis. Int J Urol 2001;8:692–696.

112. Froeling FMJA, Sorber MJG, DeLaRosette JJMCH, DeVries JDM. The nonpalpable testis and the changing role of laparoscopy. Urology 1994;43:222–227.

113. Chilvers C, Dudley NE, Gough MH, Jackson MB, Pike MC. Undescended testis: the effect of treatment on subsequent risk of subfertility and malignancy. J Pediatr Surg 1986;21:691–696.

114. Okuyama A, Nonomura N, Namiki M, et al. Surgical management of undescended testis: retrospective study of potential fertility in 274 cases. J Urol 1989;142:749–751.

115. Miller KD, Coughlin MT, Lee PA. Fertility after unilateral cryptorchidism: paternity, time to conception, pretreatment testicular location and size, hormone and sperm parameters. Horm Res 2001;55:249–253.

116. Docimo SG. The results of surgical therapy for cryptorchidism: a literature review and analysis. J Urol 1995;154:1148–1152.

117. Kirsch AJ, Escala J, Duckett JW, et al. Surgical management of the nonpalpable testis: the children's hospital of Philadelphia experience. J Urol 1998;159:1340–1343.

118. Ferro F, Inon A, Caterino S, Lais A, Inserra A. Staged orchidopexy: simplifying the second stage. Pediatr Surg Int 1990;5:10–12.

119. Kolon TF, Miller OF. Comparison of single versus multiple dose regimens for the human chorionic gonadotropin stimulatory test. J Urol 2001;166:1451–1454.

120. Tzvetkova P, Tzvetkov D. Diagnosis of abdominal bilateral cryptorchidism: HCG stimulation test. Urol Int 2001;67:46–48.

121. Bhowmick SK, Gidvani VK. Pitfalls of conventional human chorionic gonadotropin stimulation test to detect hormonally functional cryptorchid testes in midchildhood. Endocr Pract 2000;6:8–12.

122. Lee PA. Appropriate use and interpretation of human chorionic gonadotropin stimulation in prepubertal male patients. Endocr Pract 2000;6:112–114.

123. Bertelloni S, Baroncelli GI, Ghirri P, Spinelli C, Saggese G. Hormonal treatment for unilateral inguinal testis: comparison of four different treatments. Horm Res 2001;55:236–239.

124. Saggese G, Ghirri P, Gabrielli S, Cosenza GCM. Hormonal therapy for cryptorchidism with a combination of human chorionic gonadotropin and follicle-stimulating hormone. Am J Dis Child 1989;143:980–982.

125. Pyorala S, Huttunen NP, Uhari M. A review and meta-analysis of hormonal treatment of cryptorchidism. J Clin Endocrinol Metab 1995;80:2795–2799.

126. Urban MD, Lee PA, Lanes R, Migeon CJ. HCG stimulation in children with cryptorchidism. Clin Pediatr 1987;26:512–514.

127. Thorup J, Cortes D, Nielsen OH. Clinical and histopathologic evaluation of operated maldescended testes after luteinizing hormone-releasing hormone treatment. Pediatr Surg Int 1993;8 419–422.

128. Cortes D, Thorup J, Visfeldt J, Hormonal treatment may harm the germ cells in 1 to 3-year-old boys with cryptorchidism. J Urol 2000;163:1290–1292.

129. Kirk JMW, Savage MO, Grant DS, Bouloux P-M G, Besser GM. Gonadal function and response to human chorionic and menopausal gonadotropin therapy in male patients with idiopathic hypogonadotropic hypogonadism. Clin Endocrinol 1994;41:57–63.

130. Werder EA, Illig R, Torresani T, et al. Gonadal function in young adults after surgical treatment of cryptorchidism. Br J Med 1976;2:1357–1359.

131. Lee PA, Bellinger MF, Coughlin MT. Correlations between hormone levels, sperm parameters and paternity among formerly unilaterally cryptorchid men. J Urol 1998;160:1155–1157.

132. Gracia J, Sanchez Zalabardo J, Sanchez Garcia C, Ferrandez A. Clinical, physical, sperm and hormonal data in 251 adults operated on for cryptorchidism is childhood. Br J Urol Int 2000;85:1100–1103.

133. Lee PA, Coughlin MT, Bellinger MF. Inhibin B: comparison with indices of fertility among formerly cryptorchid and control men. J Clin Endocrinol Metab 2001;86:2576–2584.

134. Martinetti M, Machnie M, Salvaneschi N, et al. Immunogenetic and hormonal study of cryptorchidism. J Clin Endocrinol Metab 1992;74:39–42.

135. Bremholm Rasmussen TB, Ingerslev HJ, Hostrup H. Bilateral spontaneous descent of the testis after the age of 10: subsequent effects on fertility. Br J Urol 1988;75:820–823.

136. Nagar H, Haddad R. Impact of early orchidopexy on testicular growth. Br J Urol 1997;80:334–335.

137. Puri P, Nixon MH. Bilateral retractile testes-subsequent effects on fertility. J Pediatr Surg 1977;12:563–566.

138. Noh PH, Cooper CS, Snyder HM, 3rd, Zderic SA, Canning DA, Huff DS. Testicular volume does not predict germ cell count in patients with cryptorchidism J Urol 2000;163:593–566.

139. Lee PA, Coughlin MT. Fertility after bilateral cryptorchidism: evaluation by paternity, hormone and semen data. Horm Res 2001;55:28–32.

140. Takihara H, Baba Y, Ishizu K, Ueno T, Sakatoku J. Testicular development following unilateral orchiopexy measured by a new orchiometer. Urology 1990;36:370–372.

141. Bujan L, Mieusset R, Mansat A, Moatti JP, Mondinat C, Pontonnier F. Testicular size in infertile men: relationship to semen characteristics and hormonal blood levels. Br J Urol 1989;64:632–637.

142. Taskinen S, Wikstrom S. Effect of age at operation, location of testis and preoperative hormonal treatment on testicular growth after cryptorchidism. J Urol 1997;158:471–473.

143. Mosher WD. Infertility: why business is booming. Am Demograph 1987;9:42–43.

144. Hull MGR, Glazener CMA, Kelly NJ, et al. Population study of causes, treatment and outcome of infertility. Br Med J 1985;291:1693–1697.

145. Ribe N, Manasia P, Martinez L, Egozcue S, Pomerol JM. TESE-ICSI in the treatment of secretory azoospermia secondary to cryptorchidism. Report of a clinical case. Arch Ital Urol Androl 2001;73:45–48.

146. Cortes D, Brandt B, Thorup J. Direct mixed antiglobulin reaction (MAR) test in semen at follow-up after testicular biopsy of maldescended testes operated in puberty. Z Kinderchir 1990;45:227–228.

147. Coughlin MT, Bellinger MF, LaPorte RE, Songer NJ, Lee PA. Testicular suture: a significant risk factor for infertility among formerly cryptorchid men. J Pediatr Surg 1998;33:1–5.

148. Cortes D, Thorup J. Histology of testicular biopsies taken at operation for bilateral maldescended testes in relation to fertility in adulthood. Br J Urol 1991;68:185–291.

149. Engeler DS, Hosli PO, Hubert J, et al. Early orchiopexy: prepubertal intratubular germ cell neoplasia and fertility outcome. Urology 2000;56:144–148.

150. Gracia J, Sanchez J, Garcia C, Pueyo C, Ferrandez A. What is the relationship between spermotozoa per milliliter at adulthood and the tubular fertility index at surigcal age for patients with cryptorchidism? J Pediatr Surg 1998;33:594–596.

151. Cortes D, Thorup JM, Visfeldt J. Cryptorchidism: aspects of fertility and neoplasms. A study including data of 1,335 consecutive boys who underwent testicular biopsy simultaneously with surgery for cryptorchidism. Horm Res 2001;55:21–27.

152. Ludwig G, Potempa J. Optimal time for treating cryptorchidsm. Dutch Med Wochenschr 1975;100:680–683.

153. Puri P, O'Donnell B. Semen analysis of patients who had orchidopexy at or after seven years of age. Lancet 1988;2:1051–1052.

154. Lee PA, O'Leary LA, Songer NJ, Bellinger MF, LaPorte RE. Paternity after cryptorchidism: lack of correlation with age at orchidopexy. Br J Urol 1995;75:705–707.

155. Coughlin MT, Lee PA, Bellinger MF. Age at unilateral orchiopexy: effect on hormone levels and sperm count in adulthood. J Urol 1999;162:986–988.

156. Hadziselimovic F, Herzog B. The meaning of the Leydig cell in relation to the etiology of cryptrochidism: an experimental electron-microscopic study. J Pediatr Surg 1976;11:1–8.

157. Albescu JZ, Bergada C, Cullen M. Male fertility in patients treated for cryptorchidism before puberty. Fertil Steril 1971;22:829–833.

158. Scott LS. Unilateral cryptorchidism: subsequent effects of fertility. J Reprod Fertil 1961;2:54–60.

159. Yavetz H, Harash B, Paz G, et al. Cryptorchidism: incidence and sperm quality in infertile men. Andrologia 1992;24:293–297.

160. Grasso M, Buonaguidi A, Lania C, Bergamaschi F, Castelli M, Rigatti P. Post pubertal cryptrochidism: review and evaluation of fertility. Eur Urol 1991;20:126–128.

161. Eldrup J, Steven K. Influence of orchidopexy for cryptorchidism on subsequent fertility. Br J Surg 1980;67:269–270.

162. Alpert PF, Klein RS. Spermatogenesis in the unilateral cryptorchid testis after orchiopexy. J Urol 1983;129:301–302.

163. Lee PA, Coughlin MT. A single testis: paternity assessment after presentation as unilateral cryptorchidism. J Urol 2002;168:1680–1682.

164. Zuckerman Z, Rodriguez-Rigau LJ, Smith KD, Steinberger E. Frequency distribution of sperm counts in fertile and infertile males. Fertil Steril 1977;28:1310–1313.

165. Sheriff DS. Setting standards of male fertility I Semen analyses in 1500 patients—a report. Andrologia 1983;15:687–692.

166. The Centers for Disease Control Vietnam Experience Study. Health Status of Vietnam Veterans. II. Physical Health: JAMA 1988;259:2708–2714.
167. Hand JR. Undescended testes. report of 153 cases with evaluation of clinical findings, treatment and results followed up to 33 years. J Urol 1956;75:973–989.
168. Barcat J. L'ectopie testiculaire: statistiques, clinique et operatoire des Services de Chirurgie Infantile des Enfants-Malades de 1914 a 1950. Mem Acad Chir 1957;83:909–926.
169. Atkinson PM. A follow up study of surgically treated cryptorchid patients. J Pediatr Surg 1975;10:115–119.
170. Cendron M, Keating MA, Huff DS, Koop CE, Snyder HMcC, Duckett JE. Cryptorchidism, orchidopexy and infertility—a critical long-term retrospective analysis. J Urol 1989;142:559–562.
171. Fallon B, Kennedy TJ. Long-term follow-up fertility in cryptorchid patients. Urology 1985;25:502–504.
172. Lee PA, Bellinger MF, Songer NJ, O'Leary L, Fishbough R, LaPorte R. An epidemiologic study of paternity after cryptorchidism: initial results. Eur J Pediatr 1993;152:S25–S27.
173. Lee PA, Coughlin MT, Bellinger MF. No relationship between testicular size at orchiopexy with fertility in men who previously had unilateral cryptorchidism. J Urol 2001;166:236–239.
174. Gross RE, Jewett TC. Surgical experience from 1222 operations for undescended testes. JAMA 1956;160:634–641.
175. Coughlin MT, O'Leary LA, Songer NJ, Bellinger MF, LaPorte RE, Lee PA. Time to conception after orchidopexy for cryptorchidism: evidence for subferility? Fertil Steril 1997;67:742–746.
176. Heaton ND, Davenport M, Pryor JP. Fertility after correction of bilateral undescended testes at the age of 23 years. Br J Urol 1993;71:490–491.
177. Gondos B. Ultrastructure of developing and malignant germ cells. Eur Urol 1993;23:68–75.
178. Cortes D, Thorup J, Frisch M, Moller H, Jacobsen GK, Beck BL. Examination for intratubular germ cell neoplasia (ITGCN) at operation for undescended testis in boys. A follow-up study. J Urol 1994;151:722–725.
179. Giwercman A, Muller J, Skakkebaek NE. Cryptorchidism and testicular neoplasia. Horm Res 1988;30:157–163.
180. Cortes D. Cryptorchidism—aspects of pathogenesis, histology and treatment. Scand J Urol Nephrol 1998;32:1–54.
181. Moller H, Cortes D, Engholm G, Thorup J. Risk of testicular cancer with cryptorchidism and with testicular biopsy: cohort study. Br Med J 1998;317:729.
182. Pike MC, Chilvers C, Peckham MJ. Effect of age at orchidopexy on risk of testicular cancer. Lancet 1986;1:1246–1248.
183. United Kingdom Testicular Cancer Study Group. Aetiology of testicular cancer: association with congenital abnormalities, age at puberty, infertility, and exercise. Br Med J 1994;308:1393–1399.
184. Cortes D, Visfeldt J, Moller H, Thorup J. Testicular neoplasia in cryptorchid boys at primary surgery: case series. Br Med J 1999;319:888–889.
185. Swerdlow AJ, Higgins CD, Pike MC. Risk of testicular cancer in cohort of boys with cryptorchidism. Br Med J 1997;314:1507–1511.
186. Oh J, Landman J, Evers A, Yan Y, Kibel AS. Management of the postpubertal patient with cryptorchidism: an updated analysis. J Urol 2002;167:1329–1333.

11 Hypogonadism in Men With HIV-AIDS

Shalender Bhasin, MD

CONTENTS

Human immunodeficiency virus (HIV)-1 produces a complex, multisystem syndrome that results from the combined effects of the virus infection, progressive immunosuppression, malignancies and opportunistic infections, poor nutrition, and the complications of antiretroviral therapy. Androgen deficiency is only one facet of this highly heterogeneous syndrome. Therefore, androgen supplementation should only be viewed as an adjunctive therapy within the context of a multicomponent therapeutic strategy. Although there is increasing evidence that androgen deficiency, defined solely in terms of low testosterone levels, is highly prevalent in HIV-infected men and women and that low testosterone levels are associated with adverse disease outcomes, the long-term benefits and risks of testosterone supplementation on health-related outcomes in HIV-infected individuals have not been clearly demonstrated.

From: *Male Hypogonadism:*
Basic, Clinical, and Therapeutic Principles
Edited by: S. J. Winters © Humana Press Inc., Totowa, NJ

HIGH PREVALENCE OF ANDROGEN DEFICIENCY
IN HIV-INFECTED MEN AND WOMEN

Early studies *(1–4)* suggested that as many as 30–50% of HIV-infected men have serum testosterone levels that are below the lower limit of the normal range for healthy, young men. For instance, Dobs et al. *(1)* reported that 50% of HIV-infected men had low testosterone concentrations. Grinspoon et al. *(2)* described a reduction in free testosterone levels in 49% of HIV-infected men with AIDS wasting. In a prospective survey *(5)* conducted in 1998 during the early days of protease inhibitor therapy, we prospectively measured serum total and free-testosterone and dihydrotestosterone (DHT) levels in 148 consecutive HIV-infected men and compared the results to 42 healthy men. Thirty-one percent of HIV-infected men had serum testosterone levels less than 275 ng/dL, the lower limit of the normal male range *(5)*. Overall, serum testosterone, free-testosterone, and DHT levels were lower in HIV-infected men than in healthy men, but serum DHT-to-testosterone ratios were not significantly different between the two groups. Serum total- and free-testosterone levels were lower in HIV-infected men who had lost 5 lb or more of weight in the preceding 12 mo than in those who had not lost any weight *(5)*.

With the advent of highly active antiretroviral therapy, the prevalence of low testosterone levels has decreased. However, more recent studies *(6,7)* in patients treated with antiretroviral drug therapy suggest that androgen deficiency continues to be a significant clinical problem in HIV-infected men. For example, Rietschel et al. *(7)* reported that 21% of HIV-infected men with weight loss who were receiving highly active antiretroviral therapy had low free-testosterone levels.

Almost 80% of HIV-infected men with low testosterone levels have low or inappropriately normal luteinizing hormone (LH) concentrations *(5)*; these patients have hypogonadotropic hypogonadism, whereas the remaining 20% have high LH concentrations, consistent with primary testicular dysfunction. Thus, the pathophysiology of androgen deficiency in HIV-infection is complex and involves dysregulation at all levels of the hypothalamic–pituitary–testicular axis.

PATHOPHYSIOLOGY OF HIV-INFECTION
IN THE REPRODUCTIVE TRACT AND POTENTIAL MECHANISMS
OF GONADAL DYSFUNCTION

Testicular atrophy is a common finding in autopsy series of patients infected with HIV *(8–11)*. Histological examination of the testes reveals a spectrum of abnormalities, including hypospermatogenesis, spermatogenic arrest, and Sertoli cell-only phenotypes *(11)*. In addition to the loss of germ cells and atrophy, the seminiferous tubules exhibit basement membrane thickening and peritubular fibrosis *(8,9)*. Common abnormalities in semen include leukocytospermia, lower ejaculation volume and total sperm count, and lower percentage of rapidly progressive sperm in comparison to healthy controls *(12,13)*; however, in the majority of HIV-infected patients, these values are within the normal adult male range.

The body mass index was the best predictor of testicular atrophy in a retrospective analysis *(8)*; thus, underweight patients are at 3.5-fold higher risk for testicular atrophy than are normal weight patients. Surprisingly, in this small series, CD4+ T-lymphocyte count was not a significant predictor of testicular atrophy.

Opportunistic organisms may directly infect the testes in men with AIDS *(10)*. The common pathogens involved in testicular infection include cytomegalovirus, *Toxoplasma gondii,* and *Mycobacterium avium intracellulare.* In developing countries, infections of the reproductive tract by *M. tuberculosis* are relatively common. In addition, other sexually transmitted pathogens, such as trichomonas, chlamydia, gonococcus, and syphilis, often coexist in HIV-infected individuals because of common risk factors. The presence of Kaposi's sarcoma and some types of lymphoma in testis has also been reported.

The HIV virus is present in human semen *(14),* and sexual transmission is the major mode of HIV transmission; however, the exact source of HIV particles in the human semen is not known. The human testicular macrophages express cell surface markers CD45 and MAC387, and most also express CD4. These observations have led to the idea that macrophages in the testis may be infected by HIV and might be a site of early viral localization and a potential HIV reservoir *(15)*. The presence of HIV-1 proviral DNA has been reported in the nuclei of germ cells at all stages of differentiation *(16)*. In HIV-1-infected men who are receiving highly active antiretroviral therapy and who have undetectable viral RNA plasma levels, the virus may be still present in seminal cells and, therefore, may be transmitted by sexual contact.

HIV-related protein has been demonstrated in the prostate glands of infected individuals *(17)*. Using *in situ* real-time polymerase chain reaction analysis of prostate and testis tissues, Paranjpe et al. *(18)* reported that T lymphocytes were the predominant cells infected with HIV-1 in both tissues. Because seminal plasma is derived mostly from the secretions of accessory sex organs, such as the prostate and seminal vesicles, and cells in the semen are derived mostly from the testis and the epididymis, the presence of HIV-1 in both the seminal plasma and cells in the semen led these investigators *(18)* to propose that the HIV in semen could originate from infection in either of these two compartments. Although this issue is controversial, there is no conclusive evidence to support HIV infection of spermatozoa.

The Effects of the Mediators of Systemic Inflammatory Response on Reproductive Function

Mediators and products of the systemic inflammatory response affect the hypothalamic–pituitary–gonadal axis at multiple levels. In the testis, Leydig cells and interstitial testicular macrophages are functionally related; the interactions between these two cell types can be both beneficial and deleterious *(19)*. During development, the presence of interstitial macrophages is necessary for Leydig cell maturation *(19)*. However, inflammatory mediators produced by the activated macrophage-derived cells inhibit the production of steroid hormones by Leydig cells. Activated macrophages produce proinflammatory cytokines, such as interleukin-1 (IL-1) and tumor necrosis factor (TNF), that act as transcriptional repressors of several steroidogenic enzymes in the Leydig cell *(19,20)*. In addition, macrophages produce reactive oxygen species (ROS) that inhibit steroidogenic acute response (StAR) protein expression. The net result is decreased testosterone production by the Leydig cells.

The mediators of inflammatory and stress responses can activate the hypothalamic–pituitary–adrenal axis, which inhibits hypothalamic GnRH secretion *(21–24)*. Inputs from the cerebral cortex, subcortical systems, the sensory organs, and sensory nerves, generated in response to stress, induce corticotropin-releasing hormone (CRH) production that inhibits GnRH secretion and the LH response to gonadotropin-releasing hormone (GnRH) and increases cortisol secretion. Glucocorticoids inhibit GnRH secretion, the pituitary LH response to GnRH, and testicular steroidogenesis. In addition, several products and mediators of the systemic inflammatory response exert direct inhibitory effects on hypothalamic GnRH secretion and Leydig cell steroidogenesis. Endotoxin administration in animal models suppresses GnRH secretion, reduces pulsatile LH secretion, and attenuates the LH response to GnRH (22,23). Endotoxin administration also disrupts the estradiol-induced LH surge in the female rat by interfering with the early activating effects of the estradiol signal (24). Inhibitory effects of endotoxin on GnRH secretion are mediated partly through increased cortisol secretion; however, direct inhibitory effects of endotoxin on GnRH secretion that are independent of the activation of the hypothalamic–pituitary–adrenal axis have also been demonstrated (22).

Several proinflammatory cytokines—IL-1α, IL-1β, and TNF-α—inhibit LH secretion; of these, IL-1β is the most potent inhibitor (25). IL-1β, generated within the central nervous system (CNS) during the course of the inflammatory response, upregulates opioid and tachykinin peptides in the hypothalamus (25). These two groups of neuropeptides—the opioids and the tachykinins—convey the cytokine signal to neuroendocrine neurons and cause hypothalamic GnRH suppression.

Malnutrition and Reproduction

Normal reproductive function requires an optimal nutritional intake, and both caloric deprivation and consequent weight loss, as well as excessive food intake and obesity, are associated with impaired reproductive function (26). Sexual maturation may be substantially delayed during food deprivation (27,28); small animals with a short life span may not even achieve puberty before death during periods of food scarcity (29). Undernutrition caused by famine, eating disorders, or exercise results in weight loss and changes in body composition and the endocrine milieu that can impair reproductive function (30). As a general rule, weight loss and body composition changes resulting from undernutrition are associated with reduced GnRH secretion, and the decrease in follicle-stimulating hormone (FSH) and LH levels correlates with the amount of weight loss (30). However, both hypogonadotropic and hypergonadotropic hypogonadism have been described in cachexia associated with certain chronic illnesses, such as HIV infection (5). Collectively, these observations provide compelling evidence that energy balance is an important determinant of reproductive function in all mammals.

The precise nature of the biochemical pathways that connect these two body systems that are essential for survival is not known. It is generally believed that the regulatory signals that modulate hypothalamic GnRH secretion are mediated through leptin and neuropeptide Y (29,31–34). Leptin, the product of the obesity (ob) gene, is a circulating hormone secreted by fat cells that acts centrally to regulate the activity of CNS effector systems that maintain energy balance (35). Leptin stimulates LH secretion by activation of the nitric oxide synthase (NOS) in gonadotropes (34). Leptin inhibits neuropeptide Y secretion, which has a tonic inhibitory effect on both leptin and GnRH secretion. Leptin also stimulates nitric oxide production in the mediobasal hypothalamus; nitric oxide stimulates GnRH secretion by the hypothalamic GnRH-secreting neurons. Therefore, the net effect of leptin action is stimulation of hypothalamic GnRH secretion (31,33,34).

Caloric deprivation in experimental animals is associated with reduced leptin levels and a concomitant reduction in circulating LH levels (31). Leptin administration to calorically deprived mice reverses the inhibition of gonadotropin secretion that attends food restriction. Similarly, genetically ob/ob mice with leptin deficiency have hypogonadotropic hypogonadism and are infertile; treatment of these mice with leptin restores gonadotropin secretion and fertility. Collectively, these observations suggest that energy deficit and weight loss are associated with impaired GnRH secretion, in part, because of decreased leptin secretion and a reciprocal increase in neuropetide Y activity. Although there is agreement that leptin is an important metabolic signal that links energy balance and reproductive axis, it is doubtful that it is the primary trigger for the activation of the GnRH pulse generator at the onset of puberty. Emerging evidence suggests that leptin is essential but not sufficient for initiation of puberty.

Susser and Stein *(36,37)* studied the effects of acute food scarcity during World War II on a previously healthy and nutritionally replete population. Between October 1944 and May 1945, during the German occupation of the Netherlands, the German army restricted food supplies into certain Dutch cities, resulting in a substantial reduction in average daily energy intake to fewer than 1000 kcal. Adjacent cities, in which food supplies were not curtailed by the Germans, were not affected by the famine. Fifty percent of women who were affected by the famine developed amenorrhea. The conception rate dropped to 53% of normal (based on control cities) and correlated with the decreased caloric ration. In addition to the decrease in fertility, undernutrition resulted in an increase in perinatal mortality, congenital malformations, schizophrenia, and obesity. These observations indicate that optimal caloric intake is essential for normal fertility and prenatal growth.

The Kung San of Botswana were a tribe of hunter-gatherers until approx 20 yr ago. The body weight of the men and women in the tribe varied substantially throughout the year, depending on the availability of food. In the summer months, the food supply was more abundant, and the body weight increased, whereas the nadir of body weight was achieved in winter months. The number of births in the tribe peaked approx 9 mo after the peak of body weight. This is another example of how food availability can affect fertility patterns in nature *(38)*.

These nature experiments have led to speculation that androgen deficiency is an adaptive response to malnutrition and illness. Therefore, some investigators have questioned whether it is wise to administer anabolic/androgenic therapies to men with chronic illness.

ADVERSE CONSEQUENCES OF LOW TESTOSTERONE CONCENTRATIONS ON HEALTH-RELATED OUTCOMES IN HIV-INFECTED INDIVIDUALS

Low testosterone levels are associated with an adverse disease outcome in HIV-infected men. Serum testosterone levels are lower in HIV-infected men who have lost weight than in those whose weight has been stable *(39)*. Longitudinal follow-up of HIV-infected homosexual men revealed a progressive decrease in serum testosterone levels *(40)*. This decrease was much greater in HIV-infected men who progressed to AIDS than in those who did not. We do not know whether the decrease in testosterone levels is a consequence of weight loss or is a contributory factor that precedes muscle wasting. In a longitudinal study, Dobs et al. *(41)* measured serum testosterone levels in a cohort of HIV-infected men and reported that serum testosterone levels decline early in the course of events that culminate in wasting. Testosterone levels correlate positively with muscle mass and exercise capacity in HIV-infected men *(2)*, leading to the speculation that hypogonadism may contribute to muscle wasting and debility. Although patients with HIV infection may lose both fat and lean tissue, the loss of lean body mass is an important aspect of the weight loss associated with wasting. The magnitude of depletion of nonfat tissues is an important determinant of the time of death in AIDS *(42,43)*. In addition, fat-free mass is an important correlate of the health-related quality of life in HIV-infected individuals and in older men and women. There is also a high prevalence of sexual dysfunction in HIV-infected men *(44,45)*. With the increasing life expectancy of HIV-infected men, frailty and sexual dysfunction have emerged as important quality-of-life issues.

EVIDENCE THAT TESTOSTERONE HAS ANABOLIC EFFECTS ON MUSCLE

The anabolic effects of androgens have generated enormous controversy for more than 60 yr, in part because of flaws in the design of studies published before the 1990s. Many of the earlier studies were neither randomized nor blinded, and the doses of androgenic steroids used were relatively small. Exercise stimulus and protein and energy intakes were not standardized in many studies. Some of the studies even included competitive athletes, and failure to control exercise regimens made it difficult to separate the effects of androgens from those of resistance exercise training.

However, several recent studies have demonstrated unequivocally that testosterone supplementation in androgen-deficient men increases fat-free mass, muscle size, and maximal voluntary strength in numerous clinical paradigms. Some, but not all, testosterone replacement studies have reported loss of fat mass during testosterone replacement. Brodsky et al. *(46)* reported that testosterone replacement increases fractional muscle protein synthesis.

Conversely, lowering of serum testosterone concentrations by administration of a long-acting GnRH agonist is associated with a decline in fat-free mass and decreased muscle protein synthesis *(47)*. Furthermore, fat-free mass is lower and fat mass is higher in androgen-deficient men when compared to age-matched controls. Several epidemiological studies are in agreement that low non-sex hormone-binding globulin (SHBG) (bioavailable) testosterone levels correlate with lower whole body and appendicular fat-free mass and strength of knee flexion and extension in older men.

Supraphysiological doses of testosterone, when administered to eugonadal men, further increase fat-free mass, muscle size, and strength, when confounding variables, such as energy and protein intake and exercise stimulus, are controlled *(48–50)*. Testosterone effects on the muscle are related to testosterone dose and concentrations *(51)*. Resistance exercise training augments the anabolic response to androgen administration; thus, the combination of administration of testosterone and strength training is associated with greater increments in fat-free mass and muscle strength than either intervention alone *(52,53)*.

EFFECTS OF ANDROGEN REPLACEMENT ON BODY COMPOSITION AND MUSCLE FUNCTION IN HIV INFECTION

Several different anabolic interventions have been examined as treatments for HIV-related wasting, including appetite stimulants (such as dronabinol) *(54)* and megesterol acetate) *(55)*, anabolic hormones (such as human growth hormone *(56,57)*, insulin-like growth factor (IGF)-1 *(57)*, and androgens *(44,52,53,58–67)*; and immune response modulators, such as thalidomide. Dronabinol increases appetite but does not increase lean body mass. Similarly, megesterol acetate treatment produces a modest weight gain but no significant change in lean body mass. Importantly, this progestational agent decreases serum testosterone levels and may produce androgen deficiency symptoms.

In two recently published clinical trials, treatment of HIV-infected men with human growth hormone (hGH) was associated with a 1.5-kg increase in lean body mass *(56,57)*. Although greater gains in weight were recorded after 6 wk of hGH treatment, these gains were not sustained with continued treatment for 12 wk. The reasons for the failure to sustain weight gains during hGH treatment are not clear, although it is conceivable that weight gain early in the course of treatment results from water retention. Growth hormone (GH) administration is often associated with side effects, including edema, arthralgias, myalgias, and jaw pain. Not surprisingly, treatment-discontinuation rates were high (21–40%) in the two hGH studies. The annual cost of treating HIV-infected men with hGH is substantially greater than that of testosterone replacement therapy using any of the available androgen formulations.

Several studies of the effects of androgen supplementation in HIV-infected men have been reported and are summarized in Table 1 *(6,44,52,53,58–60,62–67)*. However, many of these studies were not controlled clinical trials. In addition, most studies were of short duration, ranging from 12 to 24 wk. Several androgenic steroids have been studied in a limited fashion, including nandrolone decanoate, oxandrolone, oxymetholone, stanozolol, testosterone cypionate, and testosterone enanthate.

Of the five placebo-controlled studies of testosterone replacement in HIV-infected men with weight loss, three (*see* Table 1) *(52,60,68)* demonstrated an increase in fat-free mass, and two *(59,62)* did not. The three studies *(60,68,69)* that showed gains in fat-free mass selected patients with low testosterone levels. Coodley et al. *(59)* examined the effects of 200-mg testosterone cypionate given every 2 wk for 3 mo to 40 HIV-seropositive patients with weight loss of greater than 5% of usual body weight and CD4 cell counts of less than 2×10^5/L in a double-blind, placebo-controlled study. Of the 35 patients who completed the first 3 mo of the study, there was no significant difference in weight gain between testosterone and placebo treatment. However, testosterone supplementation improved overall sense of well-being ($p = 0.03$). Body composition was not assessed.

In a placebo-controlled, double-blind, clinical trial, we examined the effects of physiological testosterone replacement by means of the nonscrotal patch *(60)*. Forty-one HIV-positive men with serum testosterone levels less than 400 ng/dL were randomly assigned to receive either two placebo patches nightly or two testosterone patches, designed to release 5 mg testosterone during a 24-h period. Testosterone replacement was associated with a 1.34-kg increase in lean body mass ($p = 0.02$), as well as a significantly greater reduction in fat mass than that observed with placebo treatment. There were no significant changes in liver enzymes, plasma HIV-RNA copy number, or CD4 and CD8+ T-cell counts. Both placebo and testosterone-treatment were associated with a significant increase in muscle strength. Because most of the participants in this study did not have prior weight-lifting experience, we hypothesized that the apparent increase in muscle strength in the placebo group reflected a learning

Table 1

Placebo-Controlled Studies of Androgen Supplementation in HIV-Infected Men

Study (Ref.)	Subjects	Treatment Regimen	Changes in Body Composition	Changes in Muscle Function	Comments
Bhasin et al., 1998 (60)	HIV-infected men with serum testosterone <400 ng/dL	Testosterone patch (5-mg d) vs placebo patch × 10 wk	+1.3 kg gain in FFM after testosterone replacement	Strength gains in placebo and testosterone-treated men not significantly different	Strength measurements confounded by learning effect
Grinspoon et al., 1998 (61)	HIV-infected men with AIDS wasting syndrome and free-testosterone levels <42 pmol/L	300-mg every 3 wk × 6 mo	+2 kg increase in FFM; no change in fat mass	Muscle strength not measured; no change in exercise functional capacity	Testosterone-treated patients reported feeling better, improved quality of life and appearance
Bhasin et al., 2000 (69)	HIV-infected men with >5% weight loss and serum testosterone less than 350 ng/dL	100-mg testosterone enanthate weekly × 16 wk, with or without resistance training; placebo controlled	+2.9 kg gain in testosterone-treated men	Significantly greater gains in muscle strength with testosterone treatment than with placebo	
Grinspoon et al., 2001 (72)	HIV-infected men with AIDS wasting syndrome	200-mg testosterone enanthate weekly, with or without strength training; placebo controlled × 12-wk	Greater increments in muscle mass and volume in response to testosterone and resistance exercise training as compared to placebo	Strength gains not significantly greater in testosterone or resistance training groups in comparison to placebo group	
Dobs et al., 2000 (62)	HIV-infected men with AIDS and 5–10% weight loss, and baseline testosterone <400 ng/dL or free testosterone <16 pg/mL	Testoderm 6-mg scrotal patch vs placebo patch × 12 wk	Changes in body weight or body cell mass by bioelectrical impedance not significantly different between testosterone and placebo groups	Not measured	Quality-of-life measure not changed
Coodley et al., 1995 (92a)	HIV-infected men with >5% weight loss, and CD4 counts <200/cmm	Testosterone cypionate 200 mg every 2 wk × 12 wk vs placebo in a crossover design	No significant differences in change in body weight between testosterone and placebo periods	Not measured	Testosterone treatment associated with improved well-being

214

Study	Population	Intervention	Results	Outcome	Comments
Sattler et al., 1998 (92)	HIV-infected men with CD4+ cell count <400/cmm	Nandrolone 600 mg weekly alone or nandrolone plus resistance training exercise for 12 wk	+3.9 kg gain in FFM after nandrolone treatment alone, and 5.2 kg in combined treatment group	Strength gains greater with combined treatment than with nandrolone alone	No placebo alone group
Strawford et al., 1999 (53)	HIV-infected men with weight loss >5% in the preceding 2 yr	All subjects received resistance exercise training plus testosterone enanthate 100 mg weekly, and randomized to 20-mg oxandrolone or placebo daily	+6.9 kg mean increase in LBM in oxandrolone group; 3.8 kg gain in placebo group	Greater muscle strength gains in oxandrolone group than in placebo group	Significant drop in plasma HDL cholesterol in oxandrolone
Strawford et al., 1999 (66)	HIV-infected men with AIDS wasting syndrome and borderline low testosterone concetrations	Placebo, 65 mg nandrolone weekly, or 200 mg nandrolone weekly	Greater increments in nitrogen retention in both nandrolone groups compared to placebo	LBM increased by 3.1 kg in 10 men in open-label treatment phase	
Batterham and Garsia	HIV-infected men with >5% weight loss	Randomized to nutritional supplementation alone, megesterol acetate 400 mg daily or nandrolone 100 mg every 15 d	Greater LBM gain in association with nandrolone than placebo	Muscle strength not measured	Small sample size
Hengge et al., 1996 (65)	HIV-infected men with chronic cachexia cachexia	Oxymetholone monotherapy, oxymetholone plus ketotifen, compared to historical controls	8.2 kg weight gain in the oxymetholone group, 6.1 kg gain in combination group, compared with a weight loss of 1.8 kg in historical controls	Body composition and muscle performance not measured	Controls not concurrent; no placebo group

FFM, fat free body mass; LBM, lean body mass; HDL, high-density lipoprotein

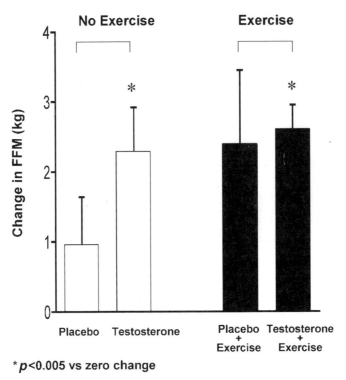

Fig. 1. Change in fat-free mass during testosterone administration with or without resistance exercise training in HIV-infected men with weight loss and low testosterone concentrations. Data are mean +/–SEM. Fat-free mass was measured by dual energy X-ray absorptiometry. *, significantly greater than placebo. (Reproduced from ref. *69.*)

effect. Most other studies of testosterone replacement in HIV-infected men have also failed to demonstrate significant increases in muscle strength.

Therefore, in a subsequent study *(52)* (*see* Figs. 1 and 2), the subjects returned to the exercise laboratory on two or more occasions until they were familiar with the equipment and technique and stability of measurement had been achieved. In this study, we determined the effects of testosterone replacement, with or without a program of resistance exercise, on muscle strength and body composition in androgen-deficient, HIV-infected men with weight loss and low testosterone levels. This was a placebo-controlled, double-blind, randomized, clinical trial in HIV-infected men with serum testosterone levels less than 350 ng/dL and weight loss of 5% or more in the previous 6 mo. Men were randomly assigned to one of four groups: placebo, no exercise; testosterone, no exercise; placebo plus exercise; or testosterone plus exercise. Placebo or 100-mg testosterone enanthate were given intramuscular weekly for 16 wk. The exercise program was a thrice weekly, progressive, supervised strength-training program. Effort-dependent muscle strength in five different exercises was measured by the 1-repetition maximum method. In the placebo alone group, muscle strength did not change for any of the five exercises (–0.3 to –4.0%). This indicates that this strategy was effective in minimizing the influence of the learning effect. Men who were treated

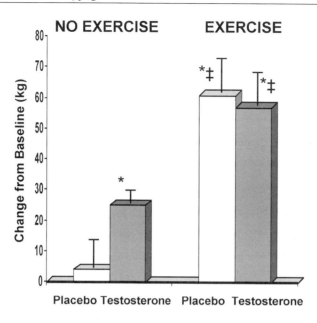

Fig. 2. Change in maximal voluntary muscle strength in the leg-press exercise during testosterone administration with or without resistance exercise training in HIV-infected men with weight loss and low testosterone concentrations. Data are mean +/–SEM. Muscle strength was measured as the 1-repetition maximum in the leg press exercise. (Reproduced from ref. *69.*)

with testosterone alone, exercise alone, or combined testosterone and exercise experienced significant increases in maximum voluntary muscle strength in the leg press (+22 to 30%) (*see* Fig. 2), leg curls (+18 to 36%), bench press (+19 to 33%), and latissimus pulls (+17 to 33%) exercises. The gains in strength in all exercises were greater in men receiving testosterone or exercise alone than in those receiving placebo alone. The change in leg press strength correlated positively with an increase in muscle volume ($r = 0.44$, $p = 0.003$) and fat-free mass ($r = 0.55$, $p < 0.001$).

We conclude that when the confounding influence of the learning effect is minimized, as in this study, and appropriate androgen-responsive measures of muscle strength are selected, testosterone replacement is associated with demonstrable increase in maximal voluntary strength in HIV-infected men with low testosterone levels.

Strength training also promotes gains in lean body mass and muscle strength *(52,70)*. Supraphysiological doses of androgens augment the anabolic effects of resistance exercise on lean body mass and maximal voluntary strength *(53,67)*.

A systematic review of the randomized, placebo-controlled trials that compared the effects of testosterone therapy with placebo in HIV patients with wasting was conducted *(71)*. This analysis showed a difference of 1.04 kg (–0.01–2.10) between the testosterone treatment group and the placebo group by random effect, and 0.63 kg (–0.01–1.28) for fixed effect models. The meta-analysis of the six trials that included measurements of lean body mass revealed a difference in lean body mass between the testosterone group and the placebo group of 1.22 kg (95% CI 0.23–2.22) for the random effect model and 0.51 kg (0.09–0.93) for fixed effect. The difference in lean body mass between the testosterone and placebo groups was much greater in the three trials that used the im route of administration (–3.34 kg) in the post hoc analysis, presumably because of the higher testosterone dose used in these trials.

These data suggest that testosterone can promote weight gain and increase in lean body mass, as well as muscle strength in HIV-infected men with low testosterone levels.

TESTOSTERONE EFFECTS ON HEALTH-RELATED OUTCOMES IN MEN WITH CHRONIC ILLNESS

The effects of testosterone supplementation on health-related outcomes in HIV-infected men have not been rigorously examined in adequately powered, prospective studies. However, in several placebo-controlled trials, testosterone administration has been associated with improvements in several subdomains of health-related quality of life. For example, testosterone administration has been reported to improve depression indices in HIV-infected men (72). In a recent study, Pope et al. (73) administered a replacement dose of a testosterone gel or placebo to men with refractory depression and low testosterone levels. Testosterone administration was associated with greater improvements in scores on the Hamilton depression scale than was placebo. These preliminary data suggest that testosterone administration might have a clinically important antidepressant effect. In open-label, studies of healthy, hypogonadal men, testosterone replacement also improved positive aspects of mood and reduced irritability and negative aspects of mood (74). Wilson et al. (75) reported that lean body mass is an important determinant of health-related quality of life. Therefore, testosterone administration by increasing lean body mass might be expected to improve health-related quality of life; this hypothesis has not been rigorously tested. We do not know, however, whether physiological androgen replacement can produce meaningful changes in the quality of life, use of health care resources, and physical function in HIV-infected men. Emerging data suggest that testosterone does not affect HIV replication, but its effects on virus shedding into the genital tract are not known.

TESTOSTERONE EFFECTS ON FAT METABOLISM

Percent body fat is increased in hypogonadal men (76). Induction of androgen deficiency in healthy men by administration of a GnRH agonist leads to an increase in fat mass (47). Some studies of young, hypogonadal men have reported a decrease in fat mass with testosterone replacement (46,76), whereas others (77,78) found no change. In contrast, long-term studies of testosterone supplementation of older men are consistent in demonstrating a significant decrease in fat mass (79). Epidemiological studies (80,81) have found lower serum testosterone levels in middle-aged men with visceral obesity. Serum testosterone levels correlate inversely with visceral fat area and directly with plasma high-density lipoprotein (HDL) levels. Testosterone replacement of middle-aged men with visceral obesity improved insulin sensitivity and decreased blood glucose and blood pressure (82). Testosterone is an important determinant of regional fat distribution and metabolism in men (82). In our dose-response study of healthy, young men, we found testosterone dose and concentrations to be inversely related to whole body fat mass. Lower doses of testosterone that reduced serum testosterone concentrations below baseline were associated with gains

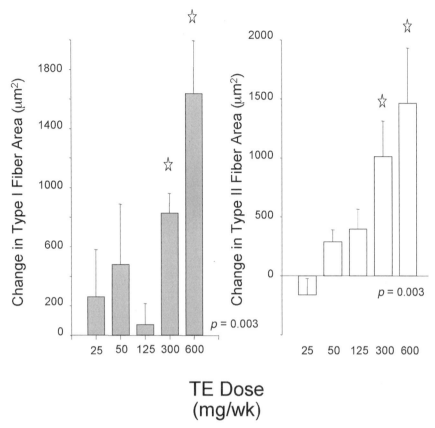

Fig. 3. Change in muscle fiber cross-sectional area in the vastus lateralis muscle of healthy, young men treated with a long-acting gonadotropin-releasing hormone agonist and graded doses of testosterone enanthate. The doses of testosterone enanthate are shown on the X-axis. Data are mean +/–SEM. (Reproduced from of ref. *84.*)

in fat mass, whereas higher doses were associated with a dose-dependent decrease in fat mass. Loss of fat mass at higher doses was distributed evenly between the abdomen and trunk. Similarly, loss of fat mass was proportionate in the superficial subcutaneous compartment and the deep intermuscular compartments of the thigh. Grinspoon *(61)* also reported that administration of a supraphysiologic dose of testosterone is associated with loss of intermuscular fat mass in HIV-infected men. It has been hypothesized that testosterone supplementation might be beneficial in HIV-infected men with the fat-redistribution syndromes; this hypothesis is being investigated in ongoing studies.

MECHANISMS OF TESTOSTERONE'S EFFECTS ON BODY COMPOSITION

The prevalent view that testosterone produces muscle hypertrophy by increasing fractional muscle protein synthesis *(46,83)* is supported by several studies. However, as discussed below, recent observations suggest that increase in muscle protein synthesis probably occurs as a secondary event and may not be the sole or the primary mechanism by which testosterone induces muscle hypertrophy (84).

To determine whether testosterone-induced increase in muscle size results from muscle fiber hypertrophy or hyperplasia, muscle biopsies were obtained from the *vastus lateralis* in 39 healthy, young men before and after 20 wk of combined treatment with GnRH agonist and weekly injections of 25-, 50-, 125-, 300-, or 600-mg testosterone enanthate (84). Graded doses of testosterone administration were associated with a testosterone dose- and concentration-dependent increase in muscle fiber cross-sectional area (*see* Fig. 3). Changes in cross-sectional areas of both type I and II fibers were dependent on testosterone dose and significantly correlated with total ($r = 0.35$ and 0.44, $p < 0.0001$ for type I and II fibers, respectively) and free ($r = 0.34$ and 0.35, $p < 0.005$) testosterone concentrations during treatment. The men receiving 300 and 600 mg of testosterone enanthate weekly experienced significant increases from baseline in areas of type I (baseline vs 20 wks, 3176 ± 163 vs 4201 ± 163 μm^2, $p < 0.05$ at 300-mg dose, and 3347 ± 253 vs 4984 ± 374 μm^2, $p = 0.006$ at 600-mg dose) muscle fibers; the men in the 600-mg group also had significant increments in cross-sectional area of type II (4060 ± 401 vs 5526 ± 544 μm^2, $p = 0.03$) fibers. The relative proportion of type I and type II fibers did not change significantly after treatment in any group. The myonuclear number per fiber increased significantly in men receiving the 300- and 600-mg doses of testosterone enanthate and was significantly correlated with testosterone concentration and muscle fiber cross-sectional area. These data demonstrate that increases in muscle volume in healthy eugonadal men rendered testosterone-deficient with a GnRH-analog and treated with graded doses of testosterone are associated with concentration-dependent increases in muscle fiber cross-sectional area and myonuclear number but not muscle fiber number. We conclude that the testosterone-induced increase in muscle volume results from muscle fiber hypertrophy. In our study, the myonuclear number increased in direct relation to the increase in muscle fiber diameter. Therefore, it is possible that muscle fiber hypertrophy and increase in myonuclear number were preceded by testosterone-induced increase in satellite cell number and their fusion with muscle fibers. The mechanisms by which testosterone might increase satellite cell number are not known. An increase in satellite cell number could occur by an increase in satellite cell replication, inhibition of satellite cell apoptosis, and/or increased differentiation of stem cells into the myogenic lineage. We do not know which of these processes is the site of regulation by testosterone. The hypothesis that testosterone promotes muscle fiber hypertrophy by increasing the number of satellite cells should be further tested. Because of the constraints inherent in obtaining multiple biopsy specimens in humans, the effects of testosterone on satellite cell replication and stem cell recruitment would be more conveniently studied in an animal model.

The molecular mechanisms, which mediate androgen-induced muscle hypertrophy, are not well understood. Urban et al. (83) proposed that testosterone stimulates the expression of IGF-I and downregulates IGF-binding protein-4 (IGFBP-4) in the muscle. Reciprocal changes in IGF-1 and its binding protein thus provide a potential mechanism for amplifying the anabolic signal.

It is also not clear whether the anabolic effects of pharmacological doses of testosterone are mediated through the androgen receptor. In vitro-binding studies (85) suggested that the maximum effects of testosterone should be manifest at serum testosterone levels of approx 300 ng/dL, i.e., levels that are at the lower end of the normal male range. Therefore, it is possible that the supraphysiological doses of androgen produce muscle hypertrophy through an androgen-receptor independent mechanism, such as through an antiglucocorticoid effect *(86)*. We cannot exclude the possibility that some androgen effects may be mediated through nonclassical binding sites. Testosterone effects on the muscle are modulated by several other factors, such as genetic background, growth hormone secretory status *(87)*, nutrition, exercise, cytokines, thyroid hormones, and glucocorticoids. Testosterone may also affect muscle function by its effects on neuromuscular transmission *(88,89)*.

The Role of 5-α Reduction of Testosterone in the Muscle

Although the enzyme 5-α-reductase is expressed at low concentrations in muscle *(90)*, it is unknown whether conversion of testosterone to DHT is required for mediating the androgen effects on the muscle. Men with benign prostatic hypertrophy who are treated with the a 5-α reductase inhibitor do not experience muscle loss. Similarly, individuals with congenital 5-α-reductase deficiency have normal muscle development at puberty. These data imply that 5-α reduction of testosterone is not obligatory for mediating its anabolic effects on the muscle cells. Because testosterone effects on the prostate involve conversion to DHT, selective androgen receptor modulators that bind the androgen receptor but are not 5-α reduced would be attractive *(91)*. Such agents could produce desirable anabolic effects on muscle without the undesirable effects on the prostate.

Sattler et al. *(92)* reported that serum DHT levels are lower and the ratio of testosterone to DHT levels is higher in HIV-infected men than in healthy men. From these data, the investigators proposed that an abnormality in the conversion of testosterone to DHT may contribute to wasting in a subset of HIV-infected men. If this hypothesis were true, then it would be rational to treat HIV-AIDS patients with DHT rather than with testosterone. A DHT gel is currently under clinical investigation. However, unlike testosterone, DHT is not aromatized to estradiol. Therefore, there is concern that suppression of endogenous testosterone and estradiol production by DHT may produce osteoporosis and other undesirable adverse effects.

SUMMARY

There is a high prevalence of low testosterone concentrations in HIV-infected individuals resulting from defects at all levels of the hypothalamic–pituitary–gonadal axis. Both hypogonadotropic and hypergonadotropic hypogonadism have been described, the former being more prevalent. Low testosterone concentrations are associated with adverse disease outcomes, including weight loss, disease progression, and decreased muscle mass and exercise capacity. Physiologic testosterone replacement increases fat-free mass and maximal voluntary strength in HIV-infected men with low testosterone concentrations. Testosterone administration also decreases whole body and visceral fat mass in middle-aged men with low normal testosterone concentrations. The effects of testosterone supplementation in HIV-associated fat redistribution syndromes are being investigated. Testosterone increases muscle mass and decreases fat mass by promoting the differentiation of pluipotent precursor cells into the myogenic lineage and inhibiting their differentiation into the adipogenic lineage. Long-term, adequately powered, randomized, placebo-controlled, studies are needed to determine the effects of testosterone replacement on health-related outcomes, such as cardiovascular event rates, health-related quality of life, and disability.

REFERENCES

1. Dobs AS, Dempsey MA, Ladenson PW, Polk BF. Endocrine disorders in men infected with human immunodeficiency virus. Am J Med 1988;84:611–616.
2. Grinspoon S, Corcoran C, Lee K, et al. Loss of lean body and muscle mass correlates with androgen levels in hypogonadal men with acquired immunodeficiency syndrome and wasting. J Clin Endocrinol Metab 1996;81:4051–4058.
3. Laudat A, Blum L, Guechot J, et al. Changes in systemic gonadal and adrenal steroids in asymptomatic human immunodeficiency virus-infected men: relationship with the CD4 cell counts. Eur J Endocrinol 1995;133:418–424.
4. Raffi F, Brisseau JM, Planchon B, Remi JP, Barrier JH, Grolleau JY. Endocrine function in 98 HIV-infected patients: a prospective study. Aids 1991;5:729–733.
5. Arver S, Sinha-Hikim I, Beall G, Guerrero M, Shen R, Bhasin S. Serum dihydrotestosterone and testosterone concentrations in human immunodeficiency virus-infected men with and without weight loss. J Androl 1999;20:611–618.
6. Berger JR, Pall L, Hall CD, Simpson DM, Berry PS, Dudley R. Oxandrolone in AIDS-wasting myopathy. Aids 1996;10:1657–1662.
7. Rietschel P, Corcoran C, Stanley T, Basgoz N, Klibanski A, Grinspoon S. Prevalence of hypogonadism among men with weight loss related to human immunodeficiency virus infection who were receiving highly active antiretroviral therapy. Clin Infect Dis 2000;31:1240–1244.
8. Mhawech P, Onorato M, Uchida T, Borucki MJ. Testicular atrophy in 80 HIV-positive patients: a multivariate statistical analysis. Int J STD AIDS 2001;12:221–224.
9. Shevchuk MM, Nuovo GJ, Khalife G. HIV in testis: quantitative histology and HIV localization in germ cells. J Reprod Immunol 1998;41:69–79.
10. Lo JC, Schambelan M. Reproductive function in human immunodeficiency virus infection. J Clin Endocrinol Metab 2001;86:2338–2343.
11. Shevchuk MM, Pigato JB, Khalife G, Armenakas NA, Fracchia JA. Changing testicular histology in AIDS: its implication for sexual transmission of HIV. Urology 1999;53:203–208.
12. Dulioust E, Du AL, Costagliola D, et al. Semen alterations in HIV-1 infected men. Hum Reprod 2002;17:2112–2118.
13. Umapathy E, Simbini T, Chipata T, Mbizvo M. Sperm characteristics and accessory sex gland functions in HIV-infected men. Arch Androl 2001;46:153–158.
14. Zhang H, Dornadula G, Beumont M, et al. Human immunodeficiency virus type 1 in the semen of men receiving highly active antiretroviral therapy. N Engl J Med 1998;339:1803–1809.
15. Habasque C, Aubry F, Jegou B, Samson M. Study of the HIV-1 receptors CD4, CXCR4, CCR5 and CCR3 in the human and rat testis. Mol Hum Reprod 2002;8:419–425.
16. Muciaccia B, Filippini A, Ziparo E, Colelli F, Baroni CD, Stefanini M. Testicular germ cells of HIV-seropositive asymptomatic men are infected by the virus. J Reprod Immunol 1998;41:81–93.
17. da Silva M, Shevchuk MM, Cronin WJ, et al. Detection of HIV-related protein in testes and prostates of patients with AIDS. Am J Clin Pathol 1990;93:196–201.
18. Paranjpe S, Craigo J, Patterson B, et al. Subcompartmentalization of HIV-1 quasispecies between seminal cells and seminal plasma indicates their origin in distinct genital tissues. AIDS Res Hum Retroviruses 2002;18:1271–1280.
19. Hales DB. Testicular macrophage modulation of Leydig cell steroidogenesis. J Reprod Immunol 2002;57:3–18.
20. Ben-Rafael Z, Orvieto R. Cytokines—involvement in reproduction. Fertil Steril 1992;58:1093–1099.
21. Torpy DJ, Chrousos GP. The three-way interactions between the hypothalamic-pituitary-adrenal and gonadal axes and the immune system. Baillieres Clin Rheumatol 1996;10:181–198.
22. Debus N, Breen KM, Barrell GK, et al. Does cortisol mediate endotoxin-induced inhibition of pulsatile luteinizing hormone and gonadotropin-releasing hormone secretion? Endocrinology 2002;143:3748–3758.
23. Williams CY, Harris TG, Battaglia DF, Viguie C, Karsch FJ. Endotoxin inhibits pituitary responsiveness to gonadotropin-releasing hormone. Endocrinology 2001;142:1915–1922.
24. Battaglia DF, Beaver AB, Harris TG, Tanhehco E, Viguie C, Karsch FJ. Endotoxin disrupts the estradiol-induced luteinizing hormone surge: interference with estradiol signal reading, not surge release. Endocrinology 1999;140:2471–2479.
25. Kalra PS, Edwards TG, Xu B, Jain M, Kalra SP. The anti-gonadotropic effects of cytokines: the role of neuropeptides. Domest Anim Endocrinol 1998;15:321–332.

26. Frisch RE, McArthur JW. Menstrual cycles: fatness as a determinant of minimum weight for height necessary for their maintenance or onset. Science 1974;185:949–951.

27. Frisch RE. Fatness and fertility. Sci Am 1988;258:88–95.

28. Frisch RE. Body weight and reproduction. Science 1989;246:432.

29. Foster DL, Nagatani S. Physiological perspectives on leptin as a regulator of reproduction: role in timing puberty. Biol Reprod 1999;60:205–215.

30. Bates GW, Bates SR, Whitworth NS. Reproductive failure in women who practice weight control. Fertil Steril 1982;37:373–378.

31. Cunningham MJ, Clifton DK, Steiner RA. Leptin's actions on the reproductive axis: perspectives and mechanisms. Biol Reprod 1999;60:216–222.

32. Aubert ML, Pierroz DD, Gruaz NM, et al. Metabolic control of sexual function and growth: role of neuropeptide Y and leptin. Mol Cell Endocrinol 1998;140:107–113.

33. Clarke IJ, Henry BA. Leptin and reproduction. Rev Reprod 1999;4:48–55.

34. McCann SM, Kimura M, Walczewska A, Karanth S, Rettori V, Yu WH. Hypothalamic control of gonadotropin secretion by LHRH, FSHRF, NO, cytokines, and leptin. Domest Anim Endocrinol 1998;15:333–344.

35. Raisz LG, Wiita B, Artis A, et al. Comparison of the effects of estrogen alone and estrogen plus androgen on biochemical markers of bone formation and resorption in postmenopausal women. J Clin Endocrinol Metab 1996;81:37–43.

36. Stein Z, Susser M, Rush D. Prenatal nutrition and birth weight: experiments and quasi-experiments in the past decade. J Reprod Med 1978;21:287–299.

37. Susser M, Stein Z. Timing in prenatal nutrition: a reprise of the Dutch Famine Study. Nutr Rev 1994;52:84–94.

38. Kirchengast S. Differential reproductive success and body size in Kung San people from northern Namibia. Coll Anthropol 2000;24:121–132.

39. Coodley GO, Loveless MO, Nelson HD, Coodley MK. Endocrine function in the HIV wasting syndrome. J Acquir Immune Defic Syndr 1994;7:46–51.

40. Salehian B, Jacobson D, Grafe M, McCutchan A, Swerdloff RS. Pituitary-testicular axis during HIV infection: A prospective study. Presented at the 18th annual meeting of the American Society of Andrology. Vol. Abstract 9. Tampa, Florida, April 15–19, 1993.

41. Dobs AS, Few WL, 3rd, Blackman MR, Harman SM, Hoover DR, Graham NM. Serum hormones in men with human immunodeficiency virus-associated wasting. J Clin Endocrinol Metab 1996;81:4108–4112.

42. Kotler DP, Tierney AR, Wang J, Pierson RN, Jr. Magnitude of body-cell-mass depletion and the timing of death from wasting in AIDS. Am J Clin Nutr 1989;50:444–447.

43. Chlebowski RT, Grosvenor MB, Bernhard NH, Morales LS, Bulcavage LM. Nutritional status, gastrointestinal dysfunction, and survival in patients with AIDS. Am J Gastroenterol 1989;84:1288–1293.

44. Rabkin JG, Rabkin R, Wagner GJ. Testosterone treatment of clinical hypogonadism in patients with HIV/AIDS. Int J STD AIDS 1997;8:537–545.

45. Meyer-Bahlburg FH. HIV positive gay men: sexual dysfunction. Proc VI Int Conf AIDS. Vol. Abstract 701, 1989.

46. Brodsky IG, Balagopal P, Nair KS. Effects of testosterone replacement on muscle mass and muscle protein synthesis in hypogonadal men—a clinical research center study. J Clin Endocrinol Metab 1996;81:3469–3475.

47. Mauras N, Hayes V, Welch S, et al. Testosterone deficiency in young men: marked alterations in whole body protein kinetics, strength, and adiposity. J Clin Endocrinol Metab 1998;83:1886–1892.

48. Griggs RC, Kingston W, Jozefowicz RF, Herr BE, Forbes G, Halliday D. Effect of testosterone on muscle mass and muscle protein synthesis. J Appl Physiol 1989;66:498–503.

49. Young NR, Baker HW, Liu G, Seeman E. Body composition and muscle strength in healthy men receiving testosterone enanthate for contraception. J Clin Endocrinol Metab 1993;77:1028–1032.

50. Bhasin S, Storer TW, Berman N, et al. The effects of supraphysiologic doses of testosterone on muscle size and strength in normal men. N Engl J Med 1996;335:1–7.

51. Bhasin S, Woodhouse L, Casaburi R, et al. Testosterone dose-response relationships in healthy young men. Am J Physiol Endocrinol Metab 2001;281:E1172–E1181.

52. Bhasin S, Javanbakht M. Can androgen therapy replete lean body mass and improve muscle function in wasting associated with human immunodeficiency virus infection? JPEN J Parenter Enteral Nutr 1999;23:S195–S201.

53. Strawford A, Barbieri T, Neese R, et al. Effects of nandrolone decanoate therapy in borderline hypogo-nadal men with HIV-associated weight loss. J Acquir Immune Defic Syndr Hum Retrovirol 1999;20:137–146.

54. Beal JE, Olson R, Laubenstein L, et al. Dronabinol as a treatment for anorexia associated with weight loss in patients with AIDS. J Pain Symptom Manage 1995;10:89–97.

55. Von Roenn JH, Armstrong D, Kotler DP, et al. Megestrol acetate in patients with AIDS-related cachexia [see comments]. Ann Intern Med 1994;121:393–399.

56. Schambelan M, Mulligan K, Grunfeld C, et al. Recombinant human growth hormone in patients with HIV-associated wasting. A randomized, placebo-controlled trial. Serostim Study Group [see com-ments]. Ann Intern Med 1996;125:873–882.

57. Waters D, Danska J, Hardy K, et al. Recombinant human growth hormone, insulin-like growth factor 1, and combination therapy in AIDS-associated wasting. A randomized, double-blind, placebo-con-trolled trial [see comments]. Ann Intern Med 1996;125:865–872.

58. Engelson ES, Rabkin JG, Rabkin R, Kotler DP. Effects of testosterone upon body composition. J Acquir Immune Defic Syndr Hum Retrovirol 1996;11:510–511.

59. Coodley GO, Coodley MK. A trial of testosterone therapy for HIV-associated weight loss. AIDS 1997;11:1347–1352.

60. Bhasin S, Storer TW, Asbel-Sethi N, et al. Effects of testosterone replacement with a nongenital, trans-dermal system, Androderm, in human immunodeficiency virus-infected men with low testosterone lev-els. J Clin Endocrinol Metab 1998;83:3155–3162.

61. Grinspoon S, Corcoran C, Askari H, et al. Effects of androgen administration in men with the AIDS wasting syndrome. A randomized, double-blind, placebo-controlled trial. Ann Intern Med 1998;129:18–26.

62. Dobs AS, Cofrancesco J, Nolten WE, et al. The use of a transscrotal testosterone delivery system in the treatment of patients with weight loss related to human immunodeficiency virus infection. Am J Med 1999;107:126–132.

63. Bucher G, Berger DS, Fields-Gardner C, Jones R, Reiter WM. A prospective study on the safety and effect of nandrolone decanoate in HIV positive patients. International Conference on AIDS. Vol. Abstract Mo.B. 423. Nov. 26, 1996.

64. Gold J, High HA, Li Y, et al. Safety and efficacy of nandrolone decanoate for treatment of wasting in patients with HIV infection. AIDS 1996;10:745–752.

65. Hengge UR, Baumann M, Maleba R, Brockmeyer NH, Goos M. Oxymetholone promotes weight gain in patients with advanced human immunodeficiency virus (HIV-1) infection. Br J Nutr 1996;75:129–138.

66. Strawford A, Barbieri T, Van Loan M, et al. Resistance exercise and supraphysiologic androgen ther-apy in eugonadal men with HIV-related weight loss: a randomized controlled trial. JAMA 1999;281:1282–1290.

67. Sattler FR, Jaque SV, Schroeder ET, et al. Effects of pharmacological doses of nandrolone decanoate and progressive resistance training in immunodeficient patients infected with human immunodefi-ciency virus. J Clin Endocrinol Metab 1999;84:1268–1276.

68. Grinspoon S, Corcoran C, Stanley T, Katznelson L, Klibanski A. Effects of androgen administration on the growth hormone-insulin-like growth factor I axis in men with acquired immunodeficiency syn-drome wasting. J Clin Endocrinol Metab 1998;83:4251–4256.

69. Bhasin S, Storer TW, Javanbakht M, et al. Testosterone replacement and resistance exercise in HIV-infected men with weight loss and low testosterone levels. JAMA 2000;283:763–770.

70. Roubenoff R, McDermott A, Weiss L, et al. Short-term progressive resistance training increases strength and lean body mass in adults infected with human immunodeficiency virus. AIDS 1999;13:231–9.

71. Kong A, Edmonds P. Testosterone therapy in HIV wasting syndrome: systematic review and meta-analysis. Lancet Infect Dis 2002;2:692–699.

72. Grinspoon S, Corcoran C, Parlman K, et al. Effects of testosterone and progressive resistance training in eugonadal men with AIDS wasting. A randomized, controlled trial. Ann Intern Med 2000;133:348–355.

73. Pope HG, Jr., Cohane GH, Kanayama G, Siegel AJ, Hudson JI. Testosterone gel supplementation for men with refractory depression: a randomized, placebo-controlled trial. Am J Psychiatry 2003;160:105–111.

74. Wang C, Swedloff RS, Iranmanesh A, et al. Transdermal testosterone gel improves sexual function, mood, muscle strength, and body composition parameters in hypogonadal men. Testosterone Gel Study Group. J Clin Endocrinol Metab 2000;85:2839–2853.

75. Wilson JD. Androgen abuse by athletes. Endocr Rev 1988;9:181–199.
76. Katznelson L, Finkelstein JS, Schoenfeld DA, Rosenthal DI, Anderson EJ, Klibanski A. Increase in bone density and lean body mass during testosterone administration in men with acquired hypogonadism. J Clin Endocrinol Metab 1996;81:4358–4365.
77. Wang C, Eyre DR, Clark R, et al. Sublingual testosterone replacement improves muscle mass and strength, decreases bone resorption, and increases bone formation markers in hypogonadal men—a clinical research center study. J Clin Endocrinol Metab 1996;81:3654–3662.
78. Bhasin S, Storer TW, Berman N, et al. Testosterone replacement increases fat-free mass and muscle size in hypogonadal men. J Clin Endocrinol Metab 1997;82:407–413.
79. Snyder PJ, Peachey H, Hannoush P, et al. Effect of testosterone treatment on body composition and muscle strength in men over 65 years of age. J Clin Endocrinol Metab 1999;84:2647–2653.
80. Seidell JC, Bjorntorp P, Sjostrom L, Kvist H, Sannerstedt R. Visceral fat accumulation in men is positively associated with insulin, glucose, and C-peptide levels, but negatively with testosterone levels. Metabolism 1990;39:897–901.
81. Barrett-Connor E, Khaw KT. Endogenous sex hormones and cardiovascular disease in men. A prospective population-based study. Circulation 1988;78:539–545.
82. Marin P, Oden B, Bjorntorp P. Assimilation and mobilization of triglycerides in subcutaneous abdominal and femoral adipose tissue in vivo in men: effects of androgens. J Clin Endocrinol Metab 1995;80:239–243.
83. Urban RJ, Bodenburg YH, Gilkison C, et al. Testosterone administration to elderly men increases skeletal muscle strength and protein synthesis. Am J Physiol 1995;269:E820–E826.
84. Sinha-Hikim I, Artaza J, Woodhouse L, et al. Testosterone-induced increase in muscle size in healthy young men is associated with muscle fiber hypertrophy. Am J Physiol Endocrinol Metab 2002;283:E154–E164.
85. Saartok T, Dahlberg E, Gustafsson JA. Relative binding affinity of anabolic-androgenic steroids: comparison of the binding to the androgen receptors in skeletal muscle and in prostate, as well as to sex hormone-binding globulin. Endocrinology 1984;114:2100–2106.
86. Konagaya M, Max SR. A possible role for endogenous glucocorticoids in orchiectomy-induced atrophy of the rat levator ani muscle: studies with RU 38486, a potent and selective antiglucocorticoid. J Steroid Biochem 1986;25:305–308.
87. Fryburg DA, Weltman A, Jahn LA, et al. Short-term modulation of the androgen milieu alters pulsatile, but not exercise- or growth hormone (GH)-releasing hormone-stimulated GH secretion in healthy men: impact of gonadal steroid and GH secretory changes on metabolic outcomes. J Clin Endocrinol Metab 1997;82:3710–3719.
88. Leslie M, Forger NG, Breedlove SM. Sexual dimorphism and androgen effects on spinal motoneurons innervating the rat flexor digitorum brevis. Brain Res 1991;561:269–273.
89. Blanco CE, Popper P, Micevych P. Anabolic-androgenic steroid induced alterations in choline acetyltransferase messenger RNA levels of spinal cord motoneurons in the male rat. Neuroscience 1997;78:873–882.
90. Bartsch W, Krieg M, Voigt KD. Quantification of endogenous testosterone, 5 alpha-dihydrotestosterone and 5 alpha-androstane-3 alpha, 17 beta-diol in subcellular fractions of the prostate, bulbocavernosus/levator ani muscle, skeletal muscle and heart muscle of the rat. J Steroid Biochem 1980;13:259–264.
91. Winters SJ. Androgens: endocrine physiology and pharmacology. NIDA Res Monogr 1990;102:113–130.
92. Sattler F, Briggs W, Antonipillai I, Allen J, Horton R. Low dihydrotestosterone and weight loss in the AIDS wasting syndrome. J Acquir Immune Defic Syndr Hum Retrovirol 1998;18:246–251.
92a. Coodley GO, Coodley MK. A trial of testosterone therapy for HIV-associated weight loss. AIDS 1997;11:1347–1352.

12 Hypogonadism in Men With Chronic Renal Failure

Peter Y. Liu, MB BS, PhD,
and David J. Handelsman, MB BS, PhD

CONTENTS

INTRODUCTION

Chronic renal failure has major detrimental effects on male reproductive function, with renal failure, dialysis, and transplantation influencing all levels of the hypothalamic–pituitary–testicular axis *(1,2)*. Although the nonreproductive clinical features of uremia usually overshadow the impaired sexual function, virilization, and infertility of chronic renal failure, comprehensive medical care requires a knowledgeable and empathetic appreciation of men's valued, but often unstated, expectations of their reproductive health. This chapter reviews the clinical basis for and role of androgen therapy as an adjunct to standard medical care in chronic renal failure.

Androgen therapy may be considered physiological (replacement therapy) or supraphysiological (pharmacological therapy). The former is restricted to the physiological androgen (testosterone) at replacement doses aiming to replicate physiological blood testosterone concentrations. By aiming to replicate and not exceed physiological endogenous androgen exposure, replacement therapy is expected to have a safety profile comparable to the lifelong experience of eugonadal men. The restriction to testosterone, in theory, precludes use of synthetic designer androgens, which feature

From: *Male Hypogonadism:*
Basic, Clinical, and Therapeutic Principles
Edited by: S. J. Winters © Humana Press Inc., Totowa, NJ

tissue-specific activation and whose spectrum of activity may differ from testosterone. In contrast, pharmacological androgen therapy aims to use any androgen with the dosage optimized to provide maximal effects on androgen-responsive tissues within acceptable safety limits, ultimately judged by the rigorous criteria of efficacy, safety, and cost-effectiveness applicable to any nonhormonal drug. Evaluating the pharmacological role of androgens requires interventional clinical studies featuring randomization, placebo controls, and key design features, such as adequate power, duration, and validated, objective end points. Few published studies fulfill these requirements, with most comprising observational and mechanistic studies so that unequivocal therapeutic implications are limited.

The goals of androgen therapy in renal failure should be considered in relation to the natural history and current standard treatment of the disorder. Because complete androgen deficiency from early life does not reduce life expectancy *(3)*, it is unrealistic to expect that physiological androgen replacement therapy *per se* can alter mortality. However, pharmacological androgen therapy may modify the natural history of chronic renal failure, and these effects may vary according to the concurrent standard therapy (e.g., renal transplantation and peritoneal vs. hemodialysis). Evidence from controlled clinical trials of androgen therapy in renal failure is highlighted with a focus on men, because pharmacological androgen therapy in women and children risks virilization or growth limitation, respectively. Currently, anemia and nutritional status are the only established indications for pharmacological androgen therapy in uremia. More recently, the availability of recombinant human erythropoietin (EPO) for treatment has greatly limited use of androgen therapy. Although there is a growing recognition of the lower costs, as well as the equivalent efficacy, and synergistic interaction with EPO has resulted in a re-examination of the role of androgen therapy in chronic renal failure. Deteriorating nutritional status in patients on dialysis, notably markers such as serum albumin (A15) and lean body mass, independently predict mortality in prospective studies *(4)*, as well as morbidity and mortality in cross-sectional studies *(5,6)*. Small retrospective *(7)* and uncontrolled *(8)* and controlled *(9)* prospective studies in patients on dialysis confirm that these markers are androgen responsive. Hence, it is possible that androgens, by increasing lean mass and promoting protein anabolism, could prolong life expectancy in patients on dialysis, particularly those undergoing peritoneal dialysis *(10)*. The longer term safety of pharmacological androgen therapy regarding the natural history of cardiovascular and prostate disease must be considered, but is beyond the scope of this review *(11)*.

REPRODUCTIVE ENDOCRINOLOGY OF CHRONIC RENAL FAILURE

Men with chronic renal failure have consistent reduction in circulating testosterone, accompanied by moderate elevations in luteinizing hormone (LH), follicle-stimulating hormone (FSH), and inhibin-α *(1,12)*. The pathophysiological interpretation of these changes is complex. *Prima facie* elevated blood gonadotropin and inhibin concentrations, together with moderate reduction in sperm and testosterone production, are indicative of primary (testicular) hypogonadism. Nevertheless, the modest elevations in peptide hormones, despite markedly impaired peptide clearance, together with direct evidence of hypothalamic dysregulation of pulsatile LH and FSH secretion *(13)*, suggest important defects in hypothalamic–pituitary regulation of gonadotropin secretion as well. This functional state of partial gonadotropin deficiency has interesting but largely unexplored therapeutic implications for adjuvant hormonal treatment. The hormonal changes of renal failure become evident with even moderate reduction in renal function (once serum creatinine is consistently elevated), and the effects progressively worsen as renal function deteriorates. The hormonal changes of uremia are minimally affected, or not improved, by dialysis, with the best results from intensive hemodialysis. Transplantation leading to restoration of normal renal function can reverse most hormonal changes of chronic renal failure, although some changes resulting from prolonged dialysis may be irreversible (14). The effects of immunosuppressive medication on human reproductive function are not well understood, because data are restricted to a few observational studies. Long-term surveillance suggests only minimal effects of conventional immunosuppressive regimens (azathioprine, prednisone, and cyclosporin) on male reproductive function (1,14,15), but further studies to clarify the effect of immunosuppressive agents on male reproductive function would be desirable.

Functional Gonadotropin Deficiency

Men with chronic renal failure have reduced circulating total and free testosterone concentrations, unchanged sex hormone-binding globulin (SHBG) and elevated immunoreactive LH, FSH, and inhibin-α; however, these changes are largely reversed after successful transplantation (1). Although this pattern is consistent with a primarily defect in testicular function, there is also strong evidence for defective neuroendocrine regulation as an important functional aspect of the reproductive dysfunction in uremia. The increase in gonadotropins is less than expected in castrated men who are nonuremic or controls with a similar degree of androgen deficiency (16), indicating a defect in neuroendocrine regulation leading to reduced LH secretion. Indeed, the increase in gonadotropins is largely explained by the substantial (~70%) reduction in renal filtration and whole-body clearance rate of LH, which, in the presence of decreased testosterone secretion, indicates significantly reduced LH secretion. Evidence supporting a hypogonadotropic state (1) includes (a) the regularity of delayed puberty in adolescents with chronic renal failure, (b) a blunted acute testosterone response to human chorionic gonadotropin (hCG) stimulation with restoration of normal circulating testosterone levels by chronic hCG treatment (17), (c) normal or low circulating estradiol levels (18) (which are more consistent with a hypogonadotropic rather than a hypergonadotropic state) because high estradiol results from enhanced LH-induced testicular estradiol secretion, (d) histological features consistent with functional gonadotropin deficiency (19), and (e) short-term responses to gonadotropin stimulation (anti-estrogens, hCG and pulsatile gonadotropin-releasing hormone (GnRH) (20). In addition to impaired LH secretion, a dialyzable gonadotropin inhibitor in uremic serum, which blocks the LH receptor, has been reported (21). As shown in Fig. 1, the pattern of pulsatile and GnRH-stimulated LH secretion also suggests a central defect in the neuroendocrine regulation of gonadotropin secretion in men with chronic renal failure (1,2). Pulsatile secretion of immunoreactive and bioactive LH is severely dampened in uremia but can be restored by renal transplantation (22–25). Using deconvolution analysis, the reduced net LH secretion is attributable to reduced LH secreted per burst with prolongation of LH clearance half-life but no reduction in LH pulse frequency (13,26). More basic and less bioactive LH isoforms (27) and degradation fragments accumulate in uremic serum according to their circulating

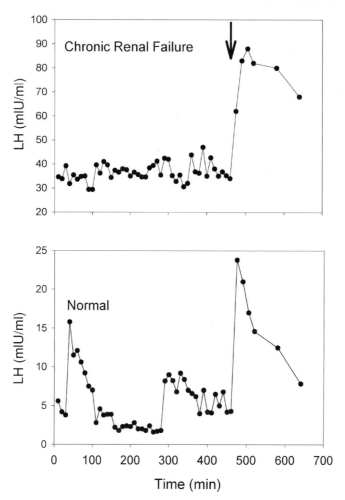

Fig. 1. Spontaneous and gonadotropin-releasing hormone (GnRH)-stimulated luteinizing hormone (LH) secretion in an adult man with chronic renal failure and in a normal adult man. Blood samples were obtained every 10 min for 8 h. The arrow indicates the administration of 100 μg iv GnRH. Note the scale for LH differs, and mean values are 36.5 and 5.41 mIU/mL, respectively, indicating the presence of Leydig cell insufficiency. In the man with chronic renal failure there are low amplitude LH secretory episodes with a normal threefold rise in LH after GnRH stimulation, implying GnRH deficiency. The delay to peak LH and the delayed downstroke are indicative of prolonged LH clearance. (Data courtesy of F. Bruns and S.J. Winters, and are unpublished.)

half-times *(28)*, resulting in a skewing of molecular microheterogeneity to less bioactive, but more immunoreactive, LH isoforms. These observations suggest that hCG therapy has considerable potential in men with uremia, but no controlled studies have been reported. The efficacy of chronic hCG treatment for reproductive dysfunction has been examined in two prospective but uncontrolled studies. Administering hCG (2–4000 units per week) for 4 mo in 13 men with uremic undergoing regular dialysis did not alter hemoglobin or postdialysis body weight *(29)*. Furthermore, semen parameters were not consistently improved in a subgroup of eight men tested *(29)*. However, in a larger study of 20 men with chronic renal failure, half treated conservatively before inception of dialysis and half having regular hemodialysis, hCG (2000 units on alternate days) treatment for 120 d markedly improved sperm output and quality but only in the group that did not receive dialysis *(30)*. Sexual function was improved, especially in men who did not receive dialysis. These studies suggest that hCG treatment may have a role in managing the reproductive effects of uremia, particularly before dialysis, but well-controlled studies of adequate power are not available. The somatic effects of hCG treatment on androgen-responsive tissues, notably bone, muscle, cognition, and quality of life in uremia, as recently studied in nonuremic older men *(31),* have not been evaluated in a well-controlled study.

Estrogen blockade, using either anti-estrogens or aromatase inhibitors, also has potential to overcome functional partial gonadotropin deficiency in men with uremia, because hypothalamic and pituitary responsiveness are preserved. This raises the possibility of using anti-estrogens to increase pituitary gonadotropin and endogenous testosterone secretion *(20)*. Short-term clomiphene citrate (100 mg/d for 7 d) treatment can normalize plasma testosterone for at least 3 d after cessation in men with uremia treated by dialysis ($n = 34$) or renal transplantation ($n = 8$) *(32)*, but the clinical consequences of increased endogenous testosterone secretion were not reported. A smaller, uncontrolled study of five men who received dialysis previously reported that hormonal responses (rise in gonadotropins and testosterone) to clomiphene citrate (100 mg/d) were sustained for 5–12 mo and led to improved libido, potency, and well-being *(20)*. No studies of aromatase inhibitors in men with chronic renal failure have been reported. Placebo-controlled studies of adequate power and duration, as well as dose optimization, would be required to properly evaluate this interesting but neglected approach to adjunctive treatment in uremia, which must be balanced against the growing understanding of the physiological importance of estrogens in men *(33)*.

Androgen Deficiency

Men with chronic renal failure exhibit features consistent with classical androgen deficiency: reproductive manifestations, including gynecomastia, impotence, testicular atrophy, impaired spermatogenesis, and infertility, as well as somatic disorders of bone, muscle, and other androgen responsive tissues *(1,2)*. However, only a single well-controlled study has examined androgen replacement therapy in men with uremia *(34)*. Nineteen men who were receiving regular hemodialysis were randomized to receive either oral testosterone undecanoate (240 mg/d) or placebo for 12 wk. Libido and sexual activity were increased, but hemoglobin was unchanged. There were no adverse clinical effects or hepatotoxicity. Effects on bone, muscle, cognition, and well-being were not reported. Further studies examining physiological androgen replacement therapy in men with chronic renal failure, notably using nonparenteral therapies in view of the increased bleeding risks in men with chronic renal failure, would be of great interest. Preliminary studies of transdermal testosterone patches demonstrate similar pharmacokinetics in uremic as in hypogonadal men *(35)*.

A recent study evaluated pharmacological androgen therapy in receiving dialysis men. Twenty-nine men requiring regular hemodialysis were randomized to weekly im injections of nandrolone decanoate (100 mg, $n = 14$) or saline placebo ($n = 15$) for 6 mo in a study examining somatic and functional endpoints *(36)*. Lean body (muscle) mass (measured by dual-energy x-ray absorptiometry) was increased and was associated with functional improvements as reflected by faster timed walking and stair climbing and a reduction in self-reported fatigue *(37)*. Peak oxygen consumption was increased at 3 mo, but declined by the sixth month. Two of the three women receiving nandrolone required dose reduction because of virilization. Although the functional improvements in a well-controlled study were impressive, whether they are sustainable and improve survival remains to be evaluated. These encouraging findings suggest that larger, placebo-controlled clinical studies of longer duration to delineate the benefits and limitations of pharmacological androgen therapy in men with uremia would be of considerable interest.

Other Potential Causes of Androgen Deficiency

Men with pre-existing testicular dysfunction (including renal failure) may be more susceptible to further impairment of steroidogenesis caused by medications or illnesses. HMG-CoA reductase inhibitors inhibit cholesterol synthesis and may, therefore, impair steroidogenesis, particularly because adverse events consistent with androgen deficiency (gynecomastia and impotence) have been reported. A prospective, open-label study of 25 nephrotic, hyperlipidemic men with moderate chronic renal failure treated for 12 mo with lovastatin (40 mg/d) showed no change in baseline and GnRH-stimulated LH, FSH, and testosterone levels *(38)*. A more discerning test of testicular steroidogenesis, such as testosterone response to submaximal hCG stimulation, was not reported. Adrenal steroidogenesis (plasma cortisol before and after adrenocorticotropic hormone [ACTH] stimulation) was comparable with age-matched healthy controls at entry and remained unchanged by lovastatin treatment. Not surprisingly, testosterone was lower and gonadotropins were higher than in 25 age-matched untreated healthy controls before and after treatment. This study suggests that concurrent use of HMG-CoA reductase inhibitors in moderate chronic renal failure is not a major contributor to androgen deficiency.

A deleterious effect of secondary hyperparathyroidism has also been postulated as a factor contributing to uremic hypogonadism. However, a recent study examining seven men with severe secondary hyperparathyroidism before and at 3 and 6 mo after subtotal parathyroidectomy *(39)* reported no change in circulating LH, FSH, or testosterone before or after acute GnRH stimulation, despite dramatic reduction in circulating parathyroid hormone concentrations. These and other findings suggest that secondary hyperparathyroidism is not a major factor in the pathogenesis of uremic hypogonadism.

EFFECT OF ANDROGENS ON RENAL FUNCTION

The androgen responsiveness of the kidney has led to speculation that androgen therapy in patients with chronic renal failure or nephrotic syndrome might improve or slow deterioration in underlying renal function. This hypothesis arose from animal experiments showing androgen-induced renal hypertrophy and protection against certain nephrotoxins *(40)*. Clinical evidence for renotrophic effects of androgen therapy has been comprehensively reviewed *(40,41)* but remains ambiguous because of the lack of adequately powered, placebo-controlled studies. The best evidence for a renotrophic effect of androgen therapy derives from two older studies with significant methodological limitations. The first was a placebo-controlled study of elderly patients without renal disease *(42)* in which indices of both glomerular and tubular function were improved by nandrolone phenylpropionate (25 mg injections weekly) after approx 40 wk. The second, but uncontrolled, study showed apparent improvements in well-being and biochemical tests of renal function in 88 patients with uremia treated with various doses of injectable testosterone propionate (50 mg/d) or cypionate (100 mg/d to monthly) and oral fluoxymesterone (5 mg/d) *(43)*, but detailed findings and analysis were lacking. Although renotrophic effects have a biological basis, the lack of adequate clinical trials precludes an established role for androgen therapy in the conservative management of chronic renal failure *per se*.

On the contrary, experimental studies of rodent kidney transplantation suggest that androgen administration may be detrimental to renal function. In rats with kidney transplants, exogenous androgen therapy increased, whereas androgen blockade or estradiol administration reduced histological and functional features of chronic allograft nephropathy *(44,45)*. Further studies of human allograft recipients are required to determine whether these findings are relevant to humans, in which case caution in the use of androgen therapy after renal transplantation might be indicated.

PUBERTY IN CHRONIC RENAL FAILURE

Disorders of puberty commonly accompany chronic renal failure and require age-appropriate medical management. Although centrally mediated precocious puberty, which is reversed by renal transplantation, has been reported *(46)*, the most characteristic feature of chronic renal failure in boys is delayed puberty with retarded bone age *(1)*. The delayed puberty usually progresses slowly to completion during dialysis, whereas transplantation accelerates maturation unless complicated by poor graft function and/or high-dose glucocorticoids *(47)*. Because puberty involves the unleashing by the hypothalamus of pulsatile GnRH secretion that subsequently entrains pituitary gonadotropin secretion, the delayed puberty is further evidence of neuroendocrine dysfunction in uremia. This is consistent with experimental models of chronic renal failure, which show a predominant defect in the regulation of hypothalamic GnRH secretion *(12)*. In concert, these findings raise the issue of gonadotropin or androgen treatment for delayed puberty in chronic renal failure.

Three available studies of androgen therapy for delayed puberty in adolescents with uremia are small and uncontrolled *(48–50)*, so they provide little evidence of efficacy or safety. Oxandrolone (0.25 mg/kg per day for 2 mo, then alternate days) therapy for an average of more than 1 yr *(48)* in nine adolescent boys undergoing regular hemodialysis produced a modest increase in growth, which was slightly greater than the concomitant advance of skeletal maturation and improved appetite and vigor. However, one boy was dismissed from the study because of oxandrolone-induced hepatotoxicity, and the remainder developed fluid overload. In another study of four boys with uremia exhibiting severe growth and pubertal delay, injections of testosterone ester (50 mg escalating to 100 mg) each third week for 9–45 mo *(49)* accelerated growth and pubertal development, but skeletal maturation was preferentially enhanced and bony deformity developed. In 11 boys with normal renal function but pubertal delay associated with steroid treatment of nephrotic syndrome, oxandrolone (2.5 mg/d) therapy for 6 mo *(50)* did not increase growth more than untreated historical controls matched for age and pubertal status. Hence, the efficacy and safety of androgen therapy for uremic pubertal delay remains inadequately demonstrated. Whether androgen sensitivity is modified by chronic renal failure, for example, remains unclear. As in other clinical circumstances, improvement of underlying renal function (e.g., transplantation) is more likely to be effective than hormonal therapy in boys with chronic renal failure.

Pulsatile GnRH stimulation (~150 ng/kg subcutaneously every 120 min) adminis-tered for 7 d produced greater LH and testosterone responses in five boys with uremia than in six nonuremic controls with equivalent pubertal delay *(51)*. This intriguing and important observation warrants further evaluation. If reproducible, this would provide further corroboration for a state of functional GnRH (and gonadotropin) deficiency in uremia and would encourage further studies of estrogen blockade or hCG treatment in adolescents with uremia with delayed puberty, none of which is yet reported.

Cystinosis is a rare autosomal recessive disease characterized by defective extrusion of cystine from lysosomes, causing lysosomal storage and crystal formation that can lead to early renal failure, with the need for dialysis and/or transplantation before puberty. Cross-sectional studies have shown marked delay in growth and pubertal development, which improves after transplantation *(52)* but that remains more severe than other patients matched for age, gender, puberty, and renal status *(53)*. This sug-gests that toxic cystine accumulation in the testis can lead to hypergonadotrophic hypogonadism when life is prolonged by transplantation. If chelation therapy does not prevent progression to renal failure with attendant growth and pubertal delay, therapeu-tic trials of androgen therapy could be useful.

GROWTH FAILURE

Short stature is common in boys with uremia, and, after transplantation, catch-up growth is impaired. A small randomized, double-blind, placebo-controlled crossover study examined the short-term effects of testosterone on growth in short-statured boys undergoing hemodialysis *(54)*. After an 8-wk run-in, eight boys with growth-retarda-tion on regular hemodialysis were randomized to receive transdermal testosterone (top-ical dose 50 mg/m^2/d) or placebo gel for 4 wk before crossover to the other treatment after a 6-wk washout period. Although a significant increase in short-term growth velocity (using knemometry) was reported, the randomization was unbalanced with a likely period effect (all boys starting on active treatment had subnormal pretreatment growth velocity, whereas those starting on placebo all had normal pretreatment growth velocity). The small sample size, period effects, and uncertain efficacy makes it diffi-cult to interpret the growth results of this short-term study. Furthermore, the clinical significance of short-term growth acceleration is uncertain, because it may represent catch-up without necessarily predicting final height gain. Two other small, uncon-trolled series do not support a therapeutic role for androgen therapy for delayed puberty in adolescents with uremia *(49,50)*. More powerful and longer placebo-con-trolled studies are needed before even low-dose androgen therapy can be considered effective or safe for routine use.

SEXUAL DYSFUNCTION

Sexual function is frequently impaired by chronic renal failure *(55)* and is only partly reversed by transplantation, although few well-controlled studies are available. Contrib-utory factors include vascular failure, pelvic autonomic neuropathy, antihypertensives (particularly centrally acting agents and beta blockers), and other medications, together with additive effects of age, depression, and general debility. Uremic sexual function is not consistently improved with androgen therapy (200–400 mg testosterone enanthate weekly) *(56–58)*. Other proposed treatments, such as zinc supplementation *(59)*, prolactin-lowering with bromocriptine *(60)*, and tricyclic antidepressants *(61)*, are equally inconsistent. Oral vitamin E supplementation (300 mg/d for 8 wk) improved self-reported sexual function (libido, erectile activity, and coitus) in a balanced randomized, double-blind, placebo-controlled study of 24 men with uremia *(62)*. The modest improvement was not associated with significant changes in reproductive hormones and, if reproducible, further studies, including dose optimization, may be worthwhile.

General debility (including anemia) may have a significant role in causation of uremic sexual dysfunction, because recombinant human EPO therapy improves reproductive function. Menstrual and male sexual function were significantly improved and blood prolactin concentrations lowered in a study that randomized 44 patients on dialysis to standard treatment with EPO (180 U/kg/wk) or no treatment *(63)*. Other cross-sectional *(64)* and uncontrolled studies *(65–67)* corroborate these findings. Nevertheless, EPO does not improve the sexual dysfunction of men with impaired renal function who do not requiring dialysis *(65)*. EPO administration reduces the endocrine abnormalities in men with uremia with lowering of the exaggerated basal and GnRH-stimulated LH and FSH concentrations and increases in blood testosterone concentrations *(67–69)*. Whether this is a specific effect of EPO or is mediated via general effects, such as improvement in anemia and nutritional status, remains to be clarified.

There is increasing experience applying the recent advances in the management of erectile dysfunction, notably pharmacotherapy and mechanical devices, to men with chronic renal failure. For men with chronic renal failure complaining of erectile dysfunction, the management involves initially optimizing conventional medical treatment for uremia, including intensive dialysis or transplantation, nutritional support (including raising hemoglobin), and medication review *(70)*. The first line of specific therapy is oral sildenafil *(71)*, which appears significantly better than placebo in a preliminary report of a randomized, placebo-controlled study *(72)*, which extends similar positive experience from uncontrolled studies of men on dialysis *(73,74)*. However, particular vigilance with sildenafil usage is required for men with chronic renal failure in view of their accelerated rates of atherogenesis. Sildenafil is absolutely contraindicated in men using nitrates for coronary artery disease (where lethal hypotension can occur), and caution is also required in men with complex antihypertensive regimes. If sildenafil is not effective or is contraindicated, additional options include mechanical devices (vacuum/constriction devices or implantable prosthesis) or cavernosal vasodilator pharmacotherapy (prostaglandin E and phentolamine, papaverine, and mixtures). One study found high rates of satisfaction with a vacuum device in a selected subset of impotent men on dialysis *(56)*, but these devices are most useful in men with only partial erectile dysfunction. Surgically implanted hydraulic cavernosal prostheses are an expensive last resort, with significant risks of mechanical failure and infection, especially in immunocompromised transplant patients. Vasodilator therapy is most effective when injected intracavernosally *(75)*, but involves significant safety concerns requiring careful monitoring, including the risks of priapism, bleeding, thrombosis, or hypertension; nevertheless, some preliminary experience is encouraging *(76,77)*. Transurethral application of prostaglandin E *(78)* has theoretical safety advantages over intracavernosal injection but has limited efficacy.

INFERTILITY

Cross-sectional studies of spermatogenesis, sperm output, and fertility in men with chronic renal failure have previously been reviewed *(1,12)*. Successful renal transplantation reverses spermatogenic depression and infertility, as shown in short-term prospective and long-term retrospective studies. Even after successful transplantation, which restores testicular endocrine function, the degree of fertility recovery may be limited by irreversible damage to spermatogenesis accrued during prolonged dialysis *(1,14)*. Spermatogenesis and fertility were examined prospectively in 19 young men during at least 6 mo of regular hemodialysis and subsequently at least 6 mo after successful transplantation *(79)*. During regular hemodialysis, there were no pregnancies and all but two had subnormal sperm output with biopsy-proven hypospermatogenesis. After living-related renal transplantation, fertility and spermatogenesis improved markedly, with five wives conceiving, 13 men normalizing sperm density and motility, and 4 of 8 men, who underwent testicular biopsy before and after transplantation, normalizing spermatogenesis. Based on the hormonal evidence for partial gonadotropin deficiency (or resistance), further well-controlled clinical studies of gonadotropin therapy (estrogen blockade, hCG, FSH, and pulsatile GnRH) on spermatogenesis in men with chronic renal failure will be of considerable interest.

Androgen therapy for men with chronic renal failure to correct anemia or nutritional status involves risk of depressing endogenous testicular steroidogenesis and spermatogenesis *(80)*. If fertility is desired, the appropriate management is to stop the exogenous androgen, which allows spermatogenesis to recover. If this is not feasible or is inadequate, hCG treatment may be useful but has not been formally evaluated. Any treatment to improve fertility can theoretically also be combined with testicular sperm extraction for intracytoplasmic sperm injection (ICSI) although the bleeding and infection risks of the large testicular biopsy required careful consideration.

ANEMIA

The anemia of end-stage renal failure has multiple contributory factors, including EPO deficiency, toxic inhibitors of EPO action, androgen deficiency, micronutrient deficiency (iron, folate, and pyridoxine), blood loss, and hemolysis *(81)*. Although the balance between these remains conjectural, EPO deficiency is a major factor *(82)*, and androgen therapy has consistent effects on EPO secretion and hemoglobin concentrations *(83)*. Endogenous testosterone is an important physiological determinant of red cell mass in men, because blockade of androgen action lowers hemoglobin levels *(84,85)*. Androgen therapy has no effect on hemoglobin after bilateral nephrectomy *(86)*, when the major source of endogenous EPO is removed and circulating EPO is not consistently increased by androgens nor related to resultant increases in hemoglobin *(87)*. Furthermore, posttransplant erythrocytosis may depend on EPO and possibly also endogenous testosterone *(88)*. These findings suggest that androgens may act predominately by enhancing EPOs effect.

Although the effect of androgens on EPO has been long recognized, it has recently become clear that EPO can directly stimulate human Leydig cell testosterone secretion (in men with normal renal function). In a study of infertile, oligozoospermic men undergoing internal spermatic vein cannulation for radiological imaging of varicocele *(89)*, five men received EPO (60 U/kg), another five GnRH (50 µg) and three saline vehicle control as an i.v. bolus into the cubital vein. Simultaneous internal spermatic and peripheral vein sampling demonstrated that EPO increased spermatic vein testosterone secretion approx 12-fold, without concurrent change in peripheral LH, FSH, or testosterone or spermatic vein LH and FSH concentrations. In men with impaired renal function, EPO increases circulating testosterone concentrations in men on dialysis *(65,69)* as well as those not yet requiring dialysis *(65)*. The clinical significance of such increases in circulating testosterone is conjectural, given the inconsistent effects of exogenous testosterone on sexual function, growth, and puberty as discussed. However, improved spermatogenesis is possible if intratesticular testosterone concentrations are sufficiently increased to promote spermatogenesis.

Two randomized controlled studies have shown that pharmacological androgen therapy increases hemoglobin in patients with end-stage renal failure. One study randomized 21 men to nandrolone (100 mg/wk) or placebo vehicle injections for 5 mo in a cross-over design *(90)*, whereas another randomized 18 patients to nandrolone decanoate (200 mg/wk) for 3 mo *(91)*. Mean hemoglobin was significantly increased in both (15 g/L and 10 g/L, respectively), with one also reporting a clinically significant reduction in transfusion requirement *(90)*. Subsequent studies have confirmed the beneficial effects of nandrolone decanoate (200 mg/wk), compared with placebo vehicle injections for 4 mo *(92)*, whereas three smaller, less well-conducted *(34,93,94)* studies using lower dose oral androgen *(34,93)* have failed to show an increase in hemoglobin. These discrepancies may be explained partly by another randomized, controlled clinical study that compared four androgen regimens in patients on dialysis *(95)*. Intramuscular testosterone enanthate (4 mg/kg/wk) and nandrolone decanoate (3 mg/kg/wk) were more effective in increasing hematocrit than oral oxymetholone (1 mg/kg/d) and fluoxymesterone (0.4 mg/kg/d). However, the relatively arbitrary doses used cause uncertainty whether these differences reflected different effective androgen doses, androgen class (17-α alkylated or not), or administration route (including pharmacokinetics). The use of the obsolete class of hepatotoxic 17-α alkylated androgens in this setting is hard to justify when equally effective, safer androgens are available.

Androgen therapy increases hemoglobin primarily by increasing circulating EPO concentration *(92)*, but also partly by augmenting EPO action *(96)*. However, a prospective but uncontrolled study of 25 men undergoing hemodialysis reported that treatment with nandrolone decanoate (200 mg/wk) for 6 mo resulted in consistent increases in hemoglobin but highly variable changes in circulating EPO. Only 60% of men on dialysis exhibited an increase in EPO and the hemoglobin increase persisted long after circulating EPO fell and androgen therapy ceased *(87)*. The same investigators have subsequently confirmed the lack of association between EPO and hemoglobin using the same study design, but examining nine men undergoing peritoneal dialysis *(8)*. These two studies suggest that the augmentation of endogenous EPO action by androgen therapy may be more important than previously accepted in men undergoing hemodialysis or peritoneal dialysis.

The role of androgen therapy relative to EPO therapy in patients with chronic renal disease remains unresolved, because direct comparisons in well-controlled studies are lacking. A retrospective analysis of 84 patients receiving androgen therapy (nandrolone decanoate 200 mg/wk) for 6 mo reported that men older than 55 yr of age had the best hemoglobin responses and that this response was comparable with those treated with EPO *(97)*. This was subsequently confirmed in two controlled prospective studies using nandrolone decanoate 200 mg/wk or EPO (6000 U/wk) for 6 mo. The first study *(98)* reported similar hemoglobin responses and safety profiles in 18 men aged older than 50 yr treated with androgen therapy (nandrolone decanoate 200 mg/wk) compared with 6 men under 50 yrs and 16 women receiving EPO (6000 U/wk), but the lack of randomization and noncomparability of groups by age and gender limit the interpretation of these findings. In the second study *(9)*, 33 patients over the age of 65 yr who were receiving maintenance EPO treatment three times weekly were assigned to receive intramuscular nandrolone decanoate (200 mg/wk, $n = 14$ men) without EPO or to continue the same EPO treatment ($n = 12$ men, 7 women) for 6 mo. Nandrolone alone was at least as effective as continued EPO treatment in maintenance of all hematological and nutritional variables, suggesting that androgen therapy may be more cost-effective than EPO, particularly in older men on dialysis. These findings were corroborated in a small, uncontrolled study of nine older (>50 yr) men undergoing peritoneal dialysis who received nandrolone decanoate (200 mg/wk) for 6 mo *(8)*. These studies highlight that intramuscular nandrolone decanoate (200 mg/wk) in older men on dialysis (>50 yr old) is as effective as EPO in maintaining hemoglobin at a much lower cost. The comparative safety of these treatments requires more detailed evaluation.

Androgen therapy may also have a role in sparing EPO dose and cost. The addition of androgen therapy to intravenous EPO administered with hemodialysis has been examined in two randomized studies *(99,100)* and one nonrandomized *(96)* study. In the largest study with the longest treatment duration *(99)*, 19 patients on dialysis were randomized to receive nandrolone (100 mg wk) plus EPO (4500 U/wk) or EPO alone for 26 wk. The addition of nandrolone to low-dose EPO (approximately equal to 60 U/kg/wk) resulted in a significantly greater rise in hematocrit. Similar significant additional increases in hemoglobin were reported in a small nonrandomized study of eight men choosing to receive nandrolone decanoate (100 mg/wk) plus intermediate-dose EPO (6000 U/wk) compared with EPO alone *(96)* for 12 wk. However, another small but randomized study employing a higher dose of EPO (120 U/kg/wk) did not detect any benefit of nandrolone decanoate (2 mg/kg/wk) for 16 wk plus EPO compared with the same dose of EPO alone in 12 on dialysis patients *(100)*. Whether these discrepancies result from study design, age, or EPO dose remains to be clarified. It is possible that androgens have greatest synergism with submaximal EPO dosage and that the higher EPO dose obviates any additional androgen effect on hemoglobin. No study has examined the effect of subcutaneous EPO, and randomized prospective studies to examine the use of low-dose subcutaneous EPO with adjunctive androgen therapy are needed *(101)*, particularly in older men.

A caveat on androgen therapy is the risk of polycythemia, which may occur in men with normal renal function who are receiving exogenous testosterone *(102)*. Testosterone-induced polycythemia may be more common in older men receiving im testosterone injections *(103)* but has been observed with all forms of exogenous androgen *(104)* (*see* Chapter 18).

In summary, although androgen therapy is considerably cheaper than EPO *(105)*, its wider use is limited by modest efficacy when used alone and by adverse effects, notably virilization of women and children, and the hepatotoxicity of 17α-alkylated androgens. Restricting use to non-17α-alkylated androgens, particularly in older men

(9,97), may avoid most of the hazards. Present practice limits the role of androgen therapy in chronic renal failure to patients in whom EPO is contraindicated or unavailable, although evidence for its use as an EPO-sparing agent is accumulating. Whether it is more effective according to the degree of androgen deficiency induced by renal failure or according to the EPO dose remains to be clarified.

SLEEP APNEA

Obstructive sleep apnea can adversely affect reproductive function *(106)*, and one study found that androgen therapy can precipitate sleep apnea *(107)*. An observational study reported a high prevalence of obstructive sleep apnea in men on hemodialysis and examined whether testosterone ester injections are causative *(108)*. Sleep apnea symptoms were common (12/29, 41%), particularly in those receiving regular testosterone enanthate injections (250 mg/wk) to stimulate erythropoiesis (9/12, 75%), compared with those not receiving testosterone (6/17, 35%). However, withdrawal of testosterone did not alter the signs or symptoms of sleep apnea in the five men studied both during and 2 mo after cessation of testosterone treatment. Further surveillance has shown that sleep apnea is common in patients with chronic renal failure even before commencement of dialysis or testosterone treatment *(109)*. Hence, the contribution of pharmacological androgen therapy to breathing while asleep (and consequently on daytime wakefulness) remains conjectural with the limited data from well-controlled studies of androgen therapy on sleep and breathing. One randomized, double-blind, placebo-controlled study examined healthy men (with normal renal function) over the age of 65 yr with low baseline serum testosterone levels. Of the 108 men randomized to receive transdermal testosterone or placebo for 36 mo, sleep breathing patterns determined by a portable device were not worsened by testosterone, but formal sleep studies were not performed *(110)*. Although this indicates that androgen replacement therapy in older men does not regularly induce severe sleep apnea, more modest, or infrequent idiosyncractic, effects are not fully excluded, nor are the effects of higher androgen doses clear *(111)*.

THE PROSTATE

The effects of exogenous androgen therapy on the prostate are not well defined. Because severe androgen deficiency prevents prostate development and disease, exposure to adult male testosterone concentrations for decades must establish the origins of prostate disease *(11)*. Yet the effects of androgen deficiency and administration during midlife on risk of late-life prostate disease is unclear. Although men who are androgen deficient have reduced prostate volume *(112,113)*, testosterone administration for androgen replacement therapy restores prostate volume, either in part *(113)* or fully *(112)*; however, even massive androgen doses don't cause significant prostatic hyperplasia at least during midlife *(114)*. Although the effects of androgen therapy on prostate size or cancer risk are not reported in men with chronic renal failure, prolonged pharmacological androgen therapy (nandrolone decanoate 200 mg/wk for up to 24 mo) had no significant effects on blood levels of prostate markers prostate-specific antigen and prostatic acid phosphatase in elderly men on hemodialysis *(115)*.

CONCLUSION

Chronic renal failure, dialysis, and transplantation cause major effects on male reproductive health, notably impairment of spermatogenesis, steroidogenesis, and sexual function, through effects at all levels of the hypothalamic–pituitary testicular axis. Delayed growth and puberty, sexual dysfunction, androgen deficiency, and infertility are the clinical consequences. This chapter reviews the basis and scope for various clinical applications of gonadotropin and androgen therapy as an adjunct to standard medical care of men with chronic renal failure. Androgen therapy is considered as either androgen replacement therapy (using testosterone doses equivalent to endogenous production rates aiming to restore but not exceed physiological testosterone exposure) or as pharmacological androgen therapy (using any androgen in doses optimized for efficacy, safety, and cost-effectiveness).

There is now convincing evidence that chronic renal failure is associated with a gonadotropin- and androgen-deficient state, providing a basis for evaluating the clinical use of androgen or gonadotropin replacement therapy. Various forms of gonadotropin therapy (estrogen blockade and gonadotropin administration) and of androgen replacement therapy have been little evaluated, so their risks and benefits remain to be clarified.

Pharmacological androgen therapy in chronic renal failure has a proven indication only for treatment of renal anemia, where it has been widely applied for more than three decades before being largely supplanted by recombinant human EPO. Although EPO is highly effective and widely used (including for women and children where androgens are best avoided), it is much more expensive. Recent studies suggest pharmacological androgen therapy is as effective as EPO in older men, and has synergistic, EPO dose- (and cost-) sparing effects in conjunction with low-dose EPO therapy. This suggests a diminished but continuing role of pharmacological androgen therapy for renal anemia. The potential for pharmacological androgen therapy to improve nutritional status and nonreproductive functions has long been considered, but the overall benefits on quality of life and survival remain to be well established. Such potential benefits would have to be weighed against potential adverse effects, including acceleration of cardiovascular or prostate disease and idiosyncratic androgen effects (polycythemia and sleep apnea).

REFERENCES

1. Handelsman DJ. Hypothalamic-pituitary gonadal dysfunction in chronic renal failure, dialysis, and renal transplantation. Endocr Rev 1985;6:151–182.
2. Handelsman DJ, Liu PY. Androgen therapy in chronic renal failure. Baillieres Clin Endocrinol Metab 1998;12:485–500.
3. Nieschlag E, Nieschlag S, Behre HM. Lifespan and testosterone. Nature 1993;366:215.
4. Anonymous. Adequacy of dialysis and nutrition in continuous peritoneal dialysis: association with clinical outcomes. Canada-USA (CANUSA) Peritoneal Dialysis Study Group. J Am Soc Nephrol 1996;7:198–207.
5. Fung L, Pollock CA, Caterson RJ, et al. Dialysis adequacy and nutrition determine prognosis in continuous ambulatory peritoneal dialysis patients. J Am Soc Nephrol 1996;7:737–744.
6. Kopple JD. Effect of nutrition on morbidity and mortality in maintenance dialysis patients. Am J Kidney Dis 1994;24:1002–1009.
7. Dombros NV, Digenis GE, Soliman G, Oreopoulos DG. Anabolic steroids in the treatment of malnourished CAPD patients: a retrospective study. Peritoneal Dialysis Int 1994;14:344–347.

8. Navarro JF, Mora-Fernandez C, Rivero A, et al. Androgens for the treatment of anemia in peritoneal dialysis patients. Adv Peritoneal Dialysis 1998;14:232–235.

9. Gascon A, Belvis JJ, Berisa F, Iglesias E, Estopinan V, Teruel JL. Nandrolone decanoate is a good alternative for the treatment of anemia in elderly male patients on hemodialysis. Geriatr Nephrol Urol 1999;9:67–72.

10. Cianciaruso B, Brunori G, Kopple JD, et al. Cross-sectional comparison of malnutrition in continuous ambulatory peritoneal dialysis and hemodialysis patients. Am J Kidney Dis 1995;26:475–486.

11. Handelsman DJ. The safety of androgens: prostate and cardiovascular disease. In: Wang C, ed. Male Reproductive Function. Kluwer Academic Publishers, Boston, 1998, pp. 227–237.

12. Handelsman DJ, Dong Q. Hypothalamo-pituitary gonadal axis in chronic renal failure. Endocrinol Metab Clin North Am 1993;22:145–161.

13. Veldhuis JD, Wilkowski MJ, Zwart AD, et al. Evidence for attenuation of hypothalamic gonadotropin-releasing hormone (GnRH) impulse strength with preservation of GnRH pulse frequency in men with chronic renal failure. J Clin Endocrinol Metab 1993;76:648–654.

14. De Celis R, Pedron-Nuevo N. Male fertility of kidney transplant patients with one to ten years of evolution using a conventional immunosuppressive regimen. Arch Androl 1999;42:9–20.

15. Ramirez G, Narvarte J, Bittle PA, Ayers-Chastain C, Dean SE. Cyclosporine-induced alterations in the hypothalamic hypophyseal gonadal axis in transplant patients. Nephron 1991;58:27–32.

16. Jecht E, Klupp E, Heidler R, Huben H, Schwarz W. Investigation of the hormonal axis hypothalamus-pituitary-gonads in 20 dialyzed men. Andrologia 1980;12:146–155.

17. Stewart-Bentley M, Gans D, Horton R. Regulation of gonadal function in uremia. Metab Clin Exp 1974;23:1065–1072.

18. Handelsman DJ, Ralec VL, Tiller DJ, Horvath JS, Turtle JR. Testicular function after renal transplantation. Clin Endocrinol 1981;14:527–538.

19. Holdsworth S, Atkins RC, de Kretser DM. The pituitary-testicular axis in men with chronic renal failure. N Engl J Med 1977;296:1245–1249.

20. Lim VS, Fang VS. Restoration of plasma testosterone levels in uremic men with clomiphene citrate. J Clin Endocrinol Metab 1976;43:1370–1377.

21. Dunkel L, Raivio T, Laine J, Holmberg C. Circulating luteinizing hormone receptor inhibitor(s) in boys with chronic renal failure. Kidney Int 1997;51:777–784.

22. Rodger R, Morrison L, Dewar J, Wilkinson R, Ward M, Kerr D. Loss of pulsatile luteinizing hormone secretion in men with chronic renal failure. Br Med J 1985;291:1598–1600.

23. Wheatley T, Clark P, Raggatt P, Evans D, Holder R. Pulsatility of luteinising hormone in men with chronic renal failure: abnormal rather than absent. Br Med J 1987;294:482.

24. Talbot JA, Rodger RSC, Robertson WR. Pulsatile bioactive luteinising hormone secretion in men with chronic renal failure and following renal transplantation. Nephron 1990;56:66–72.

25. Schaefer F, Seidel C, Mitchell R, Scharer K, Robertson WR, Cooperative Study Group on Pubertal Development in Chronic Renal Failure (CSPCRF). Pulsatile immunoreactive and bioactive luteinizing hormone secretion in adolescents with chronic renal failure. Pediatr Nephrol 1991;5:566–571.

26. Schaefer F, Veldhuis JD, Robertson WR, Dunger D, Scharer K. Immunoreactive and bioactive luteinizing hormone in pubertal patients with chronic renal failure. Kidney Int 1994;45:1465–1476.

27. Handelsman DJ, Spaliviero JA, Turtle JR. Bioactive luteinizing hormone in plasma of uraemic men and men with primary testicular damage. Clin Endocrinol 1986;24:259–266.

28. Mitchell R, Bauerfeld C, Schaefer F, Scharer K, Robertson WR. Less acidic forms of luteinizing hormone are associated with lower testosterone secretion in men on haemodialysis treatment. Clin Endocrinol 1994;41:65–73.

29. Bundschu HD, Rager K, Heller S, et al. Auswirkungen einer langdaueren exogenen Gonadotropinzufuhr auf die testikulare Insuffizienz bei Dauerdialysepatienten. Klinische Wochenschricht 1976;54:1039–1046.

30. Canale D, Barsantini S, Minervini R, Fiorentini L, Barsotti G, Menchini-Fabris GF. Human chorionic gonadotropin treatment of male sexual inadequacy in patients affected by chronic renal failure. J Androl 1984;5:120–124.

31. Liu PY, Wishart SM, Handelsman DJ. A double-blind, placebo-controlled, randomised clinical trial of recombinant human chorionic gonadotropin (r-hCG) on muscle strength and physical function and activity in older men with partial age-related androgen deficiency. J Clin Endocrinol Metab 2002;87:3125–3135.

32. Martin-Malo A, Benito P, Castillo D, et al. Effect of clomiphene citrate on hormonal profile in male hemodialysis and kidney transplant patients. Nephron 1993;63:390–394.
33. Sharpe RM. Do males rely on female hormones? Nature 1997;390:447–448.
34. van Coevorden A, Stolear JC, Dhaene M, Herweghem JLv, Mockel J. Effect of chronic oral testosterone undecanoate administration on the pituitary-testicular axes of hemodialyzed male patients. Clin Nephrol 1986;26:48–54.
35. Singh AB, Norris K, Modi N, et al. Pharmacokinetics of a transdermal testosterone system in men with end stage renal disease receiving maintenance hemodialysis and healthy hypogonadal men. J Clin Endocrinol Metab 2001;86:2437–2445.
36. Johansen KL, Mulligan K, Schambelan M. Anabolic effects of nandrolone decanoate in patients receiving dialysis: a randomized controlled trial [see comments]. JAMA 1999;281:1275–1281.
37. McNair DM, Lorr M, Droppleman LF. EITS manual for the profile of mood states. Educational and Industrial Testing Service, San Diego, 1971.
38. Segarra A, Chacon P, Vilardell M, Piera LL. Prospective case-control study to determine the effects of lovastatin on serum testosterone and cortisol concentrations in hyperlipidemic nephrotic patients with chronic renal failure. Nephron 1996;73:186–190.
39. Zofkova I, Sotornik I, Kancheva RL. Adenohypophyseal-gonadal dysfunction in male haemodialyzed patients before and after subtotal parathyroidectomy. Nephron 1996;74:536–540.
40. Kopera H. Miscellaneous uses of anabolic steroids. In: Kochakian CD, ed. Anabolic-Androgenic Steroids. Vol. 43. Springer-Verlag, Berlin, 1976, pp. 535–625.
41. Kruskemper HL. Anabolic Steroids. Academic, New York, 1968, pp. 236.
42. Dontas AS, Papanicolaou NT, Papanayiotou P, Malamos BK. Long-term effects of anabolic steroids on renal functions in the aged subject. J Gerontol 1967;22:268–273.
43. Wilkey JL, Barson LJ, Kest L, Bragagni A. The effect of testosterone on the azotemic patient: an intermediary report. J Urol 1960;83:25–29.
44. Antus B, Yao Y, Liu S, Song E, Lutz J, Heemann U. Contribution of androgens to chronic allograft nephropathy is mediated by dihydrotestosterone. Kidney Int 2001;60:1955–1963.
45. Muller V, Szabo A, Viklicky O, et al. Sex hormones and gender-related differences: their influence on chronic renal allograft rejection. Kidney Int 1999;55:2011–2020.
46. Loh KC, Salisbury SR, Accott P, Gillis R, Crocker JF. Central precocious puberty and chronic renal failure: a reversible condition post renal transplantation. J Pediatr Endocrinol Metab 1997;10:539–545.
47. Kassmann K, Arsan A, Sharer K, Broyer M. Fonction gonadique et activite genitale des malades transplantes renaux de sexe masculin. Annales de Pediatre 1991;38:405–406.
48. Jones RWA, El Bishti MM, Bloom SR, et al. The effects of anabolic steroids on growth, body composition, and metabolism in boys with chronic renal failure on regular hemodialysis. J Pediatr 1980;97:559–566.
49. Van Steenbergen MW, Wit JM, Donckerwolcke RA. Testosterone esters advance skeletal maturation more than growth in short boys with chronic renal failure and delayed puberty. Eur J Pediatr 1991;150:676–680.
50. Rees L, Greene SA, Rigden SPA, Haycock GB, Chantler C, Preece MA. Oxandrolone for delayed puberty in boys taking long-term steroid therapy for renal disease. Pediatr Nephrol 1990;4:160–162.
51. Giusti M, Perfumo F, Verrina E, et al. Delayed puberty in uremia: pituitary-gonadal function during short-term pulsatile luteinizing hormone-releasing hormone administration. J Endocrinol Invest 1992;15:709–717.
52. Winkler L, Offner G, Krull F, Brodehl J. Growth and pubertal development in nephropathic cystinosis. Eur J Pediatr 1993;152:244–249.
53. Chik CL, Friedman A, Merriam GR, Gahl WA. Pituitary-testicular function in nephropathic cystinosis. Ann Intern Med 1993;119:568–575.
54. Kassmann K, Rappaport R, Broyer M. The short-term effect of testosterone on growth in boys on hemodialysis. Clin Nephrol 1992;37:148–154.
55. Steele TE, Wuerth D, Finkelstein S, et al. Sexual experience of the chronic peritoneal dialysis patient. J Am Soc Nephrol 1996;7:1165–1168.
56. Lawrence IG, Price DE, Howlett TA, Harris KP, Fechally J, Walls J. Correcting impotence in the male dialysis patient: experience with testosterone replacement and vacuum tumescence therapy. Am J Kidney Dis 1998;31:313–319.
57. Barton CH, Mirahmadi MK, Vaziri ND. Effects of long-term testosterone administration on pituitary-testicular axis in end-stage renal failure. Nephron 1982;31:61–64.

58. Chopp RT, Mendez R. Sexual function and hormonal abnormalities in uremic men on chronic dialysis and after renal transplantation. Fertil Steril 1978;29:661–666.
59. Brook AC, Ward MK, Cook DB, Johnston DG, Watson MJ, Kerr DNS. Absence of a therapeutic effect of zinc in the sexual dysfunction of haemodialysis patients. Lancet 1980;2:618–620.
60. Bommer J, del Pozo E, Ritz E, Bommer G. Improved sexual function in male haemodialysis patients on bromocriptine. Lancet 1979;2:496–497.
61. Zetin M, Frost NR, Brumfield D, Stone RA. Amitryptiline stimulates weight gain in hemodialysis patients. Clin Nephrol 1982;18:79–82.
62. Yeksan M, Polat M, Turk S, et al. Effect of vitamin E therapy on sexual functions or uremic patients in hemodialysis. Int J Art Organs 1992;15:648–652.
63. Yeksan M, Tamer N, Cirit M, et al. Effect of recombinant human erythropoietin (r-HuEPO) therapy on plasma FT3, FT4, TSH, FSH, LH, free testosterone and prolactin levels in hemodialysis patients. Int J Art Organs 1992;5:585–589.
64. Lawrence IG, Price DE, Howlett TA, Harris KP, Feehally J, Walls J. Erythropoietin and sexual dysfunction. Nephrol Dialysis Transplant 1997;12:741–747.
65. Wu SC, Lin SL, Jeng FR. Influence of erythropoietin treatment on gonadotropic hormone levels and sexual function in male uremic patients. Scand J Urol Nephrol 2001;35:136–140.
66. Schaefer RM, Kokot F, Heidland A. Impact of recombinant erythropoietin on sexual function in hemodialysis patients. In: Baldamus CA, Scigalla P, Wieczorek L, Koch KM, eds. Erythropoietin: From Molecular Structure to Clinical Application. Vol. 76. Karger, Basel, 1989, pp. 273–282.
67. Kokot F, Wiecek A, Grzeszczak W, Klin M. Infleunce of erythropoietin treatment on follitropin and lutropin response to luliberin and plasma testosterone in haemodialysed patients. Nephron 1990;56:126–129.
68. Diez JJ, Iglesias P, Bajo MA, de Alvaro F, Selgas R. Effects of erythropoietin on gonadotropin responses to gonadotropin-releasing hormone in uremic patients. Nephron 1997;77:169–175.
69. Tokgoz B, Utas C, Dogukan A, et al. Effects of long-term erythropoietin therapy on the hypothalamo-pituitary-testicular axis in male CAPD patients. Perit Dial Int 2001;21:448–454.
70. Palmer BF. Sexual dysfunction in uremia. J Am Soc Nephrol 1999;10:1381.
71. Goldstein I, Lue TF, Padma-Nathan H, Rosen RC, Steers WD, Wicker PA. Oral sildenafil in the treatment of erectile dysfunction. Sildenafil Study Group. N Engl J Med 1998;338:1397–1404.
72. MacDougall IC, Mahon A, Muir G, Sidhu P. Randomised placebo-controlled study of sildenafil (Viagra) in peritoneal dialysis patients with erectile dysfunction. J Am Soc Nephrol 1999;10:318A.
73. Chen J, Mabjeesh NJ, Greenstein A, Nadu A, Matzkin H. Clinical efficacy of sildenafil in patients on chronic dialysis. J Urology 2001;165:819–821.
74. Turk S, Karalezli G, Tonbul HZ, et al. Erectile dysfunction and the effects of sildenafil treatment in patients on haemodialysis and continuous ambulatory peritoneal dialysis. Nephrol Dialysis Transplant 2001;16:1818–1822.
75. Linet OI, Ogrinc FG. Efficacy and safety of intracavernosal alprostadil in men with erectile dysfunction. The Alprostadil Study Group. N Engl J Med 1996;334:873–877.
76. Mansi MK, Alkhudair WK, Huraib S. Treatment of erectile dysfunction after kidney transplantation with intracavernosal self-injection of prostaglandin E1. J Urol 1998;159:1927–1930.
77. Rodriguez Antolin A, Morales JM, Andres A, et al. Treatment of erectile impotence in renal transplant patients with intracavernosal vasoactive drugs. Transplant Proc 1992;24:105–106.
78. Padma-Nathan H, Hellstrom WJ, Kaiser FE, et al. Treatment of men with erectile dysfunction with transurethral alprostadil. Medicated Urethral System for Erection (MUSE) Study Group N Engl J Med 1997;336:1–7.
79. Prem AR, Punekar SV, Kalpana M, Kelkar AR, Acharya VN. Male reproductive function in uraemia: efficacy of haemodialysis and renal transplantation. Br J Urol 1996;78:635–638.
80. Maeda Y, Nakanishi T, Ozawa K, et al. Anabolic steroid-associated hypogonadism in male hemodialysis patients. Clin Nephrol 1989;32:198–201.
81. Neff MS, Goldberg J, Slifkin RF, et al. Anemia in chronic renal failure. Acta Endocrinol 1985;271(suppl):80–86.
82. Winearls CG. Historical review of the use of recombinant human erythropoietin in chronic renal failure. Nephrol Dialysis Transplant 1995;10(suppl 2):3–9.
83. Navarro JF, Mora C. In-depth review: effect of androgens on anemia and malnutrition in renal failure: implications for patients on peritoneal dialysis. Perit Dialysis Int 2001;21:14–24.

84. Weber JP, Walsh PC, Peters CA, Spivak JL. Effect of reversible androgen deprivation on hemoglobin and serum erythropoietin in men. Am J Hematol 1991;36:190–194.

85. Teruel JL, Cano T, Marcen R, et al. Decrease in the haemoglobin level in haemodialysis patients undergoing antiandrogen therapy. Nephrol Dialysis Transplant 1997;12:1262–1263.

86. von Hartitzsch B, Kerr DNS. Response to parenteral iron with and without androgen therapy in patients undergoing regular haemodialysis. Nephron 1976;17:430–438.

87. Teruel JL, Marcen R, Navarro JF, et al. Evolution of serum erythropoietin after androgen administration to hemodialysis patients: a prospective study. Nephron 1995;70:282–286.

88. Chan PCK, Wei DCC, Tam SCF, Chan FL, Yeung WC, Cheng IKP. Post-transplant erythrocytosis: role of erythropoietin and male sex hormones. Nephrol Dialysis Transplant 1992;7:137–142.

89. Foresta C, Mioni R, Bordon P, Miotto D, Montini G, Varotto A. Erythropoietin stimulates testosterone production in man. J Clin Endocrinol Metab 1994;78:753–756.

90. Hendler ED, Goffinet JA, Ross S, Longnecker RE, Bakovic V. Controlled study of androgen therapy in anemia of patients on maintenance hemodialysis. N Engl J Med 1974;291:1046–1051.

91. Williams JS, Stein JH, Ferris TF. Nandrolone decanoate therapy for patients receiving hemodialysis. A controlled study. Arch Intern Med 1974;134:289–292.

92. Buchwald D, Argyres S, Easterling RE, et al. Effect of nandrolone decanoate on the anemia of chronic hemodialysis patients. Nephron 1977;18:232–238.

93. Bock EL, Fulle HH, Heimpel H, Pribilla W. Die Wirkung von Mesterolon bei Panmyelopathien und renalen Anaemien. Medizinische Klinik 1976;1:539–547.

94. Naik RB, Gibbons AR, Gyde OH, Harris BR, Robinson BH. Androgen trial in renal anaemia. Proc Eur Dialysis Transplant Assoc 1978;15:136–143.

95. Neff MS, Goldberg J, Slifkin RF, et al. A comparison of androgens for anemia in patients on hemodialysis. N Engl J Med 1981;304:871–875.

96. Ballal SH, Domoto DT, Polack DC, Marciulonis P, Martin KJ. Androgens potentiate the effects of erythropoietin in the treatment of anemia of end-stage renal disease. Am J Kidney Dis 1991;17:29–33.

97. Teruel JL, Aguilera A, Marcen R, Antolin JN, Otero GG, Ortuno J. Androgen therapy for anaemia of chronic renal failure. Scand J Urol Nephrol 1996;30:403–408.

98. Teruel JL, Marcen R, Navarro-Antolin J, Aguilera A, Fernandez-Juarez G, Ortuno J. Androgen versus erythropoietin for the treatment of anemia in hemodialyzed patients: a prospective study. J Am Soc Nephrol 1996;7:140–144.

99. Gaughan WJ, Liss KA, Dunn SR, et al. A 6-month study of low-dose recombinant human erythropoietin alone and in combination with androgens for the treatment of anemia in chronic hemodialysis patients. Am J Kidney Dis 1997;30:495–500.

100. Berns JS, Rudnick MR, Cohen RM. A controlled trial of recombinant human erythropoietin and nandrolone decanoate in the treatment of anemia in patients on chronic hemodialysis. Clin Nephrol 1992;37:264–267.

101. Horl WH. Is there a role for adjuvant therapy in patients being treated with epoetin? Nephrol Dialysis Transplant 1999;14:50–60.

102. Drinka PJ, Jochen AL, Cuisinier M, Bloom R, Rudman I, Rudman D. Polycythemia as a complication of testosterone replacement therapy in nursing home men with low testosterone levels. J Am Geriat Soc 1995;43:899–901.

103. Hajjar RR, Kaiser FE, Morley JE. Outcomes of long-term testosterone replacement in older hypogonadal males: a retrospective analysis. J Clin Endocrinol Metab 1997;82:3793–3796.

104. Jockenhovel F, Vogel E, Reinhardt W, Reinwein D. Effects of various modes of androgen substitution therapy on erythropoiesis. Eur J Med Res 1997;2:293–298.

105. Powe NR, Griffiths RI, Bass EB. Cost implications to Medicare of recombinant erythropoietin therapy for the anemia of end-stage renal disease. J Am Soc Nephrol 1993;3:1610–1671.

106. Grunstein RR, Handelsman DJ, Lawrence SJ, Blackwell C, Caterson ID, Sullivan CE. Hypothalamic dysfunction in sleep apnea: reversal by nasal continuous positive airways pressure. J Clin Endocrinol Metab 1989;68:352–358.

107. Sandblom RE, Matsumoto AM, Scoene RB, et al. Obstructive sleep apnea induced by testosterone administration. N Engl J Med 1983;308:508–510.

108. Millman RP, Kimmel PL, Shore ET, Wasserstein AG. Sleep apnea in hemodialysis patients: the lack of testosterone effect on its pathogenesis. Nephron 1985;40:407–410.

109. Kimmel PL, Miller G, Mendelson WB. Sleep apnea syndrome in chronic renal disease. Am J Med 1989;86:308–314.

110. Snyder PJ, Peachey H, Hannoush P, et al. Effect of testosterone treatment on bone mineral density in men over 65 years of age. J Clin Endocrinol Metab 1999;4:1966–1972.
111. Liu PY, Yee B, Wishart SM, Yang Q, Grunstein R, Handelsman DJ. The acute effects of high dose testosterone on sleep in ageing men [abstract]. US Endocrine Society, San Francisco, 2002.
112. Behre HM, Bohmeyer J, Nieschlag E. Prostate volume in testosterone-treated and untreated hypogonadal men in comparison to age-matched normal controls. Clin Endocrinol 1994;40:341–349.
113. Jin B, Conway AJ, Handelsman DJ. Effects of androgen deficiency and replacement on prostate zonal volumes. Clin Endocrinol (Oxf) 2001;54:437–445.
114. Jin B, Turner L, Walters WAW, Handelsman DJ. Androgen or estrogen effects on the human prostate. J Clin Endocrinol Metab 1996;81:4290–4295.
115. Teruel JL, Aguilera A, Avila C, Ortuno J. Effects of androgen therapy on prostatic markers in hemodialyzed patients. Scand J Urol Nephrol 1996;30:129–131.

13 Male Hypogonadism Resulting From Cancer and Cancer Treatments

Simon J. Howell, MD, MRCP
and Stephen M. Shalet, MD, FRCP

CONTENTS

INTRODUCTION
PRETREATMENT TESTICULAR DYSFUNCTION
CHEMOTHERAPY
RADIOTHERAPY
GENETIC DAMAGE FOLLOWING CYTOTOXIC THERAPY
PROTECTION OF TESTICULAR FUNCTION DURING CANCER
    TREATMENT
SUMMARY
REFERENCES

INTRODUCTION

It has been recognized for many years that testicular dysfunction is relatively common after treatment with cytotoxic chemotherapy and radiotherapy. The number of malignancies which are potentially treatable has increased during the last few decades. This increase, coupled with the improving long-term survival rates of many cancers, has meant that the number of surviving patients who have received cytotoxic therapy or radiotherapy is growing rapidly, and cancer treatment is becoming an increasingly common cause of acquired testicular dysfunction.

Spermatogenesis impairment has been demonstrated in patients with various malignancies before treatment. In addition, damage to the germinal epithelium resulting in oligospermia or azoospermia is a recognized consequence of certain chemotherapeutic agents and radiotherapy, and there is also evidence of Leydig cell dysfunction after treatment. Testicular damage is drug specific and dose related *(1–4)*. The chance of recovery of spermatogenesis after the cytotoxic insult and the extent and speed of recovery are related to the agent used and the dose received. It has also been suggested that the germinal epithelium of the adult testis is more susceptible to damage than that of the prepubertal testis *(5)*, implying that patient age or testis maturation at the time of

From: *Male Hypogonadism:*
Basic, Clinical, and Therapeutic Principles
Edited by: S. J. Winters © Humana Press Inc., Totowa, NJ

cytotoxic insult may influence the susceptibility to damage. Radiotherapy-induced testicular damage is similarly dose-dependent, with speed of onset, chance of reversal, and time to recovery, of spermatogenesis all related to the testicular irradiation dose *(6)*. However, the few data available regarding the influence of pubertal status suggest that, unlike the germinal epithelium, Leydig cell function may be more prone to damage from irradiation in prepubertal life compared with adulthood *(7)*.

PRETREATMENT TESTICULAR DYSFUNCTION

Alterations in germinal epithelial function have been demonstrated in patients with cancer before any treatment is commenced. This is particularly apparent in men with testicular cancer and Hodgkin's disease, both of which are relatively common cancers presenting during reproductive years. In addition, there are other situations in which gonadal dysfunction is associated with malignancy.

Hodgkin's Disease

Several studies have shown reduced fertility in men with Hodgkin's disease. Padron et al. *(7a)* found oligospermia (sperm count $<20 \times 10^6$/mL) in 18 of 49 (37%) patients with Hodgkin's disease who produced semen for cryopreservation before treatment. Similar rates of oligospermia were also demonstrated by Vigersky et al. *(8)* (total sperm count $<40 \times 10^6$ in 40%) and Chapman et al. *(9)* (total sperm count $<50 \times 10^6$ in 36%). In addition to reductions in sperm number, there is also evidence of abnormalities of sperm motility. When this is considered, up to 70% of men with Hodgkin's disease have abnormal semen analysis before treatment *(8,10–12)*. Because of severe debilitation or impotence, not all men can provide semen for cryopreservation before treatment. Because these reports examined only men who were able to do so, they may have selected out a slightly healthier cohort and may, thus, underestimate the extent of gonadal dysfunction before treatment.

The pathogenesis of this dyspermia is not clearly understood. It has been suggested that the general debilitation and psychological effects of the disease may account for the reductions in semen quality. However, this is not supported by the observation that the degree of gonadal involvement does not correlate with disease stage *(10,12)* and also does not explain why infertility is more common in men with Hodgkin's disease compared with other malignancies. Studies incorporating testicular biopsies have failed to find any evidence for a role of direct tumor involvement of the testes. A further possible explanation was proposed by Barr et al., who hypothesized that alterations in spermatogenesis may be immune mediated *(13)*, although clear evidence for this is lacking.

Testicular Cancer

Testicular cancer is associated with oligospermia in more than 50% of men before treatment *(11,14)*. Several possible causes have been suggested. First, local pathological change to the testis is apparent on biopsy of the contralateral testis, with 24–60% showing significant fibrosis of the seminiferous tubules, Sertoli cell only in 8%, and carcinoma *in situ* in 5–8%. Local tumor effects, including elevation of scrotal temperature, alterations in testicular blood flow, and disruption of the blood–testis barrier, may also contribute. Furthermore, sperm antibodies have been found in a high proportion of

Table 1
Gonadotoxic Drugs

Group	Definite Gonadotoxicity
Alkylating agents	Cyclophosphamide (5)
	Chlorambucil
	Mustine
	Melphalan
	Busulfan (27)
	Carmustine (68)
	Lomustine (68)
Antimetabolites	Cytarabine
Vinca alkaloids	Vinblastine (69)
Others	Procarbazine
	Cisplatin (70)

patients with testicular cancer (15). Finally, testicular cancer may be hormonally active, and local hormone production may impair spermatogenesis.

Other Associations of Cancer and Hypogonadism

Cryptorchidism is associated with spermatogenesis impairment and an increased risk of neoplastic change in the testes. Tumors arising in the region of the pituitary and hypothalamus or their treatment may result in hypopituitarism and consequent hypogonadism. Hormonally active tumors elsewhere may also inhibit hypothalamic–pituitary function. Ectopic adrenocorticotropic hormone (ACTH) secretion, most commonly from lung tumors, may cause secondary hypogonadism. Androgen-secreting tumors may suppress gonadotrophin secretion, thereby causing oligospermia or azoospermia. However, with the exception of cryptorchidism, hypogonadism would be an unusual presentation for these conditions.

CHEMOTHERAPY

Many drugs, particularly alkylating agents, are gonadotoxic, and the agents most commonly implicated are listed in table Table 1. The germinal epithelium is far more sensitive to the effects of cytotoxic drugs than are the Leydig cells, and, although complete azoospermia is not uncommon after chemotherapy, evidence of Leydig cell dysfunction is usually limited to raised luteinizing hormone (LH) levels with normal or low normal testosterone levels. Most research has focused on either cyclophosphamide given alone for immunologically mediated disease or combination chemotherapy used in the treatment of hematological malignancies and testicular cancer.

Cyclophosphamide

Rivkees and Crawford (5) published a meta-analysis of 30 studies that examined gonadal function after various chemotherapy regimens, which included 116 men who had been treated with cyclophosphamide alone. Gonadal function and/or histology were assessed by several different methods; semen analysis, basal LH and follicle-stimulating hormone (FSH) levels, and testicular biopsy were the most commonly used. Of the 116 patients, 52 (45%) had evidence of testicular dysfunction after treatment. The finding of gonadal dysfunction correlated with the total dose of cyclophosphamide, occurring in more than 80% of postpubertal patients who received more than 300 mg/kg.

Treatment of Hematological Malignancy

The effect of chemotherapy used in the treatment of lymphomas, especially Hodgkin's disease, on testicular function has been widely reported. Several studies have reported azoospermia with raised FSH levels in more than 90% of men after cyclical chemotherapy with MVPP (mustine, vinblastine, procarbazine, and prednisolone) (16,17).

In an attempt to reduce the gonadotoxic effect of MVPP by halving the alkylating drug and reducing the procarbazine dose, a hybrid combination of chlorambucil, vinblastine, prednisolone, procarbazine, doxorubicin, vincristine, and etoposide (ChlVPP/EVA) has been used. However, in a direct comparison with MVPP, hybrid chemotherapy had the same effect on gonadal function (18). However, an alternative regimen, consisting of ABVD (adriamycin, bleomycin, vinblastine, and dacarbazine) is less gonadotoxic. Viviani et al. (19) studied a total of 53 men treated with combination chemotherapy for Hodgkin's disease. Of the 29 men treated with MOPP (similar to MVPP but with vinblastine replaced by vincristine), 28 were azoospermic, at a median time of 6 mo after the completion of therapy. Of these men, 21 were retested 18 to 58 mo after the initial analysis and only in 3 was there any recovery of spermatogenesis. However, the impact of ABVD was considerably less, with a normal sperm count in 11 of 24 patients and oligospermia in a further 5. Furthermore, full recovery of spermatogenesis occurred within 18 mo of the first evaluation in all 13 men in whom the sperm count was repeated.

Other chemotherapy regimens used for the treatment of lymphomas have also been investigated. The effect on adult testicular function has been assessed in patients treated for Hodgkin's disease with ChlVPP (chlorambucil, vinblastine, procarbazine, and prednisolone) during childhood. Testicular dysfunction, as indicated by raised gonadotropin levels, was found in a significant proportion of a cohort of 46 male patients treated with ChlVPP reported by Mackie et al. (20), with 89% and 24% having raised FSH and LH levels, respectively. The use of COPP (cyclophosphamide, vincristine, procarbazine, and prednisolone), which includes the gonadotoxic agent cyclophosphamide in addition to procarbazine, is associated with even more marked gonadal dysfunction. Charak et al. (21) found azoospermia in all 92 patients after treatment with six or more COPP cycles, along with significant rises in gonadotropin levels compared with pretreatment values. Median follow-up in this study was 6 yr, with 17% of patients treated more than 10 yr previously, suggesting that germinal epithelial failure is likely to be permanent.

In addition to effects on the germinal epithelium, there is also some evidence for Leydig cell dysfunction after chemotherapy for lymphomas. Howell et al. (22) measured testosterone and LH levels in 135 men treated with either MVPP or ChlVPP/EVA hybrid. They demonstrated significantly higher LH levels in patients compared with a cohort of age-matched controls (mean LH 7.8 vs 4.1 IU/L). They suggested that this raised LH level indicated a reduction in hypothalamic–pituitary negative feedback consequent to a small reduction in testosterone production. This may still result in testosterone levels that fall in the cross-sectional normal range, and they thus defined mild Leydig cell dysfunction as a raised LH level in the presence of a testosterone level that is in the lower half of the normal range or is frankly subnormal. This combination was found in 44 men (31%) after chemotherapy with a further 10 (7%) having a raised LH level alone. This suggests that a significant proportion of men treated with cytotoxic chemotherapy have biochemical abnormalities, suggesting mild testosterone deficiency.

Chemotherapy regimens used for the treatment of non-Hodgkin's lymphoma (NHL) are generally less gonadotoxic than are those used for Hodgkin's disease. Pryzant et al. *(1)* reported on 71 patients treated with CHOP (cyclophosphamide, doxorubicin, vincristine, and prednisolone)-based chemotherapy. All men were rendered azoospermic during treatment, but by 5 yr after treatment, 67% had recovered to normospermic levels, with a further 5% to oligospermia. The reduced prevalence of permanent azoospermia in men treated for NHL compared with patients with Hodgkin's disease is probably related to the absence of procarbazine in the standard regimens used for NHL *(23)*, although the reduction in the dose of alkylating agents may also be important. The absence of procarbazine and alkylating drugs is also the likely explanation for the reduced toxicity of ABVD reported by Viviani et al. *(19)*. Other regimens not containing procarbazine, which have been used for NHL, are also less gonadotoxic. VAPEC-B (vincristine, doxorubicin, prednisolone, etoposide, cyclophosphamide, and bleomycin) *(24)*, VACOP-B (vinblastine, doxorubicin, prednisolone, vincristine, cyclophosphamide, and bleomycin) *(25)*, MACOP-B (mustine in place of vinblastine) *(25)*, and VEEP (vincristine, etoposide, epirubicin, and prednisolone) *(26)* have all been associated with normal posttreatment fertility in the majority of men.

Testicular function after high-dose chemotherapy used as preparation for bone marrow transplantation has also been studied. Sanders et al. *(27)* reported on 155 men treated with cyclophosphamide (200 mg/kg) or busulphan and cyclophosphamide (busulphan 16 mg/kg, cyclophosphamide 200 mg/kg). After an average of 2 to 3 yr after the transplant, 67 of the 109 patients who received cyclophosphamide (61%) but only 8 of the 46 (17%) patients treated with busulphan and cyclophosphamide had recovery of testicular function defined by normal LH, FSH, and testosterone levels with evidence of sperm production. The only prospective study to examine testicular function after high-dose treatment reported data in 13 men who received either BEAM (BCNU, etoposide, Ara-C, and melphalan) ($n = 11$) or melphalan and single fraction TBI ($n = 2$) *(28)*. All had previously received multiagent chemotherapy, and four had abnormal semen parameters before transplantation. All patients were azoospermic 2–3 mo posttransplantation, associated with raised FSH levels. LH levels increased and testosterone levels decreased after transplantation, indicating Leydig cell, apparent as well as germ cell failure.

These findings were also confirmed by Howell et al. *(22)* who studied 68 patients treated with high-dose chemotherapy (either cyclophosphamide, BCNU and etoposide, busulphan and cyclophosphamide or BCNU, etoposide, doxorubicin, and melphalan) as conditioning for bone marrow transplantation. They demonstrated a raised FSH in 60 patients (88%) and a raised LH level in 47 men (69%), 22 of whom (32%) also had a testosterone level in the lower half of the normal range, or frankly, subnormal.

Testicular Cancer

The other group of patients in whom the effects of chemotherapy on testicular function have been widely investigated is those with testicular cancer *(29–32)*. To attempt to delineate which abnormalities are a result of cytotoxic chemotherapy, several of these studies also examined pretreatment testicular function or compared chemotherapy-treated patients with those who underwent orchidectomy alone. Lampe et al. *(31)* analyzed data concerning 170 patients with testicular germ cell cancers, who underwent treatment with either cisplatin-based or carboplatin-based chemotherapy. Of the 170 patients, 40 (24%) were azoospermic before treatment, with a further 41 (24%) oligospermic. At a median of 30 mo after the completion of chemotherapy, only 64% of those who were normospermic before therapy remained normospermic, whereas 54 (32%) of the total cohort were azoospermic and 43 (25%) were oligospermic. The probability of recovery to a normal sperm count was higher for those men with a normal pretreatment sperm count, those who received carboplatin-based rather than cisplatin-based therapy, and in those treated with fewer than five chemotherapy cycles. Recovery continued for more than 2 yr, with the calculated chance of oligospermia or normospermia at 2 yr being 48% and 80% at 5 yr. Several authors have compared testicular function in patients after chemotherapy with that of patients treated with orchidectomy alone *(29,30,32)*. All have demonstrated greater testicular dysfunction in the cytotoxic-treated groups, with evidence of germinal epithelial damage indicated by raised FSH levels and/or reduced sperm counts. In addition, mild Leydig cell dysfunction, as indicated by a raised LH levels in the presence of a normal testosterone level, was found in 59 to 75% of men after chemotherapy, compared with 6 to 45% in those after orchidectomy alone.

Other Malignancies

Similar results have been demonstrated in men treated with cisplatin-based chemotherapy for osteosarcoma *(2,33)* and lung cancer *(34)*. However, the majority of patients treated with cytotoxic chemotherapy for leukemia do not have persistent gonadal dysfunction. Wallace et al. *(35)* found long-term germinal epithelial dysfunction in only 6 out of 36 (17%) patients treated during childhood for acute lymphocytic leukemia, although the follow-up period in this study was considerable, and the majority of patients had evidence of germinal epithelial damage on testicular biopsy immediately after chemotherapy (which included cyclophosphamide and cytosine arabinoside), a median time of 10.7 yr earlier.

RADIOTHERAPY

The testis is one of the most radiosensitive tissues, with low doses of radiation causing significant impairment of function. Damage may be caused during direct irradiation of the testis or, more commonly, from scattered radiation during treatment directed at adjacent tissues.

Spermatogenesis After Single-Dose Irradiation

The effects of relatively low-dose single fraction irradiation on spermatogenesis in healthy fertile men have been well documented *(6)* and are illustrated in Fig. 1. The more immature cells are more radiosensitive, with doses as low as 0.1 Gy causing morphological and quantitative changes to spermatogonia. Doses of 2 to 3 Gy result in overt damage to spermatocytes, leading to a reduction in spermatid numbers. At doses of 4 to 6 Gy, numbers of spermatazoa are significantly decreased, implying spermatid damage. The decline in sperm count after damage to more immature cells, with doses of up to 3 Gy, takes 60 to 70 d, with doses more than 0.8 Gy resulting in azoospermia and doses less than 0.8 Gy giving rise to oligospermia. A much faster fall in sperm concentration occurs after doses of 4 Gy and higher because of damage to spermatids.

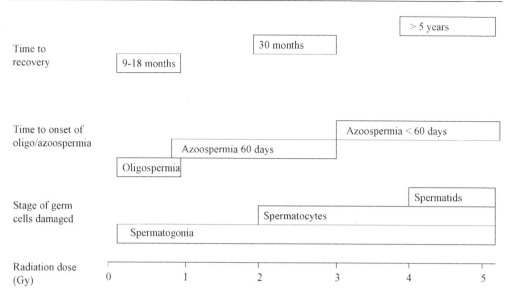

Fig. 1. Impairment of spermatogenesis after single-dose irradiation: the effect of radiation dose on stage of germ cell damage and time to onset and recovery from germ cell damage. (Adapted from ref. *6.*)

Spermatogenesis recovery occurs from surviving stem cells (type A spermatogonia) and is dependent on the radiation dose. Complete recovery, as indicated by a return to pre-irradiation sperm concentrations and germinal cell numbers, occurs within 9 to 18 mo after 1 Gy or less, 30 mo for 2 to 3 Gy, and 5 yr or more for doses of 4 Gy and above.

Spermatogenesis After Scattered Irradiation

Animal data suggest that fractionation of radiotherapy increases its gonadal toxicity, and the evidence suggests that this is also the case in humans. Speiser et al. *(36)* studied 10 patients who received a testicular dose of radiation of 1.2 to 3 Gy in 14 to 26 fractions during inverted Y-inguinal field irradiation for Hodgkin's disease. All patients were azoospermic after treatment, and recovery was not seen in a single patient, despite follow-up of more than 15 mo in 4 patients and up to 40 mo in 1 patient. An update of these data published in 1994 *(37)* revealed no recovery of spermatogenesis in patients receiving doses of 1.4 to 2.6 Gy after 17 to 43 mo follow-up, but a return of fertility in the 2 patients with testicular radiation doses of 1.2 Gy, suggesting that this may represent a threshold for permanent testicular damage. Hahn et al. *(38)* carried out serial semen analysis on 11 patients with cancer who had received large pelvic field irradiation or interstitial ^{125}I seeds implanted into the prostate gland. The dose of radiation to the testis was 1.18 to 2.28 Gy delivered in 24 to 34 fractions. All patients became azoospermic, and recovery to oligospermia (three men) or normospermia (two men) was only seen in five patients. The other six remained azoospermic during a follow-up period of 35 to 107 wk.

However, lower doses of radiation to the testes are associated with better recovery rates for spermatogenesis. Centola et al. *(37)* reported a return of spermatogenesis in all 8 patients who received radiation doses of 0.28 to 0.9 Gy for testicular seminoma, with 4 out of 5 reviewed at 12 mo having normal sperm counts. Kinsella et al. *(39)* published data concerning 17 patients who had received low-dose scattered irradiation during treatment for Hodgkin's disease. Testicular doses of less than 0.2 Gy had no significant effect on FSH levels or sperm counts, whereas doses between 0.2 Gy and 0.7 Gy caused a transient dose-dependent increase in FSH and reduction in sperm concentration, with a return to normal values within 12 to 24 mo.

Leydig Cell Function

Leydig cells are more resistant to damage from radiotherapy than is the germinal epithelium. Significant rises in LH have been demonstrated after single dose radiation doses of above 0.75 Gy *(6)* and fractionated doses above 2 Gy *(40)*. However, no change in testosterone level was seen at these doses, and LH values gradually return to normal levels during 30 mo. Higher testicular radiation doses do, however, result in more marked Leydig cell insufficiency. Giwercman et al. *(41)* studied 20 men who were previously treated with unilateral orchidectomy for testicular cancer, who received direct testicular irradiation at a dose of 20 Gy, in 10 fractions, for carcinoma *in situ* in the remaining testis. A significant increase in mean LH levels was observed in the first 3 mo (10.4 to 15.6 IU/L), with a decrease in mean serum testosterone level (13.3 to 10.8 nmol/L). Similar results were observed by Shalet et al. *(7)* in adults treated with high-dose (30 Gy) testicular irradiation after unilateral orchidectomy. Serum testosterone levels were significantly reduced (12.5 vs 16.0 nmol/L), and LH levels significantly increased (16 vs 6 IU/L), compared with a control group who had undergone unilateral orchidectomy without subsequent radiotherapy. In addition, more marked abnormalities were observed in a group of five adult men treated with the same testicular dose of irradiation during childhood. Median LH level was greater than 32 IU/L, and median testosterone level was less than 2.5 nmol/L, and there was no response to a human chorionic gonadotrophin (hCG) stimulation test, suggesting that the prepubertal testis is much more vulnerable to radiation-induced Leydig cell damage.

The Clinical Effect of Leydig Cell Dysfunction

A significant proportion of men have evidence of impairment of Leydig cell function after high-dose chemotherapy, procarbazine-containing chemotherapy, or radiation involving the testis. The biochemical abnormalities are usually mild and consist of a raised LH level associated with a low/normal testosterone level. A deleterious effect of overt testosterone deficiency and a clear benefit of androgen replacement in such patients on bone density, body composition, and quality of life, has been well demonstrated. However, there are few data concerning the effect of milder forms of testosterone deficiency.

Howell et al. *(22)* investigated a cohort of men treated with MVPP, ChlVPP/EVA hybrid, or high-dose chemotherapy for several malignancies. They identified a cohort of 35 men with biochemical evidence of mild Leydig cell insufficiency, as defined by a raised LH level and a testosterone level in the lower half of the normal range or, frankly, subnormal. They demonstrated significantly reduced bone mineral density at the hip in these men compared with a similarly treated cohort with normal hormone levels and found some evidence of altered body composition, reduced sexual activity, and mood alterations *(42,43)*. The men were then enrolled into a 12-mo randomized, single-blind placebo-controlled testosterone replacement trial *(44)*. However, during the 12-mo study period, there were no significant improvements in bone density, body composition, sexual function, energy levels, or mood in the testosterone-treated group compared with the controls.

Thus, it seems likely that the mild biochemical abnormalities (raised LH and low/normal testosterone) observed in many men after cytotoxic chemotherapy are of limited clinical importance in the majority of patients and that androgen replacement cannot be routinely recommended for such patients. However, it remains possible that a minority of men with more marked biochemical abnormalities may benefit from androgen therapy.

GENETIC DAMAGE FOLLOWING CYTOTOXIC THERAPY

In addition to impairment of steroidogenesis and sperm production, there has been concern that cytotoxic chemotherapy may also result in transmissible genetic damage. Animal studies have demonstrated untoward effects in offspring of animals treated with cytotoxic agents, but no clear evidence for this has been reported in humans. Increased aneuploid frequency has been observed in human sperm after chemotherapy for Hodgkin's disease *(45,46),* and an increase in chromosomal abnormalities has been demonstrated several years after treatment for testicular cancer *(47).* However, data concerning the outcome of pregnancies have not shown any increase in genetically mediated birth defects, altered sex ratios, or birthweight effects in offspring of cancer survivors *(48),* possibly as a result of selection bias against genetically abnormal sperm. On the evidence thus far, it is reasonable to conclude that patients treated with cytotoxic chemotherapy who remain fertile are not at increased risk of fathering children with genetic abnormalities.

PROTECTION OF TESTICULAR FUNCTION DURING CANCER TREATMENT

The deleterious effect of chemotherapy and radiotherapy on germinal epithelial function has initiated a search for possible strategies to preserve fertility in men who are undergoing therapy.

Semen Cryopreservation and Assisted Reproduction

Cryostorage of semen has become standard practice and should be offered to all men before undergoing potentially sterilizing therapy. Improvements in the techniques used to store semen *(49)* and advances in the field of assisted reproduction, such as intracytoplasmic sperm injection (ICSI), have increased the chance of successful pregnancies using cryopreserved sperm. However, there are some limitations to this method of preserving fertility. First, it is not a feasible option for prepubertal patients. Furthermore, testicular function in adult men with malignant disease is often impaired before treatment *(9)* resulting in poor sperm quality or difficulty providing semen for storage. Oligospermia is found in a third to a half of patients with Hodgkin's disease, NHL, and testicular cancer before treatment and also occurs in men with leukemia and soft-tissue cancer *(7a).* Sperm motility is also impaired in these patients, and the process of freezing and thawing semen further reduces the sperm quality. Although successful fertilization may be achieved with only a few viable sperm using ICSI, pregnancy rates using this method are lower with abnormal semen than with normal semen *(50).* As a result, methods for protecting, or enhancing the recovery of normal spermatogenesis after gonadotoxic therapy have been pursued.

Hormonal Manipulation

The belief that prepubertal boys have a lower rate of permanent chemotherapy-induced gonadal damage *(5)* has led many investigators to propose that suppression of testicular function in adult men (i.e., inducing a prepubertal state) will provide a degree of protection against cytotoxic therapy. Irrespective of the validity of the hypothesis, data derived from animal models have been encouraging, but there is presently no convincing evidence of similar success in humans. Ward et al. *(51)* demonstrated enhanced spermatogenesis recovery in procarbazine-treated rats by the administration of the gonadotropin-releasing hormone (GnRH) analog Zoladex for 2 wk before chemotherapy and during chemotherapy. Increased stem cell survival was evident by 50 d, and, at 90 d, sperm count was close to normal values and significantly higher than procarbazine-only treated rats. Similar protective effects have been described with the use of testosterone *(52)*, testosterone and estradiol *(53)*, GnRH and testosterone *(54)*, and GnRH and the antiandrogen flutamide *(55,56)* after testicular insult with procarbazine, cyclophosphamide, or radiotherapy. Pogach et al. *(54)* suggested that testosterone administered after treatment with procarbazine enhanced spermatogenesis recovery. More recently, Meistrich et al. *(57)* confirmed that treatment with either testosterone or Zoladex after irradiation with 3.5 Gy markedly improved the recovery of spermatogenesis, even if treatment was delayed for 10 wk after irradiation. The same group had previously shown that spermatogenesis did not occur after a similar dose of irradiation. Despite the presence of A spermatogonia in the seminiferous tubules *(58)*, they postulated that the role of hormonal treatments in the "protection" of germinal epithelial function, possibly to enhance recovery of surviving A spermatogonia and to facilitate their differentiation to more mature cells, rather than to protect them from damage during cytotoxic therapy or radiotherapy. They suggested that a reduction of the level of intratesticular testosterone or one of its metabolites is the mechanism by which hormone therapy stimulates spermatogenesis recovery.

In humans, attempts to reproduce the protective effects seen in animals have been unsuccessful. Several groups have used GnRH analogs, with and without testosterone replacement, to suppress testicular function during MOPP *(59)* or MVPP *(60)* chemotherapy for lymphoma, cisplatin-based chemotherapy for teratoma *(61)*, and testicular irradiation for seminoma *(62)*. None has demonstrated any significant protective effect of these therapies in spermatogenesis maintenance or increasing the rate of recovery. However, none of the studies involved the continuation of gonadal-suppressive therapy for a significant period of time after the completion of chemotherapy or radiotherapy. The most recent animal data suggest that hormonal treatment may enhance recovery of spermatogenesis from surviving stem cells rather than protect them from damage during cytotoxic or radiation insult. Thus, suppression of gonadal function with a GnRH agonist or testosterone for a fixed time after the completion of irradiation or chemotherapy may prove more successful in reducing the effect of these treatments on fertility.

This approach relies on enhancing recovery of sperm production, and, therefore, a prerequisite for its success is the survival of stem cells during the gonadotoxic insult. However, there are few data regarding testicular histology after chemotherapy or radiotherapy. After cisplatin-based chemotherapy and low-dose radiation, spontaneous spermatogenesis recovery occurs in most patients, although there is often a latent period of azoospermia, which may last several years. However, the eventual spermatogenesis recovery implies the survival of A spermatogonia. After chemotherapy for Hodgkin's disease with procarbazine-containing regimens, and high-dose radiotherapy, recovery to oligospermia or normospermia is much less common. Testicular biopsies taken after standard chemotherapy (MVPP and COPP) for Hodgkin's disease have shown complete germinal aplasia with a Sertoli cell-only pattern *(9,16,21,63–64)*, and this is also the case in men treated with 20-Gy radiotherapy *(41)*. There have been some recent reports of the isolation of mature sperm in the testicular parenchyma of some men with biopsy evidence of Sertoli cell only, suggesting that even in this situation, there may be small foci of spermatogenesis *(65)*. In addition, spermatogenesis recovery occurs in a minority of these patients, indicating that some germ cells survive in some patients. However, the absence of histological evidence of any spermatogenesis at biopsy in many men suggests that all spermatogonia may be eradicated during chemotherapy.

Hormonal manipulation after treatment to enhance the recovery of spermatogenesis is, therefore, likely to be of most benefit in those patients in whom the testicular insult is less severe, because it is these patients in whom there is significant preservation of A spermatogonia. The success of this approach in those patients who have undergone more intense gonadotoxic therapy will depend on whether any stem cells remain. Complete ablation of the germinal epithelium may occur in many men after treatment with procarbazine-based chemotherapy regimens for Hodgkin's disease, and this will clearly be irreversible.

Stem Cell Cryopreservation

Results from recent animal experiments have also indicated another possible method of preserving testicular function during gonadotoxic therapy. In 1994, Brinster et al. *(66)* demonstrated that stem cells isolated from a donor mouse could be injected into the seminiferous tubules of a sterile recipient mouse and reinitiate spermatogenesis. More recently, the same group demonstrated that spermatogenesis can be achieved in previously sterile mice after cryopreservation and subsequent then injection of donor stem cells into the testis. Potentially, therefore, stem cells could be harvested from the human testis before the start of sterilizing therapy, freeze-stored, and reimplanted at a later date, with a subsequent spermatogenesis return.

A clinical trial testing this hypothesis is currently underway in adults: 16 men have had testicular tissue harvested shortly before commencing treatment with sterilizing chemotherapy for Hodgkin's disease or NHL. In each case, a 0.5-cm cube of testicular tissue has been subjected to enzymatic digestion to produce a single cell suspension that, after equilibration in cryoprotectant, has been stored in liquid nitrogen *(67)*. Seven men have now successfully completed chemotherapy, and thawed testicular suspension has been reinjected into the donor testis. Semen analysis has demonstrated a spermatogenesis return in one man at the time of writing. However, this may simply represent spontaneous spermatogenesis recovery, as is seen in a small proportion of men after treatment, rather than repopulation from cryopreserved stem cells. The lack of greater success may relate to problems reinjecting the testicular suspension. The seminiferous tubules in adult men are too fibrous to allow direct injection, and, therefore, an indirect approach had to be used. This consisted of injecting into the rete testes and relying on retrograde flow to fill the tubules; this may not occur to a sufficient extent to allow repopulation and a return of spermatogenesis. Further studies are currently being undertaken using nondisaggregated testicular tissue, and the results are awaited with interest.

Table 2
Summary of Fertility in Adult Men After Treatment of Different Malignancies

Diagnosis	Treatment	Fertility After Treatment
Hodgkin's disease	MVPP	Azoospermia in >90%
	MOPP	Azoospermia in >90%
	ChlVPP/EVA hybrid	Azoospermia in >90%
	COPP	Azoospermia in >90%
	ABVD	Temporary azoospermia with normal sperm count in all at 18 mo
Non-Hodgkin's lymphoma	CHOP	Permanent azoospermia in approx 30%
	VAPEC-B	Normospermia in >95%
	VACOP-B	Normospermia in >95%
	MACOP-B	Normospermia in >95%
	VEEP	Normospermia in >95%
Bone marrow transplant for several malignancies	Cyclophosphamide alone	FSH raised in 40%
	Busulphan and cyclophosphamide	FSH raised in 80%
	CBV	FSH raised in >95%
	High-dose melphalan BEAM	FSH raised in >95%
Testicular cancer	Cisplatin-carboplatin-based therapy	Normospermia in 50% at 2 yr, and 80% at 5 yr

MVPP, mustine, vinblastine, procarbazine, and prednisolone; MOPP, mustine, vincristine, procarbazine, and prednisolone; ChlVPP/EVA, chlorambucil, vinblastine, prednisolone, procarbazine, doxorubicin, vincristine, and etoposide; COPP, cyclophosphamide, vincristine, procarbazine, and prednisolone; ABVD, adriamycin, bleomycin, vinblastine, and dacarbazine; CHOP, cyclophosphamide, doxorubicin, vincristine, and prednisolone; VAPEC-B, vincristine, doxorubicin, prednisolone, etoposide, cyclophosphamide, and bleomycin; VACOP-B, vinblastine, doxorubicin, prednisolone, vincristine, cyclophosphamide, and bleomycin; MACOP-B, mustine in place of vinblastine; VEEP, vincristine, etoposide, epirubicin, and prednisolone; CBV, cyclophosphamide; BCNU, and etoposide; BEAM, BCNU, etoposide, Ara-C, and melphalan.

SUMMARY

Treatment with cytotoxic chemotherapy and radiotherapy is associated with significant gonadal damage in men. Alkylating agents, such as cyclophosphamide and procarbazine, are the most common agents implicated. The majority of men receiving procarbazine-containing regimens for the treatment of lymphomas are rendered permanently infertile. Treatment with ABVD has a significant advantage in terms of testicular function, with a return to normal fertility in the majority of patients. Cisplatin-based chemotherapy for testicular cancer results in temporary azoospermia in most men, with spermatogenesis recovery in approx 50% after 2 yr and 80% after 5 yr. There is also evidence of chemotherapy-induced Leydig cell impairment in a proportion of these men, although this is of no clinical significance in the majority of patients. The germinal epithelium is sensitive to radiation-induced damage, with changes to spermatogonia after as little as 0.1 Gy and permanent infertility after fractionated doses of 2 Gy and higher, whereas clinically significant Leydig cell impairment occurs rarely with doses of less than 20 Gy. These effects are summarized in Table 2.

All men should be counseled regarding the possible effects of treatment on testicular function, and sperm banking should be offered to all patients who are undergoing potentially sterilizing therapy. Hormonal manipulation to enhance spermatogenesis recovery and cryopreservation of testicular tissue are possible future methods of preserving fertility but are currently unproven. Regular semen analyses should be offered to men after cytotoxic treatment to allow appropriate family planning. Measurement of testosterone and LH are appropriate for men with symptoms consistent with testosterone deficiency who have received significant doses of irradiation to the testes, procarbazine-containing chemotherapy, or high-dose chemotherapy. Mild LH elevations, accompanied by testosterone levels in the normal range (the most common abnormality), do not require treatment, but patients with subnormal testosterone levels and markedly elevated LH levels may benefit from androgen replacement.

REFERENCES

1. Pryzant RM, Meistrich ML, Wilson G, Brown B, McLaughlin P. Long-term reduction in sperm count after chemotherapy with and without radiation therapy for non-Hodgkin's lymphomas [published erratum appears in J Clin Oncol 1993 May;11:1007]. J Clin Oncol 1993;11:239–247.
2. Meistrich ML, Chawla SP, Da Cunha MF, et al. Recovery of sperm production after chemotherapy for osteosarcoma. Cancer 1989;63:2115–2123.
3. da Cunha MF, Meistrich ML, Fuller LM, et al. Recovery of spermatogenesis after treatment for Hodgkin's disease: limiting dose of MOPP chemotherapy. J Clin Oncol 1984;2:571–577.
4. Watson AR, Rance CP, Bain J. Long term effects of cyclophosphamide on testicular function. Br Med J Clin Res Ed 1985;291:1457–460.
5. Rivkees SA, Crawford JD. The relationship of gonadal activity and chemotherapy-induced gonadal damage. JAMA 1988;259:2123–2125.
6. Rowley MJ, Leach DR, Warner GA, Heller CG. Effect of graded doses of ionizing radiation on the human testis. Radiat Res 1974;59:665–678.
7. Shalet SM, Tsatsoulis A, Whitehead E, Read G. Vulnerability of the human Leydig cell to radiation damage is dependent upon age. J Endocrinol 1989;120:161–165.
7a. Padron OF, Sharma RK, Thomas AJ, Jr., Agarwal A. Effects of cancer on spermatozoa quality after cryopreservation: a 12-yr experience. Fertil Steril 1997;67:326–331.
8. Vigersky R, Chapman R, Berenberg J, Glass A. Testicular dysfunction in untreated Hodgkin's disease. Am J Med 1982;73:482–486.
9. Chapman RM, Sutcliffe SB, Malpas JS. Male gonadal dysfunction in Hodgkin's disease. A prospective study. JAMA 1981;245:1323–1328.
10. Viviani S, Ragni G, Santoro A, et al. Testicular dysfunction in Hodgkin's disease before and after treatment. Eur J Cancer 1991;27:1389–1392.
11. Hendry W, Stedronska J, Jones C, CA B, Barrett A, Peckham M. Semen analysis in testicular cancer and Hodgkin's disease: pre- and post-treatment findings and implications for cryopreservation. Br J Urol 1983;55:769–773.
12. Shekarriz M, Tolentino MV, Jr., Ayzman I, Lee JC, Thomas AJ, Jr., Agarwal A. Cryopreservation and semen quality in patients with Hodgkin's disease. Cancer 1995;75:2732–2736.
13. Barr RD, Clarke DA, Booth JD. Dyspermia in men with localised Hodgkin's disease. A potentially reversible, immune-mediated disorder. Med Hypoth 1993;40:165–168.
14. Meirow D, Schenker JG. Cancer and male fertility. Hum Reprod 1995;10:2017–2022.
15. Guazzieri S, Lembo A, Ferro G, et al. Sperm antibodies and infertility in patients with testicular cancer. Urology 1985;26:139–142.
16. Chapman RM, Sutcliffe SB, Rees LH, Edwards CR, Malpas JS. Cyclical combination chemotherapy and gonadal function. Retrospective study in males. Lancet 1979;1:285–289.
17. Whitehead E, Shalet SM, Blackledge G, Todd I, Crowther D, Beardwell CG. The effects of Hodgkin's disease and combination chemotherapy on gonadal function in the adult male. Cancer 1982;49:418–422.

18. Clark ST, Radford JA, Crowther D, Swindell R, Shalet SM. Gonadal function following chemotherapy for Hodgkin's disease: a comparative study of MVPP and a seven-drug hybrid regimen. J Clin Oncol 1995;13:134–139.
19. Viviani S, Santoro A, Ragni G, Bonfante V, Bestetti O, Bonadonna G. Gonadal toxicity after combination chemotherapy for Hodgkin's disease. Comparative results of MOPP vs ABVD. Eur J Cancer Clin Oncol 1985;21:601–605.
20. Mackie EJ, Radford M, Shalet SM. Gonadal function following chemotherapy for childhood Hodgkin's disease. Med Pediatr Oncol 1996;27:74–78.
21. Charak BS, Gupta R, Mandrekar P, et al. Testicular dysfunction after cyclophosphamide-vincristine-procarbazine-prednisolone chemotherapy for advanced Hodgkin's disease. A long-term follow-up study. Cancer 1990;65:1903–1906.
22. Howell SJ, Radford JA, Shalet SM. Testicular function following cytotoxic chemotherapy—evidence of Leydig cell insufficiency. J Clin Oncol 1999;17:1493–1498.
23. Bokemeyer C, Schmoll HJ, van Rhee J, Kuczyk M, Schuppert F, Poliwoda H. Long-term gonadal toxicity after therapy for Hodgkin's and non-Hodgkin's lymphoma. Ann Hematol 1994;68:105–110.
24. Radford JA, Clark S, Crowther D, Shalet SM. Male fertility after VAPEC-B chemotherapy for Hodgkin's disease and non-Hodgkin's lymphoma. Br J Cancer 1994;69:379–381.
25. Muller U, Stahel RA. Gonadal function after MACOP-B or VACOP-B with or without dose intensification and ABMT in young patients with aggressive non-Hodgkin's lymphoma. Ann Oncol 1993;4:399–402.
26. Hill M, Milan S, Cunningham D, et al. Evaluation of the efficacy of the VEEP regimen in adult Hodgkin's disease with assessment of gonadal and cardiac toxicity [see comments]. J Clin Oncol 1995;13:387–395.
27. Sanders JE, Hawley J, Levy W, et al. Pregnancies after high-dose cyclophosphamide with or without high-dose busulfan or total-body irradiation and bone marrow transplantation. Blood 1996;87:3045–3052.
28. Chatterjee R, Mills W, Katz M, McGarrigle HH, Goldstone AH. Germ cell failure and Leydig cell insufficiency in post-pubertal males after autologous bone marrow transplantation with BEAM for lymphoma. Bone Marrow Transplant 1994;3:519–522.
29. Hansen SW, Berthelsen JG, von der Maase H. Long-term fertility and Leydig cell function in patients treated for germ cell cancer with cisplatin, vinblastine, and bleomycin versus surveillance. J Clin Oncol 1990;8:1695–1698.
30. Stuart NS, Woodroffe CM, Grundy R, Cullen MH. Long-term toxicity of chemotherapy for testicular cancer—the cost of cure. Br J Cancer 1990;61:479–484.
31. Lampe H, Horwich A, Norman A, Nicholls J, Dearnaley DP. Fertility after chemotherapy for testicular germ cell cancers. J Clin Oncol 1997;15:239–245.
32. Palmieri G, Lotrecchiano G, Ricci G, et al. Gonadal function after multimodality treatment in men with testicular germ cell cancer. Eur J Endocrinol 1996;134:431–436.
33. Siimes MA, Elomaa I, Koskimies A. Testicular function after chemotherapy for osteosarcoma. Eur J Cancer 1990;26:973–975.
34. Aasebo U, Slordal L, Aanderud S, Aakvaag A. Chemotherapy and endocrine function in lung cancer. Acta Oncol 1989;28:667–669.
35. Wallace WH, Shalet SM, Lendon M, Morris Jones PH. Male fertility in long-term survivors of childhood acute lymphoblastic leukaemia. Int J Androl 1991;14:312–319.
36. Speiser B, Rubin P, Casarett G. Aspermia following lower truncal irradiation in Hodgkin's disease. Cancer 1973;32:692–698.
37. Centola GM, Keller JW, Henzler M, Rubin P. Effect of low-dose testicular irradiation on sperm count and fertility in patients with testicular seminoma. J Androl 1994;15:608–613.
38. Hahn EW, Feingold SM, Nisce L. Aspermia and recovery of spermatogenesis in cancer patients following incidental gonadal irradiation during treatment: a progress report. Radiology 1976;119:223–225.
39. Kinsella TJ, Trivette G, Rowland J, et al. Long-term follow-up of testicular function following radiation therapy for early-stage Hodgkin's disease. J Clin Oncol 1989;7:718–724.
40. Shapiro E, Kinsella TJ, Makuch RW, et al. Effects of fractionated irradiation of endocrine aspects of testicular function. J Clin Oncol 1985;3:1232–1239.
41. Giwercman A, von der Maase H, Berthelsen JG, Rorth M, Bertelsen A, Skakkebaek NE. Localized irradiation of testes with carcinoma in situ: effects on Leydig cell function and eradication of malignant germ cells in 20 patients. J Clin Endocrinol Metab 1991;73:596–603.

42. Howell SJ, Radford JA, Adams JE, Shalet SM. The impact of mild Leydig cell dysfunction following cytotoxic chemotherapy on bone mineral density (BMD) and body composition. Clin Endocrinol (Oxf) 2000;52:609–616.

43. Howell SJ, Radford JA, Smets EMA, Shalet SM. Fatigue, sexual function and mood following treatment for haematological malignancy—the impact of mild Leydig cell dysfunction. Br J Cancer 2000;82:789–793.

44. Howell SJ, Radford JA, Adams JE, Smets EMA, Warburton R, Shalet SM. Randomised placebo controlled trial of testosterone replacement in men with mild Leydig cell insufficiency following cytotoxic chemotherapy. Clin Endocrinol 2001;55:315–324.

45. Monteil M, Rousseaux S, Chevret E, Pelletier R, Cozzi J, Sele B. Increased aneuploid frequency in spermatozoa from a Hodgkin's disease patient after chemotherapy and radiotherapy. Cytogenet Cell Genet 1997;76:134–138.

46. Robbins WA, Meistrich ML, Moore D, et al. Chemotherapy induces transient sex chromosomal and autosomal aneuploidy in human sperm. Nat Genet 1997;16:74–78.

47. Genesca A, Benet J, Caballin MR, Miro R, Germa JR, Egozcue J. Significance of structural chromosome aberrations in human sperm: analysis of induced aberrations. Hum Genet 1990;85:495–499.

48. Robbins WA. Cytogenetic damage measured in human sperm following cancer chemotherapy. Mutat Res 1996;355:235–252.

49. Royere D, Barthelemy C, Hamamah S, Lansac J. Cryopreservation of spermatozoa: a 1996 review. Hum Reprod Update 1996;2:553–559.

50. Aboulghar MA, Mansour RT, Serour GI, et al. Fertilization and pregnancy rates after intracytoplasmic sperm injection using ejaculate semen and surgically retrieved sperm. Fertil Steril 1997;68:108–111.

51. Ward JA, Robinson J, Furr BJ, Shalet SM, Morris ID. Protection of spermatogenesis in rats from the cytotoxic procarbazine by the depot formulation of Zoladex, a gonadotropin-releasing hormone agonist. Cancer Res 1990;50:568–574.

52. Delic JI, Bush C, Peckham MJ. Protection from procarbazine-induced damage of spermatogenesis in the rat by androgen. Cancer Res 1986;46:1909–14.

53. Kurdoglu B, Wilson G, Parchuri N, Ye WS, Meistrich ML. Protection from radiation-induced damage to spermatogenesis by hormone treatment. Radiat Res 1994;139:97–102.

54. Pogach LM, Lee Y, Gould S, Giglio W, Huang HF. Partial prevention of procarbazine induced germinal cell aplasia in rats by sequential GnRH antagonist and testosterone administration. Cancer Res 1988;48:4354–4360.

55. Meistrich ML, Parchuri N, Wilson G, Kurdoglu B, Kangasniemi M. Hormonal protection from cyclophosphamide-induced inactivation of rat stem spermatogonia. J Androl 1995;16:334–341.

56. Kangasniemi M, Wilson G, Huhtaniemi I, Meistrich ML. Protection against procarbazine-induced testicular damage by GnRH-agonist and antiandrogen treatment in the rat. Endocrinology 1995;136:3677–3680.

57. Meistrich ML, Kangasniemi M. Hormone treatment after irradiation stimulates recovery of rat spermatogenesis from surviving spermatogonia. J Androl 1997;18:80–87.

58. Kangasniemi M, Huhtaniemi I, Meistrich ML. Failure of spermatogenesis to recover despite the presence of a spermatogonia in the irradiated LBNF1 rat. Biol Reprod 1996;54:1200–1208.

59. Johnson DH, Linde R, Hainsworth JD, et al. Effect of a luteinizing hormone releasing hormone agonist given during combination chemotherapy on posttherapy fertility in male patients with lymphoma: preliminary observations. Blood 1985;65:832–836.

60. Waxman JH, Ahmed R, Smith D, et al. Failure to preserve fertility in patients with Hodgkin's disease. Cancer Chemother Pharmacol 1987;19:159–162.

61. Kreuser ED, Hetzel WD, Hautmann R, Pfeiffer EF. Reproductive toxicity with and without LHRHA administration during adjuvant chemotherapy in patients with germ cell tumors. Horm Metab Res 1990;22:494–498.

62. Brennemann W, Brensing KA, Leipner N, Boldt I, Klingmuller D. Attempted protection of spermatogenesis from irradiation in patients with seminoma by D-Tryptophan-6 luteinizing hormone releasing hormone. Clin Invest 1994;72:838–842.

63. Ortin TT, Shostak CA, Donaldson SS. Gonadal status and reproductive function following treatment for Hodgkin's disease in childhood: the Stanford experience [see comments]. Int J Radiat Oncol Biol Phys 1990;19:873–880.

64. Das PK, Das BK, Sahu DC, Mohanty GN, Rath RN. Male gonadal function in Hodgkin's disease before and after treatment. J Assoc Physicians India 1994;42:604–605.

65. Mulhall JP, Burgess CM, Cunningham D, Carson R, Harris D, Oates RD. Presence of mature sperm in testicular parenchyma of men with nonobstructive azoospermia: prevalence and predictive factors. Urology 1997;49:91–95.

66. Brinster RL, Zimmermann JW. Spermatogenesis following male germ-cell transplantation [see comments]. Proc Natl Acad Sci U S A 1994;91:11298–11302.

67. Brook P, Radford J, Shalet S, Joyce A, Gosden R. Isolation of germ cells from human testicular tissue for low temperature storage and autotransplantation. Fertil Steril 2001;75:269–274.

68. Clayton PE, Shalet SM, Price DA, Campbell RH. Testicular damage after chemotherapy for childhood brain tumors. J Pediatr 1988;112:922–926.

69. Vilar O. Effect of cytostatic drugs on human testicular function. In: Mancini RE, Martini L, eds. Male Fertility and Sterility. Academic, London, 1974, pp. 5, 423–440.

70. Wallace WH, Shalet SM, Crowne EC, Morris Jones PH, Gattamaneni HR, Price DA. Gonadal dysfunction due to cis-platinum. Med Pediatr Oncol 1989;17:409–413.

14 An Ensemble Perspective of Aging-Related Hypoandrogenemia in Men

Johannes D. Veldhuis, MD, Ali Iranmanesh, MD, and Daniel Keenan, PhD

CONTENTS

The aging process is marked by a relatively subtle short-term decline in reproductive hormone outflow in men. However, the nominal 0.8–1.3% annual fall in systemic bioavailability of testosterone results in a reduction of 30–50% by the sixth through eighth decades of life. Low testosterone concentrations forecast relative sarcopenia, osteopenia, visceral fat accumulation, detectable cognitive impairment, and variable mood depression. Accordingly, the mechanisms driving progressive androgen deprivation are important to understand. To this end, age-associated alterations in three dominant sites of physiological control, namely the hypothalamus, pituitary gland, and testis, are highlighted. The cognate signals are gonadotropin-releasing hormone (GnRH), luteinizing hormone (LH), and testosterone, which jointly determine androgen availability via feedback and feedforward adaptations. According to this emergent notion, no single gland acts in isolation to maintain homeostasis. An integrative concept is underscored by highlighting how aging-related testosterone depletion is an ensemble outcome of deterioration of interlinked control.

From: *Male Hypogonadism:*
Basic, Clinical, and Therapeutic Principles
Edited by: S. J. Winters © Humana Press Inc., Totowa, NJ

OVERVIEW

Androgen deficiency in men is associated with reduced physical stamina, relative sarcopenia, osteopenia, visceral obesity, sexual dysfunction, depressed mood, reduced sense of well-being, and detectable cognitive impairment *(1–10)*. Impoverished testosterone production in the older male has been affirmed by (1) direct sampling of the human spermatic vein, (2) meta-analysis of cross-sectional epidemiological data *(11)*, and (3) longitudinal investigations in healthy populations *(12–15)*. For example, the European SENIEUR and Massachusetts Male Aging Cohort studies inferred that bioavailable (non-sex hormone-binding globulin [SHBG]-bound) testosterone concentrations decline by 0.8–1.3% annually *(13,16)*, and, a 15-yr prospective analysis in New Mexico observed that total testosterone concentrations fall by 110 ng/dL per decade in men after age 60 *(14,17)*. Surgery, trauma, stress, systemic illness, medication use, and chronic institutionalization exacerbate androgen depletion in elderly individuals *(6,8,13,18–21)*. However, the fundamental mechanisms that mediate waning testosterone secretion in aging men are unknown. Indeed, a unified physiological concept has been difficult to develop in this arena.

Available data point to an array of contributing mechanisms underlying relative androgen depletion in the older male *(22–33)*. Primary (nonexclusive) considerations include reduced hypothalamic GnRH outflow, limited gonadotrope secretory capacity, impaired Leydig cell steroidogenesis, and anomalous androgen-directed feedback control *(34–37)*.

As a unifying approach, the male gonadal axis is viewed as an adaptive neuroendocrine ensemble. In this broader concept, testosterone availability is adjusted on a minute-by-minute basis by repeated decremental and incremental signaling interactions among GnRH, LH, and testosterone *(see* Fig. 1). Simplified biomathematical simulations based on this network-like perspective predict that hypoandrogenemia and altered LH secretion in aging could arise singly or jointly by way of (1) attenuated hypothalamic GnRH feedforward drive (albeit not acting alone), (2) impaired Leydig cell steroidogenesis, and/or (3) reduced negative feedback by testosterone *(38–40)*. Figure 2 highlights the foregoing primary mechanistic considerations.

ROLE OF INTRINSIC GnRH DEFICIENCY IN MEDIATING LOW-AMPLITUDE LH SECRETION

Experiments in the male mouse and rat support an important, but not exclusive, role of GnRH-deficient hypogonadotropism in the hypoandrogenemia of aging *(41–44)*. Evidence to this end includes (1) decreased castration-, naloxone-, and restraint stress-induced LH release in the older rodent *(24,42,45–47);* (2) diminished in vivo LH pulse amplitude in senescent animals *(43,48);* (3) reduced in vitro hypothalamic GnRH secretion *(49,50);* (4) altered GnRH neuronal synaptology *(51);* (5) preservation of the stimulatory efficacy of GnRH *(43,52);* and (6) restoration of sexual activity in the impotent animal by fetal hypothalamic neuronal transplantation *(53)*. Although such observations afford important clues for clinical investigation, the regulation of GnRH outflow in the laboratory animal is complex, multifactorial, and incompletely defined.

The intuition that hypothalamic GnRH deficiency subserves relative hypogonadism in elderly men has not been established or refuted *(22,26,28,54–57)*. However, the

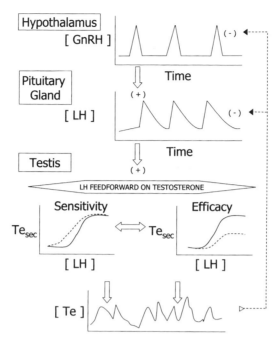

Fig. 1. Simplified schema of the gonadotropin-releasing hormone (GnRH), luteinizing hormone (LH)-testosterone (hypothalamic–pituitary–Leydig cell) axis with feedback (–, inhibitory) and feed-forward (+, stimulatory) interactions mediated via specific interface (dose-response) functions. (Unpublished line drawing.)

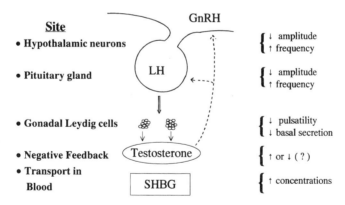

Fig. 2. Primary loci of postulated regulatory failure defects in the gonadotropin-releasing hormone (GnRH)– luteinizing hormone (LH)–testosterone ensemble axis in aging men.

notion is congruent with many clinical observations, as highlighted in Table 1. A necessary, but not sufficient, prediction is that GnRH action on gonadotropes is preserved. A recent prospectively randomized, interventional study used 14 d of pulsatile i.v. infusion of GnRH vs. saline to stimulate LH and testosterone secretion. Older and young men treated with this regimen achieved an equivalent elevation of 24-h LH concentrations (*see* Fig. 3A) consistent with retention of gonadotrope secretory responsiveness in the older male *(28)*. In young men, the increment in mean LH

Table 1
Indirect Evidence for Impaired Hypothalamic GnRH Drive in Aging Men

	References
1. Low-amplitude spontaneous LH pulses	*(23,27,28,38,55)*
2. Normal or increased (maximal) GnRH efficacy	*(28,47,54,97–98)*
3. Blunted unleashing of pulsatile LH secretion under negative-feedback withdrawal	*(26,56,57,75,76,123)*
4. More disorderly patterns of LH release	*(28,30,39,40,76)*
5. Asynchrony of central neurohormone outflow; namely, LH, FSH, PRL, sleep stage, and NPT	*(31,32,115)*
6. Increased pituitary LH stores postmortem	*(24)*
7. Neurotransmitter and sex-steroid receptor adaptations in the aged hypothalamus and pituitary gland	*(77,78)*
8. Mathematical predictions based on an ensemble concept	*(39,40,83)*

LH, luteinizing hormone; GnRH, gonadotropin-releasing hormone; FSH, follicle-stimulating hormone; PRL, prolactin; NPT, nocturnal penile tumescence.

concentrations elicited a proportionate rise in testosterone production. On the other hand, the same average increase in LH immunoreactivity in aged individuals failed to augment total (*see* Fig. 3B), as well as, bioavailable and free-testosterone concentrations equivalently. The latter age-related contrast would point to an abnormal pulsatile LH signal (of equivalent mean concentration only), relatively defective Leydig cell responsiveness, and/or accelerated testosterone metabolism in older men. The last (kinetic) consideration is excluded by the age-related fall in the metabolic clearance rate of testosterone associated with higher SHBG concentrations *(34,36,37)*.

CONTRIBUTION OF PRIMARY LEYDIG CELL STEROIDOGENIC FAILURE

Anatomical studies document an attrition of Leydig cell number in the older male *(58)*. From a functional perspective, pharmacological stimulation with human chorionic gonadotropin (hCG) does not induce maximal young-adult concentrations of testosterone in many elderly men *(19,22,59–62)*. Nonetheless, current hCG paradigms are difficult to interpret on experimental and physiological grounds; for example, (1) unequal concomitant (endogenous) LH concentrations in individuals may confound testicular responses to hCG *(12,19,24,61,62)*; (2) the half-life of circulating hCG is approx 20–30 h, compared with 0.75–1.5 h for LH; indeed, the former kinetics abrogate normal intermittent stimulation of the testis *(38,63,64)*. This distinction is relevant, because each LH pulse normally evokes a prompt burst of testosterone release, as monitored directly in the human spermatic vein *(65,66)*; (3) the nearly irreversible binding of hCG to the gonadal LH receptor downregulates steroidogenesis in vitro and in vivo *(67,68)*; and (4) the magnitude of hCG drive limits clinical evaluation to maximal Leydig cell responsivity. An equivalently sustained and potent lutropic stimulus is never achieved physiologically in vivo, except under maternal hCG exposure in the developing fetus *(34,36)*.

A second means of appraising Leydig cell responsiveness is cross-correlation analysis of LH and (time-delayed) testosterone concentrations in paired hormone time series

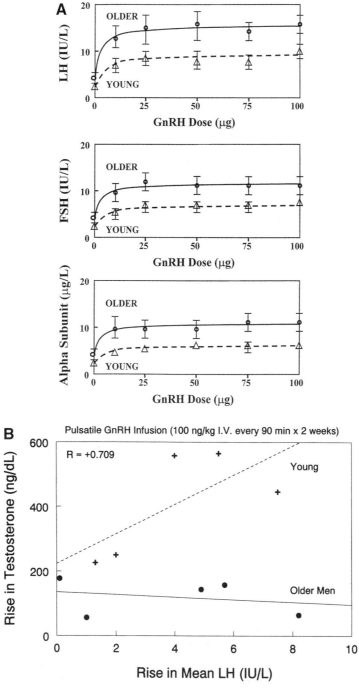

Fig. 3. (A) GnRH dose-responsive response stimulation of (2-h mean) serum concentrations of luteinizing hormone (LH) (top), follicle-stimulating hormone (FSH) (middle), and free (uncombined) alpha subunit (bottom) in young men (interrupted lines) and older volunteers (solid lines). Data are the mean ± SEM. Adapted with permission from *(96).* **(B)** Relationship between the increment in 24-h mean concentrations of LH (*x*-axis) and testosterone (*y*-axis) induced by 14 d of uninterrupted pulsatile i.v. gonadotropin-releasing hormone (GnRH) infusion (100 ng/kg every 90 min) compared with saline in young men (upper interrupted curve and plus signs). There is no correlation in older men (lower continuous line and solid circles). (Adapted from ref. *28.*)

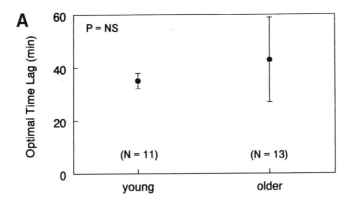

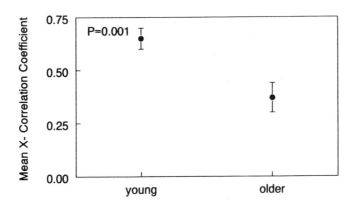

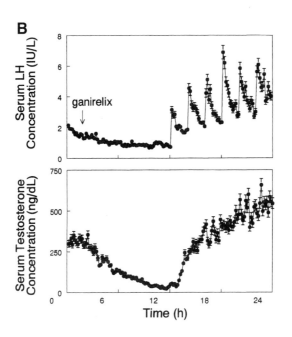

Fig. 4. (A) Cross-correlation of 10-min luteinizing hormone (LH) concentrations with (deconvolution-calculated) testosterone secretion rates sampled for 24 h in 11 young and 13 older men. The optimal time lag (upper panel) defines the latency (min) between rising LH concentrations and increasing testosterone secretion rates. The cross-correlation coefficient r (rho) quantitates the strength of feedforward coupling. Data are the mean ± SEM. **(B)** Infusion of six consecutive rh LH pulses (50 IU i.v. over 6 min every 2 h) in a healthy young man pretreated 12 h earlier with a single sc dose of the selective gonadotropin-releasing hormone (GnRH)-receptor antagonist, ganirelix. Time zero is 2000 h. Blood was withdrawn every 10 min for 2 h before ganirelix injection and for 24 h thereafter. (Unpublished plot from ref. *71.*)

(69). Comparisons by age disclose a young adult-like time lag of 30–40 min but significantly reduced feedforward coupling between LH and testosterone in older men. The latter distinction is reflected in a 50% reduction in the cross-correlation coefficient *(27,29)*, as shown in Fig. 4A.

A third experimental strategy to examine Leydig cell steroidogenic capacity is to downregulate gonadotropin secretion with a GnRH analog and then add back pulses of rh LH intravenously to emulate physiological patterns of gonadotropin stimulation. In this paradigm, LH withdrawal enforced by pituitary downregulation impairs testosterone secretory responsiveness profoundly in both age groups, albeit twofold more in elderly men *(70)*.

A fourth interventional scheme is illustrated by a recent pilot analysis in eight young and seven older volunteers. In this approach, a selective GnRH-receptor antagonist (ganirelix) was injected 10 h before infusing successive i.v. pulses of rh LH. Pulsatile injections of rh LH increased testosterone concentrations within 6–8 h from <120 ng/dL to >450 ng/dL in both age cohorts *(71)*. The response in one young subject is illustrated in Fig. 4B. This preliminary study was restricted to 14 h of LH stimulation, measurement of the total testosterone concentration, and a small number of participants. Thus, further investigations will be required to ascertain whether intermittent LH infusion will sustain young-adult production of total, non SHBG-bound, and free testosterone for prolonged intervals in healthy older men.

ALTERATIONS IN TESTOSTERONE FEEDBACK RESTRAINT

Whether or how sex-steroid negative feedback is altered in older men is controversial. For example, three clinical studies report heightened negative feedback by exogenous androgens in the aging male. These analyses were based on short-term i.v. infusion of testosterone and or dihydrotestosterone (DHT) for 4 d *(33)* or transdermal delivery of 5-α-DHT for 11 d *(72)* or testosterone for 12 mo *(73)*. Two other investigations describe reduced androgen feedback efficacy in the older male after several weeks of im injection of high-dose testosterone *(54,74)*. Two interventional studies using an estrogen- and or androgen-receptor antagonist and one biomathematical construct imply reduced LH secretory adaptations to muted sex-steroid feedback in elderly men *(56,75,76)*. From another vantage, cross-correlation analysis of 24-h (paired) LH and testosterone concentration profiles identifies impaired negative feedback by *endogenous* androgen in older volunteers *(29)*. Based on immunocytochemical detection, androgen (and estrogen) receptors may decline in the brain and pituitary gland of aged rats and in genital fibroblasts of older men *(77,78)*.

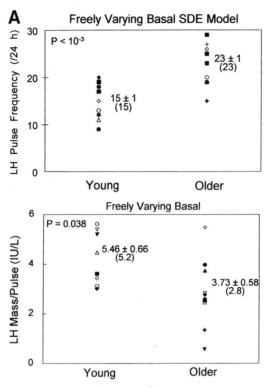

Fig. 5. Comparison of luteinizing hormone (LH) secretory attributes in young and older men based on a variable-waveform model that allows a freely varying basal secretion rate. **(A)** Impact of age on LH pulse frequency (events/day) and LH secretory-burst mass (international unit secreted per pulse per liter of distribution volume). *(Figure continues)*

Prominent adaptations to experimental androgen depletion in young men are accelerated frequency and reduced incremental amplitude of LH pulses (*see* Fig. 5A) and quantitatively irregular patterns of LH release *(76,79–81)*. The neuroendocrine phenotype in older men includes each of the foregoing feedback adjustments *(27,28,30,31,55)*. Thus, a facile hypothesis is that lower bioavailable and free-testosterone concentrations in the elderly male are the proximate cause of unleashing anomalous LH secretion patterns. However, quite unlike the feedback-deprived state, basal, pulsatile and total LH secretion remain normal in many healthy older men *(38,39)* (*see* Fig. 5B). Accordingly, an important but unresolved mechanistic issue is whether neuroendocrine disturbances in aging individuals reflect expected feedback withdrawal resulting from hypoandrogenemia *(37)*. This question becomes important, inasmuch as testosterone repletion in androgen-deficient young men reverses each of rapid-frequency, diminutive-amplitude, and disorderly LH secretion *(76,79,80)*.

REGULATION OF THE ENSEMBLE
HYPOTHALAMO–PITUITARY–LEYDIG CELL AXIS

An emergent thesis in neuroendocrine research is that early disruption of (negative) feedback and/or (positive) feedforward may be detectable without any demon-

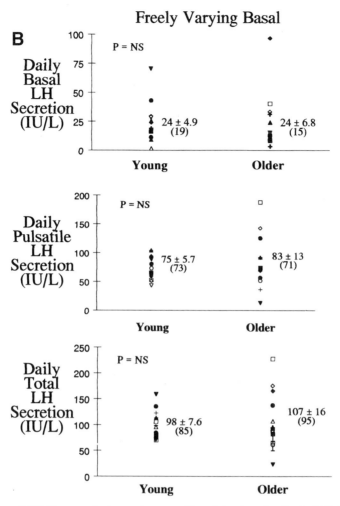

Fig. 5. *(Continued)* **(B)** Deconvolution estimates of basal (top), pulsatile (middle), and total (bottom) daily LH secretion in young and older men. Numerical values are the mean ± SEM (median). *P* values are estimated by the rank-sum test. *p* = NS denotes < 0.05. (Adapted from ref. *38.*)

strable change in overall hormone production *(28,30,35,39,40)*. The foregoing insight is relevant to understanding early disarray of the hypothalamic–pituitary–gonadal axis in aging. Therein, we adopt the basic precept that repeated, dose-dependent, time-delayed adjustments in regulatory sites govern systemic androgen availability in a homeostatic fashion *(38,66,82–89)*. To aid intuition, we have formalized core feedback connections among GnRH, LH and testosterone mathematically *(38,81–83)* A simplified model structure predicts that jointly impaired feedforward by LH and feedback by testosterone would yield a high-frequency, low-amplitude, and disorderly pattern of LH release. On the other hand, isolated failure of GnRH outflow would explain only inappropriately low LH concentrations and attendant hypoandrogenemia but not an elevated LH pulse frequency or irregular release patterns *(39,40)*. Exploration of this ensemble concept requires more focused assessment of physiological regulation, as highlighted next.

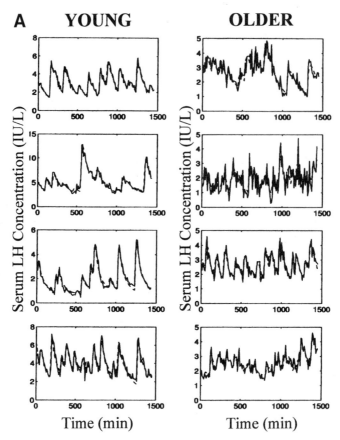

Fig. 6. Diminution in luteinizing hormone (LH) secretory-burst mass and acceleration of LH pulse frequency in aging when compared with young men inferred by two deconvolution methods *(40).* **(A)** LH concentration profiles (± sample SDs) measured in serum collected every 10 min for 24 h and analyzed by immunoradiometric assays and variable-waveform (stochastic differential equation-based) deconvolution analysis (predicted continuous curve) *(38).(Figure continues)*

Sampling and Counting of Pulses

The frequency and amplitude of LH pulses provide a window to signals from the brain and pituitary gland. Withdrawal of blood at 5- or 10-min intervals for 12–24 h will capture the majority of discrete LH release episodes in healthy men *(34,90–94).* Suitable monitoring paradigms define an accelerated frequency and attenuated amplitude of pulsatile LH release in older men by independent methods of pulse detection, in separate gonadotropin assays, and in different volunteer cohorts *(28,39,40,55,95).* Figure 6A illustrates comparisons by age of immunoradiometric LH concentration times series collected every 10 min for 24 h, and Fig. 6B presents robotics-assisted chemiluminometric LH release patterns monitored every 2.5 min over night *(27,31).* Simultaneous records of FSH, prolactin (PRL), and nocturnal penile tumescence are also shown. Some, but not all, earlier analyses using radioimmunoassay methods and/or less frequent (e.g., 20 min) blood-sampling protocols presaged the concept of lower amplitude and higher frequency LH peaks in older men *(19,34–36).* Recent biomathematical simulations establish that failure to detect either a loss of amplitude or a gain in

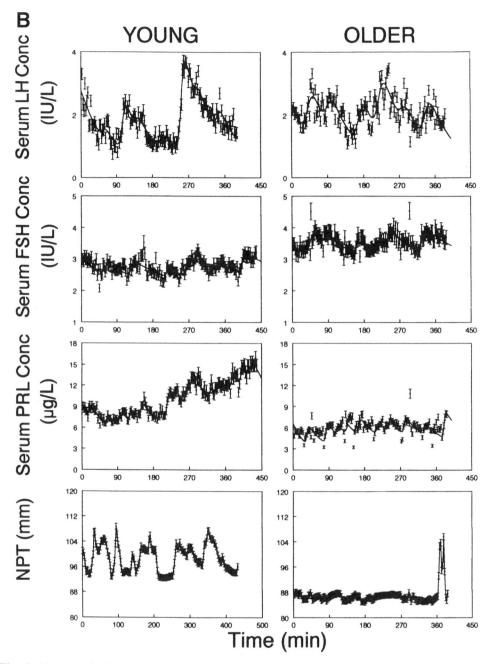

Fig. 6. *(Continued)* **(B)** LH concentrations monitored by sampling blood every 2.5 min overnight followed by chemiluminescence (robotics-assisted) assay and Gaussian secretory-burst deconvolution analysis (continuous curves [top row]). Simultaneous records of follicle-stimulating hormone (FSH) (upper middle), prolactin (PRL) (lower middle), and nocturnal penile tumescence (NPT) (bottom) are shown for comparison. (Adapted from ref. *32.*)

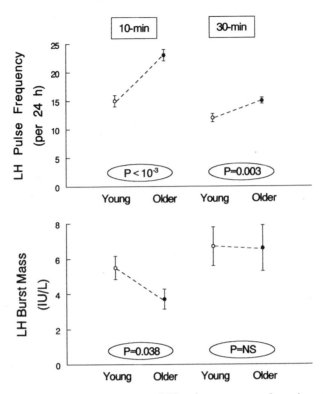

Fig. 7. Undersampling of luteinizing hormone (LH) release censors detection of LH pulses (top) and inflates estimates of LH secretory-burst mass. The resultant technical bias limits the identification of age-related contrasts in pulse frequency and size. Twenty-four LH concentration time series were edited from original 10-min sampling sets to yield 30-min daughter series (simple subsets) in 11 young and 13 older men. (Unpublished reanalysis of data in *28,29,55;* Bradford, Kuipers, and Veldhuis.)

frequency of LH pulses is a predictable technical artifact of insufficiently intensive blood sampling (*see* Fig. 7).

Gonadotrope Responsiveness to GnRH

Viewed mechanistically, a 50% reduction in incremental (peak minus nadir) LH pulse amplitude in aging men could denote a diminished amount of hypothalamic GnRH secreted per burst, an abnormal GnRH waveform, and/or impaired gonadotrope-cell responsiveness to GnRH. Recent GnRH dose-response analyses conducted in randomly assigned order on separate days establish normal maximal and enhanced submaximal acute and short-term (14-d) stimulatory effects of GnRH in the elderly male *(28,96,97).* Heightened sensitivity to small GnRH amounts would occur predictably in the presence of augmented pituitary LH stores in older individuals, as inferred postmortem *(24).* A preliminary report indicates that pituitary sensitivity to submaximal GnRH stimulation is accentuated further by short-term androgen depletion in aged volunteers *(98).* If confirmed, the latter insight would indicate that lower bioavailable testosterone concentrations in older men cause or potentiate disproportionate LH release induced by a submaximal GnRH stimulus.

Accelerated LH Pulse Frequency in the Aging Male

A basic, unresolved mechanistic issue is whether aging causes a primary hypo-thalamic disturbance that enforces a high frequency of GnRH pulses and/or whether low bioavailable testosterone concentrations elevate LH pulse frequency via feed-back withdrawal *(27,35–37,40,55)*. This query is central to contemporary physiolog-ical assessments of aging, inasmuch as earlier investigations in healthy young men document that (1) infusion of testosterone or a nonaromatizable androgen sup-presses LH pulse frequency and elevate LH peak amplitude *(24,88,99,100)* and (2) administration of ketoconazole (which depletes testosterone) or flutamide (which inhibits androgen-receptor binding) augments LH pulse frequency and reduces incremental LH peak (fractional) amplitude *(79,80,101)*. In the human, monkey, sheep, and rat, a high frequency of GnRH stimuli reduces incremental (fractional) LH pulse amplitude *(37,48)*. In view of this reciprocal control mechanism (albeit not fully understood), diminished androgen bioavailability in older men could con-tribute, in principle, to both more rapid and lower amplitude LH pulses. What remains unknown is whether hypoandrogenemia in aging fully accounts for the degree of observed neuroendocrine changes.

Monitoring Unobserved Gonadotropin Secretion

Lower incremental LH peak amplitude in older men can be dissected further mech-anistically under the premise that fluctuating hormone concentrations are driven by specific (unobserved) secretion and kinetic processes. Deconvolution analysis is a family of computer-assisted methods designed to quantitate underlying secretion and/or elimination. Some deconvolution procedures allow one to determine (1) the fre-quency of secretory bursts, (2) the amount of hormone released within each burst (mass of hormone discharged within the event normalized to unit distribution volume), (3) the subject- and condition-specific half-life of elimination of the hormone, and (4) concomitant basal or (nonpulsatile) secretion.

There are several complementary deconvolution approaches to secretion analysis. Figure 8A illustrates one basic idea, wherein an unobserved Gaussian-shaped secretory burst creates each peak in serum hormone concentrations *(102)*. In this *waveform-dependent* concept, hormone concentrations increase rapidly because of the sharp onset of an underlying secretory burst and then fall gradually after the burst as the hor-mone is eliminated slowly from the circulation. The Gaussian-burst model allows one to calculate the number, location, duration, and amplitude of secretory bursts and pre-dict the hormone half-life at the same time *(103,104)*. Application of this methodology in healthy men quantitates a lower mass and higher frequency of LH secretory events in older than young men but a comparable LH half-life *(27,35,55)*. The lower mass (IU) of LH released per secretory burst in the elderly male results from attentuation of the amplitude (maximal secretion rate attained) rather than abbreviation of the duration (min) of release episodes.

A second-generation deconvolution technology defines secretion as an admixture of unknown basal output and superimposed events of any height, width, shape, and number *(103)* (*see* Fig. 8B). This deconvolution construct is, therefore, defined as *waveform independent*. For statistical reasons, optimal analysis in this methodology requires *a pri-ori* knowledge of the two-component half-life of hormone elimination *(105)*. Because the true waveform of secretory bursts is (definitionally) unknown, definitive pulse counting is analytically difficult, unless assumptions are made about event shape, smoothness, location, or number *(104)*. However, this mathematical strategy predicts lower peak LH secretion rates in older men.

A third-generation deconvolution strategy uses coupled, stochastic differential equations to reconstruct simultaneously the number, shape, size, and timing of (unknown) secretory bursts, the basal release rate, biexponential disappearance kinetics, and random effects driving hormone release *(82,83)* (*see* Fig. 8C). This comprehensive statistical platform predicts a lower mass and higher frequency of LH secretory bursts in older than young men, with no age difference in LH kinetics *(38,40,81)*. The diminution in mass and acceleration in frequency of LH pulses counterbalance closely, thus leaving the total and pulsatile daily LH secretion rate unchanged in aging individuals.

Contemporary secretion-based insights explain some earlier observations. For example, one method of discrete hormone peak detection, cluster analysis, identifies a pulse simply as a statistical jump and drop in the hormone concentration *(34,106)*. This approach is termed model-free, because few assumptions are made in defining a pulse. Deconvolution analysis illustrates that the peak increment is proportionate to the mass of hormone secreted in the burst *ceterus paribus (104,105,107)*. This point is important, because elderly men consistently exhibit a reduced incremental LH peak amplitude compared with young counterparts *(28,81)*.

Regularity Analysis

Homeostasis in an endocrine axis requires repeated decremental and incremental adjustments in secretion *(39,82,83)*. (*see* Fig. 1). In the male gonadal axis, core homeostatic signals include (at least) GnRH, LH, and testosterone, which enforce adaptations over a rapid (minute-by-minute) time course *(108)*. Orderliness of the resultant subpatterns of hormone release can be quantitated objectively via a regularity statistic, approximate entropy (ApEn) *(30,109–111)*. ApEn is calculated on a desktop computer as a single number, which exploits accurate probabilistic accounting to quantitate the reproducibility of successive measurements in a time series *(111)* (*see* Fig. 9A). Higher ApEn denotes heightened irregularity of minute-by-minute hormone release, which, in turn, signifies deterioration or adaptation of feedback and feedforward adjustments *(110,113,114)*.

In a clinical context, ApEn identifies highly disorderly patterns of tumoral hormone release, which denotes autonomy from normal regulatory adjustments *(21,110)*. In addition, ApEn delineates irregular secretion of LH, testosterone, GH, adrenocorticotropic hormone (ACTH), cortisol, and insulin in older compared with young individuals, thus defining age-related deterioration of adaptive control *(28,30–32,35,76,115)* (*see* Fig. 9B). For example, elevated ApEn of LH and testosterone release patterns unmask disruption of one or more key signaling elements within the interlinked GnRH-LH-testosterone axis *(30,39,40,113)*. Interventional studies are necessary to localize the individual and joint sites of statistically inferred regulatory defects.

The cross-ApEn statistic extends the concept of appraising single-hormone regularity to quantitating two-hormone (pairwise) synchrony *(30)*. Cross-ApEn unveils significant loss of bihormonal synchrony between LH and testosterone secretion in

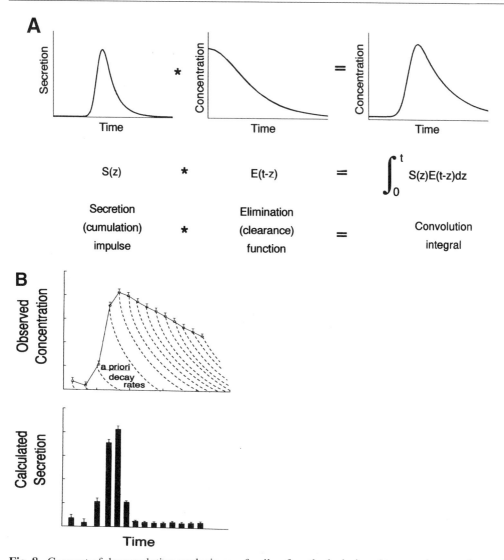

Fig. 8. Concept of deconvolution analysis as a family of methods designed to quantitate unobserved secretion and/or kinetics from fluctuating hormone concentrations. **(A)** A *Gaussian* or slightly skewed *secretory-burst model* (top left) provides estimates of time-delimited, burst-like discharge of molecules with individual release velocities driving a pulse. A secretory burst is defined by its position in time, maximum (amplitude), and half-duration (duration at half-maximal height) *(102,104).* The time integral of the convolution product of the secretory burst (left) and disappearance function (middle) yields the pulsatile hormone concentration (right). The reverse process of deducing underlying secretion and elimination from observed concentrations is termed deconvolution analysis. *(B)* A *waveform-independent approach* allows one to calculate sample secretion rates (bottom) from measured hormone concentrations (top) based on *a priori* biexponential kinetics (interrupted decay curves). Experimental errors inherent in hormone measurements and the populational half-life estimate are combined to determine statistical confidence limits for each sample secretion rate *(103,105).* *(Figure continues)*

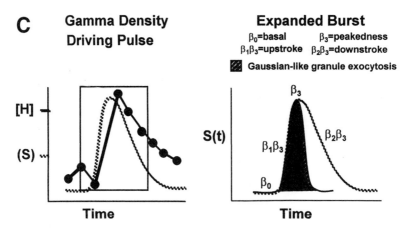

Fig. 8. *(Continued)* **(C)** Flexible deconvolution construct of a *generalized Gamma-density (variable) secretory-pulse waveform* is used to encapsulate burst timing, number, shape and size, basal secretion, and rapid and slow-phase hormone elimination kinetics simultaneously with random effects *(81,83)*. Random effects arise from sampling uncertainty, assay error, stochastic admixture of secreted hormone in the bloodstream, unpredictable pulse times, and varying effector-response interface properties *(39,82)*. (Unpublished illustrative schema.)

older men *(see* Fig. 9C). This measure further documents deterioration of coordinate patterns of LH release and oscillations of each of PRL, FSH, nocturnal penile tumescence, and sleep stage *(31,39,40)*. According to this idea, brainstem regulatory centers oversee synchronous secretion of GnRH, LH, FSH, and PRL; sleep-stage transitions, and autonomic control of NPT cycles. Thus, the foregoing findings establish multilevel disruption of central nervous system (CNS)-dependent neurohormone outflow in older men.

Appraising Testosterone Signaling

To date, the majority of clinical studies have used the total testosterone concentration to assess androgen-dependent negative feedback on the hypothalamic–pituitary unit *(36,37)*. However, in men, total testosterone is distributed in plasma as free (approx 2%), weakly albumin-bound (50–55%) and tightly globulin-bound (40–45%) steroid *(116,117)*. Rapid dissociation of testosterone from low-affinity albumin (nominal unidirectional half-time 0.2 s at 37°C) would favor effectual tissue uptake within a brief (2 to 10 s) capillary transit time, so long as reassociation is minimized *(118)*. On the other hand, slow release of testosterone from high-affinity SHBG (half-time 3.3 s at 37°C) would putatively restrict access to cells, at least when reassociation is limited. Protein-binding effects are important, because SHBG concentrations increase as much as twofold and bioavailable (non-SHBG-bound) testosterone concentrations fall by 30–50% in older individuals *(20,119–122)* *(see* Fig. 10A). Dynamic mechanisms of physiological control of free, SHBG- and Alb-bound testosterone are highlighted in the kinetic schema of Fig. 10B. Therefore, according to contemporary perspectives, carefully designed clinical studies will be needed to examine the age-dependence of free and bioavailable testosterone-mediated negative feedback on gonadotropin secretion *(37)*.

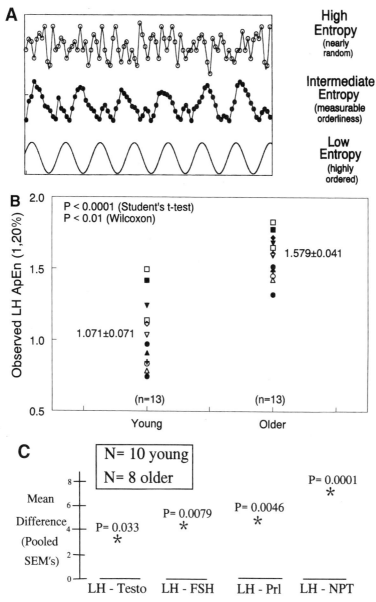

Fig. 9. (A) Notion of the approximate entropy (ApEn) statistic to quantitate relative regularity of serial (sample-by-sample) measurements. The bottom curve gives a cosine function (low ApEn) to illustrate a well-reproduced pattern, the middle curve shows partial degradation of regularity (intermediate ApEn), and the top frame depicts marked erosion of orderliness (high ApEn). **(B)** Increased ApEn of overnight (2.5-min) luteinizing hormone (LH) release profiles in healthy older compared with young men. Higher ApEn points to less orderly outflow of gonadotropin-releasing hormone (GnRH) and/or LH, or disruption of the GnRH-LH feedforward interface. Numerical values are the mean ± SEM. **(C)** Cross-approximate entropy (cross-ApEn) differences in older and young men. Differences exceeding three SEMs (older minus young) denote significant deterioration of young-adult coupling between oscillations of LH and testosterone (leftmost), LH and follicle-stimulating hormone (FSH), (left middle), LH and prolactin (PRL), (right middle), and LH and nocturnal penile tumescence (NPT) (rightmost). *P* values denote the probability of falsely rejecting the null hypothesis of equivalent two-hormone synchrony in the two age groups. (Unpublished compilation of data reported in refs. *30–32,95.*)

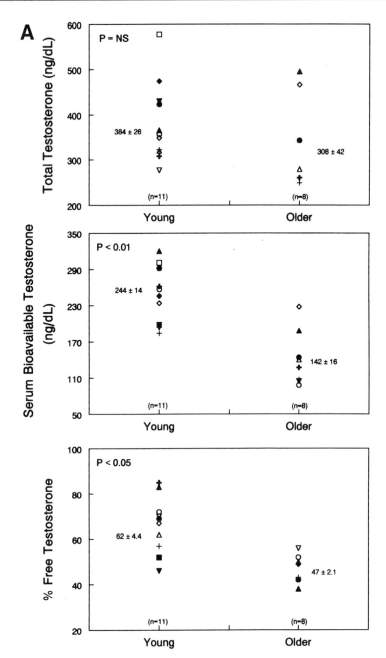

Fig. 10. (A) Comparison of serum total, non-sex hormone-binding globulin (SHBG) (bioavailable) and percentage free testosterone measurements in two cohorts of men; namely, young (n = 11) and older (n = 8). Similar mean total testosterone concentrations by age (top) belie a reduction in bioavailable and percentage non-SHBG-bound (percent free) testosterone (middle and lower) in older individuals. Adapted from ref. *32*. *(Figure continues)*

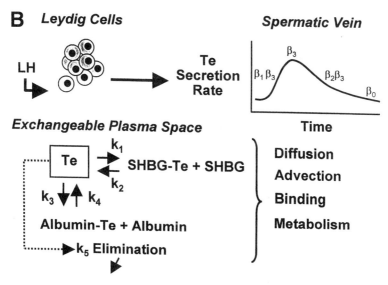

Fig. 10. *(Continued)* **(B)** Schema of fate of secreted testosterone in plasma. (Unpublished line drawing.)

SUMMARY

Developing concepts of time-adaptive control of testosterone secretion incorporate interactions among GnRH, LH, and testosterone. Homeostasis requires reversible, recurrent, and reciprocal (feedback and feedforward) adjustments to external stress (e.g., food deprivation and trauma) and internal needs (e.g., anabolism and procreation). In this ensemble perspective, no single gland acts alone. Clinical studies in the healthy aging male point to regulatory failure of GnRH-driven pulsatile LH secretion, LH-stimulated Leydig cell androgen biosynthesis, and testosterone-enforced feedback on GnRH/LH outflow. Accordingly, hypoandrogenemia in the older male is the final common consequence of a matrix of primary and secondary deficits in the hypothalamic–pituitary–gonadal ensemble.

REFERENCES

1. Stearns EL, MacDonald JA, Kaufman BJ, et al. Declining testicular function with age, hormonal and clinical correlates. Am J Med 1974;57:761–766.
2. Davidson JM, Chen JJ, Crapo L, Gray GD, Greenleaf WJ, Catania JA. Hormonal changes and sexual function in aging men. J Clin Endocrinol Metab 1983;57:71–77.
3. Wang C, Alexander G, Berman N, et al. Testosterone replacement therapy improves mood in hypogonadal men—a clinical research center study. J Clin Endocrinol Metab 1996;81:3578–3583.
4. Morley JE, Perry HM, Kaiser FE, et al. Effects of testosterone on replacement therapy in old hypogonadal males: a preliminary study. J Am Geriatr Soc 1993;41:149–152.
5. Urban RJ, Bodenburg YH, Gilkison C, et al. Testosterone administration to elderly men increases skeletal muscle strength and protein synthesis. Am J Physiol 1995;269:E280–E286.
6. Barrett-Connor E, Von Muhlen DG, Kritz-Silverstein D. Bioavailable testosterone and depressed mood in older men: the Rancho Bernardo study. J Clin Endocrinol Metab 1999;84:573–577.
7. Barrett-Connor E, Goodman-Gruen D, Patay B. Endogenous sex hormones and cognitive function in older men. J Clin Endocrinol Metab 1999;84:3681–3685.
8. Abbasi AA, Drinka PJ, Mattson DE, Rudman D. Low circulating levels of insulin-like growth factors and testosterone in chronically institutionalized elderly men. J Am Geriatr Soc 1993;41:975–982.

9. Tenover JS. Testosterone in the aging male. J Androl 1997;18:103–106.
10. Moffat SD, Zonderman AB, Metter EJ, Blackman MR, Harman SM, Resnick SM. Longitudinal assessment of serum free testosterone concentration predicts memory performance and cognitive status in elderly men. J Clin Endocrinol Metab 2002;87:5001–5007.
11. Gray A, Berlin JA, McKinlay JB, Longcope C. An examination of research design effects on the association of testosterone and male aging: results of a meta-analysis. J Clin Epidemiol 1991;44:671–684.
12. Nieschlag E, Kley HK, Wiegelmann W, Solbach HG, Kruskemper HL. Age and endocrine function of the testes in adult man. Deutsche Medizinische Wochenschrift 1973;98:1281–1284.
13. Gray A, Feldman HS, McKinlay JB, Longcope C. Age disease, and changing sex hormone levels in middle-aged men: results of the Massachusetts Male Aging Study. J Clin Endocrinol Metab 1991;73:1016–1025.
14. Morley JE, Kaiser FE, Perry HM, 3rd, et al. Longitudinal changes in testosterone luteinizing hormone and follicle-stimulating hormone in healthy older men. Metab Clin Exp 1997;46:410–413.
15. Hollander N, Hollander VP. The microdetermination of testosterone in human spermatic vein blood. J Clin Endocrinol Metab 1958;18:966–971.
16. de Lignieres B. Transdermal dihydrotestosterone treatment of andropause. Ann Med 1993;25:235–241.
17. Morley JE, Kaiser F, Raum WJ, et al. Potentially predictive and manipulable blood serum correlates of aging in the healthy human male: progressive decreases in bioavailable testosterone, dehydroepiandrosterone sulfate, and the ratio of insulin-like growth factor I to growth hormone. Proc Natl Acad Sci USA 1997;94:7537–7542.
18. Blackman MR, Weintraub BD, Rosen SW, Harman SM. Comparison of the effects of lung cancer, benign lung disease, and normal aging on pituitary-gonadal function in men. J Clin Endocrinol Metab 1988;66:88–95.
19. Deslypere JP, Vermeulen A. Leydig cell function in normal men: effect of age, lifestyle, residence, diet and activity. J Clin Endocrinol Metab 1984;59:955–962.
20. Mankin HR, Calkins JH. Decreased bioavailable testosterone in aging normal and impotent men. J Clin Endocrinol Metab 1986;63:1418–1420.
21. Bergendahl M, Aloi JA, Iranmanesh A, Mulligan T, Veldhuis JD. Fasting suppresses pulsatile luteinizing hormone (LH) secretion and enhances the orderliness of LH release in young but not older men. J Clin Endocrinol Metab 1998;83:1967–1975.
22. Winters SJ, Troen P. Episodic luteinizing hormone (LH) secretion and the response of LH and follicle-stimulating hormone to LH-releasing hormone in aged men: evidence for coexistent primary testicular insufficiency and an impairment in gonadotropin secretion. J Clin Endocrinol Metab 1982;55:560–565.
23. Vermeulen A, Deslypere JP, De Meirleir K. A new look at the andropause: altered function of the gonadotrophs. J Steroid Biochem 1989;32:163–165.
24. Baker HWG, Burger HG, de Kretser DM, et al. Changes in the pituitary-testicular system with age. Clin Endocrinol 1976;5:349–372.
25. Mitchell R, Hollis S, Rothwell C, Robertson WR. Age-related changes in the pituitary-testicular axis in normal men; lower serum testosterone results from decreased bioactive LH drive. Clin Endocrinol 1995;42:501–507.
26. Urban RJ, Veldhuis JD, Blizzard RM, Dufau ML. Attenuated release of biologically active luteinizing hormone in healthy aging men. J Clin Invest 1988;81:1020–1029.
27. Mulligan T, Iranmanesh A, Gheorghiu S, Godschalk M, Veldhuis JD. Amplified nocturnal luteinizing hormone (LH) secretory burst frequency with selective attenuation of pulsatile (but not basal) testosterone secretion in healthy aged men: possible Leydig cell desensitization to endogenous LH signaling—a clinical research center study. J Clin Endocrinol Metab 1995;80:3025–3031.
28. Mulligan T, Iranmanesh A, Kerzner R, Demers LW, Veldhuis JD. Two-week pulsatile gonadotropin releasing hormone infusion unmasks dual (hypothalamic and Leydig-cell) defects in the healthy aging male gonadotropic axis. Eur J Endocrinol 1999;141:257–266.
29. Mulligan T, Iranmanesh A, Johnson ML, Straume M, Veldhuis JD. Aging alters feedforward and feedback linkages between LH and testosterone in healthy men. Am J Physiol 1997;42:R1407-R1413.
30. Pincus SM, Mulligan T, Iranmanesh A, Gheorghiu S, Godschalk M, Veldhuis JD. Older males secrete luteinizing hormone and testosterone more irregularly and jointly more asynchronously than younger males. Proc Natl Acad Sci USA 1996;93:14100–14105.
31. Veldhuis JD, Iranmanesh A, Godschalk M, Mulligan T. Older men manifest multifold synchrony disruption of reproductive neurohormone outflow. J Clin Endocrinol Metab 2000;85:1477–1486.

32. Veldhuis JD, Iranmanesh A, Mulligan T, Pincus SM. Disruption of the young-adult synchrony between luteinizing hormone release and oscillations in follicle-stimulating hormone, prolactin, and nocturnal penile tumescence (NPT) in healthy older men. J Clin Endocrinol Metab 1999;84:3498–3505.
33. Winters SJ, Sherins RJ, Troen P. The gonadotropin-suppressive activity of androgen is increased in elderly men. Metabolism 1984;33:1052–1059.
34. Urban RJ, Evans WS, Rogol AD, Kaiser DL, Johnson ML, Veldhuis JD. Contemporary aspects of discrete peak detection algorithms. I. The paradigm of the luteinizing hormone pulse signal in men. Endocr Rev 1988;9:3–37.
35. Veldhuis JD. Recent insights into neuroendocrine mechanisms of aging of the human male hypothalamo-pituitary-gonadal axis. J Androl 1999;20:1–17.
36. Veldhuis JD. Male hypothalamic-pituitary-gonadal axis. In: Yen SSC, Jaffe RB, Barbieri RL, eds. Reproductive Endocrinology, 4th ed.: W.B. Saunders, Philadelphia, 1999, pp. 622–631.
37. Veldhuis JD, Johnson ML, Keenan D, Iranmanesh A. The ensemble male hypothalamo-pituitary-gonadal axis. In: Timiras PS, ed. Physiological Basis of Aging and Geriatrics, 3rd ed. CRC, Boca Raton, FL, 2003, pp. 213–231.
38. Keenan DM, Veldhuis JD, Yang R. Joint recovery of pulsatile and basal hormone secretion by stochastic nonlinear random-effects analysis. Am J Physiol 1998;274:R1939-R1949.
39. Keenan DM, Veldhuis JD. Hypothesis testing of the aging male gonadal axis via a biomathematical construct. Am J Physiol Reg Integr Comp Physiol 2001;280:R1755–R1771.
40. Keenan DM, Veldhuis JD. Disruption of the hypothalamic luteinizing-hormone pulsing mechanism in aging men. Am J Physiol 2001;281:R1917–R1924.
41. Chubb CE, Desjardins C. Testicular function and neuroendocrine activity in senescent mice. Am J Physiol 1984;247:E410–E415.
42. Shin SH, Howitt C. Effect of castration on luteinizing hormone and luteinizing hormone releasing hormone in the male rat. J Endocrinol 1975;65:447–448.
43. Gruenewald DA, Naai MA, Hess DL, Matsumoto AM. The Brown Norway rat as a model of male reproductive aging: evidence for both primary and secondary testicular failure. J Gerontol 1994;49:B42–B50.
44. Bonavera JJ, Swerdloff RS, Leung A, et al. In the male Brown-Norway (BN) male rat reproductive aging is associated with decreased LH-pulse amplitude and area. J Androl 1997;18:359–365.
45. Shaar CJ, Euker JS, Riegle GD, Meites J. Effects of castration and gonadal steroids on serum luteinizing hormone and prolactin in old and young rats. J Endocrinol 1974;66:45–51.
46. Mulligan T, Kuno HL, Vij S, Iranmanesh A, Veldhuis JD. Healthy older men show heightened LH secretory sensitivity and capacity to GnRH stimulation. Presented at the Annual Meeting of the American Geriatrics Society, Philadelphia, Pennsylvania, 1999.
47. Kaufman JM, Giri M, Deslypere JM, Thomas G, Vermeulen A. Influence of age on the responsiveness of the gonadotrophs to luteinizing hormone-releasing hormone in males. J Clin Endocrinol Metab 1991;72:1255–1260.
48. Karpas AE, Bremner WJ, Clifton DK, Steiner RA, Dorsa DM. Diminished luteinizing hormone pulse frequency and amplitude with aging in the male rat. Endocrinology 1983;112:788–791.
49. Jarjour LT, Handelsman DJ, Swerdloff RS. Effects of aging on the in vitro release of gonadotropin-releasing hormone. Endocrinology 1986;119:1113–1117.
50. Coquelin AW, Desjardins C. Luteinizing hormone and testosterone secretion in young and old male mice. Am J Physiol 1982;243:E257–E263.
51. Witkin JW. Aging changes in synaptology of luteinizing hormone-releasing hormone neurons in male rat preoptic area. Neuroscience 1987;22:1003–1013.
52. Kaler LW, Critchlow V. Anterior pituitary luteinizing hormone secretion during continuous perifusion in aging male rats. Mech Ageing Devel 1984;25:103–115.
53. Huang HH, Kissane JQ, Hawrylewicz EJ. Restoration of sexual function and fertility by fetal hypothalamic transplant in impotent aged male rats. Neurobiol Aging 1987;8:465–472.
54. Deslypere JP, Kaufman JM, Vermeulen T, Vogelaers D, Vandalem JL, Vermeulen A. Influence of age on pulsatile luteinizing hormone release and responsiveness of the gonadotrophs to sex hormone feedback in men. J Clin Endocrinol Metab 1987;64:68–73.
55. Veldhuis JD, Urban RJ, Lizarralde G, Johnson ML, Iranmanesh A. Attenuation of luteinizing hormone secretory burst amplitude is a proximate basis for the hypoandrogenism of healthy aging in men. J Clin Endocrinol Metab 1992;75:52–58.
56. Veldhuis JD, Urban RJ, Dufau ML. Differential responses of biologically active LH secretion in older versus young men to interruption of androgen negative feedback. J Clin Endocrinol Metab 1994;79:1763–1770.

57. Vermeulen A, Deslypere JP, Kaufman JJ. Influence of antiopioids on luteinizing hormone pulsatility in aging men. J Clin Endocrinol Metab 1989;68:68–72.

58. Kaler LW, Neaves WB. Attrition of the human Leydig cell population with advancing age. Anat Rec 1978;192:513–518.

59. Reubens R, Dhondt M, Vermeulen A. Further studies on Leydig cell response to human choriogonadotropin. J Clin Endocrinol Metab 1976;39:40–45.

60. Nankin HR, Lin T, Murono EP. The aging Leydig cell III. Gonadotropin stimulation in men. J Androl 1981;2:181–186.

61. Harman SM, Tsitouras PD. Reproductive hormones in aging men. I. Measurement of sex steroids, basal luteinizing hormone, and Leydig cell response to human chorionic gonadotropin. J Clin Endocrinol Metab 1980;51:35–40.

62. Longcope C. The effect of human chorionic gonadotropin on plasma steroid levels in young and old men. Steroids 1973;21:583–592.

63. Veldhuis JD, Fraioli F, Rogol AD, Dufau ML. Metabolic clearance of biologically active luteinizing hormone in man. J Clin Invest 1986;77:1122–1128.

64. Veldhuis JD, Johnson ML, Dufau ML. Physiological attributes of endogenous bioactive luteinizing hormone secretory bursts in man: assessment by deconvolution analysis and *in vitro* bioassay of LH. Am J Physiol 1989;256:E199–E207.

65. Winters SJ, Troen PE. Testosterone and estradiol are co-secreted episodically by the human testis. J Clin Invest 1986;78:870–872.

66. Foresta C, Bordon P, Rossato M, Mioni R, Veldhuis JD. Specific linkages among luteinizing hormone, follicle stimulating hormone, and testosterone release in the peripheral blood and human spermatic vein: evidence for both positive (feed-forward) and negative (feedback) within-axis regulation. J Clin Endocrinol Metab 1997;82:3040–3046.

67. Glass AR, Vigersky RA. Resensitization of testosterone production in men after human chorionic gonadotropin-induced desensitization. J Clin Endocrinol Metab 1980;51:1395–1400.

68. Dufau ML, Catt KJ. Gonadotropin receptors and regulation of steroidogenesis in the testis and ovary. Vitam Horm 1978;36:461–585.

69. Veldhuis JD, King JC, Urban RJ, et al. Operating characteristics of the male hypothalamo-pituitary-gonadal axis: pulsatile release of testosterone and follicle-stimulating hormone and their temporal coupling with luteinizing hormone. J Clin Endocrinol Metabolism 1987;65:929–941.

70. Mulligan T, Iranmanesh A, Veldhuis JD. Pulsatile iv infusion of recombinant human LH in leupro-lide-suppressed men unmasks Iimpoverished leydig-cell secretory responsiveness to midphysiological LH drive in the aging male. J Clin Endocrinol Metab 2001;86:5547–5553.

71. Fox CR, Mulligan T, Iranmanesh A, Veldhuis JD. A paradigm of GnRH-receptor antagonist administration followed by pulsatile I.V. recombinant human (RH) LH demonstrates equivalent acute Leydig-cell steroidogenic function in younger and older men. 84th Annual Meeting of the Endocrine Society San Francisco California June 19–22 2002.

72. Desylpere JP, Kaufman JM, Vermeulen A, Vogelaers D, Vandalem JL, Vermeulen A. Influence of age on pulsatile luteinizing hormone release and responsiveness of the gonadotrophs to sex hormone feedback in men. J Clin Endocrinol Metab 1987;64:68–73.

73. Winters SJ, Atkinson L. Serum LH concentrations in hypogonadal men during transdermal testosterone replacement through scrotal skin: further evidence that aging enhances testosterone negative feedback. Clin Endocrinol 1997;47:317–322.

74. Gentili A, Mulligan T, Godschalk M, et al. Unequal impact of short-term testosterone repletion on the somatotropic axis of young and older men. J Clin Endocrinol Metab 2002;87:825–834.

75. Veldhuis JD, Urban RJ, Dufau ML. Evidence that androgen negative-feedback regulates hypothalamic GnRH impulse strength and the burst-like secretion of biologically active luteinizing hormone in men. J Clin Endocrinol Metab 1992;74:1227–1235.

76. Veldhuis JD, Zwart A, Mulligan T, Iranmanesh A. Muting of androgen negative feedback unveils impoverished gonadotropin-releasing hormone/luteinizing hormone secretory reactivity in healthy older men. J Clin Endocrinol Metab 2001;86:529–535.

77. Haji M, Kato KI, Nawata H, Ibayashi H. Age-related changes in the concentrations of cytosol receptors for sex steroid hormones in the hypothalamus and pituitary gland of the rat. Brain Res 1980;204:373–386.

78. Roth GS, Heiss GI. Changes in the mechanisms of hormone and neurotransmitter action during aging: current status of the role of receptor and post-receptor alterations. Mech Ageing Devel 1982;20:175–194.

79. Veldhuis JD, Zwart AD, Iranmanesh A. Neuroendocrine mechanisms by which selective Leydig-cell castration unleashes increased pulsatile LH release in the human: an experimental paradigm of short-term ketoconazole-induced hypoandrogenemia and deconvolution-estimated LH secretory enhancement. Am J Physiol 1997;272:R464–R474.

80. Zwart A, Iranmanesh A, Veldhuis JD. Disparate serum free testosterone concentrations and degrees of hypothalamo-pituitary-LH suppression are achieved by continuous versus pulsatile intravenous androgen replacement in men: a clinical experimental model of ketoconazole-induced reversible hypoandrogenemia with controlled testosterone add-back. J Clin Endocrinol Metab 1997;82:2062–2069.

81. Keenan DM, Sun W, Veldhuis JD. A stochastic biomathematical model of the male reproductive hormone system. J Appl Math 2000;61:934–965.

82. Keenan DM, Veldhuis JD. Stochastic model of admixed basal and pulsatile hormone secretion as modulated by a deterministic oscillator. Am J Physiol Reg Integr Comp Physiol 1997;273:R1182–R1192.

83. Keenan DM, Veldhuis JD. A biomathematical model of time-delayed feedback in the human male hypothalamic-pituitary-Leydig cell axis. Am J Physiol 1998;275:E157–E176.

84. Davies TF, Platzer M. The perifused Leydig cell: system characterization and rapid gonadotropin-induced desensitization. Endocrinology 1981;108:1757–1762.

85. Chase DJ, Schanbacher B, Lunstra DD. Effects of pulsatile and continuous luteinizing hormone (LH) infusions on testosterone responses to LH in rams actively immunized against gonadotropin-releasing hormone. Endocrinology 1988;123:816–826.

86. Lincoln GA. Luteinizing hormone and testosterone in man. Nature 1974;252:232–233.

87. Rowe PH, Racey PA, Lincoln GA, Ellwood M, Lehane J, Shenton JC. The temporal relationship between the secretion of luteinizing hormone and testosterone in man. J Endocrinol 1975;64:17–25.

88. Bagatell CJ, Dahl KD, Bremner WJ. The direct pituitary effect of testosterone to inhibit gonadotropin secretion in men is partially mediated by aromatization to estradiol. J Androl 1994;15:15–21.

89. Snyder PJ, Reitano JF, Utiger RD. Serum LH and FSH responses to synthetic gonadotropin-releasing hormone in normal men. J Clin Endocrinol Metab 1975;41:938–945.

90. Veldhuis JD, Evans WS, Johnson ML, Rogol AD. Physiological properties of the luteinizing hormone pulse signal: impact of intensive and extended venous sampling paradigms on their characterization in healthy men and women. J Clin Endocrinol Metab 1986;62:881–891.

91. Partsch C-J, Abrahams S, Herholz N, Peter M, Veldhuis JD, Sippell WG. Variability of pulsatile LH secretion in young male volunteers. Eur J Endocrinol 1994;131:263–272.

92. Veldhuis JD, Evans WS, Rogol AD, et al. Intensified rates of venous sampling unmask the presence of spontaneous high-frequency pulsations of luteinizing hormone in man. J Clin Endocrinol Metab 1984;59:96–102.

93. Veldhuis JD, Evans WS, Rogol AD, et al. Performance of LH pulse detection algorithms at rapid rates of venous sampling in humans. Am J Physiol 1984;247:554E–563E.

94. Mulligan T, Delemarre-van de Waal HA, Johnson ML, Veldhuis JD. Validation of deconvolution analysis of LH secretion and half-life. Am J Physiol 1994;267:R202–R211.

95. Veldhuis JD, Iranmanesh A, Demers LM, Mulligan T. Joint basal and pulsatile hypersecretory mechanisms drive the monotropic follicle-stimulating hormone (FSH) elevation in healthy older men: concurrent preservation of the orderliness of the FSH release process. J Clin Endocrinol Metab 1999;84:3506–3514.

96. Mulligan T, Iranmanesh A, Veldhuis JD. Pulsatile GnRH unmasks dual (hypothalamic and Leydig cell) defects in healthy older men. Presented at the American Geriatrics Society Annual Meeting Philadelphia PA, May 1999.

97. Zwart AD, Urban RJ, Odell WD, Veldhuis JD. Contrasts in the gonadotropin-releasing dose-response relationships for luteinizing hormone, follicle-stimulating hormone, and alpha-subunit release in young versus older men: appraisal with high-specificity immunoradiometric assay and deconvolution analysis. Eur J Endocrinol 1996;135:399–406.

98. Mulligan T, Iranmanesh A, Veldhuis JD. A novel acute hypoandrogenemic clamp abolishes the age difference in GnRH's dose-dependent stimulation of LH secretion and orderliness in older men. Presented at the Endocrine Society 83rd Meeting, Denver CO, June 20–23 2001.

99. Veldhuis JD, Rogol AD, Samojlik E, Ertel N. Role of endogenous opiates in the expression of negative feedback actions of estrogen and androgen on pulsatile properties of luteinizing hormone secretion in man. J Clin Invest 1984;74:47–55.

100. Santen RJ, Bardin CW. Episodic luteinizing hormone secretion in man. J Clin Invest 1973;52:2616–2618.

101. Urban RJ, Davis MR, Rogol AD, Johnson ML, Veldhuis JD. Acute androgen receptor blockade increases luteinizing-hormone secretory activity in men. J Clin Endocrinol Metab 1988;67:1149–1155.

102. Veldhuis JD, Carlson ML, Johnson ML. The pituitary gland secretes in bursts: appraising the nature of glandular secretory impulses by simultaneous multiple-parameter deconvolution of plasma hormone concentrations. Proc Natl Acad Sci USA 1987;84:7686–7690.

103. Veldhuis JD, Johnson ML. Deconvolution analysis of hormone data. Meth Enzymol 1992;210:539–575.

104. Veldhuis JD, Johnson ML. Specific methodological approaches to selected contemporary issues in deconvolution analysis of pulsatile neuroendocrine data. Meth Neurosci 1995;28:25–92.

105. Veldhuis JD, Moorman J, Johnson ML. Deconvolution analysis of neuroendocrine data: waveform-specific and waveform-independent methods and applications. Meth Neurosci 1994;20:279–325.

106. Veldhuis JD, Johnson ML. Cluster analysis: a simple versatile and robust algorithm for endocrine pulse detection. Am J Physiol 1986;250:E486–E493.

107. Veldhuis JD, Lassiter AB, Johnson ML. Operating behavior of dual or multiple endocrine pulse generators. Am J Physiol 1990;259:E351–E361.

108. Veldhuis JD, Keenan DM, Clarke I, Alexandre S, Irvine CHG. Estimation of endogenous luteinizing hormone-testosterone secretory coupling in three mammalian species. Presented at 27th Annual Meeting of American Society of Andrology Seattle, WA, April 24–27 2002.

109. Pincus SM. Approximate entropy as a measure of system complexity. Proc Natl Acad Sci USA 1991;88:2297–2301.

110. Pincus SM, Hartman ML, Roelfsema F, Thorner MO, Veldhuis JD. Hormone pulsatility discrimination via coarse and short time sampling. Am J Physiol 1999;277:E948–E957.

111. Veldhuis JD, Johnson ML, Veldhuis OL, Straume M, Pincus S. Impact of pulsatility on the ensemble orderliness (approximate entropy) of neurohormone secretion. Am J Physiol Reg Integr Comp Physiol 2001;281:R1975–R1985.

112. Pincus SM, Keefe DL. Quantification of hormone pulsatility via an approximate entropy algorithm. Am J Physiol 1992;262:E741–E754.

113. Veldhuis JD, Straume M, Iranmanesh A, et al. Secretory process regularity monitors neuroendocrine feedback and feedforward signaling strength in humans. Am J Physiol 2001;280:R721–R729.

114. Veldhuis JD, Pincus SM. Orderliness of hormone release patterns: a complementary measure to conventional pulsatile and circadian analyses. Eur J Endocrinol 1998;138:358–362.

115. Pincus SM, Veldhuis JD, Mulligan T, Iranmanesh A, Evans WS. Effects of age on the irregularity of LH and FSH serum concentrations in women and men. Am J Physiol 1997;273:E989–E995.

116. Veldhuis JD, Faunt LM, Johnson ML. Analysis of nonequilibrium dynamics of bound, free, and total plasma ligand concentrations over time following nonlinear secretory inputs: evaluation of the kinetics of two or more hormones pulsed into compartments containing multiple variable-affinity binding proteins. Meth Enzymol 1994;240:349–377.

117. Sodergard R, Backstrom T, Shanbhag V, Carstensen H. Calculation of free and bound fractions of testosterone and estradiol-17 beta to human plasma proteins at body temperature. J Steroid Biochem 1982;16:801–810.

118. Pardridge WM, Mietus LJ. Transport of steroid hormones through the rat blood-brain barrier. Primary role of albumin-bound hormone. J Clin Invest 1979;64:145–154.

119. Nankin HR, Calkins JH. Decreased bioavailable testosterone in aging normal and impotent men. J Clin Endocrinol Metab 1986;63:1418–1423.

120. Longcope C, Goldfield SRW, Brambilla DJ, McKinlay J. Androgens, estrogens, and sex hormone-binding globulin in middle-aged men. J Clin Endocrinol Metab 1990;71:1442–1446.

121. Manni A, Pardridge WM, Cefalu W, et al. Bioavailability of albumin-bound testosterone. J Clin Endocrinol Metab 1985;61:705–710.

122. Nahoul K, Roger M. Age-related decline of plasma bioavailable testosterone in adult men. J Steroid Biochem 1990;35:293–299.

123. Veldhuis JD, Urban RJ, Beitins I, Blizzard RM, Johnson ML, Dufau ML. Pathophysiological features of the pulsatile secretion of biologically active luteinizing hormone in man. J Steroid Biochem 1989;33:739–750.

15 Environmental Causes of Testicular Dysfunction

Richard M. Sharpe, *PhD*

CONTENTS

INTRODUCTION
ENVIRONMENTAL/LIFESTYLE EFFECTS ON THE ADULT MALE
ENVIRONMENTAL/LIFESTYLE EFFECTS ON THE ADULT TESTIS
   THAT ARISE DURING FETAL DEVELOPMENT
REFERENCES

INTRODUCTION

The notion that the environment can adversely affect male reproductive development and/or function is not an idea that most clinicians take seriously. There are probably good practical reasons for this stance; for example, few clinicians will have encountered patients in whom reproductive dysfunction was diagnosed as being altered by some environmental factor. Does this mean that such causes are rare or does it mean that they go unrecognized? Unfortunately, we probably still lack sufficient understanding to definitively answer this question, but hopefully this chapter will address it.

When viewed from an evolutionary perspective, it is clear that the environment and reproductive function are inextricably linked, as evidenced by the fact that the majority of mammals (seasonal breeders) exhibit seasonal hypogonadism and infertility under the influence of daylight length and other environmental cues *(1)*. Humans are not seasonal breeders, but as we undoubtedly have seasonally breeding ancestors somewhere in our evolutionary past, residues of such effects are likely, as discussed later in this chapter. Perhaps the most important lesson is that seasonal breeding evolved to ensure that offspring are born at the optimum time of year for survival, which usually equates to the availability of a good food supply. Thus, environmental factors, of which daylight is the most invariable, were adopted as cues to regulate function of the reproductive system—this seems to work primarily via central regulation of the hypothalamic–pituitary axis *(2)*. However, effects of the environment on reproduction are far more pervasive than this. The well-established relationship between food intake/energy balance and onset of puberty/maintenance of menstrual cycling in females is another example *(3)*, and the mechanisms by which these effects occur are now being established (e.g., leptin). These examples remind us that we have evolved to be in tune with our environment, and, if we accept this premise, we must

From: *Male Hypogonadism:*
Basic, Clinical, and Therapeutic Principles
Edited by: S. J. Winters © Humana Press Inc., Totowa, NJ

also recognize that when our environment or lifestyle change dramatically, there may be health consequences. The major changes in Western diet (increased intake of refined carbohydrates and diary products/fats) and lifestyle (e.g., widespread artificial light and increased sedentary habits) during the last century are, therefore, certain to have had some impact, but the extent to which these changes may have affected our general or reproductive health is unclear, with the notable exception of obesity and obesity-related disorders.

In the past decade, the specter of more widespread environmental adverse effects on male reproductive function have arisen, fueled by the possibility of falling sperm counts and increase in other male reproductive disorders (4,5). Although this is a some-what controversial topic, some aspects, such as the increase in incidence of testicular germ cell cancer during the past 50 yr or so, are beyond dispute. This increase must have a lifestyle/environmental cause, and the various possibilities are outlined here. There are strong beliefs that testis cancer may be the tip of an iceberg, signaling us about a more fundamental underlying syndrome of disorders (testicular dysgenesis syndrome) that may have a common origin in fetal life during the sexual differentiation process (6). Much of this is still hypothesis, but the evidence in its favor continues to grow. True or not, this hypothesized syndrome has played an important part in opening our eyes to the importance of fetal and neonatal life in setting up the reproductive system for adulthood more than a decade later. This reality is still not taken seriously by many, yet it is in step with thinking in other areas of medicine in which the fetal origins of adult disease are recognized increasingly as being of major importance (7). This puts the spotlight on the pregnant woman and, with the dramatic changes that have been occurring in women's lifestyles in the past two decades or so, it is inevitable that this must have lifelong consequences for the fetus. These may be good or bad, but if they adversely affect the reproductive health of the offspring (3), such effects can remain hidden for 30 or more years, with the result that recognition of the effect and its cause are made extremely difficult.

Finally, the media have made great play of the supposed dangers to the reproductive health of humans and wildlife from so-called endocrine disruptors. This is a broad and complex area with much controversy and uncertainty, but whether endocrine disruptors exert any significant effect on our reproductive health remains to be established (4,5,8). However, we must recognize that manmade products such as dichlorodiphenyltrichloroethene (DDT) and polychlorinated biphenyls (PCBs), which undoubtedly exert a range of biological effects in wildlife, persist in us all and are, to some extent, passed from one generation to the next via breast milk and the food chain. These and numerous other manmade chemicals are part of our everyday environment, and it is more likely than not that some of these compounds will have a biological effect on some of us. Such effects may be beneficial, adverse, or benign.

ENVIRONMENTAL/LIFESTYLE EFFECTS ON THE ADULT MALE

These effects fall into four different categories, namely the effects of season, occupation, lifestyle/diet, and chemical exposure (see Fig. 1). These effects are dealt with separately, but it is emphasized that they are not independent factors and that combinations of circumstances rather than individual factors may be more important in causing reproductive health changes. Similarly, some individuals may be predisposed

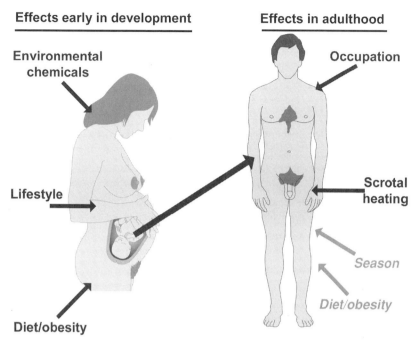

Fig. 1. Main environmental and lifestyle factors affecting testicular development and/or function. Items shown in black are probably the most important, whereas those shown in italics are probably of minor importance for most individuals.

to an adverse effect of a chemical or lifestyle factor, for example, because of their genetic background.

Seasonal Effects on Testicular Function

Although humans are considered to be nonseasonal mammals, we are undoubtedly sensitive to photoperiod *(9)*, as exemplified by seasonal affective disorder and by seasonal trends in the frequency of births and in the incidence of twins. Such effects are most obvious in northern Europe, where photoperiodic changes are most extreme *(10)*. Furthermore, both longitudinal and cross-sectional studies have demonstrated that sperm counts in men are consistently approx 30% lower in summer than in winter *(11,12)*, although not all studies have reported such effects, and they may be less apparent or absent in tropical countries *(13)*. An alternative explanation is that it is exposure to the higher summer temperature that is responsible for lowering sperm production (see section on scrotal temperature), although temperature changes do not account for all of the seasonal trends in births, especially in northern Europe *(3)*. If the reported seasonal changes in sperm counts are an echo from our seasonally breeding ancestors, then this may be variable in its effect and, in most men, is unlikely to exert any major effect on their fertility. Studies in seasonally breeding animals have established the key pathways by which daylight length can regulate the reproductive axis, and melatonin secreted by the pineal gland plays a pivotal role *(1,2)*. Therefore, it is curious that young men with hypogonadotropic hypogonadism show abnormal blood levels of melatonin, being increased in men with idiopathic hypogonadotropic hypogonadism

(IHH) and decreased in men with Kallmann syndrome, when compared with controls *(14)*. However, in both groups of patients, melatonin levels were normalized by testosterone replacement therapy, implying that the abnormal melatonin level was a consequence rather than a cause of the hypogonadotropic hypogonadism *(14)*.

Occupational Effects on Testicular Function: General Aspects

There have been numerous published studies that have retrospectively surveyed the occupations of men attending infertility clinics and/or compared occupations of fertile and infertile groups. There is some consensus in showing, for example, that farmers/agricultural workers or lorry drivers, painters, or welders may be overrepresented in infertile men *(15,16)*, but overall, the findings of such studies are inconsistent and have failed to identify common occupational causes of male infertility. Occupation is only one of a range of factors that may cause male infertility, and, therefore, searching for such factors in patients at the infertility clinic may not be the most sensitive approach. However, alternative approaches, such as direct investigation of particular working groups, also have various problems *(12)*. Low participation rates are common and may be biased toward those who have experienced, or suspect, a fertility problem *(17)*. These make interpretation of any findings difficult. Another common problem is the low numbers of workers who may eventually comprise the exposed or control groups, because many published studies involved 30–50 men or fewer per group *(12,18,19)*. As sperm counts and other semen parameters show great variation between subjects, detection of a workplace/occupational effect against such a background requires considerable numbers of subjects, otherwise, the study will lack sufficient power to detect anything other than a major change in semen parameters. For example, approx 80 control and exposed men would be required to detect a 20% fall in sperm count. Finally, there are likely to be many confounding factors in any occupational study. These may include age, ejaculatory frequency/abstinence, smoking and alcohol consumption, recreational drug use, time spent seated (see section on scrotal temperature), recent infection or febrile period, history of cryptorchidism, sexually transmitted disease, and so on *(20)*. Attempts can be made to control for some of these factors, but with the generally small numbers of subjects involved, this is inevitably less than satisfactory. Against this background, it is therefore not surprising that relatively few occupations or workplace exposures have been shown consistently to impact significantly on male reproductive health (usually on sperm counts/fertility). However, there is reasonable evidence to suggest that exposure to some solvents *(21)*, glycol ethers *(22)*, and inorganic lead *(23–25)* can affect one or more aspects of semen quality in exposed workers and, in some instances, affect fertility or miscarriage rates (although effects on the latter two parameters are small). Nevertheless, other studies that showed no significant effect of similar exposures can be found in the literature *(26,27)*. This would support the view that such workplace exposures have only minor effects on semen quality and male fertility, although in some individuals, such as those with a low sperm count for other reasons, such effects might significantly affect fertility.

Occupational/Environmental Exposure to Pesticides/Fungicides/PCBs

The occupational exposure that resulted in the greatest effect on sperm count and fertility was the workplace exposure to the nematocide dibromochloropropane (DBCP). This toxicant induced azoospermia or oligospermia in a high percentage of exposed workers, both those involved in its manufacture and those involved in its application on crops *(28–30)*. In a substantial proportion of DBCP-exposed workers who became azoospermic, no recovery of sperm counts occurred after removal from exposure *(28,29)*. This *lone* example is frequently cited as reassuring evidence of the rarity of such workplace effects on sperm counts and male fertility. In reality, this reassurance is a veil. The effects of DBCP were revealed, even though the affected workforces comprised fairly low numbers, because it had **catastrophic** effects on sperm counts/fertility. We can be reassured that similar catastrophes will also reveal themselves, but more modest effects of occupation on sperm counts/fertility will remain difficult or impossible to identify in all but large, well-controlled studies. The latter are hugely expensive and laborious, both of which act as strong deterrents to their application. In recognition of such obstacles, a multicenter European study (the Asclepios study) to investigate the effect of occupation on male reproductive health and fertility was initiated some years ago *(31)* and has been responsible for producing some of the most definitive data.

The DBCP example means that in nonscientific circles, the concept that pesticide exposure results in lowered sperm counts/infertility has become more or less accepted as dogma. In reality, there are relatively few studies that support this stance *(32–35)*, and many of these are studies in developing countries, where exposure controls may be less vigorous than in developed countries. Furthermore, there are numerous studies in which occupational pesticide exposure is associated with no change in semen quality and/or fertility and no effect on testosterone levels *(36–40)*; these include comparative studies of organic and nonorganic farmers. Although it is difficult to draw firm conclusions from these conflicting studies, it is reasonable to expect that occupational exposure to current, nonpersistent pesticides is unlikely to exert major adverse effects on semen quality and fertility in most men, but effects in individuals who might be exposed to unusually high pesticide levels should still be considered. Therefore, exposure of the general population to pesticides via contamination of food, etc. is likely to be considerably less than in men who are occupationally exposed and, consequently, risks of testicular dysfunction are extremely low. This may account for the lack of published evidence for any consistent relationship between subnormal semen quality and/or testosterone levels and pesticide exposure *(37,41,42)*, although two small recent studies have provided limited evidence for a negative relationship between semen parameters and PCB and/or dichlorodiphenylethane (DDE) levels in blood *(43,44)*.

Occupational/Lifestyle Effects on Scrotal Temperature

Another situation in which occupational effects on male reproductive function might become apparent is if the occupational effect applies to a large proportion of men. It is possible that scrotal heating may be one such example. Scrotal, and therefore testicular, temperature has to be maintained some 3–4°C lower than core body temperature if normal spermatogenesis is to occur (*see* Fig. 2), and interference with the normal scrotal cooling process can profoundly affect sperm production, quality, and fertility *(45,46)*. Interference with scrotal cooling is an effective male contraceptive *(47)*. Therefore, in theory, occupational or lifestyle factors that interfere with scrotal cooling/thermoregulation could be significant factors in lowering sperm counts *(48)*. Examples of such potential factors are exposure to radiant heat, wearing of tight trousers/underwear, time spent having hot baths, and time spent seated (*see* Fig. 2). Most of the older studies that sought to investigate such factors could rely only on establishing whether there was a

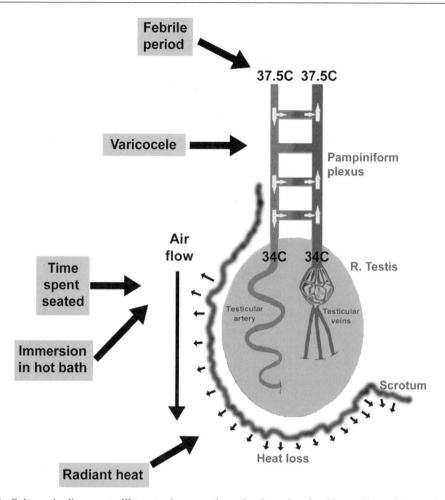

Fig. 2. Schematic diagram to illustrate the central mechanisms involved in cooling of the testis, and the various occupational or lifestyle factors that can interfere with their function. The primary mechanism of cooling the testis is by heat loss from the scrotum, and this necessitates air flow around it. The resulting cooling of the testis means that testicular venous blood is also cool when it leaves the testis and this blood is used to cool incoming warm arterial blood within the pampiniform plexus via heat exchange and via the diversion of approx 40% of incoming arterial blood into the testicular vein via numerous arteriovenous anastomoses; the presence of a varicocele may interfere with heat exchange within the pampiniform plexus. (For further details see ref. *69.*)

relationship between such factors and poor semen quality, and, perhaps not surprisingly, the evidence proved equivocal or only marginally convincing in most cases *(12)*. However, epidemiological studies did show that occupations involving prolonged sitting and, thus, reduction in air flow around the scrotum *(45,48)* were associated with significant reductions in sperm counts. An example is car or taxi driving *(49,50)*, although away from occupational situations, the worst case is probably paraplegic men who are confined to wheelchairs *(51)*.

More objective studies became possible once the technical problems relating to measurement of changes in scrotal temperature had been overcome, which enabled *quantification* of scrotal heating. Scrotal temperature was measured continuously in normal young men or in men from couples planning their first pregnancy, and a significant relationship between average daily scrotal temperature and sperm counts was established *(52)*. Moreover, the same studies linked scrotal temperature to the amount of time spent seated, i.e., the more sedentary the lifestyle/occupation, the higher the average scrotal temperature, and this has been confirmed in more extensive recent studies *(53)*. Application of continuous scrotal temperature monitoring in reasonably large numbers of healthy men has demonstrated unequivocally that increase in average scrotal temperature is clearly linked to lower sperm counts, as well as to associated changes in blood levels of follicle-stimulating hormone (FSH) and inhibin-B *(52–54)*. Such findings raised the expectation that our increasingly sedentary lifestyles in the West might induce negative effects on semen quality in a high proportion of men *(12)*, but this expectation is proving to be overly simplistic. For example, although time spent seated is an important determinant of scrotal temperature, the former has only a weak relationship with semen quality *(54)*, and other factors, such as nighttime scrotal temperature *(53)* and genetic determinants of scrotal temperature *(55)* may prove to be more important.

From a clinical perspective, the number of men in whom infertility is induced partly or totally by elevated scrotal temperature is likely to be low. However, there are three other points to keep in mind. First, even quite mild elevations in scrotal temperature in animal studies can increase miscarriage rates *(46)*, so its effects on sperm can be qualitative as well as quantitative. Second, treatment to lower overall scrotal temperature in patients who have poor semen quality, although being a shot in the dark, is relatively noninvasive and can be quite effective in some cases *(56)*—and there are no side effects! The discovery that there are genetic determinants of scrotal temperature *(55)* also reinforces the possibility that some individuals may be predisposed to adverse effects of prolonged seating or radiant heat on semen quality. Although such individuals cannot yet be recognized, careful attention to lifestyle factors to minimize scrotal heating in all men with fertility problems is therapeutically benign and can have only beneficial effects. Third, the well-established, if inconsistent, effect of a varicocele on semen quality in men may itself induce such effects by interfering with normal cooling of incoming arterial blood in the pampiniform plexus (*see* Fig. 2), and it is possible that such an effect might be exacerbated by the time spent seated or make such individuals more susceptible to effects of radiant heat than men without a varicocele.

Other Lifestyle/Dietary Factors Affecting the Adult Male

The preceding section dealing with scrotal temperature obviously applies as much to sedentary lifestyles outside, as well as inside, of the workplace. Probably the most important other factors are dietary habits, particularly obesity and alcohol intake, smoking, stress, and recreational/sporting drug use.

Unlike the well-established relationship between caloric intake and maintenance of menstrual cycles in women, there is no such clear relationship in men regarding sperm production and semen quality. However, obesity in men is clearly associated with a fall in total testosterone levels, and this may be severe in massively obese individuals *(57–60)*. One large study found no clear relationship between dietary factors and testosterone levels *(60)*, but one smaller study showed a positive relationship to carbohydrate intake *(59)*. Protein and fiber intake may also affect testosterone bioavailability via effects on sex hormone-binding globulin (SHBG) *(61)*. There is a well-established relationship between obesity, insulin resistance, and SHBG secretion *(62,63)*, but probably the most important pathways by which obesity affects testosterone levels are at the hypothalamic–pituitary level *(57)* and/or at the testicular level *(64)*. The latter study, as well as animal studies, have indicated a role for leptin in directly suppressing testosterone production by Leydig cells, so the inverse relationship between leptin and testosterone levels in obese and nonobese men *(64,65)* is perhaps indicative of cause and effect. For certain, there is an intriguing relationship emerging between sex steroids (particularly estradiol), fat stores/obesity, insulin resistance, and leptin levels *(63,65–67)*, but the precise cascade of events is unclear (*see* Chapter 17). Once this is better understood, it will hopefully shed more light on the relationship between increased abdominal obesity and lowering of testosterone levels with aging in men, as well as the ethnic differences in testosterone/SHBG/insulin levels and their relationship to adiposity and disease risk *(63)*.

Increased rates of smoking and alcohol intake are found in infertile couples *(68)*. Moreover, it is accepted that the normal testis is poised on the brink of hypoxia because of its unusual anatomy *(69)*, so, in theory, smoking is likely to compromise normal testicular function because it lowers the oxygen-carrying capacity of the blood. However, evidence to support this prediction is equivocal at best. Although smoking may sometimes emerge from epidemiology studies as a risk factor for low sperm counts or altered sperm morphology, this is an inconsistent finding *(70–72)*. Nevertheless, effects of male smoking on outcome of in vitro fertilization (IVF) have been reported *(73)*, as have effects on sperm morphology *(74)* and DNA damage *(75)*. Smoking may be associated with increased, rather than decreased, total (but not free) testosterone levels, probably through effects on SHBG *(59,76)*, and some *(77)*, but not all *(76)*, studies have reported higher estradiol levels in smokers. There is no consistent relationship between moderate alcohol intake and sperm counts in men *(59,78)*, but heavy alcohol intake is consistently associated with lowered testosterone levels *(79,80)*.

Stress arising for various reasons is frequently *(81–83)*, but not always *(84)*, associated with decrements in semen quality, with effects on both sperm counts and sperm motility. The mechanisms behind such changes are unclear. Stress is also widely considered to be associated with lowered testosterone levels in men, but the evidence to support this view is equivocal *(85–88)*. However, there is little doubt that the hypothalamic–pituitary–gonadal and hypothalamic–pituitary–adrenal axes exhibit cross-talk at various levels *(88)*, so that effects of stress on sex steroids and vice versa are expected.

Although Western men are generally less physically active today than they were 30 or so years ago, for those who do participate in sports, they are far more competitive today, and this has led to use of performance-enhancing drugs, the most common being anabolic androgenic steroids *(89–91)*. Outside of sports, the same drugs are used for improving physique and body image (*see* Chapter 16). New male contraceptive approaches also rely on systemic androgen administration (usually in combination with a progestogen) and, depending on the dose administered, it is well established that this will suppress production of endogenous testosterone and, hence, interfere with sperm production *(92)*. Similarly, individuals who use anabolic steroids are clearly at risk of hypogonadism *(90,93–95)*, but this is dependent on factors such as type of steroid, dose administered, and, perhaps, administration duration *(96)*. It is not clear how prevalent such hypogonadism may be, because much of the anabolic steroid use is

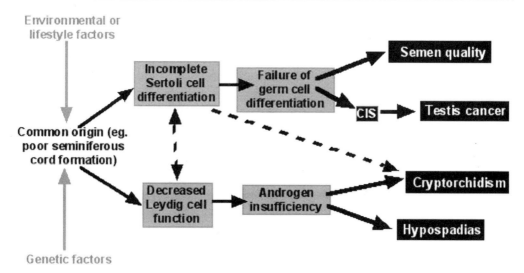

Fig. 3. Schematic diagram to illustrate the cellular basis and general pathways via which the disorders that comprise testicular dysgenesis syndrome (TDS) are likely to arise in the human. Abnormal testicular cell differentiation/function is an integral part of this syndrome of disorders, but several pathways might lead to this occurrence, including genetic, environmental, and/or lifestyle factors. Note also that the resultant disorders that arise because of TDS occur with differing frequency, varying from quite common (reduced sperm production, cryptorchidism) to rare (testis germ cell cancer). Note also that some of the disorders may occur for reasons other than TDS (e.g., low sperm counts). TDS may be associated with subnormal testosterone production and/or action, but note that neither the Sertoli cells nor germ cells are targets for testosterone action in fetal life *(104)*.

clandestine, but clinicians faced with athletic young men with hypogonadism should always consider this possibility. Similar awareness should be practiced for other nonsteroidal drugs, because we live in an age when use of a range of these recreational drugs is widespread, and some of these may adversely affect testosterone levels and/or sperm production *(97–100)*. Finally, vigorous exercise, such as long-distance running, may result in temporary suppression of testosterone levels in men and minor decrements in semen quality, but the changes are by no means as pronounced as the antireproductive effects that can occur in female athletes *(101,102)*.

ENVIRONMENTAL/LIFESTYLE EFFECTS ON THE ADULT TESTIS THAT ARISE DURING FETAL DEVELOPMENT

There is growing evidence that a syndrome of interconnected disorders affecting the human male, so-called testicular dysgenesis syndrome, may have a common origin in fetal life (Fig. 1) during the period of sexual differentiation *(68)*. Manifestations of this syndrome in adulthood can include low sperm counts/reduced fertility and/or testicular germ cell cancer, as well as a history of cryptorchidism and/or hypospadias *(see* Fig. 3); other potential aspects, such as lowered testosterone levels for life, remain to be clearly defined. Several of these disorders are increasing in incidence, with environmental/lifestyle causes implicated in this increase *(68)*. An integral part of this syndrome of disorders is evidence for impaired hormone production/action or abnormal hormone balance (e.g., between androgens and estrogens [5,8]) during the period of sexual differentiation and fetal development (see Fig. 3). These could arise for several reasons, for example because of intrauterine growth retardation (IUGR) of the affected fetus (5,8,103) or because of exposure of the mother to an environmental chemical with intrinsic hormonal activity or ones which may alter endogenous hormone levels (5,8). For numerous reasons, it is currently difficult to evaluate these various possibilities in a definitive way, so a brief overview of the available evidence that relates to environmental/lifestyle influences is presented. Further details and discussions can be found elsewhere (3,5,8).

It is perhaps not widely recognized that male reproductive development disorders are extremely common. For example, the two most common congenital malformations in children of either sex are both male sexual differentiation disorders, namely cryptorchidism and hypospadias, which affect 2–4% and 0.3–0.7% of boys at birth, respectively (8). This reminds us that development of the male reproductive system does not occur by default, as is largely the case in the female, but instead requires the timely production and action of hormones by the fetal testis—mainly testosterone but also anti-Müllerian hormone and insulin-like factor-3 (INSL-3) (5,8,104). Any dietary, lifestyle, or environmental exposures that act through the mother to affect general growth or timing of growth of the fetus or hormone production by the fetal testis can therefore potentially affect development of the reproductive system of the male fetus. For example, IUGR is associated with increased risk of both cryptorchidism and hypospadias (8,103,105). In turn, these disorders have important lifelong consequences in terms of risk of infertility/low sperm counts and of developing testicular germ cell cancer in adulthood (4,8,106,107) (see Fig. 3).

Maternal lifestyle can be an important determinant of IUGR and of fetal growth in general (3). Smoking by the pregnant mother has well-established effects on fetal growth, which can, in turn, alter risk of a range of disorders of the fetus when it has grown to adulthood (7)—these can include effects on fertility, but these are most obvious in female offspring (3). However, there is evidence that maternal smoking can adversely affect sperm counts of male offspring in adulthood (108). More generally, the trend to obesity in Western countries means that when these women become pregnant, there is increased risk of fetal growth problems, presumably resulting from the insulin resistance that accompanies obesity (3,7).

Environmental Endocrine-Active Chemicals

The issue of environmental endocrine-active chemicals has received enormous attention during the past decade, and all manner of claims made that such compounds can affect human health, particularly male reproductive health. The primary focus has been on environmental estrogens, but it is unlikely that the compounds so far identified are potent enough to affect male reproductive development because of any intrinsic estrogenicity (5,8). Whether combinations of such chemicals could affect male reproductive development is less certain and is difficult to evaluate meaningfully. However, the focus of attention has now switched to environmental chemicals that can alter endogenous hormones and, as any clinical endocrinologist will know, when endogenous hormone levels/action are disturbed, disorders invariably result. The example most relevant to male reproductive development is exposure to certain phthalate esters (104). These compounds have numerous uses and are the most ubiquitous of all environmental chemicals, so human exposure is quite high *(109)*. When rats are treated with certain phthalates during the last week of pregnancy, which encompasses the period of sexual differentiation of the fetuses, the male offspring show a high incidence of cryptorchidism and hypospadias at birth and have reduced testis size in adulthood, which result in reduced sperm production *(104,110,111)*. Although the cascade of events that leads to these disorders is not fully established, one important change is suppression of testosterone production by the fetal testis *(104,111)*. Indeed, the spectrum of changes in male offspring that is induced by phthalate treatment in pregnancy is remarkably similar to testicular dysgenesis syndrome in humans (*see* Fig. 3) and may provide a model system through which to study this hypothesized human syndrome *(104)*. Whether human exposure to phthalates causes this syndrome remains to be explored. The doses of phthalates used to induce a high prevalence of male reproductive disorders in rats certainly exceeds known human exposure levels *(104)*, but a recent study has identified a subset of humans who have considerably higher exposure to relevant phthalates, and these were predominantly women of reproductive age *(109)*. The suspicion is that the high exposure results from use of phthalates in cosmetics, shampoos, and other beauty aids. Until there are data to indicate whether humans are susceptible to similar effects of phthalates as are rats, and, our relative sensitivity to them, it is not possible to determine the risk to human health from these compounds.

Altered Estrogen Levels During Pregnancy

Another mechanism by which reproductive development of the male fetus might be adversely affected is by altered exposure to maternal/placental estrogens during pregnancy *(5)*. There is evidence that the risk of cryptorchidism and testicular germ cell cancer are both increased in twin and first pregnancies in which estrogen levels are higher and administration of the potent estrogen diethylstibestrol (DES) to pregnant women also increased risk of these disorders in the offspring *(4,5,8)*. The relationship between circulating estrogen levels in the pregnant mother and levels in target organs in the fetus is unclear, but maternal factors that could alter estrogen bioavailability could (in theory) increase fetal estrogen exposure. Therefore, dietary factors in the mother may be influential, because obesity and associated insulin resistance are well established to lower levels of SHBG, which, in turn, will affect the levels of free estrogen and androgen and influence the androgen-estrogen balance. More recently, another environmental mechanism has emerged through which maternal/fetal estrogen levels during pregnancy could be altered, at least in theory. Two classes of environmental chemicals *(112,113)* to which there is universally high human exposure are both potent suppressors of estrogen sulfotransferase (SULT1E1). The latter is the main pathway by which estrogens are inactivated as a prelude to their excretion *(114)*, so inhibition of this enzyme is likely to increase estrogen levels. The compounds in question are polyhalogenated hydrocarbons (PAHs), found in combustion/exhaust/tobacco smoke, and PCBs, which are now banned but are still widely present in the environment because of their persistence and lipophilicity *(112,113)*. The risk, if any, to humans and to the reproductive development of the fetus from exposure to such compounds remains unknown, but these examples serve as useful reminders to us that there may be other (and perhaps more important) presently unknown pathways by which environmental/lifestyle factors may affect the fetus, or even the adult male, by perturbation of endogenous hormone action.

Testicular Germ Cell Cancer and Its Fetal Origins

As evident from the discussion in the section on environmental and lifestyle effects, the importance (and mechanisms) of male fetal induction of testicular dysfunction remains speculative. This is partly because it is still a new area and partly because of the inherent difficulties in establishing cause and effect involving the human fetus, particularly when any outcome, such as infertility/low sperm counts, may not manifest for two or more decades. Nevertheless, there is a good and proven example of a major human testicular disorder that involves fetal induction and adult manifestation, and this is testicular germ cell cancer (testis cancer) *(115)*. It is now established as firmly as possible that these cancers arise from premalignant transformed fetal germ cells (primordial germ cells or gonocytes) that are termed carcinoma-in-situ (CIS) cells *(107,115–117)* (*see* Fig. 3). The latter express numerous proteins that are also expressed by fetal germ cells but not by spermatogonia and other germ cells in the adult testis *(115–117)*. For unknown reasons, affected fetal germ cells fail to differentiate normally into spermatogonia and, thus, retain many stem cell features, and their subsequent development results in their unstable transformation. These cells remain quiescent in the testis until puberty, when their multiplication is stimulated (presumably) by the same growth factors as are normal germ cells during spermatogenesis. Eventually, a germ cell tumor results. This is usually in the age range 15–45 yr, with a peak incidence at 25–30 yr *(118,119)*. In most Western countries, testis cancer is the most common cancer of young (white) men and, were it not for the tremendous success of treatment (90% success rate), it would be the biggest killer of young men after road traffic accidents *(120,121)*.

There are two particularly intriguing aspects to testis cancer that make it highly relevant to this chapter. First, its incidence in young men has increased inexorably during the past 50–65 yr at least, and this increase is clearly linked to later year of birth *(119,121)*. For example, a man born in Finland in 1965 has a more than 10-fold higher risk of developing testis cancer than a man born in Finland in 1905 *(119)*. This increase owes nothing to better diagnosis or that we are living longer (it is a cancer of young men). In most Western countries, the incidence of testis cancer has doubled every 20–35 yr and a rapid increase like this can only have an environmental or lifestyle cause. However, it is equally clear that there is a genetic or ethnic component that predetermines testis cancer risk, because American blacks have a considerably lower incidence than do American whites *(121,122)*. There are also other geographic (possibly ethnic) differences in testis cancer incidence, such as Oriental men having a lower incidence than Western Caucasian men *(4)*, Finnish men having a fourfold lower incidence than Danish men *(118,119)*. Most of the identified risk factors for testis cancer are prenatal factors *(4,6,8,123)*, and many of these factors are shared with those for cryptorchidism, hypospadias, and low sperm counts/infertility *(6,8,106,123)*, which may also be increasing in incidence *(4,8,103,124–126)*. Observations such as this give rise to the concept of a testicular dysgenesis syndrome that may have several manifestations but a common underlying mechanism *(6)* (*see* Fig. 3). Indeed, this line of thinking can also encompass the ethnic differences in testis cancer incidence, reflecting factors such as genetic differences in hormone levels during pregnancy, or other factors that affect the intrauterine environment *(8,123,127)*. Unfortunately, what is still lacking is a mechanistic appreciation of how ethnic and environmental/lifestyle factors affect the developing reproductive system of the fetus, other than knowing that effects on androgens and/or estrogens are probably involved somewhere in the chain of events

(5,8). If this was understood, then appropriate changes to lifestyle or diet could be recommended to minimize risk to the male offspring.

Future Prospects

The concept that male reproductive dysfunction in adulthood may have its origins in fetal or neonatal life is in line with the evolution in thinking about the origins of other common medical disorders, such as cardiovascular disease and type 2 diabetes. This concept is poised to grow and to embrace more aspects of male reproductive health. For example, it is notable that some ethnic groups with a low risk of developing testis cancer have a correspondingly higher risk of developing prostate cancer—this applies both to American blacks and to Finnish men *(121).* Because androgen exposure is implicated in both disorders, low exposure equating to increased risk of testis cancer and high exposure to increased risk of prostate cancer, the notion that androgen exposure of the developing male fetus (this exposure remaining to be defined) may predetermine susceptibility to reproductive dysfunction becomes attractive. This is not to imply that *all* male reproductive dysfunction has its origins in fetal life, but rather to indicate that susceptibilities are put in place that may then predispose to effects by other genetic, environmental, or lifestyle factors—these may exert their effects at various stages in life or throughout long periods of life. There is nothing remotely controversial in such thinking, because all human health disorders ultimately result from an interaction between genetic and environmental/lifestyle factors.

An important (and overlooked) aspect of the environmental/lifestyle components is that they are intrinsically preventable. However, before this possibility can be realized, the causative factor has to be identified and its mechanism established. As this chapter has hopefully demonstrated, we are a long way from achieving this for most environmental and lifestyle factors that affect male reproductive health. The exception is time spent seated and scrotal heating, and methods and studies are now in place that are defining precisely the risk to sperm counts and whether this affects fertility, sperm DNA damage, and so on. Once this is completed, a proper risk assessment can be made and appropriate action recommended—whether it will be taken or enforced remains to be seen.

REFERENCES

1. Lincoln GA, Short RV. Seasonal breeding: nature's contraceptive. Rec Progr Horm Res 1980;36:1–52.
2. Lincoln GA, Rhind SM, Pompolo S, Clarke IJ. Hypothalamic control of photoepriod-induced cycles in food intake, body weight and metabolic hormones in rams. Am J Physiol Reg Integr Comp Physiol 2001;281:R76–R90.
3. Sharpe RM, Franks S. Environment, lifestyle and human infertility—an inter-generational issue. Nature Med Cell Biol 2002;14(suppl 1):s33–s40.
4. Toppari J, Larsen JC, Christiansen P, et al. Male reproductive health and environmental xenoestrogens. Environ Health Perspect 1996;104(suppl 4):741–803.
5. Sharpe RM. The oestrogen hypothesis—where do we stand now? Int J Androl 2002;26:2–15.
6. Skakkebaek NE, Rajpert-de Meyts E, Main KM. Testicular dysgenesis syndrome: an increasingly common developmental disorder with environmental aspects. Hum Reprod 2001;16:972–978.
7. O'Brien PMS, Wheeler T, Barker DJP, (ed). Fetal Programming: Influences on Development and Disease in Later Life. Royal College of Obstetricians & Gynaecologists Press, London, 1999.
8. Sharpe RM, Skakkebaek NE. Male reproductive disorders and the role of endocrine disruption: advances in understanding and identification of areas for future research. Pure Appl Chem 2003, in press.

9. Rojansky N, Brzezinski A, Schenker JG. Seasonality in human reproduction: an update. Hum Reprod 1992;7:735–745.

10. Rojansky N, Benshushan A, Meisdorf S, Lewin A, Laufer N, Safran A. Seasonal variability in fertilization and embryo quality rates in women undergoing IVF. Fertil Steril 2000;74:476–481.

11. Jorgensen N, Andersen A-G, Eustache F, et al. Regional differences in semen quality in Europe. Hum Reprod 2001;16:1012–1019.

12. Sharpe RM. Environment, lifestyle and male infertility. Baillieres Clin Endocrinol Metab 2000;14:489–503.

13. Chia SE, Lim ST, Ho LM, Tay SK. Monthly variation in human semen quality in male partners of infertile women in the tropics. Hum Reprod 2001;16:277–281.

14. Luboshitzky R, Wagner O, Lavi S, Here P, Lavie P. Abnormal melatonin secretion in hypogonadal men: the effect of testosterone treatment. Clin Endocrinol 1997;47:463–469.

15. Henderson J, Rennie GC, Baker HWG. Association between occupational group and sperm concentration in infertile men. Clin Reprod Fertil 1986;4:275–281.

16. Kenkel S, Rolf C, Nieschlag E. Occupational risks for male fertility: an analysis of patients attending a tertiary referral centre. Int J Androl 2001;24:318–326.

17. Larsen SB, Abell A, Bonde JP. Selection bias in occupational sperm studies. Am J Epidemiol 1998;147:681–685.

18. Grajewski B, Cox C, Scrader SM, et al. Semen quality and hormone levels among radiofrequency heater operators. J Occup Environ Med 2000;42:993–1005.

19. Wang SL, Wang XR, Chia SE, et al. A study of occupational exposure to petrochemicals and smoking on semen quality. J Androl 2001;22:73–78.

20. Tas S, Lauwerys R, Lison D. Occupational hazards for the male reproductive system. Crit Rev Toxicol 1996;26:261–307.

21. Cherry N, Labreche F, Collins J, Tulandi T. Occupational exposure to solvents and male infertility. Occup Environ Med 2001;58:635–640.

22. Welch LS, Schrader SM, Turner TW, Cullen MR. Effects of exposure to ethylene glycol ethers on shipyard painters: II. Male reproduction. Am J Ind Med 1988;14:509–526.

23. Apostoli P, Kiss P, Porru S, Bonde JP, Vanhoorne M. Male reproductive toxicity of lead in animals and humans. ASCLEPIOS study group. Occup Environ Med 1998;55:364–374.

24. Sallmen M, Lindbohm ML, Anttila A, Taskinen H, Hemminski K. Time to pregnancy among the wives of men occupationally exposed to lead. Epidemiology 2000;11:141–147.

25. Bonde JP, Joffe M, Apostoli P, et al. Sperm chromatin structure in men exposed to inroganic lead: lowest adverse effect levels. Occup Environ Med 2002;59:234–242.

26. Kolstad HA, Bonde JP, Spano M, et al. Change in semen quality and sperm chromatin structure following occupational styrene exposure. ASCLEPIOS. Int Arch Occup Environ Health 1999;72:135–141.

27. Lemasters GK, Olsen DM, Yiin JH, et al. Male reproductive effects of solvent and fuel exposure during aircraft maintenance. Reprod Toxicol 1999;13:155–166.

28. Eaton M, Schenker M, Whorton MD, Samuels S, Perkins C, Overstreet J. Seven-year follow-up of workers exposed to 1,2-dibromo-3-chloropropane. J Occup Med 1986;28:1145–1150.

29. Potashnik G, Portah A. Dibromochloropropane (DBCP): a 17-year reassessment of testicular function and reproductive performance. J Occup Environ Med 1995;37:1287–1292.

30. Goldsmith JR. Dibromochloropropane: epidemiological findings and current questions. Ann N Y Acad Sci 1997;837:300–306.

31. Bonde JP, Joffe M, Danscher G, et al. Objectives, designs and populations of the European Asclepios study on occupational hazards to male reproductive capability. Scand J Work Environ Health 1999;25(suppl 1):49–61.

32. Lerda D, Rizzi R. Study of reproductive function in persons occupationally exposed to 2,4-dichlorophenoxyacetic acid (2,4-D). Mutat Res 1991;262:47–50.

33. Rupa DS, Reddy PP, Reddi OS. Reproductive performance in population exposed to pesticides in cotton fields in India. Environ Res 1991;55:123–128.

34. Abell A, Ernst E, Bonde JP. Semen quality and sexual hormones in greenhouse workers. Scand J Work Environ Helath 2000;26:492–500.

35. Padungtod C, Savitz DA, Overstreet JW, Christiani DC, Ryan LM, Xu X. Occupational pesticide exposure and semen quality among Chinese workers. J Occup Environ Health 2000;42:982–992.

36. Gerber WL, de la Pena VE, Mobley WC. Infertility, chemical exposure and farming in Iowa: absence of an association. Urology 1988;31:46–50.

37. Juhler RK, Larsen SB, Meyer O, et al. Human semen quality in relation to dietary pesticide exposure and organic diet. Arch Environ Contam Toxicol 1999;37:415–423.
38. Larsen SB, Joffe M, Bonde JP. Time to pregnancy and exposure to pesticides in Danish farmers. ASCLEPIOS study group. Occup Environ Med 1998;55:278–283.
39. Larsen SB, Spano M, Giwercman A, Bonde JP. Semen quality and sex hormones among organic and traditional Danish farmers. ASCLEPIOS study group. Occup Environ Med 1999;56:139–144.
40. Thonneau P, Abell A, Larsen SB, et al. Effects of pesticide exposure on time to pregnancy: results of a multicenter study in France and Denmark. ASCLEPIOS study group. Am J Epidemiol 1999;150:157–163.
41. Hagmar L, Bjork J, Sjodin A, Bergman A, Erfurth EM. Plasma levels of persistent organohalogens and hormone levels in adult male humans. Arch Environ Health 2001;56:138–143.
42. Martin SA, Jr, Harlow SD, Sowers MF, et al. DDT metabolite and androgens in African-American farmers. Epidemiology 2002;13:454–458.
43. Dallinga JW, Moonen EJC, Dumoulin JCM, Evers JLH, Geraedts JPM, Kleinjans JCS. Decreased human semen quality and organochlorine compounds in blood. Hum Reprod 2002;17:1973–1979.
44. Hauser R, Atlshul L, Chen Z, et al. Environmental organochlorines and semen quality: results of a pilot study. Environ Health Perspect 2002;110:229–233.
45. Mieusset R, Bujan L. Testicular heating and its possible contributions to male infertility: a review. Int J Androl 1995;18:169–184.
46. Setchell BP. Heat and the testis. J Reprod Fertil 1998;114:179–184.
47. Mieusset R, Bujan L. The potential of mild testicular heating as a safe, effective and reversible contraceptive method for men. Int J Androl 1995;17:186–191.
48. Thonneau P, Bujan L, Multigner L, Mieusset R. Occupational heat exposure and male fertility: a review. Hum Reprod 1998;13:2122–2125.
49. Figa-Talamanca I, Cini C, Varricchio GC, et al. Effects of prolonged autovehicle driving on male reproductive function: a study among taxi drivers. Am J Ind Med 1996;30:750–758.
50. Bujan L, Daudin M, Charlet J-P, Thonneau P, Mieusset R. Increase in scrotal temperature in car drivers. Hum Reprod 2000;15:1355–1357.
51. Brindley GS. Deep scrotal temperature and the effect on it of clothing, air temperature, activity, posture and paraplegia. Br J Urol 1982;54:49–55.
52. Hjollund NH, Bonde JP, Jensen TK, Olsen J. Diurnal scrotal skin temperature and semen quality. The Danish first pregnancy planner study team. Int J Androl 2000;23:309–318.
53. Hjollund NH, Storgaard L, Ernst E, Bonde JP, Olsen J. The relation between daily activities and scrotal temperature. Reprod Toxicol 2002;16:209–214.
54. Hjollund NH, Storgaard L, Ernst E, Bonde JP, Olsen J. Impact of diurnal scrotal temperature on semen quality. Reprod Toxicol 2002;16:215–221.
55. Hjollund NH, Storgaard L, Ernst E, Bonde JP, Christensen K, Olsen J. Correlation of scrotal temperature in twins. Hum Reprod 2002;17:1837–1838.
56. Jung A, Eberl M, Schill WB. Improvement of semen quality by nocturnal scrotal cooling and moderate behavioural change to reduce genital heat stress in men with oligoasthenoteratozoospermia. Reproduction 2001;121:595–603.
57. Vermeulen A. Decreased androgen levels and obesity in men. Ann Med 1996;28:13–15.
58. Bray GA. Obesity and reproduction. Hum Reprod 1997;12(suppl 1):26–32.
59. Tamimi R, Mucci LA, Spanos E, Lagiou A, Benetou V, Trichopoulos D. Testosterone and oestradiol in relation to tobacco smoking, body mass index, energy consumption and nutrient intake among adult men. Eur J Cancer Prev 2001;10:275–280.
60. Allen NE, Appleby PN, Davey GK, Key TJ. Lifestyle and nutritional determinants of bioavailable androgens and related hormones in British men. Cancer Causes Control 2002;13:353–363.
61. Longcope C, Feldman HA, McKinlay JB, Araujo AB. Diet and sex hormone-binding globulin. J Clin Endocrinol Metab 2000;85:293–296.
62. Haffner SM. Sex hormone-binding protein, hyper-insulinaemia, insulin resistance and noninsulin-dependent diabetes. Horm Res 1996;45:233–237.
63. Winters SJ, Brufsky A, Weissfeld J, Trump DL, Dyky MA, Hadeed V. Testosterone, sex hormone-binding globulin and body composition in young adult African American and Caucasian men. Metabolism 2001;50:1242–1247.
64. Isidori AM, Caprio M, Strollo F, et al. Leptin and androgen levels in male obesity: evidence for leptin contribution to reduced androgen levels. J Clin Endocrinol Metab 1999;84:3673–3680.

65. Lagiou P, Signorello LB, Manmtzoros CS, Trichopoulos D, Hsieh CC, Trichopoulou A. Hormonal, lifestyle and dietary factors in relation to leptin among elderly men. Ann Nutr Metb 1999;43:23–29.

66. Grumbach MM, Auchus RJ. Estrogen: consequences and implications of human mutations in synthesis and action. J Clin Endocrinol Metab 1999;84:4677–4694.

67. Cooke PS, Heine PA, Taylor JA, Lubahn DB. The role of estrogen and estrogen receptor-alpha in male adipose tissue. Mol Cell Endocrinol 2001;178:147–154.

68. Guzick DS, Overstreet JW, Factor-Litvack P, et al. Sperm morphology, motility and concentration in fertile and infertile men. N Engl J Med 2001;345:1388–1393.

69. Sharpe RM, Millar MR, Maddocks SM, Clegg J. Transport mechanisms for endocrine and paracrine factors in the testis. In: Desjardins C, ed. Cellular and Molecular Regulation of Testicular Cells. Springer-Verlag, New York, 1996, pp. 249–259.

70. Hughes EG, Brennan BG. Does smoking impair natural or assisted fecundity? Fertil Steril 1996;66:679–689.

71. Vine MF. Smoking and male reproduction: a review. Int J Androl 1996;19:323–337.

72. Zhang JP, Meng QY, Wang Q, Zhang LJ, Mao YL, Sun ZX. Effect of smoking on semen quality of infertile men in Shandong, China. Asian J Androl 2000;2:143–146.

73. Joesbury KA, Edirisinghe WR, Phillips MR, Yovich JL. Evidence that male smoking affects the likelihood of a pregnancy following IVF treatment: application of the modified cumulative embryo score. Hum Reprod 1998;13:1506–1513.

74. Wong WY, Thomas CM, Merkus HM, Zielhuis GA, Doesburg WH, Steegers-Theunissen RP. Cigarette smoking and the risk of male factor subfertility: minor association between cotinine in seminal plasma and semen morphology. Fertil Steril 2000;74:930–935.

75. Rubes J, Lowe X, Moore D II, et al. Smoking cigarettes is associated with increased sperm disomy in teenage men. Fertil Steril 1998;70:715–723.

76. English KM, Pugh PJ, Parry H, Scutt NE, Channer KS, Jones TH. Effect of cigarette smoking on levels of bioavailable testosterone in healthy men. Clin Sci 2001;100:661–665.

77. Barrett-Connor E, Khaw KT. Cigarette smoking and increased endogenous estrogen levels in men. Am J Epidemiol 1987;126:187–192.

78. Irvine DS. Epidemiology and aetiology of male infertility. Hum Reprod 1998;Suppl 1:33–44.

79. Castilla-Garcia A, Santolaria-Fernandez FJ, Gonzalez-Reimers CE, et al. Alcohol-induced hypogonadism: reversal after ethanol withdrawal. Drug Alcohol Depend 1987;20:255–260.

80. Emanuele MA, Emanuele N. Alcohol and the male reproductive system. Alcohol Res Health 2001;25:282–287.

81. Fenster L, Katz DF, Wyrobeck AJ, et al. Effects of psychological stress on human semen quality. J Androl 1997;18:194–202.

82. Clarke RN, Klock SC, Geoghegan A, Travassos DE. Relationship between psychological stress and semen quality among in-vitro fertilization patients. Hum Reprod 1999;14:753–758.

83. Gerhard I, Lenhard K, Eggert-Kruse W, Runnebaum B. Clinicla data which influence semen parameters in infertile men. Hum Reprod 1992;7:830–837.

84. Poland ML, Giblin PT, Ager JW, Moghissi KS. Effect of stress on semen quality in semen donors. Int J Fertil 1986;31:229–231.

85. Francis KT. The relationship between high and low trait psychological stress, serum testosterone and serum cortisol. Experientia 1981;37:1296–1297.

86. Semple CG, Gray CE, Borland W, Espie CA, Beastall GH. Endocrine effects of examination stress. Clin Sci 1988;74:255–259.

87. Schulz P, Walker JP, Peyrin L, Soulier V, Curtin F, Steimer T. Lower sex hormones in men during anticipatory stress. Neuroreport 1996;7:3101–3104.

88. Viau V. Functional cross-talk between the hypothalamic-pituitary-gonadal and -adrenal axes. J Neuroendocrinol 2002;14:506–513.

89. Lukas SE. Current perspectives on anabolic-androgenic steroid abuse. Trends Pharmacol Sci 1993;14:61–68.

90. Huhtaniemi IP. Anabolic-androgenic steroids—a double edged sword. Int J Androl 1994;17:57–62.

91. Copeland J, Peters R, Dillon P. Anabolic-androgenic steroid use disorders among a sample of Australian competitive and recreational users. Drug Alcohol Depend 2000;60:91–96.

92. Anderson RA, Baird DT. Male contraception. Endocr Rev 2002;23:735–762.

93. Turek PJ, Williams RH, Gilbaugh JH, 3rd, Lipshultz LI. The reversibility of anabolic steroid-induced azoospermia. J Urol 1995;153:1628–1630.

94. Gazvani MR, Buckett W, Luckas MJ, Aird IA, Hipkin LJ, Lewis-Jones DI. Conservative management of azoospermia following steroid abuse. Hum Reprod 1997;12:1706–1708.

95. Boyadjiev NP, Georgieva KN, Massaldjieva RI, Gueorguiev SI. Reversible hypogonadism and azoospermia as a result of anabolic-androgenic steroid use in a bodybuilder with personality disorder. A case report. J Sports Med Phys Fitness 2000;40:271–274.

96. Wu FCW. Endocrine aspects of anabolic steroids. Clin Chem 1997;43:1289–1292.

97. Ragni G, De Lauretis L, Bestetti O, Sghedoni D, Gambaro V. Gonadal function in male heroin and methadone addicts. Int J Androl 1988;11:93–100.

98. Barnett G, Chiang CW, Licko V. Effects of marijuana on testosterone in male subjects. J Theor Biol 1983;104:685–692.

99. Harclerode J. Endocrine effects of marijuana in the male: preclinical studies. NIDA Res Monogr 1984;44:46–64.

100. Maykut MO. Health consequences of acute and chronic marihuana use. Prog Neuropsychopharmacol Biol Psychiatry 1985;9:209–238.

101. Elias AN, Wilson AF. Exercise and gonadal function. Hum Reprod 1993;8:1747–1761.

102. De Souza MJ, Arce JC, Pescatello LS, Scherzer HS, Luciano AA. Gonadal hormones and semen quality in male runners. A volume threshold effect of endurance training. Int J Sports Med 1994;15:383–391.

103. Hussain N, Chaghtai A, Herndon CD, Herson VC, Rosenkrantz TS, McKenna PH. Hypospadias and early gestation growth restriction in infants. Pediatrics 2002;109:473–478.

104. Sharpe RM. Hormones and testis development and the possible adverse effects of environmental chemicals. Toxicol Lett 2001;120:221–232.

105. Weidner IS, Moller H, Jensen TK, Skakkebaek NE. Risk factors for cryptorchidism and hypospadias. J Urol 1999;161:1606–1609.

106. Moller H, Skakkebaek NE. Risk of testicular cancer in subfertile men: case-control study. Br Med J 1999;318:559–562.

107. Dieckmann KP, Skakkebaek NE. Carcinoma in situ of the testis: review of biological and clinical features. Int J Cancer 1999;83:815–822.

108. Jensen TK, Henriksen TB, Hjollund NH, et al. Adult and prenatal exposures to tobacco smoke as risk indicators of fertility among 430 Danish couples. Am J Epidemiol 1998;148:992–997.

109. Blount BC, Silva MJ, Caudhill SP, et al. Levels of seven urinary phthalate metabolites in a human reference population. Environ Health Perspect 2000;108:979–982.

110. Mylchreest E, Wallace DG, Cattley RC, Foster PMD. Dose-dependent alterations in androgen-regulated male reproductive development in rats exposed to Di(n-butyl) phthalate during late gestation. Toxicol Sci 2000;55:143–151.

111. Parks LG, Ostby JS, Lambright CR, et al. The plasticizer diethylhexyl phthalate induces malformations by decreasing fetal testosterone synthesis during sexual differentiation in the male rat. Toxicol Sci 2000;58:339–349.

112. Kester MHA, Bulduck S, Tibboel D, et al. Potent inhibition of estrogen sulfotransferase by hydroxylated PCB metabolites: a novel pathway explaining the estrogenic activity of PCBs. Endocrinology 2000;141:1897–1900.

113. Kester MHA, Bulduck S, van Toor H, et al. Potent inhibition of estrogen sulfotransferase by hydroxylated metabolites of polyhalogenated aromatic hydrocarbons reveals alternative mechanism for estrogenic activity of endocrine disrupters. J Clin Endocrinol Metab 2002;87:1142–1150.

114. Song WC. Biochemistry and reproductive endocrinology of estrogen sulfotransferase. Ann N Y Acad Sci 2001;948:43–50.

115. Skakkebaek NE, Berthelsen JG, Giwercman A, Muller J. Carcinoma-in-situ of the testis: possible origin from gonocytes and precursor of all types of germ cell tumours except spermatocytoma. Int J Androl 1987;10:19–28.

116. Rajpert-de Meyts E, Jorgensen N, Nielsen KB, Muller J, Skakkebaek NE. Developmental arrest of germ cells in the pathogenesis of germ cell neoplasia. APMIS 1998;106:198–206.

117. Rorth M, Rajpert-de Meyts E, Andersson L, et al. Carcinoma in situ of the testis. Scand J Urol Nephrol 2000;205:166–186.

118. Adami H, Bergstrom R, Mohner M, et al. Testicular cancer in nine Northern European countries. Int J Cancer 1994;59:33–38.

119. Bergstrom R, Adami H, Mohner M, et al. Increase in testicular cancer incidence in six European countries: a birth cohort phenomenon. J Natl Cancer Inst 1996;88:727–733.

120. Bray F, Sankijo R, Ferlay J, Parkin DH. Estimates of cancer incidence and mortality in Europe in 1995. Eur J Cancer 2002;38:99–166.

121. SEER (Surveillance, Epidemiology and End Results; National Cancer Institute, USA). Incidence and age-adjusted rates of testis cancer 1973–1999. Available at: http://seer.cancer.gov. 2002. Accessed April 2002.

122. Zheng T, Holford TR, Ma Z, Ward BA, Flannery J, Boyle P. Continuing increase in incidence of germ-cell testis cancer in young adults: experience from Connecticut, USA. Int J Cancer 1996;65:723–729.

123. Swerdlow AJ, De Stavola BL, Swanwick MA, Maconochie NES. Risks of breast and testicular cancers in young adult twins in England and Wales: evidence on prenatal and genetic aetiology. Lancet 1997;350:1723–1728.

124. Paulozzi LJ, Erickson JD, Jackson RJ. Hypospadias trends in two US surveillance systems. Pediatrics 1997;100:831–834.

125. Pierik FH, Burdoff A, Rien Nijman JM, de Muinck Keizer-Schrama SM, Juttmann RE, Weber RFA. A high hypospadias rate in The Netherlands. Hum Reprod 2002;17:1112–1115.

126. Toppari J, Kaleva M, Virtainen HE. Trends in the incidence of cryptorchidism and hypospadias and methodological limitations of registry-based data. Hum Reprod Update 2001;7:282–286.

127. Henderson BE, Bernstein L, Ross RK, Depue RH, Judd HL. The early in utero oestrogen and testosterone environment of blacks and whites: potential effects on male offspring. Br J Cancer 1988;57:216–218.

16 Exercise and Male Hypogonadism

Testosterone, the Hypothalamic–Pituitary–Testicular Axis, and Physical Exercise

Anthony C. Hackney, PhD, FACSM
and Jennifer Dobridge, MA

CONTENTS

INTRODUCTION

Athletes who compete in endurance-based events are swimming, running, cycling, and skating faster than ever before, and, thus, world records in many events are being broken on a nearly annual basis *(1)*. There are many factors that contribute to this improvement in human exercise performance. First, the coaches working with these athletes have improved scientific knowledge because of advances in the fields of sports medicine and exercise physiology. Second, sporting equipment changes have allowed some improvements in events *(1,2)*. Third, and perhaps most important, is the greater level of exercise training that athletes are performing in our modern era *(1–4)*. It is not uncommon, for example, for marathon runners to complete 150 to 250 km of intensive running per week or for tri athletes to spend 3 to 4 h per day in swimming, running, and cycling training. This large volume of exercise training results in physiological changes and adaptations that are highly beneficial to the human organism, such as enhanced cardiac output, enhanced arterial-venous oxygen difference, increased erythrocyte number, decreased body adiposity, and increased mitochondrial density *(3)*. However, this great volume of exercise training can also place a tremendous amount of stress on the human body and can result in unwanted

From: *Male Hypogonadism:*
Basic, Clinical, and Therapeutic Principles
Edited by: S. J. Winters © Humana Press Inc., Totowa, NJ

physiological responses and medical problems, which can potentially compromise the ability of an athlete to perform.

A physiological system that is extremely sensitive to the stress of exercise training is the endocrine reproductive system. A growing body of research during the last 25 yr reveals how chronic exposure to endurance exercise training results in the development of human endocrine reproductive dysfunction *(5–9)*. The majority of the research on exercise and endocrine reproductive dysfunction has focused on sporting women *(10–12)*. A growing number of studies, however, have begun to address the question of how exercise training affects the endocrine reproductive system in men. Comparatively, however, research reports in this area are relatively few. Nevertheless, many researchers hypothesize that the effect of endurance exercise training on the male endocrine reproductive system may be comparable to that found in sporting women, i.e., endurance exercise-trained athletes of both sexes can develop hypogonadism-like characteristics. Specifically, some men who are chronically exposed to endurance exercise training develop low basal resting levels of total and free testosterone. Most of these men display clinically normal levels of testosterone, but the levels are at the low end of normal *(13)*.

To date, no name or label has been applied to these men, other than "endurance-trained men with low resting testosterone." Although this is an accurate descriptive phrase for their condition, it is cumbersome to use. According to *Taber's Medical Dictionary, hypogonadism* can be defined as "defective internal secretion of the gonads" *(14)*. This is a simplistic definition, not giving an indication of the level of "defect" (clinical vs subclinical) or the root of the "defect" (e.g., hypergonadotropic vs hypogonadotrophic). Nonetheless, we chose to use this definition and refer to "endurance-trained men with low resting testosterone" as "exercise-hypogonadal men." This term serves as an operational definition for this special case of exercise men discussed in this chapter. These men have several common characteristics:

(1) Their low testosterone levels are not a transient phenomenon related to the immediate stress-strain of an acute exercise bout.
(2) In many cases, an adjustment in the regulatory axis (to allow a new lower set point for circulating testosterone) has occurred.
(3) They typically have a history of early involvement in organized sport and exercise training, resulting in many years of almost daily exposure to varying intensities of physical activity.
(4) The type of exercise training history most prevalent in these men is prolonged endurance-based activities, such as distance running (10 km or marathons), cycling, race walking, or triathlon.

A second endocrine reproductive disturbance also occurs in male athletic populations. This problem is a pseudohypergonadism brought about by the use of anabolic-androgenic steroid pharmaceutical agents. The term "pseudohypergonadism" is used because in reality, the usage of exogenous anabolic-androgenic steroids results in atrophy of the gonads and reduced endogenous sex-steroid hormone production because of hypothalamic–pituitary suppression. The extremely high circulating levels of anabolic-androgenic phamaceutical agents mask the endogenous hypogonadism.

Evidence points to large numbers of athletes taking anabolic-androgenic steroid agents in an attempt to stimulate muscular growth, development, and strength. The use of these agents has been a persistent occurrence in sports for approx 50 yr. Unfortunately, athletes and coaches continue to ignore the reports of serious medical side effects associated with such use.

This review presents an overview of select endocrine reproductive problems that occur in men involved in exercise training. Specifically, this review discusses (1) how endurance exercise training affects the male reproductive endocrine system to induce hypogonadal-like conditions, resulting in suppressed circulating testosterone levels (denoted here as the "exercise-hypogonadal" state), and (2) anabolic-androgenic steroid abuse and the reproductive dysfunction that is associated with the use of these pharmaceutical agents.

The following discussion is delimited to the relationship between exercise endocrinology and reproduction in men. Research in this area on women is the subject of several authoritative reviews available in the literature (12,15).

PHYSIOLOGICAL ACTIONS OF TESTOSTERONE

Testosterone is the most important sex hormone in males, and it has multiple physiological functions. These roles can be dichotomized into two major categories:

1. Androgenic effects, which are related to reproductive function and to the development of male secondary sex characteristics.
2. Anabolic effects, which are related more generally to the stimulation of tissue growth and development.

A complete discussion of these categories is beyond the scope of this chapter. What follows, instead, is a brief overview of testosterone's major androgenic and anabolic effects.

Androgenic Effects

The foremost reproductive role of testosterone is to stimulate sperm production. Activation of androgen receptors in Sertoli cells by testosterone stimulates and catalyzes the maturation and development of sperm through downstream target mechanisms that are poorly understood (16–19).

Testosterone also stimulates the development and function of the male accessory sex glands (prostate, seminal vesicles, and epididymides) that aid in sperm development and function, as well as copulation. Finally, testosterone stimulates the development of male secondary sex characteristics, such as the typical deeper male voice, increased body hair, penile growth, sex drive (libido), and male behavior patterns (17–20).

Anabolic Effects

Testosterone and 5-α dihydrotestosterone (DHT) are powerful anabolic hormones that stimulate nitrogen retention and protein synthesis (16). During puberty, testosterone acts in concert with other hormones to increase bone mass and to initiate the adolescent growth spurt. In the adult, testosterone is needed to maintain protein anabolism and, thereby, structural proteins. Athletes who use anabolic steroids (i.e., pharmacologically derived testosterone-like compounds) take advantage of this effect to facilitate the development of increased skeletal muscle mass (3,6,16,17,19). This latter action by testosterone results from androgen-receptor binding, which, in turn, increases muscle gene transcription, including that of insulin-like growth factor (IGF)-I *(21)*. In a related fashion, testosterone also decreases myostatin expression (transforming growth factor [TGF]-β family member and inhibitor of muscle development) *(21)*. Testosterone also stimulates hematopoiesis and increases sodium reabsorption in the kidney. Finally, studies in animals reveal that testosterone also plays a role in increasing skeletal muscle glycogen synthesis and storage *(17)*.

Factors Affecting Circulating Testosterone

HYPOTHALAMIC–PITUITARY–TESTICULAR AXIS

Testosterone production at by the testis is under control of the hypothalamic–pituitary unit *(22)*. The operation and components of this axis are discussed in detail elsewhere in this volume (*see* Chapters 1–3) and are not repeated here. The hypothalamic–pituitary–testicular axis hormones addressed in this discussion are luteinizing hormone (LH), follicle-stimulating hormone (FSH), inhibin, and prolactin (PRL).

CARDIOVASCULAR FACTORS

Testosterone is freely diffusible through tissues, and, thus, its secretion from the testis is directly affected by testicular blood flow. Testicular blood flow is a function of cardiac output, vascular vasoconstriction, and vasodilatation. Therefore, factors that influence vascular tone can also affect testosterone secretion (e.g., increased sympathetic nervous system activity) *(23)*.

The metabolic clearance rate (MCR) of testosterone varies in normal men but is approx 100 L/d *(16,17)*. MCR involves target-tissue uptake, as well as degradation by the liver, and is influenced by the portion of the hormone bound to carrier proteins (principally sex hormone-binding globulin [SHBG]). The degradation process involves the conversion of testosterone into functional metabolites, such as estradiol and dihydrotestosterone (DHT) and degradation products, such as 17-ketosteroids and glucuronides, which are excreted into the urine *(16,17,24)*. Hepatic clearance is primarily a function of hepatic blood flow, so that changes in the hepatic blood flow influence testosterone's removal rate *(16)*. This latter phenomenon is influenced by exercise, because hepatic blood flow is reduced during exercise when blood is shunted toward the active muscles *(3,25–27)*.

During exercise, there is the movement of plasma from the vascular space. Because testosterone is bound to carrier proteins, an increase or decrease in the plasma volume leads to dilution or concentration of the circulating testosterone level. These changes are not indicative of changes in the normal hormonal turnover rate *(25)*. For example, it is not uncommon during prolonged exercise (≥1 h) for transient plasma volume decreases of 10 to 20% to occur *(25)*. Whether these highly transient changes in the concentration of testosterone result from changes in plasma volume have a physiological effect is a point of debate and remains to be determined.

OTHER FACTORS

In addressing factors affecting blood levels of testosterone, it is important to consider the other physiological and nonphysiological factors that could account for variations in testosterone response in research studies. Examples include the blood-sampling method, diurnal variations in hormone concentrations, age, hormone detection methodology, emotional stress, diet, sleep patterns, and experimental research protocol or design. These factors are discussed in detail elsewhere *(6,24,25)*. Collectively, all of the aforementioned considerations must be carefully examined when comparing the hormonal results of research studies if a valid interpretation of the endocrine system's responses to exercise is to be made. Figure 1 illustrates some of these physiological and nonphysiological factors that affect circulating testosterone levels in exercising men.

EXERCISE AND PITUITARY–TESTICULAR FUNCTION

Normal Men—Exercise Responses

TESTOSTERONE

It is generally accepted that short-term, maximal, and anaerobic-type exercise results in an elevation of the circulating testosterone level (*see* Table 1 for definitions of exercise-types terminology) *(25,28–30)*. It is still debatable whether this effect results from solely hemoconcentration and reduced metabolic clearance or whether there is also an increase in testosterone production.

Unlike changes during maximal exercise, testosterone responses to submaximal exercise are more variable and are dependent on the duration and intensity of exercise. Progressive increases in testosterone levels during moderate intensity exercise lasting 45 to 90 min have been found *(25,31,32)*. However, 90 min of submaximal moderate intensity exercise has also been reported to produce no change or a slight decrease in testosterone concentrations *(25,31)*. Exercise of a moderate or hard intensity until exhaustion, of more than approx 2 h duration typically lowers testosterone concentrations *(25,31,32)*.

Several explanations for these dissimilar changes during short-term submaximal exercise have been proposed. Initially, hemoconcentration may increase the testosterone concentration; but as exercise continues, testicular testosterone production declines. The latter change may partly result from reduced testicular blood flow *(26,27)*. Hepatic blood flow may also decline, reducing hepatic clearance *(26,27)*. This latter change may be offset by an increased uptake of testosterone by peripheral target tissue (i.e., skeletal muscle) as exercise duration continues, gradually reducing circulating testosterone levels.

Interestingly, these acute effects of a bout of maximal and submaximal exercise on testosterone levels are transient. The changes are typically short lived and corrected during the recovery period (1 to 24 h) *(25,33–35)*.

GONADOTROPINS

Research results examining gonadotropin response to maximal and anaerobic-type exercise are contradictory *(36,37);* however, the majority of the evidence indicates there are small transient increases in the circulating gonadotropins *(35,38–44)*. In addition, the outcomes of these studies and their interpretations are subject to methodological limitations. In many cases, researchers did not obtain blood samples frequently enough to assess the highly pulsatile gonadotropin secretory profile *(12,16,24)*. Resistance-type exercise causes an increase in serum gonadotropin levels in both men and women *(43–46)*.

Likewise, the prolonged (~1–2 h) submaximal exercise responses of the gonadotropins vary considerably for both men and women *(25,41,42)*. Evidence of sig-

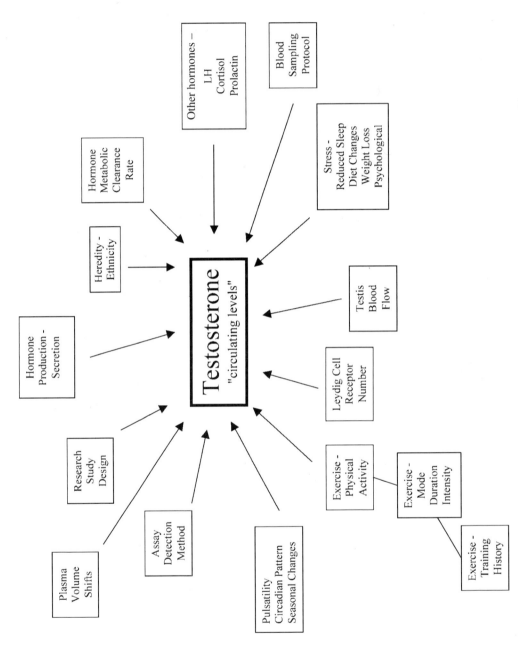

Fig. 1. Factors that influence the level of circulating testosterone in a normal, healthy man at rest and in response to a physical exercise bout. This figure is based on information from refs. *19,22,24,25.*

310

Table 1
Categorization and Definition of Exercise-Intensive and Exercise Type Relative
to Exercise Studies of Physically Fit Men

Category Term	Relative Intensity* (% VO_{2max})	Energy Pathway Predominating	Typical Duration	Other Terminology
Light or easy exercise	<35	Aerobic	>30 min	Submaximal
Moderate exercise	>35 <70	Aerobic	>30 min <180 min	Submaximal
Heavy exercise	>70	Aerobic-anaerobic	<120 min	Submaximal
Maximal exercise	100	Aerobic-anaerobic	<15 min	Maximal or Max
Supramaximal exercise	>100	Anaerobic	<1 min	Sprints, power

* In quantifying exercise intensity, it is typical to express it as a relative percentage of an individual's maximal oxygen uptake (VO_{2max}; i.e., maximal aerobic capacity). (Based on ref. *27a*.)

nificant increase, decrease, and no change has been reported *(31,35,38,39,41,42)*. If submaximal exercise is extended for extremely long periods (several hours) or until exhaustion occurs, then gonadotropin levels are suppressed *(41,47–49)*.

These exercise-induced gonadotropin disturbances are transient and last for relatively short periods into the recovery from exercise. The exception to this point is that submaximal exercise of many hours duration can produce disturbances that last several days *(48,49)*.

OTHER PITUITARY HORMONE—PROLACTIN

PRL presents an interesting paradox in reproductive physiological function. In physiological concentrations, it may be necessary for normal testicular function, whereas excessive PRL levels disrupt both central and peripheral aspects of the hypothalamic–pituitary–testicular axis *(16,50)*. Circulating PRL concentrations increase during most exercise. The magnitude of the increase is approximately proportional to the intensity of the activity *(25,41,51)*. Short-term, maximal, and anaerobic-type exercise results in increases in PRL *(25,41,51–55)*. Submaximal exercise of 30 to 60 min duration, provided it is intense enough, increases circulating PRL levels as well *(25,42,52–55)*.

Extending the duration of a submaximal exercise bout augments the magnitude of the PRL response *(24,42,51,52)*. There are several factors that further increase the PRL response to prolonged exercise: (1) consumption of a diet rich in fat, (2) fasting for an extended period of time before exercise, (3) performing exercise in conditions promoting an increase in body temperature, and (4) administration of β-adrenergic blocking agents before exercise *(25,42,52,55)*. On the other hand, PRL release is inhibited by α-adrenergic blockade *(25,42)*. Training history (i.e., training type or mode) also has a positive or negative influence on this response to submaximal exercise *(25)*.

PRL changes after maximal exercise or submaximal exercise of 1–2-h duration are short lived and transient in nature *(52–54)*. Interestingly, Hackney and associates have reported that nocturnal PRL levels are two to three times greater after 1.5 h of intensive endurance exercise than when no daytime exercise was performed *(38)*.

Exercise-Hypogonadal Males

BASAL HORMONAL RESPONSES

Retrospective comparative studies examining isolated, single blood samples have found lower testosterone levels in chronically endurance-trained males. The subjects in those studies were typically distance runners who had been involved with the physical-training aspects of their sport for 1 to 15 yr. In those studies, total and free-testosterone levels in the endurance-trained men were only 60–85% of the levels of matched sedentary controls *(7,35,54,56–58)*. Many of the early studies reporting this finding suffered from small sample sizes. However, recent work with larger numbers of subjects has substantiated the findings *(59,60)*. These low resting testosterone levels are highly reproducible and are not just an aberration of the athletes' seasonal training regime *(60)*.

Prospective studies have also been conducted in which blood samples have been collected for weeks or months during endurance training regimens. Findings thus far from such studies have been inconsistent. Some reports reveal significant reductions (decreases of 20–40%) in resting testosterone levels after 1 to 6 mo of intensive training *(60–64)*, whereas other studies have found no significant change in resting testosterone after 2 to 9 mo of training *(65–70)*. Differences in the initial training status of the subjects or the training dosage administered within these studies may explain the discrepant findings. It is also possible that some prospective studies were too brief compared to the retrospective studies in which the men with low testosterone levels had been training for many years.

Exercise-hypogonadal men also display other reproductive hormonal abnormalities in addition to low basal testosterone levels. The most frequently reported finding involves no significant elevation in resting LH to correspond with the decrease in testosterone (i.e., hypogonadotrophic-hypogonadism) *(35,58,71)*. Additionally, resting PRL levels may be decreased *(35,58)*. The findings of altered LH and PRL levels at rest in exercise-hypogonadal men have been interpreted by some researchers to indicate dysfunction of the hypothalamic–pituitary–testicular axis. These findings for LH and PRL have been reported in several retrospective and prospective based studies *(7,35,56,58,71,72)*.

There are several retrospective investigations in which basal, resting blood samples were collected (i.e., serially every 20 or 30 min for 4- to 8-h periods) in exercise-hypogonadal men and in sedentary control men. Results are similar to those of the isolated-sampling studies: resting total and free-testosterone concentrations of the exercise-trained subjects were typically only 60–80% of those found in control men *(56,73)*. As with isolated blood sampling studies, resting LH levels were not significantly elevated. Again, these findings have been cited to represent a possible dysfunction in the hypothalamic–pituitary–testicular axis.

To date, the hormonal findings described above in this section have primarily been found in endurance athletes (i.e., distance runners and triathletes). However, it is highly unlikely that these hormonal alterations are limited to this athletic-exercise group alone. The prevalence of these phenomena in endurance athletes most likely represents the tendency of researchers to focus on this group, following the initial lead of early studies conducted in the 1980s. As scientists studying exercise expand their endocrinological studies to include other athletic groups involved with endurance training, it is highly likely that comparable data will come forward.

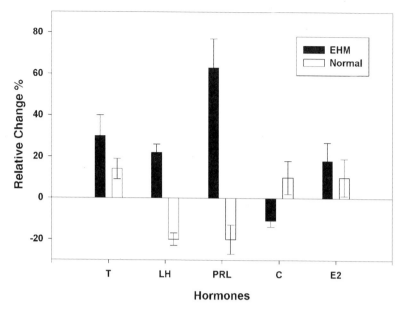

Fig. 2. Comparison of the overall percent change in hormone levels of exercise-hypogonadal men (EHM) when compared to normal, untrained men. Comparison is for a 4-h (overall mean response) period after a maximal exercise bout vs a 4-h period of rest in both groups of men. T, testosterone*; LH, lutropin*; PRL, prolactin*; C, cortisol; E2, estradiol. The * denotes significance differences between the groups ($p < 0.05$). The data are based on the findings in ref. *35*.

EXERCISE RESPONSES—TESTOSTERONE, GONADOTROPINS, AND OTHER HORMONES

Few studies have compared how exercise-hypogonadal men and normal untrained men respond differently to exercise. Evidence suggests that in response to a single exercise bout (maximal or submaximal) the direction of the hormonal changes is similar. Testosterone and PRL are increased, whereas the gonadotropin responses are variable in both groups of men *(35,72)*. However, in the recovery from exercise, the two groups differ. In normal men, the reproductive hormones display some degree of negative feedback "rebound" inhibition during the hours of recovery after exercise *(35,53)*. In exercise-hypogonadal men, this rebound effect is diminished or eliminated. Currently, it is unclear whether this represents an adjustment in regulatory aspects of the controlling axis or a temporal displacement shift in the axis of the exercise-hypogonadal men. Obviously, the resting basal levels of the hormones in each of these groups are different; therefore, relative changes in response to exercise must be compared. Figure 2 displays recovery hormonal responses of exercise-hypogonadal men and normal men as relative change after an identical exercise bout *(35)*.

MECHANISTIC STUDIES

Some studies have attempted to elucidate the mechanism for the proposed hypothalamic–pituitary–testicular axis dysfunction in exercise-hypogonadal men. These studies have focused on examining whether the dysfunction is central (hypothalamic or pituitary) or peripheral (testicular) in nature.

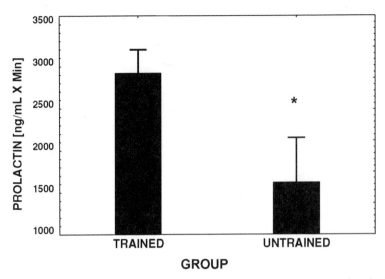

Fig. 3. Mean (±SEM) integrated area under the response curve 3-h for prolactin after the injection of a dopamine antagonist (metoclopramide hydrochloride). This challenge to the pituitary was performed in groups of endurance exercise-trained male runners and age-matched sedentary controls. The significant between group difference ($p < 0.05$) is denoted with an asterisk. The data are based on the findings in ref. *74.*

Several investigators have reported that exercise-hypogonadal men have altered PRL and LH release when either a pharmacological stimulus or an exercise bout are used to provoke the hypothalamus–pituitary *(35,47,71,74).* Figures 3 and 4 illustrate an augmented PRL response to metoclopramide and a reduced LH response to GnRH in exercise-hypogonadal men vs sedentary controls *(74).* Hyperprolactinemia is associated with decreased circulating testosterone levels *(16).* However, although the PRL response to an exogenous stimulus was augmented, there is no evidence that exercise-hypogonadal men are hyperprolactinemic. The converse has been demonstrated (see earlier discussion in section on Basal Hormonal Responses). The reduction in LH release could also reduce testosterone levels. Reports indicate that testicular sensitivity and response to exogenous stimuli are comparable in exercise-hypogonadal men and sedentary males *(35,74,75).* In contrast, Kujala et al. reported that the testicular response to a stimulus is attenuated after 4 h of exhaustive exercise *(47).*

Collectively, these findings suggest the development of both a central and a peripheral problem in the hypothalamic–pituitary–testicular axis; however, data in this area are limited and not yet definitive.

CORTISOL

Researchers have demonstrated that acute pharmacological or pathological increases in cortisol secretion are associated with a decrease in circulating testosterone levels *(33,76).* Several investigators have alluded to these hormonal changes as a potential mechanism for the low testosterone levels in exercise-hypogonadal men *(6,24,33,76).* A single, acute exercise bout at high intensity (>60% of maximal aerobic capacity) could induce transient increases in circulating cortisol, which could bring about the

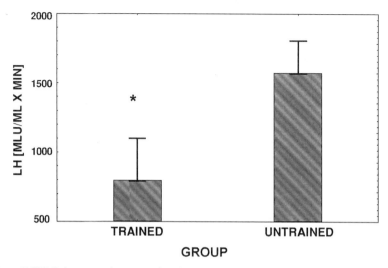

Fig. 4. Mean (±SEM) integrated area under the response curve 3-h for luteinizing hormone (LH) after the injection of gonadotropin-releasing hormone (GnRH) (gonadorelin hydrochloride). This challenge to the pituitary was performed in groups of endurance exercise-trained male runners and age-matched sedentary controls. A significant between group difference ($p < 0.05$) is denoted with an asterisk. The data are based on the findings in ref. *74.*

observed reductions in testosterone via the inhibitory effects on GnRH and LH. However, current evidence suggests that hypercortisolemia is an unlikely mechanism for exercise-hypogonadism. There are relatively small, transient changes in cortisol levels in response to exercise *(38,44,45,50,53,77–80)*. In contrast, low testosterone levels are associated with the chronic high cortisol levels of Cushing's syndrome resulting from pituitary or adrenal tumors *(16,76)*. On the other hand, the exercise-induced changes in cortisol are well within the normal range for this hormone, regardless of whether the exercise is of moderate or high intensity. This point is illustrated in Fig. 5 *(81)*. Nevertheless, systematic research examining the role of exercise-induced cortisol changes on testosterone production remains inadequate.

PHYSIOLOGICAL CONSEQUENCES OF LOW TESTOSTERONE LEVELS

There is evidence that the low resting testosterone levels in men doing endurance training have detrimental effects on testosterone-dependent physiological processes. However, the extent of evidence is limited. Currently, only a few reports of decreased spermatogenesis or oligospermia in exercise-hypogonadal men have been published *(18,82–85)*. One of the best controlled studies was by Arce et al. *(83)*. Some of the key findings from that study are displayed in Table 2. Other investigators have reported that endurance-trained men may have a lowered sex drive, but a direct cause-and-effect link between a lower sex drive and circulating testosterone levels was not found in those reports *(75,84,86–89)*. Accordingly, other factors may be affecting the libido of these athletes (e.g., overall fatigue and psychological stress) *(19,86)*. Additionally, some evidence exists that there is no influence of endurance training on sperm characteristics and the spermatogenesis process *(68)*. Relative to the androgenic-anabolic actions of

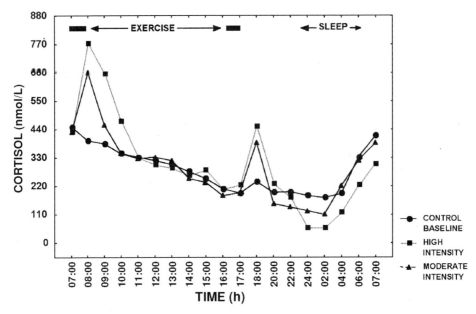

Fig. 5. Mean cortisol levels over 24-h in endurance athletes on three separate occasions; (1) control—baseline day with no exercise, (2) exercise day involving two moderate intensity exercise sessions, morning and afternoon, and (3) exercise day involving two high-intensity exercise sessions, morning and afternoon. Exercise sessions produced dose-dependent rises in serum cortisol levels lasting for 3–4 h. The data are based on the findings in ref. *81.*

Table 2
Semen Characteristics of Endurance-Trained Runners, Resistance-Trained Weight Lifters, and Sedentary Controls (values are means ± SEM)

	Runners (N = 10)	*Weight Lifters (N = 8)*	*Controls (N = 10)*	*P*
Totals				
Volume (mL)	4.2 ± 0.5	3.0 ± 0.5	2.5 ± 0.5	0.09
Sperm density ($\times 10^6 \cdot ml^{-1}$)	78 ± 12*	122 ± 15	176 ± 25	<.01
Total sperm count ($\times 10^6$)	332 ± 74	342 ± 36	376 ± 59	0.86
Normal motile count ($\times 10^6$)	55 ± 11	104 ± 20	107 ± 22	.09
Motility				
Forward progressive	40.8 ± 4.7**	58.0 ± 4.6	58.7 ± 2.4	<.01
Nonprogressive	5.0 ± 1.0	2.8 ± 1.5	2.0 ± 1.0	.17
Nonmotile	54.2 ± 4.9**	39.2 ± 3.9	39.3 ± 1.9	0.01
Morphology				
Normal (%)	40.2 ± 2.1***	54.8 ± 2.9	47.0 ± 3.3	<.01
Large (%)	2.7 ± 0.8	1.7 ± 0.9	2.3 ± 1.0	.76
Small (%)	4.3 ± 0.8	2.6 ± 0.7	2.4 ± 0.5	.10
Amorphous (%)	34.1 ± 2.5	30.1 ± 2.6	37.4 ± 2.8	.19
Immature (%)	17.2 ± 2.4**	10.5 ± 2.1	10.9 ± 1.2	.03
Round cells ($\times 10^6$)	8.3 ± 1.7**	0.6 ± 0.4	2.5 ± 0.9	<.01
In vitro sperm penetration of CM—Penetrak (mm)	22 ± 5*	–	43 ± 7	.04

* $p < 0.05$ for runners vs controls. ** $p < 0.05$ for runners vs weight lifters and controls. ***$p < 0.05$ for runners vs weight lifters. The data are based on the findings in ref. *83.*

testosterone, there are no documented detrimental effects of the lower testosterone levels (i.e., decreased protein synthesis and muscle mass development). However, this area has not been examined thoroughly. An additional area in need of research concerns the effect of the exercise-associated decline in testosterone levels on bone demineralization in trained men. Currently, there are no conclusive findings that endurance training results in mineral content changes in men *(90)*. Clinically, however, there is strong evidence that men with low testosterone concentrations have osteopenia *(91)*. Additionally, several compelling case reports have described male athletes with low testosterone levels and excessively low bone mineral density *(92,93)*.

Thus, the question arises is it necessary for endurance-trained males to supplement with testosterone-like substances to safeguard against loss of androgenic-anabolic processes. This question has not been addressed thoroughly in the literature. In one case study, Burge et al. *(75)* described a male runner with hypogonadotrophic hypogonadism who responded to clomiphene citrate treatment during a 5-mo period. Testosterone and gonadotropin concentrations increased into the normal range, and the subject's sexual function improved. Whether treatment was necessary is debatable. There is little evidence that disruptions in testosterone-dependent processes in exercise-hypogonadal men are sufficient to warrant action, but physicians must use their own medical judgement on a case-by-case basis. In extreme cases, especially in men with a low body mass index, such steps may be necessary, and a well-developed pharmacological course of therapy could be highly advantageous and efficacious.

Conversely, there may be beneficial physiologic adaptations from lowered testosterone levels. Some research indicates that lowering testosterone levels may have cardiovascular protective effects and decrease the risk of coronary heart disease *(94)*. A study from Germany demonstrated that pharmacologically induced reduction in endogenous testosterone levels resulted in significant increases in high-density lipoprotein (HDL) in men *(95)*. Whether the lowering of testosterone directly contributed to the exercise-related increase in HDL remains to be determined. Nonetheless, it is important to recognize that increased physical activity promotes a healthy cardiovascular risk profile, including increased circulating HDL *(96)*.

THE OVERTRAINING SYNDROME

Several researchers have suggested that reproductive hormones in exercise-hypogonadal men are suppressed because they are "overtraining," or are developing the "overtraining syndrome." This terminology can be confusing to non exercise physiology researchers; hence, some explanation is warranted. The terms "overtraining syndrome" and "overtraining" frequently are used interchangeably. The term "overtraining" refers to the *process* of heavier-than-usual exercise training, whereas the term "overtraining syndrome" refers to the *product* of too much of the overtraining process *(2,4,7–9,97–101)*. The overtraining syndrome is a pathological condition in which an athlete experiences consistent and persistent exercise performance incompetence that does not reverse itself after a few days of rest and recovery. Furthermore, there is no underlying medical reason or explanation for the declining performance. This exercise performance impairment can manifest itself within athletic competition as well as during exercise training. Concurrent with the declining physical performance is a host of other psychophysiological consequences that are adverse and negative. Some of the most general and commonly reported consequences and symptoms are listed in Table 3.

Table 3
Consequences and Symptoms
of the Overtraining Syndrome (*see* refs. *2,4,102*).

↓ Physical performance
Severe constant fatigue
Persistent muscle soreness
Overuse musculoskeletal injuries
Reduced appetite
Lethargy
Depression
Disturbed sleep patterns
Overall mood disturbances—shifts
Immune system deficits
Mental concentration difficulties
Δ Submaximal—maximal heart rate responses to
exercise
↓ Maximal oxygen uptake
Δ Submaximal—maximal lactate response to exercise

↓ = Decrease

Δ = Change decrease and/or increase.

One commonly reported endocrine change in overtrained athletes is suppressed or extremely low circulating testosterone levels *(2,4,7,9,99–101)*. Furthermore, in some cases, suppressed LH, FSH, and inhibin levels have been reported *(24,97,100–102)*. Although these changes are nearly identical to those reported for exercise-hypogonadal men, it does not represent the same phenomena. The hormone changes that are found in overtraining athletes are only temporary. When the exercise-training load of these overtraining athletes is reduced, or increased periods of rest are incorporated into the training program, their hormonal profiles return to normal *(102)*. Incorporation of more rest into the training of exercise-hypogonadal men has no substantial effect on their resting hormone levels. Neither do exercise-hypogonadal men display overtraining syndrome symptoms (*see* Table 3). Furthermore, most researchers studying the exercise-hypogonadal issue have been careful to ensure that their subjects under investigation are not going through periods of intensive training, and, that when they are evaluated, they are well rested.

Thus, the hormonal changes found in exercise-hypogonadal men are a more stable accommodation in the hypothalamic–pituitary–testicular axis, whereas those in overtraining athletes are transient and are associated with a declining physical performance.

ATHLETES AND ANABOLIC-ANDROGENIC STEROIDS

Anabolic-androgenic steroids are pharmacological agents that are structured similarly to testosterone *(103,104)*. They have anabolic-androgenic actions like testosterone; however, these agents have been chemically modified to enhance their anabolic actions. Athletes use anabolic-androgenic steroids to facilitate physiological development beyond that achieved with exercise training alone (e.g., increased body weight;

muscular strength, power, and speed; or endurance) *(103,104)*. These agents are used by athletes involved in many sports. However, sports such as track and field (mostly in the throwing events), weight lifting, bodybuilding, and football report the highest prevalence of use *(104–106)*. For the remainder of the discussion, anabolic-androgenic steroids will be referred to as anabolic steroids.

Physiologic Adaptation and Exercise Performance

It is now clearly established that testosterone and anabolic steroid supplementation increase muscle mass and maximal voluntary muscle strength *(105–108)*. Early studies suggested equivocal effects of anabolic steroid use on athletic or exercise performance *(105)*. However, it is important to recognize that because of ethical reasons, most of those sanctioned studies did not administer anabolic steroids at the high dosages used by athletes. This prompted researchers to report no effects, whereas anecdotal reports by individual users touted large, substantial effects. Those anecdotal reports were tainted by their lack of scientific control for confounding factors, such as extent of training and "the placebo effect." Nonetheless, the findings in those "nonexperimental" studies suggested body mass gains of 10 or 20 kg, as well as up to a 30% increase in muscle strength *(106)*. Several well-controlled short-term studies have found smaller, but significant, increases in body mass, lean body mass, muscular strength, and concurrent reductions in fat mass *(105,106)*.

Anabolic steroid usage is not limited to "weight-lifting-power" athletes. Endurance athletes (e.g., distance runners and triathletes) have also used anabolic steroids. However, most studies have failed to demonstrate a substantial, beneficial effect of anabolic steroids on maximal oxygen consumption (i.e., key determinate to aerobic-endurance capacity) *(103–105)*. It has been proposed that endurance athletes who use anabolic steroids choose to do so because they recover from exercise training bouts more rapidly. This idea seems logical, because performing more exercise training is a major stimulus to improve the cardiovascular-respiratory system and, thereby, aerobic performance, and androgen treatment should negate the decline in testosterone that normally follows heavy exercise.

Mechanism of Actions

Anabolic steroids are believed to affect athletes by mechanisms that are both physiological and psychological *(106)*. These proposed mechanisms include (1) activating steroid hormone receptors in skeletal muscle cells, (2) producing an anticatabolic effect in the skeletal muscle, and (3) inducing motivational psychological effects. It is presently unclear to what extent each of these mechanisms contributes to the overall physiological adaptation and performance changes found in anabolic steroid users. Most likely, these elements combine synergistically to bring about the changes noted.

STEROID HORMONE RECEPTORS

Anabolic steroids activate androgen receptors in skeletal muscle cells, which stimulate the promoters of specific genes and induce protein synthesis *(105,106)*. Of these proteins, one that is important in increased muscle mass and strength is IGF-1 *(109)*. IGF-1 mRNA in skeletal muscle is increased by testosterone treatment in older men *(110)* and is reduced in testosterone deficiency *(111)*. In certain cells, most notably prostate epithelium, testosterone's action is amplified by its irreversible bioconversion to 5-α dihydrotesterone by the enzyme 5-α-reductase. In skeletal muscle cells, how-ever, the activity of this enzyme is weak (112). The number of muscle androgen recep-tors is increased by androgens in certain experimental models (113,114). Several transcription factors interact with androgen receptors and upregulate androgen receptor function (115). Of these factors, supervillin, a 205-kDa actin-binding protein, was recently shown to be androgen regulated (116).

Interestingly, exercise training is necessary for anabolic steroids to exert any benefi-cial effect on performance. As an illustration, research has shown that a greater exer-cise performance improvement with anabolic steroid use has occurred in experienced weight lifters than in novice subjects (103,105,106). The experienced weight lifters were capable of training with heavier weights and of producing relatively greater mus-cle tension during exercise. Anabolic steroid effectiveness is also dependent on the number of unbound steroid hormone receptor sites in skeletal muscle, and resistance exercise training (i.e., intensive) may increase the number of unbound receptor sites (43,46,105,106).

ANTI-CATABOLIC ACTIONS

There is evidence that a portion of the anabolic effect of testosterone and anabolic steroids is via an antiglucorticoid action. Cortisol is catabolic, because one of its actions is to induce protein breakdown (25,31,50). Cortisol is secreted in large amounts in response to exercise, which may provide proteins for energy metabolism and deplete the free amino acid pool of proteogenesis precursors (25,31,50). Cortisol receptors are found in skeletal muscle cells, and anabolic steroids bind to these recep-tors (117,118) to block cortisol from binding. This prevents cortisol from inducing muscle protein breakdown and depleting the free amino acid pool (31,103,106). For example, in men with severe burn injury, testosterone treatment markedly reduced pro-tein breakdown (119). A similar effect could enhance recovery from exercise training by allowing amino acid precursors to be available for tissue repair and regeneration. Interestingly, athletes have indicated that anabolic steroids help them train more intensely and recover faster (103,106).

PSYCHOLOGICAL EFFECTS

An important aspect of the anabolic steroid effect may be enhancement of the ath-lete's "motivational psychological state" (106,120). This belief is supported by the notion that athletes indicate their emotional sense of well-being; euphoria, aggressive-ness, and tolerance to stress, are all enhanced when they are using these agents. These emotions are positive motivators and allow the athlete to train harder and to perform more intensive exercise training. This, in turn, would allow a greater exercise stimulus to be presented to muscle cells, thus resulting in improved adaptation.

Side Effects of Use

There are a large number of side effects associated with anabolic steroid usage. Some of these effects are transient in nature; however, other effects are more perma-nent and persist long after usage has stopped. Table 4 lists those side effects that have been reported in the literature. Brooks and associates (106) categorized and subdivided the principal side effects into those attributable to (1) normal physiological actions of male sex steroid hormones that are inappropriate in the recipient, and (2) toxic effects

Table 4
Major Side Effects Associated With Anabolic Steroid
Use in Athletes (*see* refs. *106* and *121*).

Acne
Aggressiveness
Altered electrolyte balance
Alterations in clotting factors
Altered thyroid function tests
Alterations in libido
Clitoral enlargement (women)
Depressed spermatogenesis
Decreased endogenous testosterone production
Decreased gonadotropin production
Dizziness
Depressed immune function
Decreased high-density lipoprotein
Edema
Elevated creatine kinase and lactate dehydrogenase
Elevated total cholesterol
Elevated triglycerides
Elevated blood glucose
Elevated blood pressure
Gastrointestinal distress
Gynecomastia and breast tenderness
Increase apocrine sweat gland activity
Increased nervous tension
Liver toxicity
Lower voice (women)
Masculinization (women)
Muscle cramps—spasms
Nosebleeds
Polyuria
Prostatic hypertrophy (and perhaps cancer)
Premature closure of epiphyses (children)
Psychosis
Wilm's tumor

caused by the chemical structure of the drug (principally C-17 α-alkylated oral anabolic steroids).

One extremely important area concerning side effects involves the greater risk of cardiovascular disease associated with anabolic steroid use. For example, during anabolic steroid use, total cholesterol increases, whereas HDL cholesterol (HDL-C) demonstrates a marked decline *(121)*. Anabolic steroids influence hepatic triglyceride lipase (HTL) and lipoprotein lipase (LPL). HTL is primarily responsible for the clearance of HDL-C, whereas LPL facilitates the cellular uptake of free fatty acids and glycerol. Androgens and anabolic steroids stimulate HTL, presumably resulting in decreased serum levels of HDL-C *(121,122)*. Anabolic steroid use may also provoke a transient hypertensive state. Data suggest that high-dose use significantly increases diastolic blood pressure. The increases in diastolic blood pressure typically subside after abstinence from anabolic steroids *(121,123,124)*.

There is evidence that anabolic steroid use elicits structural changes in the heart and that myocardial ischemic tolerance is decreased after use *(121,125,126)*. Echocardiographic studies in body builders using anabolic steroids reported a mild hypertrophy of the left ventricle with decreased diastolic relaxation, resulting in decreased diastolic filling *(121,124)*. Some investigators have associated cardiomyopathy, myocardial infarction, and cerebrovascular accidents with anabolic steroid abuse *(125,126)*. However, a possible causal relationship has not been proved. Such physiological effects have negative influences on cardiovascular risk factors; unfortunately, no data appear ethically available because of the risks associated with the long-term use.

Prevalence of Anabolic Steroid Use

Use of anabolic steroids by athletes is illegal and often has negative ramifications on athletic eligibility (see discussion below in section on Anabolic Steroids—A Banned Substance). As a consequence, the number of athletes using these agents is difficult to determine (i.e., most individuals are unwilling to admit use). Mistakenly, body builders are often cited for prevalent use of anabolic steroids. In self-report studies, estimate use rates range from 5 to 30% of the professional and amateur athletic populations *(120,127,128)*. This even includes high school athletes and recreational athletes. For example, Buckley and associates *(128)* studied a North American sample of 3400 high school seniors, and found that more than 6% periodically used anabolic steroids. In that study, the majority of the users were sports athletes. Interestingly, 35% were nonathletes, who cited improved appearance as their main reason for taking the drugs. Regrettably, 20% of anabolic steroid users in that study had obtained their drugs from a health care professional. Research by Yesalis et al. in the 1990s put the total number of users in the United States at more than 1 million *(129)*. There is no evidence that the number has declined, despite the warnings issued by health care providers of the dangers of usage *(120,127–130)*.

Other Anabolic Substances

There are many other anabolic agents an athlete can use for supplementation. One that has received a large amount of press coverage is androstenedione, a precursor for both androgens and estrogens (testosterone and estradiol). Androstenedione is a weak androgen and is poorly converted to more potent androgen forms. Instead, most orally administered androstenedione is metabolized to testosterone glucuronide and other metabolites before being released into the general circulation *(131)*. Several well-controlled studies have been conducted to examine the effects of androstenedione use *(105,132,133)*. Collectively, based on evaluations of circulating androgen levels, muscle strength, or morphology, these studies suggest that no credible evidence exists for an enhanced anabolic effect.

Dehydroepiandrosterone (DHEA) and its sulfate (DHEA-S) are the most abundant circulating steroid hormones in humans. As with androstenedione, DHEA may serve as a precursor for androgens and estrogens, although direct actions have also been claimed. Theoretically, DHEA or DHEA-S use as a supplement could have beneficial anabolic effects. In older adults, its use increased circulating androgen levels and subjective ratings of physical and psychological well-being *(134)*. It is perhaps most beneficial to those with adrenal insufficiency and those on high-dose glucocorticoid therapy *(105)*. Its effects on muscle strength and performance in athletes remain unproven *(104,105)*.

Recombinant growth hormone is used by some weight-lifting and power athletes to increase muscle mass and strength. Growth hormone (GH) is a powerful endogenous anabolic hormone. It facilitates amino acid uptake and protein synthesis in many body tissues of which skeletal muscle is strongly influenced. GH also stimulates IGF-1 production, which is also anabolic. In addition, GH has metabolic effects, such as stimulating glucose uptake, free fatty acid mobilization, and lipolysis *(25,31,50)*. Human studies examining the efficacy of GH use in exercising men are limited *(135,136)*. Muscle hypertrophy has been demonstrated, but the effects on muscular strength are equivocal. Conversely, there are negative consequences to GH supplementation. Large dosages can result in cardiomegaly, acromegaly, diabetes, atherosclerosis, peripheral neuropathy, arthritis, and heart disease *(106)*. The risk for developing some of these side effects is enhanced when GH is used in conjunction with anabolic steroids.

Anabolic Steroids—A Banned Substance

The International Olympic Committee (IOC) and all major sports-governing organizations throughout the world have banned the use of substances taken for the purpose of artificially improving performance in competition. Included on the banned substance list are varieties of anabolic steroids and similar agents.

In an attempt to deter use by athletes, it is typical for major sporting events (Olympics and international and national championship competitions) to have drug-testing programs (doping control) to determine if any banned substance has been used to enhance performance. Furthermore, sports-governing organizations perform randomized testing of national-level athletes annually. Unfortunately, the logistical and financial considerations of such banned substance testing make frequent, large scale examination of all athletic competitions impossible. Therefore, many violators go undetected. Furthermore, the allure of sports fame and fortune are so strong in many societies that athletes are willing to risk being detected to gain a competitive edge. For example, anabolic steroids have been on the IOC list of banned substances since 1975 *(120)*. Since that time, 15 total winter and summer Olympic Games have occurred. Every one of these Olympic Games has involved a doping scandal of some type, in which athletes were caught using banned substances. Many of these cases involved anabolic steroid use.

CONCLUSIONS

Endurance exercise training does have significant effects on the major male reproductive hormone, testosterone, and the hypothalamic–pituitary–axis that regulates testicular function. A growing body of evidence suggests that testosterone is chronically lowered in endurance exercise-trained men, and we have referred to this condition as exercise hypogonadism. Although the mechanism of this testosterone lowering is currently unclear, it may be related to a dysfunction or a readjustment in the hypothalamic–pituitary–testicular regulatory axis brought about by years of endurance training. Currently, the time course of these changes, including their reversibility, remains unresolved and is in need of further scientific investigation *(137)*. The lowered testosterone levels of the exercise-hypogonadal male could potentially disrupt anabolic or androgenic testosterone-dependent processes. Conversely, the alterations in testosterone levels brought about by endurance training could have cardiovascular protective effects and may, thus, be beneficial to these men.

Similar reproductive hormonal profiles exist in exercise-hypogonadal men and in men who are undergoing overtraining who develop the overtraining syndrome. However, the hormonal changes with the overtraining syndrome are transient and reflect the stress of excessive physical training. An increase in the rest and recovery portions of training regimens eliminates any hormonal abnormalities in overtraining men but not in exercise-hypogonadal men.

Some athletes are using anabolic-androgenic steroid agents to induce muscular growth, development, and strength gains. Current evidence suggests that they are effective in producing the outcomes that athletes desire. Unfortunately, athletes are ignorant of, or are willing to ignore, the serious medical side effects and health consequences associated with using these agents. Unfortunately, their use has been a persistent occurrence and problem in sports for the last 50 yr.

Although there is a large volume of literature concerning the reproductive endocrine dysfunction in exercising women, the number of studies in males is relatively small. Thus, many questions regarding the male reproductive adaptive process to exercise training remain unanswered. Consequently, this area of exercise endocrinology is in need of continued study and investigation.

ACKNOWLEDGMENT

This work is dedicated to those colleagues who have inspired us with their work, and have shown themselves to be the utmost of professionals—Dr. Stanley Hauerwas, Dr. Robert G. McMurray, Dr. Wayne E. Sinning, Dr. Atko Viru, and the late Dr. Manfred Lehmann.

REFERENCES

1. Raglin J, Barzdukas A. Overtraining in athletes: the challenge of prevention – a consensus statement. Health Fitness J 1999;3:27.
2. Lehmann M, Foster C, Keul J. Overtraining in endurance athletes: a brief review. Med Sci Sports Exerc 1993;25:854–862.
3. Brooks GA, Fahey TD, White TP. Neural-endocrine control of metabolism. Exercise physiology: human bioenergetics and its application, 2nd ed. Mayfield, Toronto, 1996, pp. 144–172.
4. Hackney AC, Pearman SN, Nowacki JM. Physiological profiles of overtrained athletes: a review. J Appl Sport Psych 1990;2:21–29.
5. Fry RW, Morton AR, Keast D. Overtraining in athletes. An update. Sports Med 1991;12:32–65.
6. Hackney AC. Endurance training and testosterone levels. Sports Med 1989;8:117–127.
7. Hackney AC, Dolny DG, Ness RJ. Comparison of resting reproductive hormonal profiles in select athletic groups. Biol Sport 1988;4:200–208.
8. Kenttä G, Hassmén P. Overtraining and recovery—a conceptual model. Sports Med 1998;26:1–16.
9. Kuipers H, Keizer HA. Overtraining in elite athletes—review and directions for the future. Sports Med 1988;6:79–92.
10. Boyden TW, Paramenter R, Stanforth P, Rotkis TC, Wilmore J. Impaired gonadotropin responses to gonadotropin-releasing hormone stimulation in endurance-trained women. Fertil Steril 1984;41:359–363.
11. Dale E, Gerlach D, Whilhite AL. Menstrual dysfunction in distance runners. Obstet Gynecol 1974;54:47.
12. Loucks AB. Exercise training in the normal female: effects of exercise stress and energy availability on metabolic hormones and LH pulsatility. In: Warren MP, Constantini NW, eds. Sports Endocrinology. Humana, Totowa, 2000, pp. 165–180.

13. Tietz NW. Clinical guide to laboratory tests. Saunders, Philadelphia, 1990, pp. 284, 314–345.
14. Taber's Medical Dictionary, 14th ed. F A Davis Co., Philadelphia, 1983.
15. Petit MA, Prior JC. Exercise and the hypothalamus: ovulatory adaptations. In: Warren MP, Constantini NW, eds. Sports Endocrinology. Humana, Totowa, 2000, pp. 133–163.
16. Griffin JE, Wilson JD. Disorders of the testes and the male reproductive tracts. In: Wilson JD, ed. Williams Textbook of Endocrinology. Saunders, Philadelphia, 1992, pp. 799–852.
17. Newshole EA. Biochemistry for the medical sciences. Wiley & Son, London, 1983, pp. 711–733.
18. Arce JC, DeSouza MJ. Exercise and male factor infertility. Sports Med 1993;15:146–169.
19. Zitzmann M, Nieschlag E. Testosterone levels in healthy men in relation to behavioural and physical characteristics: facts and constructs. Eur J Endocrinol 2001;144:183–197.
20. Christiansen K. Behavioral effects of androgen in men and women. J Endocrinol 2001;170:39–48.
21. Marcell TJ, Harman SM, Urban RJ, Metz DD, Rodgers BD, Blackman MR. Comparison of GH, IGF-I, and testosterone with mRNA of receptors and myostatin in skeletal muscle in older men. Am J Physiol Endocrinol Metab 2001;281:E1159–E1164.
22. Widmaier EP. Metabolic feedback in mammalian endocrine systems. Horm Metab Res 1992;24:147–53.
23. Eik-Nes KB. On the relationship between testicular blood flow and the secretion of testosterone. Can J Physiol Pharmacol 1964;42:671.
24. Hackney AC. The male reproductive system and endurance exercise. Med Sci Sports Exerc 1996;28:180–189.
25. Viru A. Hormonal Ensemble in Exercise—Hormones in Muscular Activity, Vol. 1. CRC, Boca Raton, FL, 1985, pp. 7–88.
26. Cadoux-Hudson TA, Few JD, Imms FJ. The effect of exercise on the production and clearance of testosterone in well trained young men. Eur J Appl Physiol 1995;54:321–325.
27. Keizer HA, Poortman J, Bunnik GS. Influence of physical exercise on sex-hormone metabolism. J Appl Physiol 1980;48:765–769.
27a. Bouchard C, ed. Exercise, fitness, and health: a consensus of current knowledge. Human, Kinetics. Champaign, IL, 1990.
28. Kuoppasalmi K, Maveri H, Rehunen S, Harkonen M, Adlercreutz H. Effect of strenuous anaerobic running on plasma growth hormone, cortisol, luteinizing hormone, testosterone, androstenedione and estrone and estradiol. J Steroid Biochem 1976;7:823–829.
29. Schmid P, Pusch PP, Wolf WW, et al. Serum FSH, LH and testosterone in humans after physical exercise. Int J Sports Med 1982;384–389.
30. Metivier G, Gauthier R, de la Chevotriere J, Grymala D. The effect of acute exercise on the serum levels of testosterone and luteinizing (LH) hormone in human male athletes. J Sports Med Phys Fit 1980;20:235–237.
31. McMurray RG, AC Hackney. Endocrine responses to exercise and training. In: Garrett W, DT Kirkendall eds. Exercise and Sport Science. Lippincott, Williams & Wilkins, Philadelphia, 2000, pp. 135–162.
32. Hackney AC. Testosterone, the hypothalamo-pituitary-testicular axis and endurance exercise training: a review. Biol Sport 1996;13:85–98.
33. Cumming DC. The male reproductive system, exercise and training. In: Warren MP, Constantini NW, eds. Sports Endocrinology. Humana, Totowa, 2000, pp. 119–132.
34. Aakvaag A, Sand T, Opstad PK, Fonnum F. Hormonal changes in serum in young men during prolonged physical strain. Eur J Appl Physiol Occup Physiol 1978;39:283–291.
35. Hackney AC, Fahrner CL, Stupnicki R. Reproductive hormonal responses to maximal exercise in endurance-trained men with low resting testosterone levels. Exp Clin Endocrinol Diabetes 1997;105:291–295.
36. Kuopposalmi K, Naveri H, Harkonen N, Adlerkreutz H. Plasma cortisol, androstenedione, testosterone and luteinizing hormone in running exercise of various intensities. Scand J Clin Lab Invest 1980;40:403–409.
37. DiLuigi L, Guidetti L, Baldari C, Fabbri A, Moretti C, Romanelli F. Physical stress and qualitative gonadotropin secretion: LH biological activity ar rest and after exercise in trained and untrained men. Int J Sports Med 2002;23:307–312.
38. Hackney AC, Ness RJ, Schrieber A. Effects of endurance exercise on nocturnal hormone concentrations in males. Chronobiol Int 1989;6:341–346.
39. Viru A. Plasma hormones and physical exercise. Int J Sports Med 1992;13:201–209.

40. Kindermann W, Schnabel A, Schmitt WM, Biro G, Cassens J, Weber F. Catecholamines, growth hormone, cortisol, insulin and sex hormones in aerobic and anaerobic exercise. Eur J Appl Physiol 1982;49:389–399.

41. Galbo H, Hummer L, Peterson IB, et al. Thyroid and testicular hormonal responses to graded and prolonged exercise in men. Eur J Appl Physiol 1977;36:101–106.

42. Galbo H, Kjaer M, Mikines KJ. Neurohormonal system. In: Skinner J. Corbin CB, Landers DM, et al. eds. Future Directions in Exercise and Sport Science Research. Human Kinetics, Champaign, IL, 1989:339–345.

43. Kraemer WJ. Patton JF, Knuttgen HG, et al. Hypothalmic-pituitary-adrenal responses to short-duration high-intensity cycle exercise. J Appl Physiol 1989;66:161–166.

44. Cumming DC, Wall SR, Galbraith MA, Belcastro A. Reproductive hormone responses to resistance exercise. Med Sci Sports Exerc 1987;19:234–238.

45. Guezennec Y, Leger F, Hostr FL, Aymonud M, Pesquies PC. Hormone and metabolite response to weight-lifting training sessions. Int J Sports Med 1986;7:100–105.

46. Kraemer WJ. Endocrine response to resistance exercise. Med Sci Sports Exerc 1988;20:S152–S157.

47. Kujala UM, Alen M, Huhtaniemi IT. Gonadotrophin-releasing hormone and human chronic gonadotrophin tests reveal that both hypothalamic and testicular endocrine functions are suppressed during acute prolonged physical exercise. Clin Endocrinol 1990;33:219–225.

48. Opstad PK. Androgenic hormones during prolonged physical stress, sleep and energy deficiency. J Clin Endocrinol Metab 1992;74:1176–1183.

49. Opstad PK. The hypothalamic-pituitary regulation of androgen secretion in young men after prolonged physical stress combined with energy and sleep deprivation. Acta Endocrinol 1992;127:231–236.

50. Galbo H. Hormonal and Metabolic Adaptation to Exercise. Verlag, Georg Thieme, Stuttgart, 1983, pp. 2–117.

51. Gawel MJ, Alaghband-Zadeh J, Park DM, Rose FC. Exercise and hormonal secretion. Postgrad Med J 1979;55:373–376.

52. Brisson G, Nolle MA, Desharnaris D, Tanka M. A possible submaximal exercise-induced hypothalamo-hypophyseal stress. Horm Metab Res 1980;12:201–205.

53. Hackney AC, Premo MC, McMurray RG. Influence of aerobic versus anaerobic exercise on the relationship between reproductive hormones in men. J Sports Sci 1995;13:305–311.

54. Hackney AC, Sharp RL, Runyon W, et al. Effects of intensive training on the prolactin response to submaximal exercise in males. J Iowa Acad Sci 1989;96:52–53.

55. Noel GL, Suh HK, Stone JG, Frantz AG. Human prolactin and growth hormone release during surgery and other conditions of stress. J Clin Endocrinol Metab 1972;35:840–851.

56. Hackney AC, Sinning WE, Bruot BC. Reproductive hormonal profiles of endurance-trained and untrained males. Med Sci Sports Exerc 1988;20:60–65.

57. Hackney AC. 2002; Personal communication.

58. Wheeler GD, Wall SR, Belcastro AN, Cumming DC. Reduced serum testosterone and prolactin levels in male distance runners. JAMA 1984;252:514–516.

59. Hackney AC, Fahrner CL, Gulledge TP. Basal reproductive hormonal profiles are altered in endurance trained men. J Sports Med Phys Fitness 1998;38:138–141.

60. Gullege TP, Hackney AC. Reproducibility of low resting testosterone concentrations in endurance trained men. Eur J Appl Physiol 1996;73:582–583.

61. Hackney AC, Sharp RL, Runyan WS, Ness RJ. Relationship of resting prolactin and testosterone in males during intensive training. Br J Sport Med 1989;23:194.

62. Wheeler GD, Singh M, Pierce WD, Epling WF, Cumming DC. Endurance training decreases serum testosterone levels in men without change in luteinizing hormone pulsatile release. J Clin Endocrinol Metab 1991;72:422–425.

63. Obminski Z, Szczypaczewska M, Tomaszewski W. Resting concentrations of cortisol and testosterone in blood of cyclists in the training and competitive periods. Medycyna Sportowa 2001;114:23–26.

64. Urhausen A, Kullmer T, Kindermann W. A 7-week follow-up study of the behaviour of testosterone and cortisol during the competition period in rowers. Eur J Appl Physiol 1987;56:528–533.

65. Alen A, Parkarinen A, Hakkinen K, Komi P. Responses of serum androgenic-anabolic and catabolic hormones to prolonged strength training. Int J Sports Med 1988;9:229–233.

66. Bonifazi M, Bela E, Carl G, et al. Influence of training on the response of androgen plasma concentrations to exercise in swimmers. Eur J Appl Physiol 1995;70:109–114.

67. Fellmann N, Coudert J, Jarrige J, et al. Effects of endurance training on the androgenic response to exercise in man. Int J Sports Med 1985;6:215–219.

68. Lucia A, Chicharro JL, Perez MM, Serratosa L, Bandres F, Legido JC. Reproductive function in male endurance athletes: sperm analysis and hormonal profile. J Appl Physiol 1996;81:2627–2636.

69. Lehmann M, Knizia K, Gastmann U, et al. Influence of 6-week, 6 days per week, training on pituitary function in recreational athletes. Br J Sports Med 1993;27:186–192.

70. Winder WW, Hagberg JM, Hickson RR, Ehsani AA, McLane JA. Time course of sympathoadrenal adaptation to endurance exercise training in man. J Appl Physiol 1978;45:370–374.

71. MacConnie S, Barkan A, Lampman R.M, Schork M, Beitins IZ. Decreased hypothalamic gonadotropin-releasing hormone secretion in male marathon runners. N Engl J Med 1986;315:411–417.

72. Duclos M, Corcuff JB, Rashedi M, Fougere B. Does functional alteration of the gonadotropic axis occur in endurance trained athletes during and after exercise? A preliminary study. Eur J Appl Physiol 1996;73:427–433.

73. McColl EM, Wheeler GD, Bhambhani Y, Cumming DC. The effects of acute exercise on pulsatile LH release in high-mileage male runners. Clin Endocrinol (Oxf) 1989;31:617–621.

74. Hackney AC, Sinning WE, Bruot BC. Hypothalamic-pituitary-testicular axis function in endurance-trained males. Int J Sports Med 1990;11:298–303.

75. Burge MR, Lanzi RA, Skarda ST, Eaton RP. Idiopathic hypogonadotropic hypogonadism in a male runner is reversed by clomiphene citrate. Fertil Steril 1997;68:745.

76. Cumming DC, Quigley ME, Yen SS. Acute suppression of circulating testosterone levels by cortisol in men. J Clin Endocrinol Metab 1983;57:671–673.

77. Dessypris A, Kuoppasalmi H, Adlercreutz HJ. Plasma cortisol, testosterone, androstenedione and luteinizing hormone (LH) in a non-competitive marathon run. J Steroid Biochem 1976;7:33–37.

78. Urhausen A, Gabriel H, Kindermann W. Blood hormones as markers of training stress and overtraining. Sports Med 1995;20:251–276.

79. Urhausen A, Kindermann W. Biochemical monitoring of training. Clin J Sports Med 1992;2:52–61.

80. Wittert GA, Livesey J, Espiner E, Donald R. Adaptation of the hypothalamopituitary adrenal axis to chronic exercise stress in humans. Med Sci Sports Exerc 1996;28:1015–1019.

81. Hackney AC, Viru A. Twenty-four-hour cortisol response to multiple daily exercise sessions of moderate and high intensity. Clin Physiol 1999;19:178–182.

82. Ayers JWT, Komesu V, Romani T, Ansbacher R. Anthropomorphic, hormonal, and psychologic correlates of semen quality in endurance-trained male athletes. Fertil Steril 1985;43:917–921.

83. Arce JC, DeSouza J, Pescatello LS, Luciano AA. Subclinical alterations in hormone and semen profile in athletes. Fertil Steril 1993;59:398–404.

84. Skarda S, Burge MR. Prospective evaluation of risk factors for exercise-induced hypogonadism in male runners. West J Med 1998;169:9–12.

85. Roberts AC, McClure RD, Weiner RL, Brooks GA. Overtraining affects males reproductive status. Fertil Steril 1993;60:686–692.

86. McGrady, AV. Effects of psychological stress on male reproduction: a review. Arch Androl 1984;13:1–7.

87. Baker ER, Leuker R, Stumpf PG. Relationship of exercise to semen parameters and fertility success of artificial insemination donors [abstract]. Fertil Steril 1984;41:107S.

88. Baker ER, Stevens C, Leuker R. Relationship of exercise to semen parameters and fertility success of artificial insemination donors. JSC Med Assoc 1988;84:580–582.

89. Special survey: running and sex [editorial]. The Runner 1982;May:26–35.

90. MacDougall JD, Webber CE, Martin J, et al. Relationship among running mileage, bone density, and serum testosterone in male runners. J Appl Physiol 1992;73:1165–1170.

91. Behre H, Kliesch S, Leifke E, Link T, Nieschlag NJ. Long-term effect of testosterone therapy on bone mineral density in hypogonadal men. J Clin Endocrinol Metab 1997;82:2386–2290.

92. Riggs BL, Eastell R. Exercise, hypogonadism, and osteopenia. JAMA 1986;256:392–393.

93. Rigotti NA, Roberts N, Jameson L. Osteopenia and bone fractures in a man with anorexia nervosa and hypogonadism. JAMA 1986;256:385–388.

94. Blair SN, Kampert JB, Kohl HW, 3rd, et al. Influences of cardiorespiratory fitness and other precursors on cardiovascular disease and all-cause mortality in men and women. JAMA 1996;276:205–210.

95. von Eckardstein A, Kliesch S, Nieschlag E, Chirazi A, Assmann G, Behre H. Suppression of endogenous testosterone in young men increases serum levels of high density lipoprotein subclass lipoprotein A-I and lipoprotein (a). J Clin Endocrinol Metab 1997;82:3367–3372.

96. Taylor AJ, Watkins T, Bell D, et al. Physical activity and the presence and extent of calcified coronary atherosclerosis. Med Sci Sports Exerc 2002;34:228–233.

97. Lehmann M, Lormes W, Opitz-Gress A, et al. Training and overtraining: an overview and experimental results in endurance sports. J Sports Med Phys Fitness 1997;37:7–17.

98. Fry AC, Kraemer W. Resistance exercise overtraining and overreaching. Neuroendocrine responses. Sports Med 1997;23:106–129.

99. Fry RW, Morton AR, Garcia-Webb P, Keast D. Monitoring exercise stress by changes in metabolic and hormonal responses over a 24-h period. Eur J Appl Physiol 1991;63:228–234.

100. Fry RW, Morton AR, Garcia-Webb P, Crawford GPM, Keast D. Biological responses to overload training in endurance sports. Eur J Appl Physiol 1992;64:335–344.

101. Hackney AC. Neuroendocrine system, exercise overload and regeneration. In: Lehmann M, et al. eds. Overload, Performance Incompetence, and Regeneration in Sport. Kluwer Academic-Plenum, Stuttgart, 1999, pp. 173–187.

102. Barron JL, Noakes TD, Levy W, Smith C, Millar RP. Hypothalamic dysfunction in overtrained athletes. J Clin Endocrinol Metab 1985;60:803–806.

103. American College of Sports Medicine. Position statement on the use of anabolic steroids. ACSM, Indianapolis, 1990.

104. Rogol AD, Yesalis CE. Clinical review—anabolic-androgenic steroids and athletes: what are the issues? J Clin Endocrinol Metab 1992;74:465–469.

105. Rogol A. Sex steroid and growth hormone supplementation to enhance performance in adolescent athletes. Curr Opin Pediatr 2000;12:382–387.

106. Brooks GA, Fahey TD, White TP. Ergogenic aids. Exercise Physiology: Human Bioenergetics and Its Application, 2nd ed. Mayfield, Mountain View, CA:1996 pp. 617–630.

107. Bhasin S, Storer TW, Berman N, et al. Testosterone replacement increases fat-free mass and muscle size in hypogonadal men. J Clin Endocrinol Metab 1997;82:407–413.

108. Bhasin S, Woodhouse L, Casaburi R, et al. Testosterone dose-response relationship in healthy young men. Am J Physiol Endocrinol Metab 2001;281:E1172–E1181.

109. Arnold AM, Peralta JM, Thonney ML. Ontogeny of growth hormone, insulin-like growth factor-I, estradiol and cortisol in the growing lamb: effect of testosterone. J Endocrinol 1996;150:391–399.

110. Urban RJ, Bodenburg YH, Gilkison C, et al. Testosterone administration to elderly men increases skeletal muscle strength and protein synthesis. Am J Physiol 1995;269:E820–E826.

111. Mauras N, Hayes V, Welch S, et al. Testosterone deficiency in young men: marked alterations in whole body protein kinetics, strength, and adiposity. J Clin Endocrinol Metab 1998;83:1886–1892.

112. Wilson JD. The role of 5 alpha-reduction in steroid hormone physiology. Reprod Fertil 2001;13:673–678.

113. Inoue K, Yamasaki S, Fushiki T, Okada Y, Sugimoto E. Androgen receptor antagonist suppresses exercise-induced hypertrophy of skeletal muscle. Eur J Appl Physiol 1994;69:88–91.

114. Sheffield-Moore M, Urban RJ, Wolf SE, et al. Short-term oxandrolone administration stimulates net muscle protein synthesis in young men. J Clin Endocrinol Metab 1999;84:2705–2711.

115. Heinlein CA, Chang C. Androgen receptor (AR) coregulators: an overview. Endocr Rev. 2002;23:175–200.

116. Ting HJ, Yeh S, Nishimura K, Chang C. Supervillin associates with androgen receptor and modulates its transcriptional activity. Proc Natl Acad Sci 2002;99:661–666.

117. Danhaive PA, Rousseau CG. Evidence for sex-dependent anabolic response to androgenic steroids medicated by muscle glucocorticoid receptors in the rat. J Steroid Biochem 1988;29:575–581.

118. Ferrando AA, Stuart CA, Sheffield-Moore M, Wolfe RR. Inactivity amplifies the catabolic response of skeletal muscle to cortisol. J Clin Endocrinol Metab 1999;84:3515–3521.

119. Ferrando AA, Sheffield-Moore M, Wolf SE, Herndon DN, Wolfe RR. Testosterone administration in severe burns ameliorates muscle catabolism. Crit Care Med 2001;29:1936–1942.

120. Mottram DR, George AJ. Anabolic steroids. Baillieres Best Pract Res Clin Endocrinol Metab 2000:14:55–69.

121. Kuipers H. Anabolic steriods: side effects. In: Fahey TD, ed. Encyclopedia of Sports Medicine and Science. Internet Society for Sport Science. Available at: http://sportsci.org. Accessed 2003.

122. Alen M, Rahkila P. Anabolic-androgenic steroids effects on endocrinology and lipid metabolism in athletes. Sports Med 1988;6:327–332.

123. Cohen JC, Hickman R. Insulin resistance and diminished glucose tolerance in power lifters ingesting anabolic steroids. J Clin Endocrinol Metab 1987;64:960–963.

124. DePiccoli B, Giada F, Benettin A, Sartori E, Piccolo E. Anabolic steroid use in body builders: an echocardiographic study of left ventricular morphology and function. Int J Sports Med 1991;12:408–412.
125. Haupt HA. Anabolic steroids and growth hormone. Am J Sports Med 1993;21:468–474.
126. Wilson JD. Androgen abuse in athletes. Endocr Rev 1988;9:181–191.
127. Laure P. Epidemiological approach of doping in sport. J Sports Med Phys Fitness 1997;37:218–224.
128. Buckley WE, Yasalis CE, Friedl KE, Anderson WA, Streit A, Wright JE. Estimated prevalence of anabolic steroid use among male high school seniors. JAMA 1988;260:3441–3445.
129. Yesalis CE III, Kennedy NJ, Kopstein AN, Bahrke MS. Anabolic-androgenic steroid use in the United States. JAMA 1993;270:1217–1221.
130. Bamberger M, Yaeger D. Over the edge. Sports Illustrated 1997;86:60–70.
131. Leder BZ, Catlin DH, Longcope C, Ahrens B, Schoenfeld DA, Finkelstein JS. Metabolism of orally administered androstenedione in young men. J Clin Endocrinol Metab 2001;86;3654–3658.
132. King D, Sharp RL, Vukovich MD, et al. Effects of oral androstenedione on serum testosterone and adaptations to resistance training in young men. JAMA 1999;281:2020–2028.
133. Leder BZ, Longcope, Catlin DH, Ahrens B, Schoenfeld DA, Finkelstein JS. Oral androstenedione administration and serum testosterone concentrations in young men. JAMA 2000;283:779–782.
134. Yen SS, Morales AJ, Khorram O. Replacement of DHEA in aging men and women: potential remedial effects. Ann N Y Acad Sci 1995;774:128–142.
135. Deyssig R, Frisch H, Blum WF, Waldhor T. Effect of growth hormone treatment on hormonal parameters, body composition, and strength in athletes. Acta Endocrinologica 1993;128:313–318.
136. Yarasheski KE, Cambell JA, Smith K, Rennie MJ, Holloszy OJ, Bier DM. Effect of growth hormone and resistance exercise on muscle growth in young men. Am J Physiol Endocrinol Metab 1992;25:E261–E267.
137. Viru A, Viru M. Biochemical Monitoring of Sport Training. Human Kinetics, Champaign, IL, 2001, pp. 5–192.

Testosterone, SHBG, and the Metabolic Cardiovascular Syndrome

Joseph M. Zmuda, PhD,
and Stephen J. Winters, MD

Contents

INTRODUCTION

Cardiovascular disease is more common in men than in menstruating women, and more common in women with elevated serum androgen levels, as in polycystic ovary syndrome (PCOS) *(1)* or type 2 diabetes *(2)* than in normal women. Interest in the relationship between androgens and cardiovascular disease has been stimulated further by the emerging use of testosterone replacement for older men because of concern that cardiovascular risk might increase as a side effect of therapy. The relationship between circulating androgens and the cardiovascular syndrome is intimately related to sex hormone-binding globulin (SHBG) and its downregulation in obesity and by insulin. In fact, SHBG is an indicator of the association between sex hormones and plasma lipids, and low levels of SHBG predict the development of type 2 diabetes. Thus, low testosterone and low SHBG are a part of the metabolic cardiovascular syndrome, and, therefore, testosterone replacement has been advocated in these men to reduce their risk for developing coronary vascular disease. In this chapter, the endocrine regulatory mechanisms that provide insight into this controversy, the epidemiological studies that evaluated the relationship between circulating testosterone levels and risk factors for

From: *Male Hypogonadism:*
Basic, Clinical, and Therapeutic Principles
Edited by: S. J. Winters © Humana Press Inc., Totowa, NJ

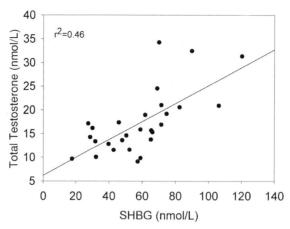

Fig. 1. Relationship between sex hormone-binding globulin and total testosterone levels in normal men.

atherosclerotic cardiovascular disease, measures of subclinical atherosclerosis, and cardiovascular disease end-points are reviewed. Also reviewed are recent animal and laboratory experiments that provide insight into how testosterone may influence the atherosclerotic disease process.

SEX HORMONE-BINDING GLOBULIN

Of the circulating testosterone in adult men, approx 45% is bound with high affinity to SHBG, 50% is loosely bound to albumin (Alb), 1–2% is bound to cortisol-binding globulin, and less than 4% is free (not protein bound) *(3)*. SHBG is a carbohydrate-rich β-globulin produced by hepatocytes. It is a 100,000-kDA dimer, with protomers of 48–52 kDA that convert to a single 39 kDA species when deglycosylated and fractionated on a polyacrylamide gel *(4)*. SHBG binds testosterone and other steroids with high affinity and prolongs their metabolic clearance *(5)*. Because of SHBG's role as a plasma testosterone binding protein, there is a positive correlation between its level and the level of testosterone in human adult male plasma, such that total testosterone levels are low when SHBG levels are low *(see* Fig. 1). The general view is that SHBG reduces the cellular uptake of androgens from the plasma compartment *(6)* and negatively regulates availability to target cells *(7)*. On the other hand, the finding of membrane binding sites for SHBG in testis, prostate, and other tissues *(8)* and the identification of SHBG mRNA and protein in human prostate cancer cell lines and cultured human prostate epithelial and stromal cells *(9)* suggest a paracrine function of SHBG after ligand activation that could directly influence androgen action.

The SHBG Gene

The human gene that encodes SHBG is found on the short arm of chromosome 17, comprises 8 exons, and spans 3 kb of genomic DNA *(10)* and is expressed at high levels in the liver. SHBG gene expression in testicular Sertoli cells produces androgen-binding protein (ABP), with an identical AA sequence but variant glycosylation. SHBG is also expressed in placenta, endometrium, brain, and prostate. So far, not

Table 1
Factors That Influence Circulating Sex Hormone-Binding
Globulin Levels

Increase	Decrease
Aging	Prepubertal development
Growth hormone deficiency	Obesity
Estrogens	Hyperinsulinema
Androgen deficiency	Glucocorticoids
Hyperthyroidism	Androgens
Hepatitis	Progestins
Porphyria	Hypothyroidism
	Growth hormone excess
	Familial

much is known about the regulation of the SHBG promoter. Hammond and coworkers reported that the proximal promoter contains a sequence partially homologous with the consensus binding-site for hepatic nuclear transcription factors (hNF). Members of this family are highly expressed in the liver, and the SHBG promoter is activated by HNF-4 in HEPG2 hepatoma cells (11).

SHBG Regulation

The hormonal control of SHBG in plasma is complex. Table 1 lists those factors that are known to decrease or increase plasma SHBG levels. Only insulin (12–14) and thyroxine (15) influence SHBG levels through effects on steady state mRNA levels. One study examined SHBG mRNA levels in orchidectomized monkeys treated with testosterone (16). Whereas testosterone lowered circulating SHBG levels, SHBG mRNA rose, indicating posttranscriptional control. How other factors increase or decrease circulating SHBG levels remains unknown.

SHBG is developmentally regulated, with high levels in newborns that decline in childhood to pubertal levels in both sexes (17,18). Growth hormone (GH) is unlikely to be responsible for this regulation, because an age-related decline, albeit across higher levels, was observed in children with idiopathic hypopituitarism (19). SHBG also declined with age in two siblings with complete androgen insensitivity, implying that the change with maturation is not androgen dependent (20).

Plasma SHBG levels are lower in adult men than in women, presumably because of suppression by androgens and stimulation by estrogens. SHBG levels increase as men grow older (21,22) but are reduced in elderly women (23). The rise in SHBG in elderly men has been attributed to GH deficiency (24), and the decline through menopause has been attributed to a predominating effect of estrogen deficiency.

TESTOSTERONE, SHBG, AND OBESITY

Glass et al. (25) first reported that circulating testosterone levels are reduced in obese men, and many subsequent studies have confirmed that total testosterone levels decrease as body mass index increases. Because men and women who are hyperandrogenic gain weight predominantly in the abdomen, it is mechanistically interesting to

Table 2
Correlations Between Sex Hormone-Binding Globulin and Measures of Adiposity in Men

		Relation Between Sex Hormone-Binding Globulin and	
Author	No. of Men	Body Mass Index	Waist-to-Hip Ratio
Stefanick (177)	73	−0.26	−0.37
Seidell (50)	23	−0.33	−0.54
Haffner (14)	178	−0.18	0.03
Longcope (60)	1563	−0.26	−0.22
Tchernof (178)	80	−0.42	−0.32

determine whether visceral fat is more closely linked to low testosterone than is total body fat, but results have been conflicting (26). Glass et al. (25) also first noted that low testosterone levels in obese men could be partly explained by a decrease in SHBG, but whether SHBG is more highly correlated with abdominal obesity or with body mass index remains controversial. A summary of several studies reporting cross-sectional correlations between SHBG and body mass index and waist-to-hip ratio (WHR) is found in Table 2. In massively obese men, weight loss after bariatric surgery can reverse the SHBG abnormalities when near-normal body weight is achieved (27).

Whereas a low level of SHBG is the major reason for low testosterone levels in mild to moderately obese men, free and non-SHBG-bound testosterone levels are also reduced in massive obesity (28,29) and correlate inversely with body mass index (30). The testosterone response to human chorionic gonadotropin (hCG) stimulation is normal in obesity (25), implying that Leydig cell function is impaired because of gonadotropin insufficiency. Blood sampling every 10 min for 12 h in 8 massively obese men revealed lower mean luteinizing hormone (LH) levels and pulse amplitude than in controls, whereas pulse frequency (6.3/12h) was comparable in both groups (31). In moderately obese men (mean 127% above ideal body weight), by contrast, 24-h mean LH levels were similar, and follicle-stimulating hormone (FSH) levels were lower than in controls (32).

Reduced LH pulse amplitude may be explained by decreased gonadotropin-releasing hormone (GnRH) production or by reduced pituitary responsiveness to GnRH. A leading hypothesis is that reduced LH pulse amplitude in obesity results from increased estrogen production, because estradiol suppresses the pituitary LH response to GnRH stimulation in males (33). Testosterone is converted to estradiol by aromatase P450, the product of the CYP19 gene (34). Aromatase is expressed in Leydig cells where it is upregulated by LH/hCG (35); however, most of the estrogen in men is from aromatase in adipose and skin stromal cells, with a lesser contribution from aortic smooth muscle cells, kidney, skeletal cells, and the brain. The promoter sequences of the P450 aromatase genes are tissue specific because of differential splicing, but the translated protein is the same in all tissues. The conversion of androstenedione to estrone was more than 10-fold greater in the upper thigh, buttock, and flank than in the breast, lower thigh, abdomen, or omentum (36). Thus, aromatase may be increased in obesity because of increased subcutaneous adipose tissue mass, or adipose-derived factors could upregulate aromatase in selected tissues. Through either mechanism, increased bioconversion of androgens to estrogens could cause LH pulse amplitude to decrease.

The plasma concentration of estradiol in normal adult men is 20–40 pg/mL, and its production rate in blood is 25–40 μg/24 h; both of these values are higher than in postmenopausal women. Mean serum estrone and estradiol levels are elevated in obese men *(29,37)*, and urinary estrone and estradiol production rates were positively correlated to percent above ideal body weight *(37)*. Moreover, FSH, LH, and testosterone levels rose normally when obese men were treated with the antiestrogen clomiphene for 5 d *(37)*. However, in the aforementioned study showing reduced LH pulse amplitude in massive obesity, estradiol levels were comparable in men with mild and moderate obesity *(38)*.

In addition, Stanik et al. *(39)* found that circulating estrone levels fell and total testosterone levels increased in obese men with weight loss, although another study did not confirm these results *(26)*. In the study by Stanik et al. *(39)*, obese men lost weight because they consumed a 320-kCal liquid diet. With prolonged dieting, the free testosterone concentration declined and SHBG was unchanged. Gonadotropins were not studied, and this research is open to various interpretations insofar as caloric deprivation also reduces LH secretion in men *(40)*, which would affect testosterone and estradiol production.

Men with Cushing's syndrome have central obesity and are generally hypogonadal *(41)*. Glucocorticoids suppress GnRH transcription *(42)*, suggesting that the hypogonadotropic hypogonadism of obese men could also be explained by hypercortisolemia. However, studies of cortisol production in obese men have produced mixed results *(43)*. Leptin, a cytokine-like product of adipocytes, is secreted into the circulation in proportion to the body mass index. Gonadotropin deficiency in leptin-deficient mice and humans, together with gonadotropin stimulation by leptin treatment, is consistent with an action of leptin to stimulate GnRH. On the other hand, leptin suppressed testosterone secretion by testicular slices and blocked hCG upregulation of SF-1, StAR, and P450scc *(44)*. Excess leptin could contribute to low testosterone levels in obesity through the latter mechanism.

The relationship between low testosterone and obesity is bidirectional. Bjorntorp *(43)* has proposed that hypogonadism predisposes to central obesity and insulin resistance in men. In support of this idea, Becker et al. *(45)* reviewed the clinical records of 50 hypogonadal men with Klinefelter syndrome seen at the Mayo Clinic, and reported in 1966 that 50% were obese as adults. Furthermore, men with prostate cancer who were receiving androgen deprivation therapy with GnRH analogs had a higher fat mass by dual energy x-ray absorptiometry (DEXA) scan than did age-matched men with nonmetastatic prostate cancer who were postprostatectomy and/or radiotherapy or age-matched normal men *(46)*. In a longitudinal study, fat mass increased 5% (from 20.2 + 9.4 to 21.9 + 9.6 kg) after 3 mo of androgen-deprivation therapy *(47)*. In a study of healthy Japanese American men, lower baseline total testosterone predicted an increase in intraabdominal fat *(48)*. Finally, testosterone replacement of middle-aged men with central obesity reduced visceral fat measured by computed tomography scan without affecting subcutaneous fat *(49)*.

Although there are many studies of low testosterone, only one study *(32)* includes data on sperm output in obese men. In that study, a semen sample was provided by 16 obese men who were 52–332% above ideal body weight. Ejaculate volumes ranged from 0.5 to 4.0 mL. The mean sperm count was 46 million/mL (95% confidence limits 10–200 million), and the percent motile forms was 69% ± 18%. The authors concluded that spermatogenesis is normal in obese men.

TESTOSTERONE, SHBG, AND INSULIN

The mechanism for the association between obesity and low testosterone and SHBG has received considerable attention. Many studies have shown that testosterone levels are inversely correlated with insulin and c-peptide concentrations *(50,51)*. This association is partly through SHBG, because fasting insulin likewise correlates negatively with SHBG levels *(52)*, and insulin infusion lowered circulating SHBG, albeit slighty *(53)*. Moreover, lowering circulating insulin levels with diazoxide increased plasma SHBG in men *(54)* and in obese women with PCOS *(55)*. The regulation of SHBG expression by insulin has been studied directly using cultures of HepG2 hepatoma cells that express the SHBG gene *(56)*. In these cells, adding insulin reduced SHBG mRNA levels *(13)* and protein secretion *(12)*. As noted in the section on the SHBG gene, this insulin effect may be mediated by the liver-enriched transcription factor HNF-4 (hepatocyte nuclear factor-4) that transactivates the SHBG promoter *(57)*. Interestingly, maturity onset diabetes of the young (MODY-1) is caused by mutation in HNF-4α.

In men with type 2 diabetes, in whom insulin sensitivity was estimated using the hyperinsulinemic euglycemic glucose clamp technique, there was a strong positive correlation between SHBG level and insulin sensitivity *(58,59)*. In the latter study, SHBG levels were comparable in men with type 2 diabetes mellitus and weight-matched controls and correlated negatively with all measures of adiposity in the groups as a whole. However, only fasting insulin levels were similar, whereas glucose-stimulated insulin secretion was reduced in the men with diabetes *(59)*. These findings and imperfect correlations between insulin levels and SHBG in obese men suggest that other factors related to obesity and insulin resistance, including GH and IGFs and their binding proteins, glucocorticoids, or adipose-derived factors may contribute to low SHBG as well. In the Massachussetts Male Aging Study, fiber and protein intakes were positively correlated with SHBG levels *(60)*. In a second study, a high-fat diet was associated with decreased SHBG, whereas a weight-reducing high-protein diet increased SHBG levels in normal men *(24)*.

LOW TESTOSTERONE, SHBG, AND DIABETES MELLITUS

Total testosterone levels are lower than normal in men with type 2 diabetes even when controlling for body mass index *(2,61–63)*. Much of this difference may result from lower SHBG, because the calculated value for free testosterone was not different from controls *(2)*, although another study found lower levels of free testosterone using an analog assay *(63)*. Several prospective studies found that low SHBG levels predict the development of type 2 diabetes *(64–66)*. This finding follows logically from the inverse correlation between SHBG and obesity *(25)* and insulin resistance *(50)* and the propensity for obese and insulin-resistant individuals to develop type 2 diabetes. In the Massachusetts Male Aging Study *(66)*, not only total but also free-testosterone levels were 17% lower in men who developed type 2 diabetes 7–10 yr later than in those with no diabetes. Free-testosterone levels that were 10% lower at baseline were also found in men in the Multiple Risk Factor Intervention Trials (MRFIT) who developed diabetes at follow-up 5 yr later *(65)*.

Testosterone levels in men with type 1 diabetes mellitus have been alternatively reported to be normal or reduced and are partly influenced by the disruption of GnRH secretion that occurs in illness *(67,68)*. In one study of adult men with type 1 diabetes mellitus, total testosterone and SHBG were higher, whereas the calculated free testosterone was lower than in healthy controls *(69)*, but in a study of adolescents with type 1 diabetes mellitus, SHBG levels were normal *(70)*.

CROSS-SECTIONAL AND PROSPECTIVE STUDIES RELATING TESTOSTERONE TO CARDIOVASCULAR DISEASE END-POINTS

There has been considerable interest during the past two decades regarding the importance of endogenous testosterone to the development of cardiovascular disease in middle-aged and elderly men *(71–77)*. Studies evaluating the relationship between endogenous testosterone and cardiovascular morbidity and mortality in men have yielded inconclusive results. Most of these studies were hospital-based, case-control studies, in which cases were either men with acute myocardial infarction or men who had survived an infarction. Of the 31 cross-sectional studies, 19 (61%) found lower plasma total or free-testosterone levels in men with myocardial infarction or coronary artery disease compared with controls *(21,78,79–95)*, whereas the remaining studies reported no significant difference in hormone levels between cases and controls *(96–107)*. Cross-sectional studies have also analyzed the relationship between endogenous testosterone levels and the presence of angiographically defined coronary artery stenosis. Of these 13 studies, 9 (69%) found significantly decreased total or free testosterone in patients with coronary artery disease compared with controls *(79–82,85,86,89,90,95)*, whereas four found no significant difference *(97,99,103,107)*. An inverse correlation with the extent of angiographically defined coronary disease was stronger for free than for total testosterone, was independent of the possible confounding effects of age and body mass, and persisted after excluding men with diabetes in one report *(92)*. Only a single cross-sectional study has analyzed the relationship between non-SHBG (bioavailable) testosterone levels and cardiovascular disease *(95)*. That study reported significantly lower (~20%) age-adjusted and body mass index-adjusted levels of bioavailable but not total or free testosterone in men with coronary artery disease (>75% occlusion in ≥ 1 major coronary artery) compared to men with normal coronary angiograms *(95)*.

Cross-sectional studies are limited in their ability to infer a causal relationship between hormone levels and cardiovascular disease. For example, hospitalization, lifestyle changes, or medication use after a cardiovascular event might have altered hormone levels in these previous case-control studies. There have been relatively few prospective epidemiologic studies of testosterone and cardiovascular disease events in men. Five prospective studies did not observe a significant relationship between total testosterone *(65,108–111)* free testosterone *(65,108,111)*, or SHBG *(65,109,111,112)* and cardiovascular disease morbidity or mortality in middle-aged and elderly men. The number of clinical events in these studies was often small, although one report had sufficient statistical power to detect a difference in total testosterone as little as 100 ng/dL between myocardial infarction cases and controls *(108)*. The relationship between bioavailable testosterone and clinical cardiovascular disease in men has not been evaluated in prospective cohort studies.

The basis for the discrepancies in previous case-control and prospective studies of cardiovascular disease remains unresolved. The majority of previous studies measured testosterone at a single point in time, which may not accurately reflect cumulative exposure to testosterone that may be important in atherosclerosis. Testosterone levels vary widely between men, and values for individual men are subject to diurnal variation, such that a single sample may characterize an individual rather poorly *(113)*. Some authors have suggested collecting multiple samples for an individual to improve the accuracy of steroid hormone measurements *(114)*. Furthermore, circulating testosterone measurements do not characterize androgen sensitivity or metabolism in the arterial wall. Such misclassification of exposure in past studies may have reduced the likelihood of detecting an association between testosterone and cardiovascular disease.

The strength of association between established risk factors and coronary artery disease in epidemiologic studies is affected by the control group *(115)*, and controls were often poorly characterized in past studies of myocardial infarction. A more stringent angiographic control group (0–24% maximal stenosis) produced much stronger associations of established risk factors with coronary artery disease than a broadly defined control group (0–49% maximal stenosis) in one report *(115)*. Thus, the strength of relationship between testosterone and cardiovascular disease may have been weakened in some studies by the inclusion of men with moderate, subclinical atherosclerosis in the control group. It is also possible that testosterone is more strongly related to the development and progression of atherosclerosis than to the incidence of clinical cardiovascular events (i.e., myocardial infarction or sudden coronary heart disease death).

MEASURES OF SUBCLINICAL ATHEROSCLEROSIS

Research in the field of atherosclerosis and cardiovascular disease has changed substantially in recent years because of the development of noninvasive methods of measuring the extent of atherosclerosis, including ultrasound measures of carotid intima-media wall thickness, CT measures of coronary artery and aortic calcification, ankle-brachial blood pressure assessments of lower extremity peripheral arterial disease, and measures of vascular stiffness, compliance, and pulse characteristics and endothelial function *(116)*. These newer techniques provide a means of studying the determinants of atherosclerosis in vivo and the progression of atherosclerotic vascular disease over time. Relatively few studies have examined the relationship between endogenous testosterone and these contemporary measures of atherosclerosis.

Numerous studies have shown that carotid intima-media wall thickness predicts coronary atherosclerosis and the incidence of clinical cardiovascular disease *(116)*. Lower total testosterone levels were associated with greater carotid atherosclerosis in 297 elderly Dutch men independent of body mass index, WHR, hypertension, diabetes, cigarette smoking, and serum cholesterol levels in one recent report *(117)*. A similar inverse association between testosterone and carotid artery wall thickness was observed in men with and without prevalent cardiovascular disease.

More recently, Hak et al. *(118)* demonstrated a relationship between endogenous testosterone levels and both the prevalence and the progression of atherosclerosis in a population-based study of 504 nonsmoking men aged 55 yr and older. The extent of arterial calcification in the abdominal aorta was measured with lateral radiographs at a baseline examination and after an average of 6.5 yr. Progression of aortic atherosclerosis was defined as the occurrence of new arterial calcifications or enlargement of preexisting calcifications. Aortic atherosclerosis was present in 175 men (35%), whereas severe atherosclerosis was present in 47 men (9%). Men with total testosterone levels

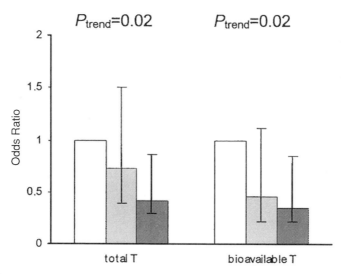

$P_{trend}=0.02$ $P_{trend}=0.02$

Fig. 2. Age-adjusted odds ratio for any progression of aortic atherosclerosis over an average of 6.5 yr in nonsmoking men. White, light gray, and darker gray columns indicate first, second, and third tertiles of baseline levels of testosterone. (Adapted from ref. *118*.)

in the lowest tertile (≤9.8 nmol/L) had 2.5-fold greater age-adjusted risk (95% confidence interval, 1.1, 5.0) of severe aortic atherosclerosis compared with men with the highest testosterone levels (>12.6 nmol/L). Men with bioavailable testosterone levels in the lowest tertile (≤5.6 nmol/L) had a fivefold greater age-adjusted risk (95% confidence interval, 1.4-10.0) of severe aortic atherosclerosis compared with those with bioavailable testosterone levels in highest tertile (>7.5 nmol/L). Additional adjustments for body mass (or central adiposity), blood pressure, total and HDL cholesterol levels, diabetes (or postload insulin), history of smoking, and alcohol intake did not appreciably alter these results. Men with total and bioavailable testosterone levels in the lowest tertile were also significantly more likely to experience progression of aortic atherosclerosis compared with men with higher testosterone levels (*see* Fig. 2). These findings raise the possibility that relatively low total, particularly bioavailable, testosterone may be related to the development or progression of atherosclerosis in men independent of established risk factors for cardiovascular disease. Additional longitudinal studies are needed to confirm the relationship between bioavailable testosterone levels and the development and progression of atherosclerosis in different vascular beds.

Arterial endothelium dysfunction is an early manifestation of subclinical atherosclerosis and contributes to myocardial ischemia, plaque instability and rupture, and myocardial infarction during the later stages of atherosclerosis *(119–121)*. Endothelial function can be assessed noninvasively in the brachial artery with high-resolution ultrasound *(121)*. This technique assesses endothelial function by measuring the arterial diameter of the brachial artery at rest and during reactive hyperaemia, a flow-mediated, endothelium-dependent vasodilatory response *(121)*. Brachial artery flow-mediated vasodilation is impaired in individuals with atherosclerosis, and these measures correlate with coronary endothelial dysfunction and atherosclerosis *(120)*.

Studies evaluating the effects of testosterone on brachial artery endothelial function in men have been inconclusive. Some reports found improved brachial artery endothelial function after acute i.v. *(122)* and short-term (12 wk) oral *(123)* testosterone administration in men with coronary artery disease. On the other hand, brachial artery endothelial function was unchanged after 12 mo of transdermal testosterone treatment *(124)* or was decreased after 3 mo of intramuscular testosterone enanthate *(125)* in men with low testosterone levels and unknown coronary artery disease status. Interpretation of these conflicting reports is difficult because of the heterogeneous and relatively small patient populations and the different testosterone formulations and dosages that were studied. There are fewer data on the relationship between endogenous testosterone and endothelial function in men. Total testosterone levels were significantly and inversely correlated with the extent of brachial artery endothelial dysfunction in 36 hypogonadal men, whereas no association was observed in the eugonadal range in 113 healthy men aged 20–69 yr *(125)*. Larger population studies are needed to evaluate the relationship between total and bioavailable testosterone levels and endothelial function in men.

There have been few studies concerning the effects of testosterone on atherogenesis in animal models. An inhibitory effect of testosterone on neointimal plaque formation was reported in a rabbit aorta culture model *(126)*. Studies in cholesterol-fed male rabbits also showed that testosterone inhibited atherosclerosis in vivo *(127,128)* although these findings have not been universal *(129)*. In one placebo-controlled study of cholesterol-fed rabbits, orchidectomy produced a 100% increase in aortic atherosclerosis compared with sham operation, whereas testosterone enanthate markedly inhibited atherosclerosis in the castrated animals *(128)*. The inhibitory effect of testosterone on atherosclerotic plaque development is at least partly independent of blood lipid changes *(127,128)*. Castration increased the extent of fatty streak formation in the aorta of male mice fed a cholesterol-rich diet *(130)*. Testosterone supplementation reduced atherosclerotic lesion formation in these animals, which was prevented by inhibiting the aromatization of testosterone to estradiol *(130)*. These provocative findings raise the possibility that testosterone may inhibit early atherogenesis in males through conversion to estrogen.

The biological mechanisms by which testosterone might influence atherosclerosis in men are unclear. A direct effect of testosterone on the arterial wall is plausible, given the presence of androgen receptors in vascular smooth muscle *(131)* and endothelial *(132)* cells. The early development of atherosclerotic lesions involves the adherence of monocytes to the vascular endothelium via cellular adhesion molecules, such as vascular cell adhesion molecule-1 (VCAM-1), differentiation of monocytes to macrophages, and subsequent accumulation of lipids to generate foam cells and fatty streaks *(133)*. Recent in vitro experiments indicate that testosterone decreases VCAM-1 expression in human endothelial cells, providing a cellular mechanism by which testosterone may attenuate atherogenesis *(132,134)*. Testosterone also upregulates the expression of HDL receptors in macrophages and promotes the efflux of cholesterol from these cells *(135)*. Thus, testosterone may directly facilitate the transport of excess cholesterol from atherosclerotic plaques of the arterial wall *(135)*. Finally, testosterone may indirectly influence the atherosclerotic disease process by modulating cardiovascular disease risk factors, such as blood lipid and lipoproteins and coagulation and fibrinolytic proteins.

TESTOSTERONE AND CARDIOVASCULAR DISEASE RISK FACTORS

Blood Lipids and Lipoproteins

HDL is a powerful independent risk factor for atherosclerotic cardiovascular disease. HDL influences atherosclerosis, in part, by promoting the efflux of cholesterol from macrophages in the arterial wall and returning this cholesterol to the liver for excretion, a process referred to as reverse cholesterol transport *(136)*. In observational studies, every 1-mg/dL increment in HDL cholesterol (HDL-C) is associated with a 2% decreased risk of coronary artery disease in men *(137)*.

Most studies that have included 100 or more adult men have found a positive association between testosterone or SHBG and HDL-C levels *(14,87,138–147)*. Although it has been less well studied, there is evidence that the age-related decline in testosterone may be associated with decreases in HDL-C in middle-aged men *(148)*. The relationship between endogenous testosterone and HDL-C has been observed in different ethnic groups *(142,143)* and is linear throughout the physiologic range of testosterone concentrations, such that HDL-C increases by 1-mg/dL with every 100 ng/dL increase in total testosterone *(143)*.

The association of testosterone with HDL-C is statistically independent of several possible confounding factors, including age, obesity, alcohol consumption, cigarette smoking, use of medications, triglyceride levels, and glucose and insulin concentrations *(14,87,139,140,143,144)*. The mechanisms by which testosterone may influence HDL-C levels are unclear. One possibility is that testosterone increases the synthesis of apolipoprotein A-I *(149)*, the major protein component of nascent HDL particles. There is also recent evidence that testosterone regulates expression of HDL receptors *(135)*.

Low HDL-C is often found in individual patients in association with other metabolic risk factors, including elevated very low-density lipoprotein (VLDL) and small, dense low-density lipoprotein (LDL), hypertriglyceridemia, and glucose intolerance *(136)*. Insulin resistance may underlie this clustering of metabolic abnormalities, which has been referred to as the metabolic syndrome *(150)*. Many of these metabolic changes promote the development of atherosclerosis and risk of cardiovascular events. All components of the metabolic syndrome have been related to low testosterone and SHBG in epidemiologic studies *(14,65,87,138–140,142–144,146)*. Whether these relationships are truly causal or indirect must be evaluated further. An association of testosterone and SHBG with at least some components of the metabolic syndrome has been attributed to insulin resistance *(65)*.

Blood Coagulation and Fibrinolytic Proteins

Testosterone may influence the risk of cardiovascular disease by affecting hemostatic function and thrombosis. Fibrinogen is the primary coagulation protein, and through conversion to fibrin, it promotes thrombus formation *(151)*. Thrombosis is a major precipitating factor in the onset of cardiovascular events, and prospective studies have shown that increased fibrinogen levels are an independent risk factor for clinical cardiovascular disease *(152)*. The few population studies that have examined the relationship between endogenous testosterone and hemostatic factors have produced inconsistent results. Lower levels of total testosterone were associated with higher concentrations of fibrinogen independent of obesity and other cardiovascular risk factors in one small cross-sectional study of middle-aged and elderly men *(153,154)* but not in another *(155)*. Bonithon-Kopp et al. *(156)* examined the cross-sectional relationships between endogenous testosterone and hemostatic factors in 251 middle-aged men without ischemic heart disease who were not taking medications that influence sex steroid hormones or hemostatic function. There was no association between total testosterone and fibrinogen concentrations in multivariate analyses that controlled for body mass, cigarette smoking, alcohol consumption, and other cardiovascular risk factors. On the other hand, lower levels of total testosterone were associated with higher concentrations of another key component of the blood coagulation system factor VII. In another report of 64 healthy men aged 18 to 45 yr, lower levels of free testosterone were associated with higher concentrations of fibrinogen and factor VII, independent of age, central obesity, fasting insulin and glucose, and other cardiovascular risk factors *(157)*.

Several studies have also reported an association between endogenous levels of testosterone and plasminogen-activator inhibitor type 1 (PAI-1), a major inhibitor of fibrinolysis. High PAI-1 plasma levels have been related to coronary atherosclerosis and myocardial infarction *(158)*. Several cross-sectional studies *(106,154,157,159)*, but not all *(153)*, observed an inverse relationship between endogenous testosterone and PAI-1 in older men. Increased PAI-1 levels are closely related to obesity, body fat distribution, and insulin resistance *(158)*, and it is unclear if endogenous testosterone levels are directly related to PAI-1 or reflect an underlying association with adiposity and insulin sensitivity. PAI activity was positively correlated with body mass, triglycerides, and fasting insulin and inversely correlated with total testosterone and SHBG in a study of 42 men with myocardial infarction and 72 healthy controls *(106)*. However, in multivariate analyses, only triglycerides, fasting insulin, and SHBG remained significant independent correlates of PAI activity, explaining nearly 27% of variation in PAI activity. In another study of 64 otherwise healthy men aged 18 to 45 yr, lower free-testosterone and SHBG concentrations were both associated with greater PAI-I antigen, independent of age, central obesity, fasting insulin and glucose, and other cardiovascular risk factors *(157)*. These observations must be confirmed in larger cohorts of middle-aged and elderly men, but they raise the possibility that lower levels of testosterone may be associated with a prothrombotic state.

Lipoprotein(a) [Lp(a)] is a lipoprotein complex in which apolipoprotein(a) is linked by a disulfide bridge to LDL particles *(160)*. Lp(a) has both proatherogenic and prothrombotic properties, and high Lp(a) levels are an independent risk factor for coronary heart disease in prospective studies *(161)*. Although serum concentrations of Lp(a) are largely under genetic control *(162)*, there is some evidence that androgens influence circulating Lp(a). For instance, suppression of endogenous testosterone levels by a GnRH antagonist *(163)* or after orchidectomy *(164)* increased Lp(a) concentrations, whereas parenteral administration of testosterone decreased Lp(a) concentrations in men *(165–167)*. These results are consistent with studies demonstrating that testosterone reduces apolipoprotein(a) gene expression in mice *(168)*. On the other hand, levels of total and free testosterone within the eugonadal range and SHBG have not correlated significantly with Lp(a) *(106,169,170)*. These population studies included fewer than 200 subjects and may have had insufficient power to detect a modest correlation between testosterone and Lp(a). Moreover, the association between endogenous testosterone and Lp(a) in the population may be nonlinear and only present at the extremes of the testosterone distribution. None of the population studies had an ade-

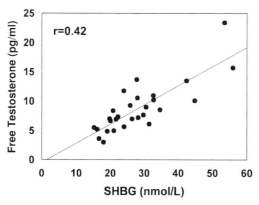

Fig. 3. Relationship between sex hormone-binding globulin and free testosterone levels estimated using an analog assay from Diagnostic Systems Laboratories (Webster, TX) in normal men.

quate sample size to analyze if a nonlinear relationship exists between endogenous testosterone and serum Lp(a).

MEASURES OF ANDROGENICITY IN MEN AT RISK FOR CORONARY ARTERY DISEASE

Because the portion of circulating testosterone that is not bound to SHBG is generally believed to represent the biologically active fraction, many laboratory methods for determining non-SHBG-bound testosterone or free testosterone have been developed. Because SHBG levels are low with obesity or hyperinsulinemia, established risk factors for the development of coronary artery disease, such methods are essential for research seeking to link testosterone to cardiovascular endpoints. Of the methods available, there is a high positive correlation between the level of free testosterone by equilibrium dialysis, the gold-standard, non-SHBG testosterone (bioavailable testosterone), and the free-testosterone level calculated from the levels of total testosterone and SHBG *(171,172)*.

The direct free-testosterone assay was developed as a single-step, nonextraction method *(125)* in which an I^{125}-labeled testosterone analog competes with free testosterone in plasma for binding to a testosterone-specific antiserum that has been immobilized on a polypropylene assay tube. The majority of commercial laboratories measure free testosterone using analog assay kits. These assays propose to adjust the total testosterone level for the effect of a high or a low level of SHBG. However, with current direct free-testosterone assay kits, the percentage of free testosterone is unrelated to the level of SHBG in normal men. Moreover, as shown in Fig. 3, like total testosterone, free-testosterone levels in serum samples from adult men measured with analog methods correlate positively with the SHBG level *(173)*. Age-related reference ranges for men have been reported for analog assays *(174)*; however, the free-testosterone level determined with analog assays provides essentially the same information as the total testosterone level in men, and these assays are not, in theory, appropriate for research on the metabolic cardiovascular syndrome.

Using an analog assay, free testosterone, like total testosterone, has been inversely correlated with insulin levels (fasting and 2-h postprandial) *(175)*. Furthermore, free-testosterone levels by analog methods were reduced in men with type 2 diabetes *(63)*, as well as in men who subsequently developed diabetes *(14,64)*. Another study found that free-, as well total, testosterone levels were reduced in men with hypertension *(176)*. De Pergola et al. *(157)* found that the thrombotic factors PAI-1 antigen, fibrinogen, and factor VII were inversely associated with free-testosterone levels. Although the method for free-testosterone measurement in that study was not stated, the range of values suggests that an analog method was used. Overall, results for free testosterone must be evaluated, with attention to methodology, and the conclusions of some studies will require confirmation with more specific methods.

CONCLUSIONS

Total testosterone and SHBG levels are reduced in men who are obese and hyperinsulinemic, and men with type 2 diabetes. Men with lower levels of testosterone have lower levels of HDL-C and triglycerides and higher levels of the thrombotic factors, tissue PAI, fibrinogen, and factor VII. Low testosterone increases the risk for developing type 2 diabetes and, perhaps, hypertension. Each of these factors predisposes to atherosclerosis and coronary vascular disease, whereas the contribution of low testosterone to the metabolic-cardiovascular syndrome is less certain. More studies are needed to examine the contribution of low SHBG levels when total testosterone or analog methods for free testosterone were used to assess androgenicity in men who are at risk for cardiovascular disease. Furthermore, prospective trials to determine whether testosterone replacement protects against the development of coronary vascular disease are justified.

REFERENCES

1. Talbott E, Guzick D, Clerici A, et al. Coronary heart disease risk factors in women with polycystic ovary syndrome. Arterioscler Thromb Vasc Biol 1995;15:821–826.
2. Andersson B, Marin P, Lissner L, Vermeulen A, Bjorntorp P. Testosterone concentrations in women and men with NIDDM. Diabetes Care 1994;17:405–411.
3. Dunn JF, Nisula BC, Rodbard D. Transport of steroid hormones: binding of 21 endogenous steroids to both testosterone-binding globulin and corticosteroid-binding globulin in human plasma. J Clin Endocrinol Metab 1981;53:58–68.
4. Joseph DR. Structure, function, and regulation of androgen-binding protein/sex hormone-binding globulin. PG – 197-280. Vitam Horm 1994;49:197–280.
5. Hammond G. Potential functions of plasma steroid-binding proteins. Endocrinol Metab 1995;6:298–304.
6. Damassa DA, Lin TM, Sonnenschein C, Soto AM. Biological effects of sex hormone-binding globulin on androgen-induced proliferation and androgen metabolism in LNCaP prostate cells. Endocrinology 1991;129:75–84.
7. Raivio T, Palvimo JJ, Dunkel L, Wickman S, Janne OA. Novel assay for determination of androgen bioactivity in human serum. J Clin Endocrinol Metab 2001;86:1539–1544.
8. Hryb DJ, Khan MS, Romas NA, Rosner W. Solubilization and partial characterization of the sex hormone-binding globulin receptor from human prostate. J Biol Chem 1989;264:5378–5383.
9. Hryb DJ, Nakhla AM, Kahn SM, et al. Sex hormone-binding globulin in the human prostate is locally synthesized and may act as an autocrine/paracrine effector. PG – 26618-22. J Biol Chem 2002;277:26618–26622.
10. Hammond GL, Underhill DA, Rykse HM, Smith CL. The human sex hormone-binding globulin gene contains exons for androgen-binding protein and two other testicular messenger RNAs. PG. Mol Endocrinol 1989;3:1869–1876.
11. Janne M, Hammond GL. Hepatocyte nuclear factor-4 controls transcription from a TATA-less human sex hormone-binding globulin gene promoter. J Biol Chem 1998;273:34105–34114.

12. Plymate SR, Matej LA, Jones RE, Friedl KE. Inhibition of sex hormone-binding globulin production in the human hepatoma (Hep G2) cell line by insulin and prolactin. J Clin Endocrinol Metab 1988;67:460–464.

13. Loukovaara M, Carson M, Adlercreutz H. Regulation of production and secretion of sex hormone-binding globulin in HepG2 cell cultures by hormones and growth factors. J Clin Endocrinol Metab 1995;80:160–164.

14. Haffner SM, Mykkanen L, Valdez RA, Katz MS. Relationship of sex hormones to lipids and lipoproteins in nondiabetic men. J Clin Endocrinol Metab 1993;77:1610–1615.

15. Raggatt LE, Blok RB, Hamblin PS, Barlow JW. Effects of thyroid hormone on sex hormone-binding globulin gene expression in human cells. J Clin Endocrinol Metab 1992;75:116–120.

16. Kottler ML, Dang CD, Salmon R, Counis R, Degrelle H. Effect of testosterone on regulation of the level of sex steroid-binding protein mRNA in monkey (Macaca fascicularis) liver. J Mol Endocrinol 1990;5:253–257.

17. Belgorosky A, Rivarola MA. Progressive decrease in serum sex hormone-binding globulin from infancy to late prepuberty in boys. J Clin Endocrinol Metab 1986;63:510–512.

18. Bartsch W, Horst HJ, Derwahl DM. Interrelationships between sex hormone-binding globulin and 17 beta-estradiol, testosterone, 5 alpha-dihydrotestosterone, thyroxine, and triiodothyronine in prepubertal and pubertal girls. J Clin Endocrinol Metab 1980;50:1053–1056.

19. Belgorosky A, Martinez A, Domene H, Heinrich JJ, Bergada C, Rivarola MA. High serum sex hormone-binding globulin (SHBG) and low serum non-SHBG-bound testosterone in boys with idiopathic hypopituitarism: effect of recombinant human growth hormone treatment. PG – 1107-11. J Clin Endocrinol Metab 1987;65:1107–1111.

20. Cunningham SK, Loughlin T, Culliton M, McKenna TJ. Plasma sex hormone-binding globulin levels decrease during the second decade of life irrespective of pubertal status. J Clin Endocrinol Metab 1984;58:915–918.

21. Gray A, Feldman HA, McKinlay JB, Longcope C. Age, disease, and changing sex hormone levels in middle-aged men: results of the Massachusetts Male Aging Study. J Clin Endocrinol Metab 1991;73:1016–1025.

22. Anderson DC. Sex-hormone-binding globulin. Clin Endocrinol (Oxf) 1974;3:69–96.

23. Burger HG, Dudley EC, Cui J, Dennerstein L, Hopper JL. A prospective longitudinal study of serum testosterone, dehydroepiandrosterone sulfate, and sex hormone-binding globulin levels through the menopause transition. J Clin Endocrinol Metab 2000;85:2832–2838.

24. Vermeulen A, Kaufman JM, Giagulli VA. Influence of some biological indexes on sex hormone-binding globulin and androgen levels in aging or obese males. J Clin Endocrinol Metab 1996;81:1821–1826.

25. Glass AR, Swerdloff RS, Bray GA, Dahms WT, Atkinson RL. Low serum testosterone and sex-hormone-binding-globulin in massively obese men. J Clin Endocrinol Metab 1977;45:1211–1219.

26. Leenen R, van der Kooy K, Seidell JC, Deurenberg P, Koppeschaar HP. Visceral fat accumulation in relation to sex hormones in obese men and women undergoing weight loss therapy. J Clin Endocrinol Metab 1994;78:1515–1520.

27. Pasquali R, Vicennati V, Scopinaro N, et al. Achievement of near-normal body weight as the prerequisite to normalize sex hormone-binding globulin concentrations in massively obese men. Int J Obes Relat Metab Disord 1997;21:1–5.

28. Amatruda JM, Hochstein M, Hsu TH, Lockwood DH. Hypothalamic and pituitary dysfunction in obese males. Int J Obes 1982;6:183–189.

29. Kley HK, Deselaers T, Peerenboom H. Evidence for hypogonadism in massively obese males due to decreased free testosterone. Horm Metab Res 1981;13:639–641.

30. Zumoff B, Strain GW, Miller LK, et al. Plasma free and non-sex-hormone-binding-globulin-bound testosterone are decreased in obese men in proportion to their degree of obesity. J Clin Endocrinol Metab 1990;71:929–931.

31. Vermeulen A, Kaufman JM, Deslypere JP, Thomas G. Attenuated luteinizing hormone (LH) pulse amplitude but normal LH pulse frequency, and its relation to plasma androgens in hypogonadism of obese men. J Clin Endocrinol Metab 1993;76:1140–1146.

32. Strain GW, Zumoff B, Kream J, et al. Mild Hypogonadotropic hypogonadism in obese men. Metabolism 1982;31:871–875.

33. Santen RJ. Is aromatization of testosterone to estradiol required for inhibition of luteinizing hormone secretion in men? J Clin Invest 1975;56:1555–1563.

34. Simpson ER, Zhao Y, Agarwal VR, et al. Aromatase expression in health and disease. Recent Prog Horm Res 1997;52:185–213; discussion 213-4.

35. Inkster S, Yue W, Brodie A. Human testicular aromatase: immunocytochemical and biochemical studies. J Clin Endocrinol Metab 1995;80:1941–1947.

36. Killinger DW, Perel E, Danilescu D, Kharlip L, Lindsay WR. Influence of adipose tissue distribution on the biological activity of androgens. Ann N Y Acad Sci 1990;595:199–211.

37. Schneider G, Kirschner MA, Berkowitz R, Ertel NH. Increased estrogen production in obese men. J Clin Endocrinol Metab 1979;48:633–638.

38. Vermeulen A. Decreased androgen levels and obesity in men. Ann Med 1996;28:13–15.

39. Stanik S, Dornfeld LP, Maxwell MH, Viosca SP, Korenman SG. The effect of weight loss on reproductive hormones in obese men. J Clin Endocrinol Metab 1981;53:828–832.

40. Cameron JL, Weltzin TE, McConaha C, Helmreich DL, Kaye WH. Slowing of pulsatile luteinizing hormone secretion in men after forty-eight hours of fasting. J Clin Endocrinol Metab 1991;73:35–41.

41. Luton JP, Thieblot P, Valcke JC, Mahoudeau JA, Bricaire H. Reversible gonadotropin deficiency in male Cushing's disease. J Clin Endocrinol Metab 1977;45:488–495.

42. Chandran UR, Attardi B, Friedman R, Zheng Z, Roberts JL, DeFranco DB. Glucocorticoid repression of the mouse gonadotropin-releasing hormone gene is mediated by promoter elements that are recognized by heteromeric complexes containing glucocorticoid receptor. J Biol Chem 1996;271:20412–20420.

43. Bjorntorp P. Neuroendocrine factors in obesity. J Endocrinol 1997;155:193–195.

44. Tena-Sempere M, Manna PR, Zhang FP, et al. Molecular mechanisms of leptin action in adult rat testis: potential targets for leptin-induced inhibition of steroidogenesis and pattern of leptin receptor messenger ribonucleic acid expression. J Endocrinol 2001;170:413–423.

45. Becker KL, Hoffman DL, Underdahl LO, Mason HL. Klinefelter's syndrome. Clinical and laboratory findings in 50 patients. Arch Intern Med 1966;118:314–321.

46. Basaria S, Lieb J, 2nd, Tang AM, et al. Long-term effects of androgen deprivation therapy in prostate cancer patients. Clin Endocrinol (Oxf) 2002;56:779–786.

47. Smith JC, Bennett S, Evans LM, et al. The effects of induced hypogonadism on arterial stiffness, body composition, and metabolic parameters in males with prostate cancer. J Clin Endocrinol Metab 2001;86:4261–4267.

48. Tsai EC, Boyko EJ, Leonetti DL, Fujimoto WY. Low serum testosterone level as a predictor of increased visceral fat in Japanese-American men. Int J Obes Relat Metab Disord 2000;24:485–491.

49. Marin P, Holmang S, Jonsson L, et al. The effects of testosterone treatment on body composition and metabolism in middle-aged obese men. Int J Obes Relat Metab Disord 1992;16:991–997.

50. Seidell JC, Bjorntorp P, Sjostrom L, Kvist H, Sannerstedt R. Visceral fat accumulation in men is positively associated with insulin, glucose, and C-peptide levels, but negatively with testosterone levels. Metabolism 1990;39:897–901.

51. Haffner SM, Karhapaa P, Mykkanen L, Laakso M. Insulin resistance, body fat distribution, and sex hormones in men. Diabetes 1994;43:212–219.

52. Toscano V, Balducci R, Bianchi P, Guglielmi R, Mangiantini A, Sciarra F. Steroidal and non-steroidal factors in plasma sex hormone binding globulin regulation. J Steroid Biochem Mol Biol 1992;43:431–437.

53. Ebeling P, Stenman UH, Seppala M, Koivisto VA. Androgens and insulin resistance in type 1 diabetic men. Clin Endocrinol (Oxf) 1995;43:601–607.

54. Pasquali R, Casimirri F, De Iasio R, et al. Insulin regulates testosterone and sex hormone-binding globulin concentrations in adult normal weight and obese men. J Clin Endocrinol Metab 1995;80:654–658.

55. Nestler JE, Powers LP, Matt DW, et al. A direct effect of hyperinsulinemia on serum sex hormone-binding globulin levels in obese women with the polycystic ovary syndrome. J Clin Endocrinol Metab 1991;72:83–89.

56. Rosner W, Aden DP, Khan MS. Hormonal influences on the secretion of steroid-binding proteins by a human hepatoma-derived cell line. J Clin Endocrinol Metab 1984;59:806–808.

57. Oyadomari S, Matsuno F, Chowdhury S, et al. The gene for hepatocyte nuclear factor (HNF)-4alpha is activated by glucocorticoids and glucagon, and repressed by insulin in rat liver. FEBS Lett 2000;478:141–146.

58. Birkeland KI, Hanssen KF, Torjesen PA, Vaaler S. Level of sex hormone-binding globulin is positively correlated with insulin sensitivity in men with type 2 diabetes. J Clin Endocrinol Metab 1993;76:275–278.

59. Abate N, Haffner SM, Garg A, Peshock RM, Grundy SM. Sex steroid hormones, upper body obesity, and insulin resistance. J Clin Endocrinol Metab 2002;87:4522–4527.

60. Longcope C, Feldman HA, McKinlay JB, Araujo AB. Diet and sex hormone-binding globulin. J Clin Endocrinol Metab 2000;85:293–296.

61. Barrett-Connor E, Khaw KT, Yen SS. Endogenous sex hormone levels in older adult men with diabetes mellitus. Am J Epidemiol 1990;132:895–901.

62. Chang TC, Tung CC, Hsiao YL. Hormonal changes in elderly men with non-insulin-dependent diabetes mellitus and the hormonal relationships to abdominal adiposity. Gerontology 1994;40:260–267.

63. Defay R, Papoz L, Barny S, Bonnot-Lours S, Caces E, Simon D. Hormonal status and NIDDM in the European and Melanesian populations of New Caledonia: a case-control study. The CALedonia DIAbetes Mellitus (CALDIA) Study Group. Int J Obes Relat Metab Disord 1998;22:927–934.

64. Tibblin G, Adlerberth A, Lindstedt G, Bjorntorp P. The pituitary-gonadal axis and health in elderly men: a study of men born in 1913. Diabetes 1996;45:1605–1609.

65. Haffner SM, Laakso M, Miettinen H, Mykkanen L, Karhapaa P, Rainwater DL. Low levels of sex hormone-binding globulin and testosterone are associated with smaller, denser low density lipoprotein in normoglycemic men. J Clin Endocrinol Metab 1996;81:3697–3701.

66. Stellato RK, Feldman HA, Hamdy O, Horton ES, McKinlay JB. Testosterone, sex hormone-binding globulin, and the development of type 2 diabetes in middle-aged men: prospective results from the Massachusetts male aging study. Diabetes Care 2000;23:490–494.

67. Distiller LA, Sagel J, Morley JE, Seftel HC. Pituitary responsiveness to luteinizing hormone-releasing hormone in insulin-dependent diabetes mellitus. Diabetes 1975;24:378–380.

68. Valimaki M, Liewendahl K, Nikkanen P, Pelkonen R. Hormonal changes in severely uncontrolled type 1 (insulin-dependent) diabetes mellitus. Scand J Clin Lab Invest 1991;51:385–393.

69. Christensen L, Hagen C, Henriksen JE, Haug E. Elevated levels of sex hormones and sex hormone binding globulin in male patients with insulin dependent diabetes mellitus. Effect of improved blood glucose regulation. Dan Med Bull 1997;44:547–550.

70. Holly JM, Dunger DB, al-Othman SA, Savage MO, Wass JA. Sex hormone binding globulin levels in adolescent subjects with diabetes mellitus. Diabet Med 1992;9:371–374.

71. Eldrup E, Lindholm J, Winkel P. Plasma sex hormones and ischemic heart disease. Clin Biochem 1987;20:105–112.

72. Godsland IF, Wynn V, Crook D, Miller NE. Sex, plasma lipoproteins, and atherosclerosis: prevailing assumptions and outstanding questions. Am Heart J 1987;114:1467–1503.

73. Kalin MF, Zumoff B. Sex hormones and coronary disease: a review of the clinical studies. Steroids 1990;55:330–352.

74. Phillips GB. Relationship of serum sex hormones to coronary heart disease. Steroids 1993;58:286–290; discussion 291-2.

75. Alexandersen P, Haarbo J, Christiansen C. The relationship of natural androgens to coronary heart disease in males: a review. Atherosclerosis 1996;125:1–13.

76. English KM, Steeds R, Jones TH, Channer KS. Testosterone and coronary heart disease: is there a link? Qjm 1997;90:787–791.

77. Rosano GM. Androgens and coronary artery disease. A sex-specific effect of sex hormones? Eur Heart J 2000;21:868–871.

78. Poggi UL, Arguelles AE, Rosner J, de Laborde NP, Cassini JH, Volmer MC. Plasma testosterone and serum lipids in male survivors of myocardial infarction. J Steroid Biochem 1976;7:229–231.

79. Barth JD, Jansen H, Hugenholtz PG, Birkenhager JC. Post-heparin lipases, lipids and related hormones in men undergoing coronary arteriography to assess atherosclerosis. Atherosclerosis 1983;48:235–241.

80. Mendoza SG, Zerpa A, Carrasco H, et al. Estradiol, testosterone, apolipoproteins, lipoprotein cholesterol, and lipolytic enzymes in men with premature myocardial infarction and angiographically assessed coronary occlusion. Artery 1983;12:1–23.

81. Hromadova M, Hacik T, Riecansky I. Concentration of lipid, apoprotein-B and testosterone in patients with coronarographic findings. Klin Wochenschr 1985;63:1071–1074.

82. Breier C, Muhlberger V, Drexel H, et al. Essential role of post-heparin lipoprotein lipase activity and of plasma testosterone in coronary artery disease. Lancet 1985;1:1242–1244.

83. Aksut SV, Aksut G, Karamehmetoglu A, Oram E. The determination of serum estradiol, testosterone and progesterone in acute myocardial infarction. Jpn Heart J 1986;27:825–837.

84. Sewdarsen M, Jialal I, Vythilingum S, Desai R. Sex hormone levels in young Indian patients with myocardial infarction. Arteriosclerosis 1986;6:418–421.

85. Hamalainen E, Tikkanen H, Harkonen M, Naveri H, Adlercreutz H. Serum lipoproteins, sex hormones and sex hormone binding globulin in middle-aged men of different physical fitness and risk of coronary heart disease. Atherosclerosis 1987;67:155–162.

86. Chute CG, Baron JA, Plymate SR, et al. Sex hormones and coronary artery disease. Am J Med 1987;83:853–859.

87. Lichtenstein MJ, Yarnell JW, Elwood PC, et al. Sex hormones, insulin, lipids, and prevalent ischemic heart disease. Am J Epidemiol 1987;126:647–657.

88. Swartz CM, Young MA. Low serum testosterone and myocardial infarction in geriatric male inpatients. J Am Geriatr Soc 1987;35:39–44.

89. Sewdarsen M, Jialal I, Naidu RK. The low plasma testosterone levels of young Indian infarct survivors are not due to a primary testicular defect. Postgrad Med J 1988;64:264–266.

90. Slowinska-Srzednicka J, Zgliczynski S, Ciswicka-Sznajderman M, et al. Decreased plasma dehydroepiandrosterone sulfate and dihydrotestosterone concentrations in young men after myocardial infarction. Atherosclerosis 1989;79:197–203.

91. Sewdarsen M, Vythilingum S, Jialal I, Desai RK, Becker P. Abnormalities in sex hormones are a risk factor for premature manifestation of coronary artery disease in South African Indian men. Atherosclerosis 1990;83:111–117.

92. Phillips GB, Pinkernell BH, Jing TY. The association of hypotestosteronemia with coronary artery disease in men. Arterioscler Thromb 1994;14:701–706.

93. Rice T, Sprecher DL, Borecki IB, Mitchell LE, Laskarzewski PM, Rao DC. Cincinnati myocardial infarction and hormone family study: family resemblance for testosterone in random and MI families. Am J Med Genet 1993;47:542–549.

94. Zhao SP, Li XP. The association of low plasma testosterone level with coronary artery disease in Chinese men. Int J Cardiol 1998;63:161–164.

95. English KM, Mandour O, Steeds RP, Diver MJ, Jones TH, Channer KS. Men with coronary artery disease have lower levels of androgens than men with normal coronary angiograms. Eur Heart J 2000;21:890–894.

96. Phillips GB. Evidence for hyperoestrogenaemia as a risk factor for myocardial infarction in men. Lancet 1976;2:14–18.

97. Luria MH, Johnson MW, Pego R, et al. Relationship between sex hormones, myocardial infarction, and occlusive coronary disease. Arch Intern Med 1982;142:42–44.

98. Labropoulos B, Velonakis E, Oekonomakos P, Laskaris J, Katsimades D. Serum sex hormones in patients with coronary disease and their relationship to known factors causing atherosclerosis. Cardiology 1982;69:98–103.

99. Zumoff B, Troxler RG, O'Connor J, et al. Abnormal hormone levels in men with coronary artery disease. Arteriosclerosis 1982;2:58–67.

100. Heller RF, Miller NE, Wheeler MJ, Kind PR. Coronary heart disease in 'low risk' men. Atherosclerosis 1983;49:187–193.

101. Phillips GB, Castelli WP, Abbott RD, McNamara PM. Association of hyperestrogenemia and coronary heart disease in men in the Framingham cohort. Am J Med 1983;74:863–869.

102. Franzen J, Fex G. Low serum apolipoprotein A-I in acute myocardial infarction survivors with normal HDL cholesterol. Atherosclerosis 1986;59:37–42.

103. Hauner H, Stangl K, Burger K, Busch U, Blomer H, Pfeiffer EF. Sex hormone concentrations in men with angiographically assessed coronary artery disease—relationship to obesity and body fat distribution. Klin Wochenschr 1991;69:664–668.

104. Hautanen A, Manttari M, Manninen V, et al. Adrenal androgens and testosterone as coronary risk factors in the Helsinki Heart Study. Atherosclerosis 1994;105:191–200.

105. Mitchell LE, Sprecher DL, Borecki IB, et al. Evidence for an association between dehydroepiandrosterone sulfate and nonfatal, premature myocardial infarction in males. Circulation 1994;89:89–93.

106. Marques-Vidal P, Sie P, Cambou JP, Chap H, Perret B. Relationships of plasminogen activator inhibitor activity and lipoprotein(a) with insulin, testosterone, 17 beta-estradiol, and testosterone binding globulin in myocardial infarction patients and healthy controls. J Clin Endocrinol Metab 1995;80:1794–1798.

107. Kabakci G, Yildirir A, Can I, Unsal I, Erbas B. Relationship between endogenous sex hormone levels, lipoproteins and coronary atherosclerosis in men undergoing coronary angiography. Cardiology 1999;92:221–225.

108. Cauley JA, Gutai JP, Kuller LH, Dai WS. Usefulness of sex steroid hormone levels in predicting coronary artery disease in men. Am J Cardiol 1987;60:771–777.

109. Barrett-Connor E, Khaw KT. Endogenous sex hormones and cardiovascular disease in men. A prospective population-based study. Circulation 1988;78:539–545.

110. Phillips GB, Yano K, Stemmermann GN. Serum sex hormone levels and myocardial infarction in the Honolulu Heart Program. Pitfalls in prospective studies on sex hormones. J Clin Epidemiol 1988;41:1151–1156.

111. Contoreggi CS, Blackman MR, Andres R, et al. Plasma levels of estradiol, testosterone, and DHEAS do not predict risk of coronary artery disease in men. J Androl 1990;11:460–470.

112. Goodman-Gruen D, Barrett-Connor E. A prospective study of sex hormone-binding globulin and fatal cardiovascular disease in Rancho Bernardo men and women. J Clin Endocrinol Metab 1996;81:2999–3003.

113. Feldman HA, Longcope C, Derby CA, et al. Age trends in the level of serum testosterone and other hormones in middle-aged men: longitudinal results from the Massachusetts male aging study. J Clin Endocrinol Metab 2002;87:589–598.

114. Brambilla DJ, McKinlay SM, McKinlay JB, et al. Does collecting repeated blood samples from each subject improve the precision of estimated steroid hormone levels? J Clin Epidemiol 1996;49:345–350.

115. Fried LP, Pearson TA. The association of risk factors with arteriographically defined coronary artery disease: what is the appropriate control group? Am J Epidemiol 1987;125:844–853.

116. Greenland P, Abrams J, Aurigemma GP, et al. Prevention Conference V: Beyond secondary prevention: identifying the high-risk patient for primary prevention: noninvasive tests of atherosclerotic burden: Writing Group III. Circulation 2000;101:E16–E22.

117. van den Beld AW, Bots ML, Janssen JA, Pols HA, Lamberts SW, Grobbee DE. Endogenous hormones and carotid atherosclerosis in elderly men. Am J Epidemiol 2003;157:25–31.

118. Hak AE, Witteman JC, de Jong FH, Geerlings MI, Hofman A, Pols HA. Low levels of endogenous androgens increase the risk of atherosclerosis in elderly men: the Rotterdam study. J Clin Endocrinol Metab 2002;87:3632–3639.

119. Celermajer DS. Endothelial dysfunction: does it matter? Is it reversible? J Am Coll Cardiol 1997;30:325–333.

120. Behrendt D, Ganz P. Endothelial function. From vascular biology to clinical applications. Am J Cardiol 2002;90:40L–48L.

121. Verma S, Anderson TJ. Fundamentals of endothelial function for the clinical cardiologist. Circulation 2002;105:546–549.

122. Ong PJ, Patrizi G, Chong WC, Webb CM, Hayward CS, Collins P. Testosterone enhances flow-mediated brachial artery reactivity in men with coronary artery disease. Am J Cardiol 2000;85:269–272.

123. Kang SM, Jang Y, Kim JY, et al. Effect of oral administration of testosterone on brachial arterial vasoreactivity in men with coronary artery disease. Am J Cardiol 2002;89:862–864.

124. Kenny AM, Prestwood KM, Gruman CA, Fabregas G, Biskup B, Mansoor G. Effects of transdermal testosterone on lipids and vascular reactivity in older men with low bioavailable testosterone levels. J Gerontol A Biol Sci Med Sci 2002;57:M460–M465.

125. Zitzmann M, Brune M, Nieschlag E. Vascular reactivity in hypogonadal men is reduced by androgen substitution. J Clin Endocrinol Metab 2002;87:5030–5037.

126. Hanke H, Lenz C, Hess B, Spindler KD, Weidemann W. Effect of testosterone on plaque development and androgen receptor expression in the arterial vessel wall. Circulation 2001;103:1382–1385.

127. Bruck B, Brehme U, Gugel N, et al. Gender-specific differences in the effects of testosterone and estrogen on the development of atherosclerosis in rabbits. Arterioscler Thromb Vasc Biol 1997;17:2192–2199.

128. Alexandersen P, Haarbo J, Byrjalsen I, Lawaetz H, Christiansen C. Natural androgens inhibit male atherosclerosis: a study in castrated, cholesterol-fed rabbits. Circ Res 1999;84:813–819.

129. Larsen BA, Nordestgaard BG, Stender S, Kjeldsen K. Effect of testosterone on atherogenesis in cholesterol-fed rabbits with similar plasma cholesterol levels. Atherosclerosis 1993;99:79–86.

130. Nathan L, Shi W, Dinh H, et al. Testosterone inhibits early atherogenesis by conversion to estradiol: critical role of aromatase. Proc Natl Acad Sci USA 2001;98:3589–3593.

131. Fujimoto R, Morimoto I, Morita E, Sugimoto H, Ito Y, Eto S. Androgen receptors, 5 alpha-reductase activity and androgen-dependent proliferation of vascular smooth muscle cells. J Steroid Biochem Mol Biol 1994;50:169–174.

132. Hatakeyama H, Nishizawa M, Nakagawa A, Nakano S, Kigoshi T, Uchida K. Testosterone inhibits tumor necrosis factor-alpha-induced vascular cell adhesion molecule-1 expression in human aortic endothelial cells. FEBS Lett 2002;530:129–132.

133. Blake GJ, Ridker PM. Novel clinical markers of vascular wall inflammation. Circ Res 2001;89:763–771.

134. Mukherjee TK, Dinh H, Chaudhuri G, Nathan L. Testosterone attenuates expression of vascular cell adhesion molecule-1 by conversion to estradiol by aromatase in endothelial cells: implications in atherosclerosis. Proc Natl Acad Sci USA 2002;99:4055–4060.

135. Langer C, Gansz B, Goepfert C, et al. Testosterone up-regulates scavenger receptor BI and stimulates cholesterol efflux from macrophages. Biochem Biophys Res Commun 2002;296:1051–1057.

136. Rader DJ. High-density lipoproteins and atherosclerosis. Am J Cardiol 2002;90:62i–70i.

137. Maron DJ. The epidemiology of low levels of high-density lipoprotein cholesterol in patients with and without coronary artery disease. Am J Cardiol 2000;86:11L–14L.

138. Lindholm J, Winkel P, Brodthagen U, Gyntelberg F. Coronary risk factors and plasma sex hormones. Am J Med 1982;73:648–651.

139. Heller RF, Wheeler MJ, Micallef J, Miller NE, Lewis B. Relationship of high density lipoprotein cholesterol with total and free testosterone and sex hormone binding globulin. Acta Endocrinol (Copenh) 1983;104:253–256.

140. Gutai J, LaPorte R, Kuller L, Dai W, Falvo-Gerard L, Caggiula A. Plasma testosterone, high density lipoprotein cholesterol and other lipoprotein fractions. Am J Cardiol 1981;48:897–902.

141. Dai WS, Gutai JP, Kuller LH, Laporte RE, Falvo-Gerard L, Caggiula A. Relation between plasma high-density lipoprotein cholesterol and sex hormone concentrations in men. Am J Cardiol 1984;53:1259–1263.

142. Miller GJ, Wheeler MJ, Price SG, Beckles GL, Kirkwood BR, Carson DC. Serum high density lipoprotein subclasses, testosterone and sex-hormone-binding globulin in Trinidadian men of African and Indian descent. Atherosclerosis 1985;55:251–258.

143. Freedman DS, O'Brien TR, Flanders WD, DeStefano F, Barboriak JJ. Relation of serum testosterone levels to high density lipoprotein cholesterol and other characteristics in men. Arterioscler Thromb 1991;11:307–315.

144. Khaw KT, Barrett-Connor E. Endogenous sex hormones, high density lipoprotein cholesterol, and other lipoprotein fractions in men. Arterioscler Thromb 1991;11:489–494.

145. Yarnell JW, Beswick AD, Sweetnam PM, Riad-Fahmy D. Endogenous sex hormones and ischemic heart disease in men. The Caerphilly prospective study. Arterioscler Thromb 1993;13:517–520.

146. Gyllenborg J, Rasmussen SL, Borch-Johnsen K, Heitmann BL, Skakkebaek NE, Juul A. Cardiovascular risk factors in men: The role of gonadal steroids and sex hormone-binding globulin. Metabolism 2001;50:882–888.

147. Van Pottelbergh I, Braeckman L, De Bacquer D, De Backer G, Kaufman JM. Differential contribution of testosterone and estradiol in the determination of cholesterol and lipoprotein profile in healthy middle-aged men. Atherosclerosis 2003;166:95–102.

148. Zmuda JM, Cauley JA, Kriska A, Glynn NW, Gutai JP, Kuller LH. Longitudinal relation between endogenous testosterone and cardiovascular disease risk factors in middle-aged men. A 13-year follow-up of former Multiple Risk Factor Intervention Trial participants. Am J Epidemiol 1997;146:609–617.

149. Tang JJ, Krul ES, Schonfeld G. In vivo regulation of apolipoprotein A-I gene expression by estradiol and testosterone occurs at the translational level in inbred strains of mice. Biochem Biophys Res Commun 1991;181:1407–1411.

150. Grundy SM. Hypertriglyceridemia, insulin resistance, and the metabolic syndrome. Am J Cardiol 1999;83:25F–29F.

151. Juhan-Vage I. Haemostatic parameters and vascular risk. Atherosclerosis 1996;124(Suppl)S49–S55.

152. Kannel WB. Influence of fibrinogen on cardiovascular disease. Drugs 1997;54(Suppl 3):32–40.

153. Glueck CJ, Glueck HI, Stroop D, Speirs J, Hamer T, Tracy T. Endogenous testosterone, fibrinolysis, and coronary heart disease risk in hyperlipidemic men. J Lab Clin Med 1993;122:412–420.

154. Yang XC, Jing TY, Resnick LM, Phillips GB. Relation of hemostatic risk factors to other risk factors for coronary heart disease and to sex hormones in men. Arterioscler Thromb 1993;13:467–471.

155. Yang XC, Jing TY, Resnick LM, Phillips GB. Relation of hemostatic risk factors to other risk factors for coronary heart disease and to sex hormones in men. Arteriosclerosis Thrombosis 1993;13:467–471.

156. Bonithon-Kopp C, Scarabin PY, Bara L, Castanier M, Jacqueson A, Roger M. Relationship between sex hormones and haemostatic factors in healthy middle-aged men. Atherosclerosis 1988;71:71–76.

157. De Pergola G, De Mitrio V, Sciaraffia M, et al. Lower androgenicity is associated with higher plasma levels of prothrombotic factors irrespective of age, obesity, body fat distribution, and related metabolic parameters in men. Metabolism 1997;46:1287–1293.

158. Kohler HP, Grant PJ. Plasminogen-activator inhibitor type 1 and coronary artery disease. N Engl J Med 2000;342:1792–1801.

159. Caron P, Bennet A, Camare R, Louvet JP, Boneu B, Sie P. Plasminogen activator inhibitor in plasma is related to testosterone in men. Metabolism 1989;38:1010–1015.

160. Marcovina SM, Koschinsky ML. Lipoprotein(a) as a risk factor for coronary artery disease. Am J Cardiol 1998;82:57U-66U;discussion 86U.

161. Danesh J, Collins R, Peto R. Lipoprotein(a) and coronary heart disease. Meta-analysis of prospective studies. Circulation 2000;102:1082–1085.

162. Boerwinkle E, Leffert CC, Lin J, Lackner C, Chiesa G, Hobbs HH. Apolipoprotein(a) gene accounts for greater than 90% of the variation in plasma lipoprotein(a) concentrations. J Clin Invest 1992;90:52–60.

163. von Eckardstein A, Kliesch S, Nieschlag E, Chirazi A, Assmann G, Behre HM. Suppression of endogenous testosterone in young men increases serum levels of high density lipoprotein subclass lipoprotein A-I and lipoprotein(a). J Clin Endocrinol Metab 1997;82:3367–3372.

164. Henriksson P, Angelin B, Berglund L. Hormonal regulation of serum Lp (a) levels. Opposite effects after estrogen treatment and orchidectomy in males with prostatic carcinoma. J Clin Invest 1992;89:1166–1171.

165. Zmuda JM, Thompson PD, Dickenson R, Bausserman LL. Testosterone decreases lipoprotein(a) in men. Am J Cardiol 1996;77:1244–1247.

166. Marcovina SM, Lippi G, Bagatell CJ, Bremner WJ. Testosterone-induced suppression of lipoprotein(a) in normal men;relation to basal lipoprotein(a) level. Atherosclerosis 1996;122:89–95.

167. Berglund L, Carlstrom K, Stege R, et al. Hormonal regulation of serum lipoprotein (a) levels: effects of parenteral administration of estrogen or testosterone in males. J Clin Endocrinol Metab 1996;81:2633–2637.

168. Frazer KA, Narla G, Zhang JL, Rubin EM. The apolipoprotein(a) gene is regulated by sex hormones and acute-phase inducers in YAC transgenic mice. Nat Genet 1995;9:424–431.

169. Haffner SM, Mykkanen L, Gruber KK, Rainwater DL, Laakso M. Lack of association between sex hormones and Lp(a) concentrations in American and Finnish men. Arterioscler Thromb 1994;14:19–24.

170. Denti L, Pasolini G, Ablondi F, Valenti G. Correlation between plasma lipoprotein Lp(a) and sex hormone concentrations: a cross-sectional study in healthy males. Horm Metab Res 1994;26:602–608.

171. Vermeulen A, Verdonck L, Kaufman JM. A critical evaluation of simple methods for the estimation of free testosterone in serum. J Clin Endocrinol Metab 1999;84:3666–3672.

172. Morley JE, Patrick P, Perry HM, 3rd. Evaluation of assays available to measure free testosterone. Metabolism 2002;51:554–559.

173. Winters SJ, Kelley DE, Goodpaster B. The analog free testosterone assay: are the results in men clinically useful? Clin Chem 1998;44:2178–2182.

174. Ooi DS, Innanen VT, Wang D, et al. Establishing reference intervals for DPC's free testosterone radioimmunoassay. Clin Biochem 1998;31:15–21.

175. Haffner SM, Valdez RA, Mykkanen L, Stern MP, Katz MS. Decreased testosterone and dehydroepiandrosterone sulfate concentrations are associated with increased insulin and glucose concentrations in nondiabetic men. Metabolism 1994;43:599–603.

176. Phillips GB, Jing TY, Resnick LM, Barbagallo M, Laragh JH, Sealey JE. Sex hormones and hemostatic risk factors for coronary heart disease in men with hypertension. J Hypertens 1993;11:699–702.

177. Stefanick ML, Williams PT, Krauss RM, Terry RB, Vranizan KM, Wood PD. Relationships of plasma estradiol, testosterone, and sex hormone-binding globulin with lipoproteins, apolipoproteins, and high density lipoprotein subfractions in men. J Clin Endocrinol Metab 1987;64:723–729.

178. Tchernof A, Despres JP, Belanger A, et al. Reduced testosterone and adrenal C19 steroid levels in obese men. Metabolism 1995;44:513–519.

18 Androgen Replacement Therapy in Hypogonadal Men

Christina Wang, MD
and Ronald S. Swerdloff, MD

CONTENTS

INTRODUCTION

In Chapters 4 to 17, hypogonadism resulting from various etiologies was described. In this chapter, we discuss the criteria for embarking on androgen replacement, the benefits and potential adverse effects of androgen replacement, and the current and future treatment options. There has been a wealth of information on androgen replacement in hypogonadal men in recent years *(1–4)*. This arose from the development and marketing of new testosterone preparations for hypogonadal men and age-related androgen deficiency in older men.

WHO SHOULD RECEIVE ANDROGEN REPLACEMENT THERAPY?

Men with androgen deficiency may have symptoms that include decreased libido, impaired erectile function, decreased body and facial hair, easy fatigability, decreased muscle mass and strength, increased body fat, bone pain or fractures resulting from low

From: *Male Hypogonadism:*
Basic, Clinical, and Therapeutic Principles
Edited by: S. J. Winters © Humana Press Inc., Totowa, NJ

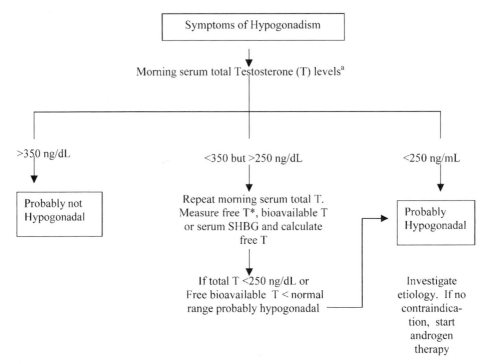

Symptoms of Hypogonadism

Morning serum total Testosterone (T) levels[a]

>350 ng/dL

Probably not
Hypogonadal

<350 but >250 ng/dL

Repeat morning serum total T.
Measure free T*, bioavailable T
or serum SHBG and calculate
free T

If total T <250 ng/dL or
Free bioavailable T < normal
range probably hypogonadal

<250 ng/mL

Probably
Hypogonadal

Investigate
etiology. If no
contraindica-
tion, start
androgen
therapy

[a]Based on a reference range of serum T levels of between 300 to 1000 ng/dL

Fig. 1. Who should be treated with androgen replacement therapy?

bone mineral density (BMD), and increased negative mood parameters, such as irritability, nervousness, inability to concentrate, and poor quality of life. Many of these symptoms are also observed in aging men.

For confirmation of the diagnosis of male hypogonadism, the total serum testosterone testosterone level should be measured, preferably in the morning, because of the known diurnal variation of serum testosterone concentrations. It should be noted that some clinical laboratories use testosterone assays with testosterone or a testosterone analog as the assay standard, using chemiluminence methods on automated platforms *(5)*. These newer assays might give a testosterone reference range for adult men, which is quite different from those obtained using traditional radioimmunoassays. The clinician must carefully review the reference range quoted by each laboratory to accurately diagnose hypogonadism *(5)*. The reference range generally is based on serum values from healthy young adult men. Serum total testosterone assays in which the reference ranges differ from approx 300–1000 ng/dL may be suspect. Based on a reference range of serum testosterone levels in healthy adult young men of 300 to 1000 ng/dL, if the serum testosterone level is less than 250 ng/dL, the patient is most likely hypogonadal. Causes for the hypogonadism should be identified, and the patient should be considered for androgen replacement therapy *(see* Fig. 1). If the serum testosterone exceeds 350 ng/mL, the patient is not biochemically hypogonadal. Other causes of his symptoms should be investigated. If a total serum testosterone level is in the lower normal or slightly below the normal range (250 to 350 ng/dL), a repeat morning serum testosterone level, together with a measurement of free or bioavailable testosterone may be helpful *(6–9)*. The free testosterone should be measured by equilibrium dialysis *(9)*, or the level of sex hormone-binding globulin (SHBG) should be measured to calculate the free testosterone according to an established formula *(10)*. Most clinical laboratories currently measure serum free testosterone using analog displacement assays on automated platforms with chemiluminescent-labeled reagents. Such assays of free testosterone do not accurately assess the free testosterone fraction, and are not recommended *(11,12)*. Bioavailable testosterone (non-SHBG testosterone) is the fraction of testosterone in the serum that is free and albumin (Alb) bound. This is usually measured after ammonium sulfate treatment of the serum. The SHBG-bound hormone is in the precipitate, and the supernatant contains the free and Alb-bound fraction *(7–8)*. Assays for bioavailable testosterone are not available in many laboratories, and reference ranges have to be established by each laboratory. If the repeat morning serum testosterone levels or the serum free testosterone or bioavailable testosterone levels are below the reference range of the laboratory, the patient may be considered for testosterone replacement therapy. The finding of an elevated serum luteinizing hormone (LH) level established the diagnosis of primary testicular hypogonadism in men with borderline low serum testosterone levels. Patients with functional or structural etiologies for hypogonadotropic hypogonadism will have low or inappropriately normal serum LH concentration coupled with low serum testosterone.

WHAT ARE THE CONTRAINDICATIONS TO ANDROGEN REPLACEMENT THERAPY IN HYPOGONADAL MEN?

The absolute contraindications to androgen replacement therapy are carcinoma of the prostate and breast. These are androgen-dependent tumors. Another contraindication includes an elevated hematocrit or hemoglobulin level (e.g., hematocrit >53%). Androgen treatment may cause fluid retention and, in unusual circumstances, may precipitate or aggravate heart failure. In older patients with symptoms or signs of moderate or severe of congestive heart failure, androgens should not be used until the heart failure has been treated. Although there is minimal evidence to implicate testosterone in the development or aggravation of benign prostate hyperplasia (BPH), if a patient has lower urinary tract obstructive symptoms of BPH, then the symptoms should be controlled before institution of testosterone replacement. Obese and older subjects who may be at risk of sleep apnea should be carefully questioned about their ventilatory disturbances during sleep. Such symptoms should be appropriately treated before the start of testosterone-replacement therapy.

WHAT TESTS SHOULD BE DONE BEFORE STARTING ANDROGEN REPLACEMENT?

A digital rectal examination and a serum prostate-specific antigen (PSA) test should be performed by the physician to assess prostate abnormalities before a middle-aged or older patient is started on androgen treatment. If the serum PSA is elevated or nodules or irregularities are found, the patient should be referred for urological assessment. A complete blood count, liver function tests, and a lipid panel should be performed to ensure that the subject does not have an elevated hemoglobin or hematocrit, and to assess the baseline liver enzymes and serum total, low-density lipoprotein (LDL), and high-density lipoprotein (HDL) cholesterol.

Table 1
Androgen Therapy

Benefits	Risks
• Improves sexual function • Maintains secondary sex characters • ↑ Bone mass, muscle mass, and strength • Improves mood in hypogonadal men • Cognitive function? • Coronary vasodilation?	• Acne, oily skin • Gynecomastia, decreased testis volume, and suppressed spermatogenesis • Weight gain, fluid retention • ↓ HDL, ↑ LDL: HDL ratio • Prostate dysfunction (CAP, BPH) • ↑ Hematocrit/hemoglobin • Sleep apnea

HDL, high-density lipoprotein; LDL, low-density lipoprotein; CAP, carcinoma of the prostate; BPH, benign prostate hyperplasia.

WHAT ARE THE BENEFITS AND RISKS OF ANDROGEN REPLACEMENT THERAPY?

Androgen administration induces pubertal changes in patients who have not undergone puberty. In adult subjects, androgen replacement maintains and restores secondary sex characteristics, including facial, body, and pubic hair; the lower tone voice; external genitalia appearance; and the growth of the prostate. The risks and benefits of testosterone replacement therapy are summarized in Table 1.

Sexual Function

It is well known that androgen replacement restores sexual function in hypogonadal men. These include sexual desire (libido), sexual fantasies, sexual enjoyment and frequency of sexual thoughts, sexual activities, and erectile function. In younger hypogonadal men, sexual performance, including erectile dysfunction, is improved by androgen replacement therapy (13–17). In older men, erectile dysfunction is usually multifactorial; other causes, such as vascular, neurogenic, psychogenic, medication-induced, and cavernosal problems may predominate. Improvement in erectile function by testosterone treatment of androgen-deficient older men may be minimal or not as significant as in younger subjects (18–20). Although objective data are limited, it is possible that in androgen-deficient older men whose erectile dysfunction has been improved by phosphodiesterase V inhibitors (e.g., Sildenafil, Vardenafil, and Tadalfil) sexual performance may benefit by cotreatment with testosterone through improvement in libido. It should be noted that androgen replacement to restore serum testosterone to the low normal range induces maximum sexual function improvement in men who are hypogonadal (13,14,17,21). Once a threshold level of serum testosterone is achieved with androgen replacement therapy, further increases in serum testosterone levels do not increase sexual motivation or performance (21).

Mood and Well-Being

Anecdotal reports have indicated that androgen treatment may cause increased anger and "rage" attacks in men. Moreover, higher testosterone salivary levels were found in athletes and other subjects who were engaged in more competitive activities (22). By contrast, studies of men who were hypogonadal administered different preparations of testosterone have demonstrated enhanced positive mood parameters, such as well-being, energy, friendliness, and reduction in negative mood parameters, including anger, fatigue, irritability, and nervousness *(23–26)*. In a placebo-controlled study in normal men administered testosterone in a supraphysiological dose, there was no significant change in aggression, and mood parameters were not changed in the testosterone treated group *(26)*. Thus, in contrast to anecdotal reports, testosterone replacement in hypogonadal men improves mood.

Whether quality-of-life measures improve after androgen replacement in young or elder hypogonadal men has not been studied systematically in randomized controlled clinical trials. Improvement in sexual function, mood, and increased vigor working in synchrony would most likely improve quality of life in hypogonadal men.

Cognitive Function

Studies of changes in cognitive function in hypogonadal younger men are lacking except for uncontrolled studies in men with Klinefelter syndrome in whom testosterone replacement improved verbal skills *(27–29)*. In younger eugonadal men rendered hypogonadal by exogenous administration of a progestin, verbal memory was reduced, which was corrected when testosterone was added to the progestin administration *(30)*. In older hypogonadal men, several well-controlled studies with limited numbers of subjects reported better performances on spatial ability, and, in some studies, verbal memory was also improved after androgen replacement *(31–35)*.

Body Composition

It is well established that androgens cause nitrogen retention in the body. Androgens increase the lean body mass and muscle mass by increasing muscle protein synthesis *(36)*. A recent study showed that testosterone treatment induces muscle fiber hypertrophy *(37)*. Androgens administered as sublingual tablets, injections, and transdermals increased muscle mass assessed by dual-energy X-ray absorptiometry (DEXA) scans in hypogonadal men *(16,17,38–40)*. This increase in muscle mass is observed not only in younger but also in older men with partial androgen deficiency *(18,20)*. The increase in muscle mass was associated with increased muscle strength in both the upper and the lower limbs in younger hypogonadal men assessed by several different techniques *(16,17,38–40)*. In older men, assessment of muscle strength is more difficult *(41)* and improvement in strength has not been always demonstrated *(18,20)*. Moreover, it is not clear whether the increase in muscle strength will be functionally important in older men. The increase in muscle mass is directly related to the amount of testosterone administered and to the serum testosterone concentration. This dose–response relationship is also observed between changes in muscle strength and serum testosterone concentrations achieved *(21)*.

Concomitant with the increases in muscle mass after androgen substitution in hypogonadal men, there are decreases in fat mass and percent fat measured by DEXA or visceral fat measured by abdominal computed tomography (CT) or magnetic resonance imaging (MRI) scan. The decreases in fat mass have been demonstrated with injectables and transdermals but not with the sublingual testosterone *(16,17,38–40)*, which may be related to the amount of testosterone delivered to the body. A dose-response study showed that the decrease in fat mass is inversely related to the serum testosterone level and the dose of testosterone administered *(21)*. Decreases in fat mass are also observed in middle-aged or older men administered testosterone *(18,30,42)*. The decrease in visceral fat observed in some studies has been suggested to result in decrease in insulin resistance. Testosterone and its esters have no significant effects on glucose metabolism and insulin sensitivity in younger men *(43)*. In older men, whether androgen replacement has any effect on insulin resistance, and, if so, whether it acts through visceral fat decreases has not been clarified *(42,43)*.

Bone Mineral Density

Androgens are required to achieve peak bone mass in adolescence and are responsible for the higher BMD in men compared to women. Hypogonadism is associated with a decrease in bone mass and is one cause of osteoporosis in men. With aging, progressive loss of BMD is associated with increased fracture rates. Interestingly, the BMD in older men is more significantly correlated with serum free estradiol than with serum free testosterone levels *(44,45)*. The few case reports of estrogen-receptor mutations and aromatase deficiency in males were all associated with severe osteoporosis *(46–48)*. Thus, the current hypothesis is that estrogens are required for maintaining peak BMD in men. The concentration of serum E_2, or the level of estrogen activity in the target tissues, that is required to maintain BMD is not known. Although it is apparent that some estrogenic action is required for normal BMD, it is probable that testosterone also directly effects bone mass through androgen receptors.

Hypogonadal men have lower BMD. Androgen replacement by injections or oral or transdermal preparations increases BMD in younger hypogonadal men *(17,38,49)*. The androgen-induced increase in BMD is accompanied by initial elevations of bone formation markers and decreases in bone resorption markers *(16,17,38,50)*. In older men, androgen administration increased BMD in some studies *(18)*, but other studies showed no effect *(51)*. In general, the lower the BMD and the lower the serum testosterone level before treatment, the greater the improvement in BMD after testosterone replacement *(17,51)*. Although significant changes in BMD have occurred in hypogonadal men after long-term administration of androgen replacement, randomized controlled studies to examine whether androgens prevent fractures have not been performed.

Lipids and Coronary Artery Disease Risk

Supraphysiological doses of testosterone esters administered to normal men suppressed serum HDL cholesterol levels by 13%, but LDL-cholesterol (LDL-C) and triglyceride levels were unchanged *(52)*. On the other hand, in hypogonadal men administered transdermal testosterone in patches or gels, serum HDL-cholesterol (HDL-C) levels were not significantly changed *(17,53–55)*. The decrease in serum HDL-C was dependent on the dose of testosterone administered and serum testosterone achieved *(43)*. Thus, in androgen replacement of hypogonadal men with near physiological doses of testosterone, significant changes of serum lipid levels are uncommon.

As discussed more thoroughly in Chapter 17, epidemiological studies have shown that men with lower serum total testosterone levels are at higher risk for cardiovascular events *(56,57)*. In men undergoing coronary angiograms, those with evidence for coronary artery disease had significantly lower serum free androgen index and bioavailable testosterone levels than did those without apparent coronary artery disease *(58,59)*. Older studies described a lessening of ST segment depression and reduced anginal symptoms in men with coronary artery disease after testosterone treatment *(60,61)*. Acute administration of testosterone in men with exercise-induced myocardial ischemia reduced ST segment depression and increase exercise testing time compared to placebo *(62,63)*. Because of this acute action of testosterone, the effect may be ascribed to a direct coronary vasodilatory effect of the steroid. A subsequent study confirmed this hypothesis by showing that acute testosterone infusion increased coronary artery diameter coronary blood flow in men with established coronary artery disease compared to vehicle administration *(64)*. Others failed to demonstrate a beneficial effect on acute stress-induced myocardial ischemia *(65)*. In summary, these studies indicate that testosterone administration does not have an adverse effect on coronary artery disease. Whether testosterone administration has beneficial effects on coronary artery disease needs to be addressed in randomized controlled clinical studies.

Prostate Disease

Normal prostate growth and development requires the presence of androgens from childhood to adolescence and adulthood. In younger hypogonadal men in whom prostate diseases are uncommon, androgen replacement increases the size of the prostate from the smaller volumes at baseline to the expected range for eugonadal men *(66)*. However, progressive increases in prostate volume do not occur with continued testosterone replacement *(66,67)*. Serum PSA levels may increase significantly with testosterone replacement but generally remain within the normal range *(15,18,55,67)*. In middle-aged and older men, androgen replacement has resulted, in a few instances, in lower urinary tract obstructive symptoms and increased serum PSA levels, resulting in urological referral and ultrasound-guided prostate biopsy *(17,20)*. In most reports, prostate-related adverse events have occurred rather early in the course of androgen replacement, suggesting that such treatment may have unmasked existing latent or histological cancer. In those men, increasing serum PSA levels to values exceeding the reference range triggered an early prostate biopsy and a cancer diagnosis.

Most urologists believe that androgens do not induce BPH, but androgens should not be used in subjects with lower urinary tract obstructive symptoms until these symptoms have been treated. There is no direct evidence in hypogonadal young or older men that androgen replacement will induce the formation of prostate cancer or convert a latent, histological prostate cancer to a clinically significant or metastatic cancer *(68)*. However, androgens should not be used in a hypogonadal man who has had prostate cancer. There are possible rare exceptions, e.g., a patient with a distant completely resected intraprostatic cancer and long-standing near-undetectable PSA levels who is suffering from severe symptoms and signs of testosterone deficiency. Treatment of such a patient may be justified but only with careful surveillance and well-documented informed consent. It is not known whether testosterone treatment, together with the 5-α reductase inhibitor finasteride or an androgen that cannot be converted to dihydrotestosterone (DHT) will have sparing effect on prostate growth. A prostate cancer primary preventive trial using a 5-α reductase inhibitor (finasteride) showed that it prevented or delayed prostate cancer but may increase the risk of high grade cancer *(68a)*. A randomized, prospective study of androgen-replacement in androgen-deficient older men is urgently required to address the concerns of whether testosterone replacement to older hypogonadal men will increase the risk of development of clinical prostate cancer.

Hematocrit, Hemoglobin, and Liver Function Tests

Androgens increase erythropoiesis (EPO) by acting directly on stem cell proliferation and through its action on the kidneys to stimulate EPO production *(69)*. Androgen therapy in hypogonadal and eugonadal men results in elevation of hematocrit and hemoglobin *(17,40,55)*. The increases in hemoglobin and hematocrit occur within 3 mo, but progressive increases are uncommon, unless the dose of testosterone is adjusted upward or another cause for polycythemia is also present. Direct dose-response relationships have been shown between testosterone and hematocrit and hemoglobin concentrations *(21)*. Thus, androgen therapy must be used with caution in subjects with baseline hematocrit of 50% or higher. When the hematocrit rises above 53%, the subject must be carefully monitored and the dose of testosterone replacement adjusted downward to ensure that hyperviscosity with increased risk of thrombosis does not occur.

Abnormal liver function tests have been reported with orally administered 17 alkylated androgens *(70,71)*. Because of the possibility of liver toxicity and the increase in LDL and decrease in HDL-C associated with 17 alkylated androgens, they are not recommended for use as androgen replacement. It should be noted that native testosterone and testosterone esters administered as replacement therapy do not result in abnormalities of liver function, nor do they affect glucose or insulin concentrations *(16,17,40,55)*.

Other Possible Adverse Effects

Increased oiliness of skin and acne are common complaints after testosterone treatment, especially if high doses of testosterone are used. These conditions can be treated by topical measures, the testosterone dose can be reduced, or the testosterone preparation can be changed. Because testosterone esters and native testosterone are aromatized to estrogens, changes in the androgen to estrogen balance may occur after testosterone replacement, which may cause gynecomastia. Testosterone replacement also causes fluid retention during the early weeks of treatment and should be used with caution in older patients with congestive heart failure or poor myocardial function.

Sleep-related breathing disorders may be aggravated by testosterone replacement *(72)*. Thus, a detailed history for symptoms of sleep apnea before and during testosterone treatment must be obtained. Patients at high risk for sleep apnea (obese and elderly) should be investigated and treated for sleep apnea before beginning androgen-replacement therapy.

Testosterone administration results in suppression of the gonadotropins and intratesticular testosterone production and spermatogenesis. Prolonged testosterone administration will decrease the size of the testes and suppress spermatogenesis. These changes are reversible after stopping testosterone replacement.

WHAT ARE THE AVAILABLE ANDROGEN PREPARATIONS?

Table 2 shows the currently available androgen preparations and those under development. Until a decade ago, the only available effective androgen replacement treatment was testosterone enanthate or cypionate administered intramuscularly. In the past 15 yr, several transdermal preparations were tested and then marketed. Future goals of the pharmaceutical industry are to develop modified androgens and synthetic androgen-receptor modulators to avoid the potential adverse effects (e.g., stimulatory effects

Table 2
Androgen Preparations and Delivery System

	Currently Available	Under Development
Injectables	Testosterone enanthate Testosterone cypionate	Testosterone undecanoate Testosterone decanoate Testosterone microspheres
Oral	Testosterone undecanoate (not available in United States, but available in Canada, Mexico, Europe, Asia, and South America)	Buccal adhesive tablets Sublingual testosterone cyclodextrin Buccal testosterone Selective androgen receptor modulators (SARMS)
Trandermals	Testosterone nonscrotal patch Testosterone gel	Other testosterone gels, creams DHT gel
Implants	Testosterone pellets (available as 75 mg in United States; 100 or 200 mg in Europe or Australia)	7α-methyl 19 nor-testosterone (MENT)

DHT, dihydrotestosterone.

of androgens on prostate growth) while maintaining the beneficial effects on muscle, masss, sexual function, and mood.

Injectables

Testosterone enanthate (TE) and cypionate are testosterone esters administered by biweekly or triweekly deep im injection. The usual recommended dose for hypogonadal men is 200 mg in 1 mL oil administered every 2 wk. The pharmacokinetics (PK) of injectable testosterone preparations have been carefully studied *(73,74),* and the PK of TE is shown in Fig. 2. Serum testosterone levels peak within 1 to 3 d after administration, and gradually decline to a trough after 2 to 3 wk. In many subjects, the peak level of serum testosterone achieved in the first few days after an injection may reach a concentration that is higher than the normal adult male reference range. In some patients, the high peaks and low troughs of serum testosterone levels may result in mood swings and acne. In such patients, the dose may be decreased and frequency of the injections increased, for example, testosterone enanthate may be administered at a dose of 100 mg every 7 to 10 d. Most patients can be taught to self-administer injections.

Several other injectable testosterone preparations are in different stages of development. Testosterone undecanoate was developed and is currently marketed in China for the treatment of hypogonadism *(75).* The preparation (testosterone undecanoate, 200 mg/mL, 1000 mg per injection) has been used in clinical studies for androgen replacement in hypogonadal men in Europe. After administration of 1000 mg testosterone undecanoate, the peak serum testosterone level occurred in the first or second week and remained within the normal range for as long as 12 wk *(76,77).* We speculate that if available worldwide, it will be a more acceptable injection for most hypogonadal men than TE or testosterone cypionate. Testosterone microspheres are testosterone incorporated in biodegradable polylactide glycolide. When administered

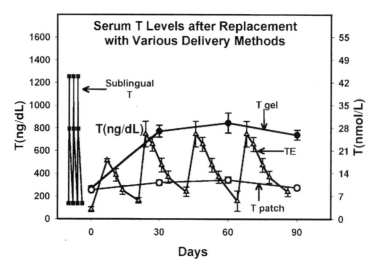

Fig. 2. Pharmacokinetic profiles of different testosterone preparations. (TE, testosterone enanthate 200 mg im once every 3 wk; T patch, trough levels after application of 5-mg T patch the day before; T gel, trough levels after application of 10-g T gel the day before; sublingual T, levels in a day after taking 5-mg sublingual T 3 times a day). (Data from refs. *84* and *92.)*

as a single injection, testosterone microspheres can maintain serum testosterone within the normal range for 10 wk in hypogonadal men *(78)*. Recent studies reaffirmed the long-acting properties of testosterone microsphere injections, with a brief pronounced early peak of serum testosterone followed by low normal testosterone levels for 10 to 11 wk *(79)*.

Oral Androgens

The oral 17 alkylated testosterone derivates, methyltestosterone and fluoxymesterone, are not recommended for long-term androgen replacement because of potential adverse effects on liver function and lipid levels. Testosterone undecanoate is a testosterone ester with a long fatty acid side chain. When administered by mouth, testosterone is absorbed by lymphatics and must be administered after ingestion of food. Serum testosterone levels rose to peak levels 4 to 5 h after administration and remained in low normal range 8 to 12 h after oral administration *(80,81)*. When testosterone undecanoate is administered in the fasting state, serum testosterone levels remained low. Testosterone undecanoate has long-term safety data *(82)*. There are marked intersubject as well as intrasubject variations in the peak serum testosterone levels achieved after oral administration. The usual dose is testosterone undecanoate 80 mg bid or 40 mg tid. This oral preparation is not available in the United States but is available in Canada, Mexico, Europe, Asia, and Australia.

Several new oral preparations are being developed for the U.S. market but have not been approved by the Food and Drug Administration (FDA). Buccal administration of testosterone *(83)* and sublingual testosterone cyclodextrin *(84)* result in high peaks and troughs lasting for approx 2 h. The PKs are represented as the sharp peaks and troughs in Fig. 2. Although sublingual testosterone improved sexual function, mood, and muscle mass, this preparation is not available for androgen replacement *(16)*. A more recent development is a buccal tablet, which, after application to the gum, gels and results in steady serum testosterone levels. The buccal bioadhesive tablet has to be administered twice per day, does not appear to cause gum irritation, and delivers steady serum testosterone levels (85).

Transdermals

Steady serum testosterone levels in the low normal range mimicking circadian variation are attained after testosterone transdermal patch application (Fig. 2). The scrotal testosterone patch was the first to become available in the early 1990s, but this patch has been superseded by other transdermals. The scrotal testosterone patch is 60 cm in diameter and requires shaving or clipping of scrotal skin hair (86,87). There are two nonscrotal skin patches available in the United States. The smaller permeation-enhanced patch (Androderm) delivers 5 mg testosterone per day and produces serum testosterone in the low normal range (86–90). This smaller testosterone patch has a major side effect of causing skin irritation in up to 60% of subjects, leading to discontinuation in up to 10 to 15% of subjects (86–90). Preapplication of corticosteroid cream may reduce the skin irritation. The larger non-scrotal testosterone patches (Testoderm TTS) produce much less skin irritation but may not adhere well to the skin.

The most recent development in transdermal delivery are testosterone gels. Androgel and Testim are 1% testosterone hydroalcoholic gels that dry in a few minutes after application. The daily dose varies between 5 and 10 g, delivering 5 to 10 mg testosterone per day (~10 to 14% is bioavailable). Application of testosterone gels result in dose-dependent increase in serum testosterone levels. With gels, the levels of serum testosterone are relatively steady after a few days of application (91,92a). As with other testosterone preparations, positive effects on libido, mood, muscle size and strength and body fat have been demonstrated in hypogonadal men with testosterone gels. In addition, positive effects on BMD have been shown (93) and the effects persist for at least 3 yr. Because of the ease of application and flexibility of dosing, this method of testosterone replacement is acceptable to many hypogonadal men. A potential problem is the possibility of transfer of testosterone to women and children during close contact of skin surfaces. This can be avoided by wearing clothing or removing the residual testosterone on the skin with showering. Several other testosterone gels and creams are being developed.

In addition to testosterone gels, the potent androgen DHT gel has been studied as a treatment for hypogonadal younger (94) and older men (95–98). DHT improved sexual dysfunction in older partially androgen-deficient men but had minimal effect on muscle mass and strength (95,96). It is controversial whether DHT has significant benefits over testosterone as an androgen replacement therapy. DHT is not converted to estradiol (nonaromatizable androgen). Because some of the beneficial (and adverse effects) of testosterone have been attributed, at least in part, to its metabolite estradiol, it is not clear whether DHT will have a positive effect on bone mass, cognitive function, and fat mass (99) or be free from the problem of testosterone-induced gynecomastia.

Implants

Crystalline testosterone in pellets had been inserted into the abdominal subcutaneous fat for androgen replacement in hypogonadal men. In Europe and Australia, where testosterone pellets are available in 100- and 200-mg doses, they are frequently used to treat hypogonadal men *(100,101)*. Four 200-mg implants maintain testosterone levels for 16 to 20 wk. Insertion of the pellets requires a minor surgical procedure under local anesthesia. Extrusion of the testosterone pellets is observed in approx 8 to 11% of subjects *(102)*, although our experience with insertion by a skilled operative is much lower. This method has not been widely used and is not routinely offered by physicians as androgen-replacement modality in the United States.

Selective Androgen Receptor Modulators (SARMs)

SARMs act via androgen receptor signaling and may be androgen agonists or antagonists, depending on the target tissues and their modulating effects on the coactivators or coinhibitors of the androgen receptor. An example of a steroid SARM is 7α-methyl 19 nor-testosterone (MENT). MENT is believed to be aromatized to an active estrogen but is not converted to a 5-α-reduced product. In rodents and monkeys, MENT has a greater stimulatory effect on skeletal muscle relative to the prostate *(103–104)*. A clinical study showed that MENT could maintain sexual function and muscle mass in hypogonadal men. MENT is being developed as a long-acting implant *(105)*. Other nonsteroidal orally active SARMs, which have potent actions on muscle and brain but little or substantially lower stimulatory effect on the prostate, are being developed by several pharmaceutical companies *(106,107)*. SARMs may inhibit the synthesis and secretion of the gonadotropins, and, thereby, testosterone production will be markedly reduced. If so, after SARMs administration serum testosterone levels may be low, and clinicians may encounter difficulty in assessing adequate androgen replacement in the absence of measurable serum testosterone concentrations.

HOW DO WE MONITOR ANDROGEN REPLACEMENT THERAPY?

In hypogonadal men, most of the symptoms of androgen deficiency are alleviated with androgen replacement. To determine the dose of testosterone to be administered, serum testosterone levels should be measured at appropriate times after drug administration, based on the PK characteristics of the specific preparation. For example, serum testosterone levels peak 12–16 h after application of testosterone patches and return toward baseline by 24 h. Monitoring is thus done approx 12 h after application, and levels should be in the mid-normal range. Because serum T levels are maintained in a steady state by the transdermal gels (*see* Fig. 2), serum testosterone can be measured at any time. Because the injectable testosterone preparations, such as testosterone enanthate and cypionate, result in early peaks (i.e., 2–3 d) and troughs (10–14 + d), serum testosterone is measured at day 7 to ensure that serum testosterone levels are within normal limits. Once a stable dose of testosterone replacement is determined, then measuring serum testosterone levels is often unnecessary unless dose adjustments are made.

Because administration of testosterone may unmask histological prostate cancers by increasing serum PSA levels, measuring PSA early after beginning treatment, e.g., 1 to 3 mo is recommended. Thereafter, PSA should be checked yearly according to the urological practice applicable to each man. Hemoglobin and hematocrit should be checked at 3 mo and after each dose adjustment, followed by yearly intervals. Subjects whose hemoglobin level is high before treatment should be monitored more carefully. As with other patients on replacement therapy, a yearly liver function test and lipid profile should be done.

CONCLUSIONS

Androgen replacement therapy should be prescribed for all hypogonadal men. Before commencement of replacement, contraindications to androgen treatment should be identified. In hypogonadal men, androgens improve sexual function, energy, and mood; increase muscle mass and strength; and increase BMD. Androgen therapy can be tailored to each patient's needs and preferences. There are many new androgen delivery systems introduced in the past few years, and many others are in development. SARMs may have the potential of optimizing beneficial effects while minimizing potential adverse effects. In older men, monitoring of prostate dysfunction and red-cell indexes are necessary and important. With care, androgens can be used efficaciously and with minimal potential side effects.

ACKNOWLEDGMENT

This work was supported by NIH grants M01 RR00425 and T32 DK07571 and by the CONRAD Program.

REFERENCES

1. Bhasin S, Gabelnick HL, Spieler JM, Swerdloff RS, Wang C. Pharmacology, Biology and Clinical Applications of Androgen. New York, Wiley Liss, 1996.
2. Nieschlag E, Behre HM. Testosterone: Action, Deficiency, Substitution, 2nd ed. Springer, Berlin, 1998.
3. Wang C, Swerdloff RS. Androgen replacement therapy. Ann Med 1997;29:365–370.
4. Wang C, Swerdloff RS. Androgen replacement therapy, risks and benefits. In: Wang C, ed. Male Reproductive Function. Norwell, Kluwer Academic Publishers, 1999, pp. 157–172.
5. Steinberger E, Ayala C, His B, et al. Utilization of commercial laboratory results in management of hyperandrogenism in women. Endocr Pract 1998;4:1–10.
6. Vermeulen A, Verdonck L, Kaufman JM. A critical evaluation of simple methods for the estimation of free testosterone in serum. J Clin Endocrinol Metab. 1999;84:3666–3672.
7. O'Connor S, Baker HWG, Dulmanis A, Hudson B. The measurement of sex steroid binding globulin by differential ammoniumsulfate precipitation. J Steroid Biochem 1973;4:331–339.
8. Cumming DC, Wall SR. Non sex hormone binding globulin bound testosterone as a marker of hyperandrogenism. J Clin Endocrinol Metab 1985;61:873–876.
9. Sinha-Hikim I, Arver S, Beall G, et al. The use of a sensitive equilibrium dialysis method for the measurement of free testosterone levels in healthy cycling women and in human immunodeficiency virus-infected women. J Clin Endocrinol Metab 1998;83:1312–1318.
10. Sodergard R, Backstrom T, Shanbhag V, Carstensen H. Calculation of free and bound fractions of testosterone and estradiol 17β to human plasma protein at body temperature. J Steroid Biochem 1982;26:801–810.
11. Rosner W. Errors in the measurement of plasma free testosterone. J Clin Endocrinol Metab 1997;82:2014–2015.
12. Winters SJ, Kelly DE, Goodpaster B. The analog free testosterone assay: are the results in men clinically useful? Clin Chem 1998;44:2178–2182.
13. Davidson JM, Camargo CA, Smith ER. Effects of androgen on sexual behavior in hypogonadal men. J Clin Endocrinol Metab 1979;48:955–958.
14. Skakkebaek NE, Bancroft J, Davidson DW, Warner P. Androgen replacement with oral testosterone undecanoate in hypogonadal men: a double-blind controlled study. Clin Endocrinol (Oxf) 1981;14:49–61.
15. Burris AS, Banks SM, Carter CS, Davidson JM, Sherins RJ. A long-term, prospective study of the physiologic and behavioral effects of hormone replacement in untreated hypogonadal men. J Androl 1992;13:297–304.

16. Wang C, Eyre DE, Clark R, et al. Sublingual testosterone replacement improves muscle mass and strength and decrease bone resorption and increases bone formation markers in hypogonadal men: a Clinical Research Center Study. J Clin Endocrinol Metab 1996;81:3654–3662.

17. Wang C, Swerdloff RS, Iranmanesh A, et al. and the Testosterone Gel Study Group. Transdermal testosterone gel improves sexual function, mood, muscle strength, and body composition parameters in hypogonadal men. J Clin Endocrinol Metab 2000;85:2839–2853.

18. Tenover JL. Male senescence. In: Wang C, ed. Male Reproductive Function. Boston, Kluwer Academic Publishers, 1999, pp. 139–156.

19. Hajjar RR, Kaiser FE, Morley JE. Outcomes of long-term testosterone replacement in older hypogonadal males: a retrospective analysis. J Clin Endocrinol Metab 1997;82:3793–3796.

20. Snyder PJ, Peachy H, Hannoush P, et al. Effect of testosterone treatment on body composition and muscle strength in men over 65 years of age. J Clin Endocrinol Metab 1999;84:2647–2653.

21. Bhasin S, Woodhouse L, Casaburi R, et al. Testosterone dose-response relationships in healthy young men. Am J Phys 2001;281:E1172–E1181.

22. Dabbs JM, Jr. Salivary testosterone measurements in behavioral studies. Ann N Y Acad Sci. 1993;694:177–183.

23. Anderson RA, Bancroft J, Wu FC. The effects of exogenous testosterone on sexuality and mood of normal men. J Clin Endocrinol Metab 1992;75:1503–1507.

24. Wang C, Alexander G, Berman N, et al. Testosterone replacement therapy improves mood in hypogonadal men—a clinical research center study. J Clin Endocrinol Metab 1996;81:3578–3583.

25. Anderson RA, Martin CW, Kung AWC, et al. 7α-Methyl-19-Nortestosterone maintains sexual behavior and mood in hypogonadal men. J Clin Endocrinol Metab 1999;84:3556–3562.

26. O'Connor DB, Archer J, Hair WM, Wu FC. Activational effects of testosterone on cognitive function in men. Neuropsychologia 2001;39:1385–1394.

27. Patwardhan AJ, Eliez S, Bender B, Linden MG, Reiss AL. Brain morphology in Klinefelter syndrome: extra X chromosome and testosterone supplementation. Neurology 2000;54:2218–2223.

28. Alexander GM, Swerdloff RS, Wang C, et al. Androgen-behavior correlations in hypogonadal men and eugonadal men. II. Cognitive abilities. Horm Behav 1998;33:85–94.

29. Boone KB, Swerdloff RS, Miller BL, et al. Neuropsychological profile of adults with Klinefelter Syndrome. J Int Neuropsychol Soc 2001;7:446–456.

30. Cherrier MM, Anawalt BD, Herbst KL, et al. Cognitive effects of short-term manipulation of serum sex steroids in healthy young men. J Clin Endocrinol Metab 2002;87:3090–3096.

31. Janowsky JS, Oviatt SK, Orwoll ES. Testosterone influences spatial cognition in older men. Behav Neurosci. 1994;108:325–332.

32. Janowsky JS, Chavez B, Orwoll E. Sex steroids modify working memory. J Cogn Neurosci 2000;12:407–414.

33. Kenny AM, Bellantonio S, Gruman CA, Acosta RD, Prestwood KM. Effects of transdermal testosterone on cognitive function and health perception in older men with low bioavailable testosterone levels. J Gerontol A Biol Sci Med Sci 2002;57:M321–M325.

34. Yaffe K, Lui LY, Zmuda J, Cauley J. Sex hormones and cognitive function in older men. J Am Geriatr Soc 2002;50:707–712.

35. Cherrier MM, Asthana S, Plymate S, et al. Testosterone supplementation improves spatial and verbal memory in healthy older men. Neurology 2001;57:80–88.

36. Brodsky IG, Balagopal P, Nair KS. Effects of testosterone replacement on muscle mass and muscle protein synthesis in hypogonadal men—a clinical research center study. J Clin Endocrinol Metab 1996;81:3469–3475.

37. Sinha-Hikim I, Artaza J, Woodhouse L, et al. Testosterone-induced increase in muscle size in healthy young men is associated with muscle fiber hypertrophy. Am J Physiol Endocrinol Metab 2001;283:E154–E164.

38. Katznelson L, Finkelstein JS, Schoenfeld DA, Rosenthal DJ, Anderson EJ, Klinbanski A. Increase in bone density and lean body mass during testosterone administration in men with acquired hypogonadism. J Clin Endocrinol Metab 1996;81:4358–4365.

39. Snyder PJ, Peachey H, Berlin JA, et al. Effects of testosterone replacement in hypogonadal men. J Clin Endocrinol Metab 2000;85:2670–2677.

40. Bhasin S, Storer TW, Berman N, et al. Testosterone replacement increases fat-free mass and muscle size in hypogonadal men. J Clin Endocrinol Metab 1997;82:407–413.

41. Clague JE, Wu FC, Horan MA. Difficulties in measuring the effect of testosterone replacement therapy on muscle function in older men. Int J Androl 1999;22:261–265.

42. Marin P, Holmang S, Jonsson L, et al. The effects of testosterone treatment on body composition and metabolism in middle aged obese men. Int J Obes 1992;16:991–997.

43. Singh AB, Hsia S, Alaupovic P, et al. The effects of varying doses of T on insulin sensitivity, plasma lipids, apolipoproteins, and C-reactive protein in healthy young men. J Clin Endocrinol Metab 2002;87:136–143.

44. Greendale G, Edelstein S, Barrett-Connor E. Endogenous sex steroids and bone mineral density in older women and men. The Rancho Bernardo Study. J Bone Miner Res 1997;12:1833–1841.

45. Khosla S, Melton LJ, Atkinson EJ, O-Fallon WM, Klee GG, Riggs BL. Relationship of serum sex steroid levels and bone turnover markers with bone mineral density in men: a key role for bio-available estrogen. J Clin Endocrinol Metab 1998;83:2266–2275.

46. Smith EP, Boyd J, Frank GR, et al. Estrogen resistance caused by a mutation in the estrogen-receptor gene in a man. N Engl J Med 1994;331:1056–1061.

47. Morishima A, Grumback MM, Simpson ER, Fisher C, Qui K. Aromatase deficiency in male and female siblings caused by a novel mutation and the physiological role of estrogens. J Clin Endocrinol Metab 1995;80:3689–3698.

48. Carani C, Oin K, Simoni M, et al. Effect of testosterone and estradiol in a man with aromatase deficiency. N Engl J Med 1997;337:91–95.

49. Behre HM, Kliesch S, Leifke E, Link TM, Nieschlag E. Long-term effect of testosterone therapy on bone mineral density in hypogonadal men. J Clin Endocrinol Metab 1997;82:2386–2390.

50. Kenny AM, Prestwood KM, Raisz LG. Short-term effects of intramuscular and transdermal testosterone on bone turnover, prostate symptoms, cholesterol, and hematocrit in men over age 70 with low testosterone levels. Endocr Res 2000;26:153–168.

51. Snyder PJ, Peachey H, Berlin JA, et al. Effects of testosterone replacement in hypogonadal men. J Clin Endocrinol Metab 2000;85:2670–2677.

52. Bagatell C, Heiman JR, Matsumoto AM, Rivier JE, Bremner WJ. Metabolic and behavioral effects of high-dose, exogenous testosterone in healthy men. J Clin Endocrinol Metab 1994;79:561–567.

53. Friedl KE, Hannan CJJ, Jones RE, Plymate SR. High-density lipoprotein cholesterol is not decreased if an aromatizable androgen is administered. Metabolism 1990;39:69–74.

54. Dobs AS, Bachorik PS, Arver S, et al. Interrelationships among lipoprotein levels, sex hormones, anthropometric parameters, and age in hypogonadal men treated for 1 year with a permeation-enhanced testosterone transdermal system. J Clin Endocrinol Metab 2001;86:1026–1033.

55. Arver S, Dobs AS, Meikle AW, et al. Long-term efficacy and safety of a permeation-enhanced testosterone transdermal system in hypogonadal men. Clin Endocrinol (Oxf) 1997;47:727–737.

56. Barrett-Connor E, Khaw K. Endogenous sex hormones and cardiovascular disease in men. Circulation 1988;78:539–545.

57. Simon D, Charles A, Nahoul K, et al. Association between plasma total testosterone and cardiovascular risk factors in healthy adult men: The Telecom Study. J Clin Endocrinol Metab 1992;82:682–685.

58. Phillips GB, Pinkernell BH, Jing TY. The association of hypotestosteronemia with coronary artery disease in men. Arterioscler Thromb 1994;14:701–706.

59. Zhao SP, Li XP. The association of low plasma testosterone level with coronary artery disease in Chinese men. Int J Cardiol 1998;63:161–164.

60. Jaffe MD. Effect of testosterone cypionate on post-exercise ST segment depression. Br Heart J 1977;39:1217–1222.

61. Wu S, Weng X. Therapeutic effects of an androgen preparation on myocardial ischemia in 62 elderly male coronary heart disease patients. Chin Med J 1993;106:415–418.

62. English KM, Mandour O, Steeds RP, Diver MJ, Jones TH, Channer KS. Men with coronary artery disease have lower levels of androgens than men with normal coronary angiograms. Eur Heart J 2000;21:890–894.

63. Rosano GM, Leonardo F, Pagnotta P, et al. Acute anti-ischemic effect of testosterone in men with coronary artery disease [erratum appears in Circulation 2000 Feb 8;101:584]. Circulation 1999;99:1666–1670.

64. Webb CM, McNeill JG, Hayward CS, de Zeigler D, Collins P. Effects of testosterone on coronary vasomotor regulation in men with coronary heart disease. Circulation 1999;100:1690–1696.

65. Thompson PD, Ahlberg AW, Moyna NM, et al. Effect of intravenous testosterone on myocardial ischemia in men with coronary artery disease. Am Heart J 2002;143:249–256.

66. Behre HM, Bohmeyer J, Nieschlag E. Prostate volume in testosterone-treated and untreated hypogonadal men in comparison to age-matched normal controls. Clin Endocrinol (Oxf) 1994;40:341–349.

67. Meikle AW, Arver S, Dobs AS, et al. Prostate size in hypogonadal men treated with a nonscrotal permeation-enhanced testosterone transdermal system. Urology 1997;49:191–196.
68. Handelsman DJ. The safety of androgens: prostate and cardiovascular disease. In: Wang C, ed. Male Reproductive Function. Boston, Kluwer Academic Publishers, 1999, pp. 173–189.
68a. Thompson IM, Goodman PJ, Tangen CM, et al. The influence of finasteride on the development of prostate cancer. NJ Engl Med 2003;349:215–224.
69. Renericca NJ, Solomon J, Fimian WJ Jr, Howard D, Rizzoli V, Stohlman F Jr. The effect of testosterone on erythropoiesis. Scand J Haematol 1969;6:431–439.
70. De Lorimier AA, Gordon GS, Lower RC, Carbone JV. Methyltestosterone, related steroids, and liver function. Arch Int Med 1965;116:289–294.
71. Nadell J, Kosek J. Peliosis hepatis. Twelve cases associated with oral androgen therapy. Arch Pathol Lab Med 1977;101:405–410.
72. Matsumoto AM, Sandblom RE, Schoene RB, et al. Testosterone replacement in hypogonadal men: effects on obstructive sleep apnoea, respiratory drives, and sleep. Clin Endocrinol (Oxf) 1985;22:713–721.
73. Snyder PJ, Lawrence DA. Treatment of male hypogonadism with testosterone enanthate. J Clin Endocrinol Metab 1980;51:1335–1339.
74. Sokol RZ, Palacios A, Campfield LA, Saul C, Swerdloff RS. Comparison of the kinetics of injectable testosterone in eugonadal and hypogonadal men. Fertil Steril 1982;37:425–430.
75. Zhang GY, Gu YO, Wang XH, Cui YG, Bremner WJ. Pharmacokinetic study of injectable testosterone undecanoate in hypogonadal men. J Androl 1998;19:761–768.
76. Behre HM, Abshagen K, Oettel M, Hubler D, Nieschlag E. Intramuscular injection of testosterone undecanoate for the treatment of male hypogonadism: phase I studies. Eur J Endocrinol 1999;140:414–419.
77. Nieschlag E, Buckter D, von Eckardstein S, Abshagen K, Simoni M, Behre HM. Repeated intramuscular injections of testosterone undecanoate for substitution therapy in hypogonadal men. Clin Endocrinol 1999;51:757–763.
78. Bhasin S, Swerdloff RS, Steiner B, et al. A biodegradable testosterone microcapsule formulation provides eugonadal levels of testosterone for 10–11 weeks in hypogonadal men. J Clin Endocrinol Metab 1992;74:75–83.
79. Amory JK, Anawalt BD, Blaskovich PD, Gilchriest J, Nuwayan ES, Matsumoto AM. Testosterone release from a subcutaneous, biodegradable microcapsule formulation (Viatrel) in hypogonadal men. J Androl 2002;23:84–91.
80. Nieschlag E, Mauss J, Coert A, Kicovic PM. Plasma androgen levels in men after oral administration of testosterone or testosterone undecanoate. Acta Endocrinol (Copenh) 1975;79:366–374.
81. Schumeyer T, Wickings E, Freischem C, Nieschlag E. Saliva and serum testosterone following oral testosterone undecanoate administration in normal and hypogonadal men. Acta Endocrinol (Copenh) 1983;102:456–462.
82. Gooren LJ. A ten-year safety study of the oral androgen testosterone undecanoate. J Androl 1994;15:212–215.
83. Dobs AS, Hoover DR, Chen M-C, Allen R. Pharmacokinetic characteristics, efficacy, and safety of buccal testosterone in hypogonadal males: a pilot study. J Clin Endocrinol Metab 1998;83:330–339.
84. Salahian B, Wang C, Alexander G, et al. Pharmacokinetics, bioefficacy, and safety of sublingual testosterone cyclodextrin in hypogonadal men: comparison to testosterone enanthate. J Clin Endocrinol Metab 1995;80:3567–3575.
85. Wang C, Kipnes M, Matsumoto A, et al. Novel testosterone bioadhesive buccal table—pharmacokinetics and safety evaluation. Abstract. 84th Annual Meeting of Endocrine Society, San Francisco, 2002.
86. Findlay JC, Place V, Snyder PJ. Treatment of primary hypogonadism in men by the transdermal administration of testosterone. J Clin Endocrinol Metab 1989;68:369–373.
87. Cunningham GR, Cordero E, Thornby JI. Testosterone replacement with transdermal therapeutic systems. Physiological serum testosterone and elevated dihydrotestosterone levels. JAMA 1989;261:2525–2530.
88. Meikle AW, Mazer NA, Moellmer JF, et al. Enhanced transdermal delivery of testosterone across nonscrotal skin produces physiological concentrations of testosterone and its metabolites in hypogonadal men. J Clin Endocrinol Metab 1992;74:623–628.
89. Meikle AW, Arver S, Dobs AS, Sanders SW, Rajaram L, Mazer NA. Pharmacokinetics and metabolism of a permeation-enhanced testosterone transdermal system in hypogonadal men: influence of application site: a Clinical Research Center Study. J Clin Endocrinol Metab 1996;81:1832–1840.

90. Brocks DR, Meikle AW, Boike SC, et al. Pharmacokinetics of testosterone in hypogonadal men after transdermal delivery: influence of dose. J Clin Pharmacol 1996;36:732–739.

91. Wang C, Berman N, Longstreth JA, et al. Pharmacokinetics of transdermal testosterone gel in hypogonadal men: application of gel at one site versus four sites. J Clin Endocrinol Metab 2000;85:964–969.

92. Swerdloff RS, Wang C, Cunningham G, et al. Comparative pharmacokinetics of two doses of transdermal testosterone gel versus testosterone patch after daily application for 180 days in hypogonadal men. J Clin Endocrinol Metab 2000;85:4500–4510.

92.a Steidle C, Schwartz S, Jacoby K, et al. North American AA2500 T Gel Study Group. AA2500 testosterone gel normalizes androgen levels in aging males with improvements in body composition and sexual function. J Clin Endocrinol Metab 2003;88(6):2673–2681.

93. Wang C, Swerdloff RS, Iranmanesh A, et al. and the Testosterone Gel Study Group. Effects of transdermal testosterone gel on bone tunrover markers and bone mineral density. Clin Endocrinol 2001;54:739–750.

94. Schaison G, Nahonl K, Couzinet B. Percutaneous dihydrotestosterone (DHT) treatment. In: Nieschlag E, Behre HM, eds. Testosterone: action deficiency, substitution. Springer Verlag, Berlin, 1990, pp. 155–164.

95. De Lignieres B. Transdermal dihydrotestosterone treatment of andropause. Ann Med 1993;25:235–241.

96. Ly LP, Jimenez M, Zhuang TN, Celermajer DS, Conway AJ, Handelsman DJ. A double-blind, placebo-controlled, randomized clinical trial of transdermal dihydrotestosteronegel on muscular strength, mobility and quality of life in older men with partial androgen deficiency. J Clin Endocrinol Metab 2001;86:4078–4088.

97. Kunelius P, Lukkainen O, Hannuksela ML, Itkonen O, Tapanaimen JS. The effects of transdermal dihydrotestosterone in the aging male: a prospective, randomized, double blind study. J Clin Endocrinol Metab 2000;87:1467–1472.

98. Wang C, Iranmanesh A, Berman N, et al. Comparative pharmacokinetics of three doses of percutaneous dihydrotestosterone gel in healthy elderly men; A Clinical Research Center Study. J Clin Endocrinol Metab 1998;83:2749–2757.

99. Wang C, Swerdloff RS. Should the non-aromatizable androgen dihydrotestosterone be considered as an alternative to testosterone in the treatment of andropause? J Clin Endocrinol Metab 2002;87:1462–1466.

100. Handelsman DJ, Conway AJ, Boylan LM. Pharmacokinetics and pharmacodynamics of testosterone pellets in man. J Clin Endocrinol Metab 1990;71:216–222.

101. Handelsman DJ, Mackey MA, Howe C, Turner L, Conway AJ. An analysis of testosterone implants for androgen replacement therapy. Clin Endocrinol (Oxf) 1997;47:311–316.

102. Kelleher S, Turner L, Howe C, Conway AJ, Handelsman DJ. Extrusion of testosterone pellets: a randomized controlled clinical study. Clin Endocrinol (Oxf) 1999;51:469–1471.

103. Kumar N, Didolkar AK, Monder C, Bardin DW, Sundaram K. The biological activity of 7 alpha-methyl-19-nortestosterone is not amplified in male reproductive tract as is that of testosterone. Endocrinology 1992;130:3677–3683.

104. Cummings DE, Kumar N, Bandin CW, Sundaram K, Bremner WJ. Prostate-sparing effects in primates of the potent androgen 7α-methyl-19nortestosterone: a potential alternative to testosterone for androgen replacement and male contraception. J Clin Endocrinol Metab 1998;83:4212–4219.

105. Anderson RA, Martin CW, Kung AWC, et al. 7α-Methyl-19-Nortestosterone maintains sexual behavior and mood in hypogonadal men. J Clin Endocrinol Metab 1999;84:3556–3562.

106. Edwards JP, Zhi L, Poolay CL, et al. Preparation, resolution, and biological evaluation of 5-aryl-1, 2-dihydro-5H-chromeno [3,4-f] quinolines:potent, orally active, nonsteroidal progesterone receptor agonists. J Med Chem 1998;41:2779–2785.

107. Hamann LG, Higuchi RI, Zhi L, et al. Syntheses and biological activity of a novel series of nonsteroidal, peripherally selective androgen receptor antagonists derived from 1,2-dihydropyridono [5,6-g] quinolines. J Med Chem 1998;41:623–639.

19 Stimulation of Spermatogenesis in Hypogonadotropic Men

Marion Depenbusch, MD
and Eberhard Nieschlag, MD

THE HYPOTHALAMIC–PITUITARY–TESTICULAR AXIS

The hypothalamic–pituitary–testicular axis coordinates two principal functions that are essential for reproduction in males: the production of physiologic quantities of sex steroid hormones, primarily testosterone, and the generation of spermatogenic cells that become mature gametes capable of fertilizing oocytes. Gonadotropin-releasing hormone (GnRH) is the primary regulator of this system. It is released into the portal blood in discrete pulses and binds to specific receptors on gonadotropic cells, where it stimulates the synthesis and release of luteinizing hormone (LH) and follicle-stimulating hormone (FSH). LH and FSH, in turn, control development, maturation, and function of the gonad through interaction with specific membrane receptors *(1)*. To induce and maintain quantitatively normal spermatogenesis in humans, both gonadotropins are required *(2)*. LH binds to Leydig cells to initiate testosterone synthesis and secretion, whereas FSH binds to Sertoli cells and stimulates the production of several factors that, together with testosterone from Leydig cells, induce and maintain spermatogenesis *(1)*.

From: *Male Hypogonadism:*
Basic, Clinical, and Therapeutic Principles
Edited by: S. J. Winters © Humana Press Inc., Totowa, NJ

Underlying Cause

Treatment

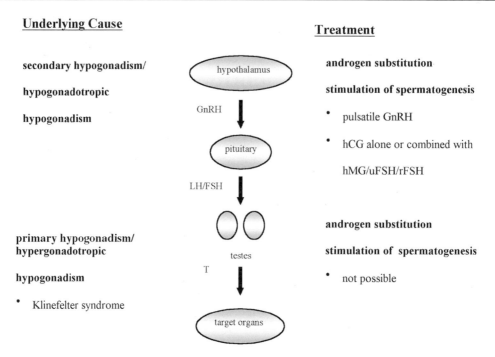

secondary hypogonadism/

hypogonadotropic

hypogonadism

androgen substitution

stimulation of spermatogenesis

* pulsatile GnRH

* hCG alone or combined with

   hMG/uFSH/rFSH

primary hypogonadism/
hypergonadotropic

hypogonadism

* Klinefelter syndrome

androgen substitution

stimulation of spermatogenesis

* not possible

Fig. 1. Treatment of hypogonadism according to pathogenesis.

HYPOGONADISM

Male hypogonadism is characterized by low testosterone levels in serum, accompanied by androgen deficiency symptoms, which depend on the time of manifestation. When hypogonadism begins before adolescence, it results in a failure to undergo puberty, whereas postpubertal hypogonadism causes a regression of reproductive function, with impaired libido and impotence, diminished body hair, soft skin, weakness and muscle atrophy, anemia, and osteoporosis. Low testosterone levels, in combination with high gonadotropin levels, indicate a testicular origin (hypergonadotropic or primary hypogonadism), whereas in combination with low gonadotropin levels, the cause is central (hypogonadotropic or secondary hypogonadism) *(3)*. In both primary and secondary hypogonadism, androgen deficiency symptoms can be treated by testosterone substitution (*see* Chapter 18). In most causes of primary testicular failure, improvement of fertility is not possible, whereas in secondary hypogonadism, fertility may be initiated or restored (*see* Fig. 1).

Hypogonadotropic Hypogonadism

Hypogonadotropic hypogonadism is a clinical syndrome resulting from a disorder of the pituitary gland, or hypothalamus, or from systemic factors that suppress GnRH production. Hypogonadotropic hypogonadism can be congenital, i.e., Kallmann syndrome, or acquired, which most often results from a pituitary tumor. Head trauma, central nervous system (CNS) infections, hemochromatosis, radiotherapy, and vascular disorders can also lead to pituitary insufficiency *(4)*. Hypogonadotropic hypogonadism can occur together with other endocrine deficiencies or can be selective.

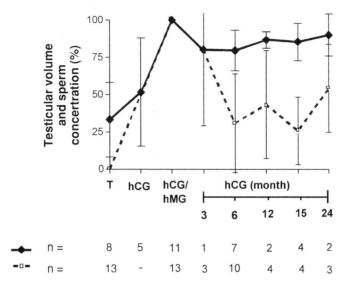

Fig. 2. Bitesticular volume (—) and sperm concentration (– – –) in men with hypogonadotropic hypogonadism during continuation treatment with human chorionic gonadotropin (hCG) alone expressed as a percentage of the final value during hCG/human menopausal gonadotropin treatment. (Data modified from ref. *9.*)

Treatment goals include the maintenance of androgen levels in the normal adult male range to allow full virilization and prevention of androgen deficiency symptoms. Furthermore, the initiation or restoration of spermatogenesis is often an integral part of the treatment plan.

TREATMENT OF PATIENTS WITH
HYPOGONADOTROPIC HYPOGONADISM

In patients with hypogonadism of prepubertal onset, treatment is initiated with testosterone to induce pubertal development and to achieve normal virilization. Subsequently, spermatogenesis can be stimulated with GnRH or with gonadotropins, because exogenous testosterone will not initiate spermatogenesis *(5,6)* (*see* Fig. 1). This treatment approach is recommended, even if fertility is not initially desired, because spermatogenesis, once driven to full maturation, can be readily restimulated when fertility is desired later in life *(5,7)*. In patients with hypogonadism that began after puberty, treatment can be initiated either with testosterone for androgen substitution or with GnRH or gonadotropins if fertility is desired immediately. Because GnRH and gonadotropins are both costly, they are justified only when fertility is desired or in the initial phase of treatment, when spermatogenesis is to be stimulated to the point of sperm production. Treatment may be required for 2 or more years, until sperm appear in the ejaculate or a pregnancy has been induced. Once it is initiated, sperm production can often be maintained with human chorionic gonadotropin (hCG) alone *(5,8,9)* (*see* Fig. 2); therefore, we continue hCG treatment until delivery, because miscarriage could occur. Thereafter, if the couple does not want to conceive additional offspring immediately, testosterone therapy is resumed, because it is less costly and easier to administer.

Table 1
Therapeutic Options for Spermatogenesis Stimulation

Drug	Trade Name	Application	Dose
Pulsatile gonadotropin-releasing hormone (GnRH)	Factrel Lutrepulse	Subcutaneous, external minipump	4–20 µg per pulse every 120 min
Human chorionic gonadotropin (hCG)	Profasi Pregnyl Novarel	Subcutaneous or intramuscular	1000–2500 IU twice per week (Monday and Friday)
In combination with			
Human menopausal gonadotropin (hMG)	Pergonal Reponex	Subcutaneous or intramuscular	75–150 IU three times weekly (Monday, Wednesday, and Friday)
Human urinary follicle-stimulating hormone (FSH), highly purified (uhFSH-HP)	Fertinex	Subcutaneous or intramuscular	75–150 IU three times weekly (Monday, Wednesday, and Friday)
Recombinant FSH (rFSH)	Follistim Gonal F	Subcutaneous or intramuscular	75–300 IU three times weekly (Monday, Wednesday, and Friday)

Spermatogenesis Stimulation

The induction of spermatogenesis in patients with hypogonadotropic hypogonadism requires testicular stimulation with GnRH or gonadotropins. Various preparations are available (see Table 1) to reach this goal, each with advantages and disadvantages. Because the maturation of spermatogonia to mature sperm takes approx 70 d, the first sperm usually do not appear in the ejaculate for at least 3 mo, but it may take 2 yr for patients with congenital hypogonadotropic hypogonadism to become sperm positive. The huge variation in individuals can be explained by the diversity of hypogonadotropic hypogonadism and depends on whether spermatogenesis previously progressed to full maturation. There are several other factors that influence the success of stimulation therapy in patients with hypogonadotropic hypogonadism which are discussed later in this chapter.

PULSATILE GnRH THERAPY

Pulsatile GnRH therapy can be used to stimulate spermatogenesis in men with GnRH deficiency and normal pituitary function (10), whereas continuous stimulation with GnRH is unsuccessful because it downregulates GnRH receptors and disrupts GnRH-R signal transduction, leading to a decrease in gonadotropin synthesis and secretion and gonadal suppression (11).

The pulsatile application of GnRH using a portable minipump most closely simulates normal physiology. The pump needle is usually placed in the subcutaneous tissue of the abdomen and is changed regularly (every 2 d). The pump is programmed to deliver a small bolus of GnRH every 120 min, because this frequency was most effective (12). A starting dose of 4 µg per pulse is often selected, with increases of 2 µg every 2 wk if LH secretion does not rise. Maximum doses are 20 µg per pulse. The dose of GnRH that is required to achieve testosterone levels in the normal adult male range and to stimulate spermatogenesis varies considerably in men with hypogonadotropic hypogonadism ranging from 5 to 20 µg/120 min or 25–600 ng/kg per bolus. The therapeutic dose correlates positively with body weight and negatively with pretreatment testicular size *(12)*. Serum testosterone levels usually normalize within 1–2 mo, and the testes increase in size within 3–6 mo after therapy begins. For adjustments, serum testosterone, gonadotropins, and testicular volume should be monitored closely at 2- to 4-wk intervals. Most patients should be treated for up to 2 yr to maximize testicular growth and achieve spermatogenesis, because it has been shown that the time until appearance of sperm in the ejaculate is quite variable, ranging from 2 to 22 mo of therapy *(7)*.

GnRH is not an appropriate treatment for patients with pituitary disease and will be ineffective in men with CHH resulting from GnRH receptor mutations. These mutations produce a variable degree of resistance to GnRH. According to our experience, GnRH-R mutations are rare, and we found none in approx 50 patients diagnosed as IHH or Kallmann syndrome (data unpublished). However, a few cases have been described *(13–15)* (*see* Chapter 5). Because these cases are rare, PCR testing of the GnRH receptor gene sequence is recommended only if a patient fails to respond to pulsatile GnRH treatment. In our view, screening before beginning pulsatile GnRH treatment is not currently necessary. Gordon Holmes spinocerebellar ataxia and X-linked adrenohypoplasia congenita are two other forms of inherited HH in which responsiveness to GnRH is impaired *(16)*. The formation of antibodies to GnRH or its receptor seldom occurs but can lead to a failure of pulsatile GnRH therapy *(17,18)*. These patients should be treated with gonadotropins to induce spermatogenesis rather than with pulsatile GnRH.

GONADOTROPIN THERAPY

Gonadotropin therapy is generally effective in achieving fertility in cases of pituitary insufficiency or GnRH resistance but is also an option for patients with hypothalamic disorders. Since the 1960s, hCG and human menopausal gonadotropin (hMG) that are purified from the urine of pregnant and menopausal women, respectively, have proven to be an effective treatment for spermatogenesis stimulation *(5,7,19–21)*. hCG is used as the source of LH activity, because both hormones have structurally similar subunits and activate the same Leydig cell receptor. hMG has been used as the source of FSH, but it also contains LH activity. However, the LH activity is too low to maintain Leydig cell function, so a combination of hMG with hCG is required to achieve fertility *(12)*. In the early 1980s, a purified preparation of urinary FSH (uFSH) and a highly purified preparation of urinary FSH (uFSH-HP), both from the urine of menopausal women, which are practically devoid of LH activity, were produced. uFSH-HP is prepared using specific anti- FSH monoclonal antibodies. Although in the original preparations of FSH the gonadotropin content represented less than 5% of the total protein, increased purity of more than 95% is achieved with uFSH-HP, with a 60-fold increase in specific activity *(22)*. Recently, recombinant preparations of human FSH, hCG, and LH, which represent the purest gonadotropin preparations, have become available. These preparations are compared in detail in the following paragraphs.

Initiation of Gonadotropin Therapy With Human Chorionic Gonadotropin. Therapy is initiated by administration of hCG, which stimulates testicular testosterone production and the synthesis of other Leydig cell products that are required for spermatogenesis and testicular growth. With a dose of 1000–2500 IU twice per week (e.g., Monday and Friday), serum testosterone levels usually normalizes within 1–2 mo, otherwise, the dose is increased. Higher doses of hCG also increase plasma estradiol levels, however, and may cause gynecomastia. The development of anti-hCG antibodies is rare but may be considered if there is resistance to GnRH therapy (23). Both intramuscular and sc adminstration of hCG are effective. Intramuscular administration is often more painful and may require medical/paramedical assistance for injections. Compliance is greater when the sc route of administration is chosen, as this can be done by self-injection comparable to insulin injection in patients with diabetes.

In patients with adult-onset (acquired) hypogonadism or incomplete congenital gonadotropin deficiency, spermatogenesis may be induced with hCG alone (19,20,24), probably because of sufficient endogenous production of FSH. Responsiveness to hCG alone may be predicted by the presence of testes that exceed prepubertal size (4 mL and larger) before therapy is initiated (20).

In patients with congenital complete forms of hypogonadotropic hypogonadism the addition of an FSH-containing preparation is usually necessary to stimulate spermatogenesis, and, therefore, the induction phase with hCG alone is followed by coadministration of an FSH-containing preparation after 8–12 wk. This regimen is also advisable for patients with hypogonadotropic hypogonadism in whom spermatogenesis had been successfully induced with hCG alone, because the addition of an FSH-containing preparation to hCG increased testicular volume, sperm concentration, and pregnancy outcome (5,24).

Alternatives to hCG: Recombinant hCG (rhCG) or LH (rhLH). Recombinant preparations of hCG and LH might be advantageous over the existing products derived from urine because they have higher purity and consistency. However, there are no data so far available concerning the efficiency of rhLH or rhCG for stimulation of spermatogenesis in patients with hypogonadotropic hypogonadism. The administration of rhCG to older men with age-related androgen deficiency produced androgenic effects on hormones and muscle mass (25). In women undergoing in vitro fertilization, rhLH and rhCG were well tolerated and as effective as urinary hCG in inducing final follicular maturation and ovulation (26,27).

Treatment With hCG and Human Menopausal Gonadotropin. hMG is purified from the urine of menopausal women. The usual starting dose is 75 IU three times weekly (e.g., Monday, Wednesday, and Friday), intramuscularly or subcutaneously, in combination with 1000–2500 IU hCG twice weekly subcutaneously. To minimize the number of injections, hCG and hMG can be mixed in the same syringe. The treatment is generally well tolerated, but because hMG preparations contain LH activity in addition to FSH activity, increased Leydig cell stimulation may occur, leading to higher plasma levels of testosterone and increased conversion to estradiol, compared with treatment with hCG alone. As a result, patients may develop gynecomastia, which is usually reversible if the dose of hCG is reduced, but may be permanent. On average, sperm appear in the ejaculate after 5 mo of therapy, and maximum sperm counts are achieved after approx 2 yr (28). Sperm quality (motility and morphology) is usually normal during treatment with hCG/hMG. If azoospermia persists beyond 6 mo of combination treatment, the hMG dose can be increased to 150 IU three times a week, with the hCG dose remaining unchanged. Approximately 10% of patients fail to produce sperm in the ejaculate *(7,28)*.

Therapy With hCG/Urinary or Highly Purified Urinary Human FSH. Urinary FSH, as well as the highly purified preparation, are effective alternatives to hMG for the initiation and maintenance of spermatogenesis in patients with hypogonadotropic hypogonadism. In comparison to hMG, uFSH-HP has enhanced specific activity (10,000 IU/mg of protein vs 150 IU/mg of protein for hMG) and negligible LH activity (<0.1 IU LH/1000 IU FSH). Administration of 75–150 IU uFSH or uFSH-HP three times weekly, in combination with 1000–2500 IU hCG twice weekly (both subcutaneously), increases testicular size, and spermatogenesis is usually induced after 5–9 mo. These preparations are generally well tolerated, and no antibody to FSH has so far been detected during or after therapy *(29–32)*.

hCG/Human Recombinant FSH Therapy. Human recombinant FSH (rhFSH) is prepared using DNA technology from Chinese Hamster Ovary (CHO) cells that are transfected with FSH subunit genes. The two preparations available contain different isoforms, follitropin α (Gonal-F) and follitropin β (Follistim). Although there are minor differences between these isoforms, they are equivalent for clinical purposes *(33)*. rhFSH has a high specific activity and contains no LH activity. It is well tolerated, and no serum antibodies to FSH or CHO proteins have yet been detected *(34,35)*. A dose of 150 IU rhFSH three times weekly (e.g., Monday, Wednesday, and Friday) or 225 IU twice weekly in combination with 1000–2500 IU hCG twice weekly (both subcutaneously) was sufficient to induce testicular growth and spermatogenesis after 6–9 mo. This regimen was successful in inducing spermatogenesis in approx 90% of patients with hypogonadotropic hypogonadism. However, if azoospermia persists, the dose of rhFSH may be increased to a maximum dose of 300 IU three times a week *(34–37)*. Testosterone levels usually show only a minor increase after rhFSH has been added to hCG. Likewise, estradiol and SHBG levels remain constant, whereas inhibin B levels increase to values typical of normozoospermic men *(34)*.

Outlook: Long-Acting rhFSH. Because of the short half-life of currently available FSH preparations, multiple injections (usually three times weekly) are necessary to produce sufficient FSH concentrations for induction of spermatogenesis in patients with hypogonadotropic hypogonadism. FSH-CTP is a long-acting recombinant FSH-like substance produced by CHO-cells transfected with the genes of the alpha subunit of human FSH and a hybrid beta subunit. In a clinical study in patients with hypogonadotropic hypogonadism, the half-life of FSH-CTP was increased two to three times compared with rhFSH. A clear rise in serum inhibin B levels was observed, and no FSH antibodies were detected. Therefore, FSH-CTP might represent a new convenient FSH preparation for the treatment of male infertility resulting from hyogonadotropic hypogonadism in the future *(38)*.

IMPACT OF BASELINE TESTICULAR VOLUME

As a result of GnRH or gonadotropin therapy, testicular volume increases, with the final testicular size depending on the initial testicular size. The testicular volume at the beginning of therapy was also a good predictor for the length of treatment necessary until spermatogenesis is induced *(7,34)*, i.e., length of treatment is inversely correlated with testicular volume. During therapy, testicular volume should be monitored carefully by ultrasonography, because an increase precedes the first appearance of sperm and the patient can be apprised of the potential for success of treatment *(39)*. Patients with a testicular volume of less than 4 mL have been classified as completely gonadotropin deficient and respond less well to stimulation therapy than do those men with a testicular volume above 4 mL as a sign of partial gonadotropin deficiency *(28,40)*. However, spermatogenesis can be induced even in patients with a testicular volume of less than 3 mL, but this may require treatment for 18–24 mo *(7,28)*.

IMPACT OF MALDESCENDED TESTES

Another predictive indicator of response to hCG/hMG or GnRH is a history of maldescended testes, because the patients often remain below the normal adult testicular volume during stimulation therapy and need extended therapy until spermatogenesis is induced. The average time of treatment for induction of spermatogenesis in patients with hypogonadotropic hypogonadism with bilateral maldescent was 13 mo compared with 4.5 mo in patients with hypogonadotropic hypogonadism with no history of maldescent *(7)*. This difference can probably be explained by damage to testicular tissue resulting from maldescent, as judged by histological evaluation *(21,41)*. Nevertheless, cryptorchidism does not preclude patients from gaining fertility, especially if it is unilateral *(7)*.

MONITORING TESTICULAR VOLUME AND LABORATORY PARAMETERS

To optimize the potential for success, as well as to achieve sufficient androgen substitution and safe treatment with minimum side effects, regular examination of the testes and selected laboratory parameters is mandatory. Because the duration of treatment with GnRH or gonadotropins necessary to induce spermatogenesis is dependent on the initial testicular size, and as an increase in testicular volume may precede sperm appearance, testicular size should be monitored by palpation or ultrasonography every 3–6 mo. Furthermore, increased echodensity, indicative of increased tissue density, results from stimulated sperm production and is, therefore, a favorable sign. Testicular volume should also be monitored regularly if a pregnancy has occurred, and spermatogenesis should be maintained with hCG alone until delivery. If spermatogenesis can be maintained with hCG alone, testicular volume decreases only slightly *(9)* (*see* Fig. 2).

To avoid androgen deficiency symptoms, such as loss of libido and potency, anemia, and osteoporosis on the one hand and side effects resulting from elevated testosterone levels, such as polycythemia on the other hand, serum testosterone levels should be checked at frequent intervals at the beginning of therapy until the correct treatment dose is identified. Subsequently, 6–12 mo for monitoring testosterone levels is usually sufficient. Serum estradiol levels should be checked at the same intervals, because elevated levels increase the risk of gynecomastia. Furthermore, hemoglobin and hematocrit should be monitored, because these parameters are dependent on testosterone levels.

IMPACT OF SEXUAL DEVELOPMENT

Patients with acquired forms of hypogonadotropic hypogonadism usually respond better to treatment than do those with congenital forms of hypogonadotropic hypogonadism. However, the time of onset (prepubertal vs. postpubertal) and the degree of gonadotropin deficiency (complete vs. partial) are important predictive factors. Patients with postpubertal hypogonadotropic hypogonadism have undergone spontaneous puberty with functioning tubules and spermatogenesis, and they may retain some

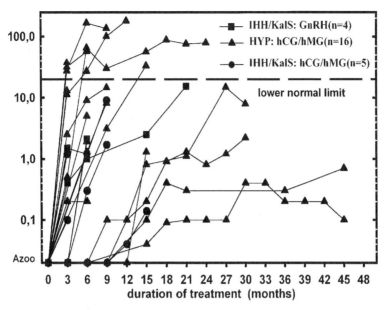

Fig. 3. Development of sperm production in patients with secondary hypogonadism during treatment with gonadotropin-releasing hormone (GnRH) or human chorionic gonadotropin (hCG)/human menopausal gonadotropin (hMG) until induction of pregnancy. (Data from ref. *117.*)

gonadotropin secretion, which is able to partially maintain seminiferous tubular function *(19,31,32)*. Likewise, patients with partial congenital gonadotropin deficiency may have residual gonadotropin secretion. However, in patients with prepubertal onset of hypogonadotropic hypogonadism the degree of sexual development, as mirrored by gonadal size, may range from complete absence of sexual maturation to partial puberty. Familial cases most often have no pubertal development (95%) and a high prevalence of cryptorchidism (71%). Those men who are most severely affected are familial cases with X-linked Kallmann syndrome *(42)*.

Pregnancy Outcome

Fertility is restored in most patients with hypogonadotropic hypogonadism during gonadotropin or pulsatile GnRH treatment, with pregnancy rates varying between 50 and 90%. Surprisingly, these pregnancies occur with sperm concentrations as low as 1–5 million/mL *(7,24,28)* (*see* Fig. 3), which is well below the normal range (>20 million/mL). Cryptorchidism or markedly subnormal testicular volume, which predict a poorer response to treatment, do not represent absolute contraindications to therapy.

Because the sperm concentration usually remains below the normal range, evaluation, and optimization of the female partner's reproductive functions is indispensable, because the fecundity of a couple is dependent on both male and female reproductive function *(43)*. An evaluation of the female cycle quality should be performed, and if pregnancy is not achieved after 6 mo, tubal function should be checked. Furthermore, hormonal disturbances such as polycystic ovary syndrome (PCOs), endometriosis, and other gynecological or systemic diseases can lead to female infertility *(44)*. It is also well-known that the time span within which a couple will conceive ("time to preg-

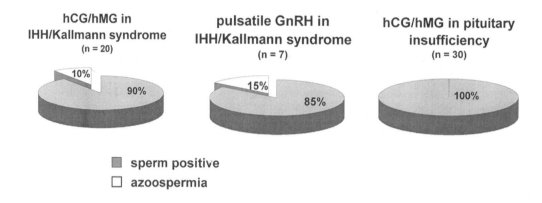

Fig. 4. Effectiveness of gonadotropin-releasing hormone (GnRH) or human chorionic gonadotropin (hCG)/human menopausal gonadotropin (hMG) treatment in patients with hypogonadotropic hypogonadism. (Data from ref. *117*.)

nancy") increases with advancing female age even in otherwise normal women. Moreover, the time of coitus is important, because most conceptions occur on the day of ovulation and the 2 preceding days *(44)*. If pregnancy fails to occur after 1 yr of regular unprotected intercourse, techniques of assisted reproduction may be employed.

COMPARISON BETWEEN THERAPIES

GnRH vs hCG/hMG

On theoretical grounds, pulsatile GnRH treatment is more physiologic because it reproduces the normal pulsatile pattern of LH and FSH release from the pituitary in patients with GnRH deficiency. Interestingly, although GnRH must be administered in a pulsatile pattern, spermatogenesis can be induced and maintained if gonadotropins are given in a nonpulsatile pattern. A direct comparison between GnRH and hCG/hMG regimens revealed that during GnRH treatment a larger testis size was achieved and spermatogenesis was induced more rapidly compared with gonadotropin therapy *(10)*. However, that study was not randomized, and the results could not be confirmed by others *(7,45)*. In all three studies, there was no significant difference in efficacy of induction of spermatogenesis or the number of pregnancies *(7,10,45)* (see Fig. 4). The patients treated with gonadotropins had a significantly greater increase in estradiol levels than those treated with GnRH, leading to the development of gynecomastia in only the gonadotropin-treated patients (28%) *(10)*.

From the data available, GnRH and hCG/hMG are probably of equal value in their efficiency to induce spermatogenesis in patients with hypogonadotropic hypogonadism. However, GnRH therapy requires good patient compliance and technical understanding because patients have to self-manage most of the technical component of the therapy. Therefore, not all patients are able or willing to use an infusion pump for approx 1 yr or more. Because hMG/hCG need not be injected intramuscularly, but can be self-injected subcutaneously, this treatment approach is more practical than the GnRH pump and is our preference.

FSH-Containing Gonadotropin Preparations and hMG

Because different FSH preparations are available, the question of variability in their potency to induce sperm production and paternity arises. Unfortunately, no direct comparison between hMG, highly purified preparations, and recombinant FSH in the treatment of male hypogonadism is available. Analysis of the studies that have been performed using individual preparations in the past is complicated by the fact that different therapeutic regimens were used.

Both hMG and uFSH contain urinary protein contaminants, which are believed to contribute to hypersensitivity reactions and reduce their purity to less than 5%. Through the application of immunochromatography with monoclonal antibodies against FSH, increased purity of more than 95% is achieved in uFSH-HP, but the purest preparation available is recombinant FSH. Furthermore, batch-to-batch consistency and the potential for limitless quantities is advantageous for rhFSH *(46)*. On the other hand, the cost of rhFSH is three times as high as the price of the earlier FSH preparations.

Recently, the potential risks of transmission of prion disease from urinary-derived gonadotropin preparations have been discussed. Because prion disease is believed to be transmitted predominantly by the ingestion of infected nervous tissue, and urine is believed not to be infective according to current advice from the World Health Organization, precautions concerning the application of uFSH are not advised. Furthermore, the urinary preparations have been widely used for 40 yr, and no infections have been described. Because rhFSH is not of human or animal origin, the potential for infections that are transmitted from living organisms is believed to be absent, but because the cell culture medium includes fetal calf serum, it could potentially be infected.

Nevertheless, all of the gonadotropin preparations have a good safety record without evidence of contamination, and there is no need to change current prescribing habits *(47)*. A pharmacokinetic-pharmacodynamic study with rhFSH in patients with hypogonadotropic hypogonadism showed dose linear serum FSH levels *(48)*, and the pharmacokinetics of recombinant and urinary FSH are similar *(49)*.

The efficiency of rhFSH compared to uFSH or hMG has been evaluated by different meta-analyses, based on pregnancy rates in in vitro fertilization cycles. Reports are contradictory, with two demonstrating an increase in pregnancy rates in the order of 5% in favor of rhFSH *(50,51)*, whereas the other showed no treatment benefit *(52)*. Although these data refer to ovarian and not to testicular stimulation, taking all information available, there is no convincing advantage of the recombinant preparations compared to the highly purified or original urinary preparations that justify the higher cost of rhFSH *(2)*.

USE OF RECOMBINANT HUMAN GROWTH HORMONE TO STIMULATE SPERMATOGENESIS

Various direct or indirect effects of growth hormone (GH) and other growth factors on the process of sexual maturation have been postulated because deprivation of GH during maturation leads to impaired or absent spermatogenesis in male rats *(53)*. Furthermore, GH and growth factors, such as insulin-like growth factor-1 (IGF-1), epidermal growth factor (EGF), and transforming growth factor (TGF), influence testicular steroid production and secretion *(54–56)*. In mice, the testicular steroidogenic response to chorionic gonadotropins stimulation was increased by GH and IGF-1 treatment *(54)*, and an effect of GH on Leydig cell function was also shown in prebubertal boys *(57)*. Because testosterone secretion by Leydig cells is necessary for spermatogenesis, a complementary or permissive role of GH in the induction of spermatogenesis by gonadotropins in patients with hypogonadotropic hypogonadism who failed gonadotropin therapy alone has been suggested. Indeed, in an open trial, in three of four patients with hypogonadotropic hypogonadism who remained azoospermic during treatment with hCG/hMG for 12 wk, spermatogenesis was induced after GH was added for a further 12 wk. Additionally, serum IGF-1 and testosterone levels rose *(58)*. However, these patients had a pretreatment testicular volume of less than 4 mL, and sperm production may have occurred if gonadotropin treatment had been prolonged without added GH. Further studies of combined gonadotropin/GH treatment of patients with hypogonadotropic hypogonadism who remained azoospermic during gonadotropin treatment confirmed the increase in IGF-1 and testosterone levels, but, although testicular volume increased, spermatogenesis was not induced *(59)*. Similarly, in 11 adult men who were gonadotropin deficient because of surgery for a pituitary lesion, treatment with recombinant GH increased IGF-1 and testosterone levels and seminal plasma volume, but sperm count and motility did not change *(60)*. Taken together, the addition of GH to gonadotropin treatment has no convincing beneficial effect on spermatogenesis in patients with hypogonadotropic hypogonadism and is, therefore, not recommended.

TRANSMISSIBILITY OF CONGENITAL HYPOGONADOTROPIC HYPOGONADISM

Patients with congenital hypogonadotropic hypogonadism are usually infertile, and most cases, therefore, occur sporadically, presumably as a result of *de novo* mutation. Because of the therapeutic use of pulsatile GnRH or gonadotropins, however, these patients may become fertile, and vertical disease transmission may increase. Segregation analysis has demonstrated X-linked, autosomal recessive and autosomal dominant inheritance patterns, suggesting the existence of several genes regulating GnRH secretion *(61–63)*. Genes currently recognized to be involved in congenital hypogonadotropic hypogonadism include *KAL (64)*, the *GnRH receptor (13–15,65,66)*, *DAX 1 (67,68)*, and *PROP 1 (69)*. Furthermore, sporadic cases of mutations in *ANK 1* gene *(70)*, SF-1 gene, *LHX 3* gene *(71)*, *HESX 1* gene *(72)* and *leptin (Ob)* gene *(73)*, *leptin receptor (Ob R)* gene *(74)*, and *prohormone convertase 1 (PC 1)* gene *(75)* have been reported. However, a genetic basis for IHH has been established in less than 20% of cases, leaving several autosomal and X-linked genes to await description *(42)* (*see* Chapter 5).

In clinical studies, there was evidence of familial transmission in approx 25% of cases, whereas the majority of cases (approx 75%) were sporadic *(42,76)*. In familial and sporadic cases the X-linked mode of inheritance, characterized clinically by the predominance of males affected, the presence of unaffected female carriers and absent male-to-male transmission, accounted for the minority of patients *(42,77)*. A few patients with IHH who received treatment for induction of ovulation or spermatogenesis and transmitted the condition to their offspring have been reported (76,78).

Given that the genetic basis of the majority of IHH patients remains unknown, it is difficult to provide accurate pretreatment counselling on the risk of the condition being inherited by the offspring. Nevertheless, the existence of a defined risk should be specifically discussed with all patients before fertility treatment *(76)*.

REFERENCES

1. Weinbauer GF, Gromoll J, Simoni M, Nieschlag E. Physiology of testicular function. In: Nieschlag E, Behre HM, eds. Andrology: Male Reproductive Health and Dysfunction, 2nd ed. Springer, Berlin, 2000, pp. 23–61.
2. Nieschlag E, Simoni M, Gromoll J, Weinbauer GF. Role of FSH in the regulation of spermatogenesis: clinical aspects. Clin Endocrinol 1999;51:139–146.
3. Behre HM, Yeung CH, Holstein AF, Weinbauer GF, Gassner P, Nieschlag E. Diagnosis of male infertility and hypogonadism. In: Nieschlag E, Behre HM, eds. Andrology: Male Reproductive Health and Dysfunction, 2nd ed. Springer, Berlin, 2000, pp. 89–124.
4. Behre HM, Nieschlag E, Meschede D, Partsch CJ. Diseases of the hypothalamus and the pituitary gland. In: Nieschlag E, Behre HM, eds. Andrology: Male Reproductive Health and Dysfunction, 2nd ed. Springer, Berlin, 2000, pp. 125–143.
5. Ley SB, Leonard JM. Male hypogonadotropic hypogonadism: factors influencing response to human chorionic gonadotropin and human menopausal gonadotropin, including prior exogenous androgens. J Clin Endocrinol Metab 1985;61:746–752.
6. Schaison G, Young J, Pholsena M, Nahoul K, Couzinet B. Failure of combined follicle-stimulating hormone-testosterone administration to initiate and/or maintain spermatogenesis in men with hypogonadotropic hypogonadism. J Clin Endocrinol Metab 1993;77:1545–1549.
7. Buechter D, Behre HM, Kliesch S, Nieschlag E. Pulsatile GnRH or human chorionic gonadotropin/human menopausal gonadotropin as effective treatment for men with hypogonadotropic hypogonadism: a review of 42 cases. Eur J Endocrinol 1998;139:298–303.
8. Johnsen SG. Maintenance of spermatogenesis induced by hMG treatment by means of continuous hCG treatment in hypogonadotropic men. Acta Endocrinol 1978;89:763–769.
9. Depenbusch M, von Eckardstein S, Simoni M, Nieschlag E. Maintenance of spermatogenesis in hypogonadotropic hypogonadal men with hCG alone. Eur J Endocrinol 2002;147:617–624.
10. Schopohl J, Mehltretter G, von Zumbusch R, Eversmann T, von Werder K. Comparison of gonadotropin-releasing hormone and gonadotropin therapy in male patients with idiopathic hypothalamic hypogonadism. Fertil Steril 1991;56:1143–1150.
11. Conn PM, Crowley JR. Gonadotropin-releasing hormone and its analogs. N Engl J Med 1991;324:93–103.
12. Whitcomb RW, Crowley WF. Clinical review 4: diagnosis and treatment of isolated gonadotropin-releasing hormone deficiency in men. J Clin Endocrinol Metab 1990;70:3–7.
13. Caron P, Chauvin S, Christin-Maitre S, et al. Resistance of hypogonadic patients with mutated GnRH receptor genes to pulsatile GnRH administration. J Clin Endocrinol Metab 1999;84:990–996.
14. De Roux N, Young J, Misrahi M, et al. A family with hypogonadotropic hypogonadism and mutations in the gonadotropin-releasing hormone receptor. N Engl J Med 1997;337:1597–1602.
15. Layman LC, Cohen DP, Jin M, et al. Mutations in the gonadotropin-releasing hormone receptor gene cause hypogonadotropic hypogonadism. Nat Genet 1998;18:14–15.
16. Quinton R, Barnett P, Coskeran P, Bouloux PM. Gordon Holmes spinocerebellar ataxia: a gonadotropin deficiency syndrome resistant to treatment with pulsatile gonadotropin-releasing hormone. Clin Endocrinol 1999;51:525–529.
17. Morris DV, Adeniyi-Jones R, Wheeler M, Sonksen P, Jacobs HS. The treatment of hypogonadotropic hypogonadism in men by the pulsatile infusion of luteinizing hormone-releasing hormone. Clin Endocrinol 1984;21:189–200.
18. Blumenfeld Z, Frisch L, Conn PM. Gonadotropin-releasing hormone (GnRH) antibodies formation in hypogonadotropic azoospermic men treated with pulsatile GnRH-diagnosis and possible alternative treatment. Fertil Steril 1988;50:622–629.

19. Finkel DM, Phillips BA, Snyder PJ. Stimulation of spermatogenesis by gonadotropins in men with hypogonadotropic hypogonadism. N Engl J Med 1985;313:651–655.

20. Burris AS, Rodbard HW, Winters SJ, Sherins RJ. Gonadotropin therapy in men with isolated hypogonadotropic hypogonadism: the response to human chorionic gonadotropin is predicted by initial testicular size. J Clin Endocrinol Metab 1988;66:1144–1151.

21. Kirk JMW, Savage MO, Grant DB, Bouloux P-MG, Besser GM. Gonadal function and response to human chorionic and menopausal gonadotropin therapy in male patients with idiopathic hypogonadotropic hypogonadism. Clin Endocrinol 1994;41:57–63.

22. Simoni M, Nieschlag E. FSH in therapy: physiological basis, new preparations and clinical use. Reprod Med Rev 1995;4:163–177.

23. Sokol RZ, McClure RD, Peterson M, Swerdloff RS. Gonadotropin therapy failure secondary to human chorionic gonadotropin-induced antibodies. J Clin Endocrinol Metab 1981;52:929–933.

24. Vicari E, Mongioi A, Calogero AE, et al. Therapy with human chorionic gonadotropin alone induces spermatogenesis in men with isolated hypogonadotropic hypogonadism—long-term follow-up. Int J Androl 1992;15:320–329.

25. Liu PY, Wishart SM, Handelsman DJ. A double-blind placebo-controlled, randomized clinical trial of recombinant human chorionic gonadotropin on muscle strength and physical function and activity in older men with partial age-related androgen deficiency. J Clin Endocrinol Metab 2002;87:3125–3135.

26. The European Recombinant LH Study Group. Human recombinant luteinizing hormone is as effective as, but safer than, urinary human chorionic gonadotropin in inducing final follicular maturation and ovulation in in vitro fertilization procedures: results of a multicenter double-blind study. J Clin Endocrinol Metab 2001;86:2607–2618.

27. Choung P, Kenley S, Burns T, et al. Recombinant human chorionic gonadotropin (rhCG) in assisted reproductive technology: results of a clinical trial comparing two doses of rhCG (Ovidrel) to urinary hCG (Profasi) for induction of final follicular maturation in in vitro fertilization-embryo transfer. Fertil Steril 2001;76:67–74.

28. Burris AS, Clark RV, Vantman DJ, Sherins RJ. A low sperm concentration does not preclude fertility in men with isolated hypogonadotropic hypogonadism after gonadotropin therapy. Fertil Steril 1988;50:343–347.

29. Barrio R, de Luis D, Alonso M, Lamas A, Moreno JC. Induction of puberty with human chorionic gonadotropin and follicle-stimulating hormone in adolescent males with hypogonadotropic hypogonadism. Fertil Steril 1999;71:244–248.

30. European Metrodin HP Study Group. Efficacy and safety of highly purified urinary follicle-stimulating hormone with human chorionic gonadotropin for treating men with isolated hypogonadotropic hypogonadism. Fertil Steril 1998;70:256–262.

31. Mastrogiacomo I, Motta RG, Botteon S, Bonanni G, Schiesaro M. Achievement of spermatogenesis and genital tract maturation in hypogonadotropic subjects during long-term treatment with gonadotropins or LHRH. Andrologia 1991;23:285–289.

32. Burgués S, Calderón MD, the Spanish Collaborative Group on Male Hypogonadotropic Hypogonadism. Subcutaneous self-administration of highly purified follicle-stimulating hormone and human chorionic gonadotropin for the treatment of male hypogonadotropic hypogonadism. Hum Reprod 1997;12:980–986.

33. Harlin J, Csemiczky G, Wramsby H, Fried G. Recombinant follicle-stimulating hormone in in-vitro fertilization treatment—clinical experience with follitropin alpha and follitropin beta. Hum Reprod 2000;15:239–244.

34. Bouloux P, Nieschlag E, Burger HG, et al. Induction of spermatogenesis by recombinant follicle-stimulating hormone (Puregon) in hypogonadotropic azoospermic men who failed to respond to human chorionic gonadotropin alone. J Androl 2003;24:604–611.

35. Liu PY, Turner L, Rushford D, et al. Efficacy and safety of recombinant human follicle-stimulating hormone (Gonal-F) with urinary human chorionic gonadotropin for induction of spermatogenesis and fertility in gonadotropin-deficient men. Hum Reprod 1999;14:1540–1545.

36. Bouloux PMG, Warne DW, Loumaye E. Efficacy and safety of recombinant human follicle-stimulating hormone in men with isolated hypogonadotropic hypogonadism. Fertil Steril 2002;77:270–273.

37. O'Dea L, Hemsey G, Brentzel J, Bock D, Matsumoto AM. Long-term treatment with follitropin Alfa (Gonal-F®) in male hypogonadotropic hypogonadism (HH). Endocrine Society, San Francisco, 2002, (Abstract) pp. 2–661.

38. Bouloux P, Handelsman DJ, Jockenhövel F, et al. FSH-CTP study group. First human exposure to FSH-CTP in hypogonadotropic hypogonadal males. Hum Reprod 2001;16:1592–1597.
39. Zitzmann M, Nieschlag E. Hormone substitution in male hypogonadism. Mol Cell Endocrinol 2000;161:73–88.
40. Spratt DI, Carr DB, Merriam GR, Scully RE, Rao PN, Crowley WF. The spectrum of abnormal patterns of gonadotropin-releasing hormone secretion in men with idiopathic hypogonadotropic hypogonadism: clinical and laboratory correlations. J Clin Endocrinol Metab 1987;64:283–291.
41. Mengel W, Hienz HA, Sippe WG, Hecker WC. Studies on cryptorchidism: a comparison of histological findings in the germinative epithelium before and after the second year of life. J Pediatr Surg 1974;9:445–450.
42. Pitteloud N, Hayes FJ, Boepple PA, et al. The role of prior pubertal development, biochemical markers of testicular maturation, and genetics in elucidating the phenotypic heterogeneity of idiopathic hypogonadotropic hypogonadism. J Clin Endocrinol Metab 2002;87:152–160.
43. Nieschlag E. Scope and goals of andrology. In: Nieschlag E, Behre HM, eds. Andrology: Male Reproductive Health and Dysfunction, 2nd ed. Springer, Berlin, 2000, pp. 1–8.
44. Knuth UA, Schneider HPG, Behre HM. Gynecology relevant to andrology. In: Nieschlag E, Behre HM, eds. Andrology: Male Reproductive Health and Dysfunction, 2nd ed. Springer, Berlin, 2000, pp. 271–309.
45. Liu L, Chaudhari N, Corle D, Sherins RJ. Comparison of pulsatile subcutaneous gonadotropin-releasing hormone and exogenous gonadotropins in the treatment of men with isolated hypogonadotropic hypogonadism. Fertil Steril 1988;49:302–308.
46. Zwart-van Rijkom JEF, Broekmans FJ, Leufkens HGM. From hMG through purified urinary FSH preparations to recombinant FSH: a substitution study. Hum Reprod 2002;17:857–865.
47. Debate group: "Bye-bye urinary gonadotropins?" Matorra R, Rodriguez-Escudero F. "The use of urinary gonadotropins should be discouraged." Crosignani PG. "Risk of infection is not the main problem." Balen A. "Is there a risk of prion disease after the administration of urinary-derived gonadotropins?" Dyer J. "The conflict between effective and affordable health care—a perspective from the developing world." Hum Reprod 2002;17:1675–1683.
48. Mannaerts B, Fauser B, Lahlou N, et al. Serum hormone concentrations during treatment with multiple rising doses of recombinant follicle stimulating hormone (Puregon) in men with hypogonadotropic hypogonadism. Fertil Steril 1996;65:406–410.
49. Le Cotonnec JY, Porchet HC, Beltrami V, Khan A, toon S, Rowland M. Clinical pharmacology of recombinant human follicle-stimulating hormone (FSH). I. comparative pharmacokinetics with urinary human FSH. Fertil Steril 1994;61:669–678.
50. Out HJ, Driessen SGAJ, Mannaerts BMJL, Coelingh Bennink HJT. Recombinant follicle-stimulating hormone (follitropin beta, Puregon) yields higher pregnancy rates in in vitro fertilization than urinary gonadotropins. Fertil Steril 1997;68:138–142.
51. Daya S, Gunby J. Recombinant versus urinary follicle-stimulating hormone for ovarian stimulation in assisted reproduction. Hum Reprod 1999;14:2207–2215.
52. Agrawal R, Holmes J, Howard SJ. Follicle-stimulating hormone or human menopausal gonadotropin for ovarian stimulation in in vitro fertilization cycles: a meta-analysis. Fertil Steril 2000;73:338–343.
53. Arsenijevic Y, Wehrenberg WB, Conz A, Eshkol A, Sizonenko PC, Aubert NL. Growth hormone (GH) deprivation induced by passive immunization against rat GH-releasing factor delays sexual maturation in the male rat. Endocrinology 1989;124:3050–3059.
54. Chatelain PG, Sanchez P, Saez JM. Growth hormone and insulin-like growth factor I treatment increases testicular luteinizing hormone receptor and steroidogenic responsiveness of growth hormone deficient dwarf mice. Endocrinology 1991;128:1857–1862.
55. Syed V, Khan SA, Nieschlag E. Epidermal growth factor stimulates testosterone production on human Leydig cells in vitro. J Endocrinol Invest 1991;14:93–97.
56. Bebaker M, Honour JW, Foster D, Liu YL, Jacobes HS. Regulation of testicular function by insulin and transforming growth factor-β. Steroids 1990;55:266–270.
57. Kulin HE, Samojlik E, Santen R, Santner S. The effect of growth hormone on the Leydig cell response to chorionic gonadotropin in boys with hypopituitarism. Clin Endocrinol 1981;15:463–472.
58. Shoham Z, Conway GS, Ostergaard H, Lahlou N, Bouchard P, Jacobs HS. Cotreatment with growth hormone for induction of spermatogenesis in patients with hypogonadotropic hypogonadism. Fertil Steril 1992;57:1044–1051.

59. Giagulli VA. Absence of effect of recombinant growth hormone to classic gonadotropin treatment on spermatogenesis of patients with severe hypogonadotropic hypogonadism. Arch Androl 1999;43:47–53.
60. Carani C, Granata AR, De Rosa M, et al. The effect of chronic treatment with GH on gonadal function in men with isolated GH deficiency. Eur J Endocrinol 1999;140:224–230.
61. White BJ, Rogol AD, Brown KS, Lieblich JM, Rosen SW. The syndrome of anosmia with hypogonadotropic hypogonadism: a genetic study of 18 new families and a review. Am J Med Genet 1983;15:417–435.
62. Dean JCS, Johnston AW, Klopper AI. Isolated hypogonadotropic hypogonadism: a family with autosomal dominant inheritance. Clin Endocrinol 1990;32:341–347.
63. Chaussian JL, Toublanc JE, Feingold J, Naud C, Vassal J, Job JC. Mode of inheritance in familial cases of primary gonadotropic deficiency. Horm Res 1988;29:202–206.
64. Franco B, Guioli S, Pragliola A, et al. A gene deleted in Kallmann's syndrome shares homology with neural cell adhesion and axonal path-finding molecules. Nature 1991;353:529–536.
65. Pralong FP, Gomez F, Castillo E, et al. Complete hypogonadotropic hypogonadism associated with a novel inactivating mutation of the gonadotropin-releasing hormone receptor. J Clin Endocrinol Metab 1999;84:3811–3816.
66. De Roux N, Young J, Brailly-Tabard S, Misrahi M, Milgrom E, Schaison G. The same molecular defects of the gonadotropin-releasing hormone receptor determine a variable degree of hypogonadism in affected kindred. J Clin Endocrionl Metab 1999;84:567–572.
67. Zanaria E, Muscatelli F, Bardoni B, et al. An unusual member of the nuclear hormone receptor superfamily responsible for X-linked adrenal hypoplasia congenita. Nature 1994;372:635–641.
68. Habiby RL, Boepple P, Nachtigall L, Sluss PM, Crowley WF, Jameson JL. Adrenal hypoplasia congenita with hypogonadotropic hypogonadism: evidence that the DAX-1 mutations lead to combined hypothalamic and pituitary defects in gonadotropin production. J Clin Invest 1996;98:1055–1062.
69. Wu W, Cogan JD, Pfaeffle RW, et al. Mutations in PROP 1 cause familial combined pituitary hormone deficiency. Nat Genet 1998;18:147–149.
70. Vermeulen S, Messiaen L, Scheir P, De Bie S, Speleman F, De Paepe A. Kallmann syndrome in a patient with congenital spherocytosis and an interstitial 8p11.2 deletion. Am J Med Genet 2002;108:315–318.
71. Netchine I, Sobrier ML, Krude H, et al. Mutations in LHX 3 result in a new syndrome revealed by combined pituitary hormone deficiency. Nat Genet 2000;25:182–186.
72. Dattani MT, Martinez-Barbera JP, Thomas PQ, et al. Mutations in the homebox gene HESX1/Hesx1 associated with septo-optic dysplasia in human and mouse. Nat Genet 1998;19:125–133.
73. Strobel A, Issad T, Camoin L, Ozata M, Strosberg AD. A leptin missense mutation associated with hypogonadism and morbid obesity. Nat Genet 1998;18:213–215.
74. Clément K, Vaisse C, Lahlou N, et al. A mutation in the human leptin receptor gene causes obesity and pituitary dysfunction. Nature 1998;392:398–401.
75. Jackson RS, Creemers JW, Ohagi S, et al. Obesity and impaired prohormone processing associated with mutations in the human prohormone convertase 1 gene. Nat Genet 1997;16:303–306.
76. Quinton R, Duke VM, Robertson A, et al. Idiopathic gonadotropin deficiency: genetic questions addressed through phenotypic characterization. Clin Endocrinol 2001;55:163–174.
77. Georgopoulos NA, Pralong FP, Seidman CE, Seidman JG, Crowley WF, Vallejo M. Genetic heterogeneity evidenced by low incidence of KAL-1 gene mutations in sporadic cases of gonadotropin-releasing hormone deficiency. J Clin Endocrinol Metab 1997;82:213–217.
78. Merriam GR, Beitins IZ, Bode HH. Father-to-son transmission of hypogonadism with anosmia: Kallmann's syndrome. Am J Dis Child 1977;131:1216–1219.

INDEX

A

Acromegaly, 143–147
ACTH, Adrenocorticotropic hormone (ACTH)
Activin
  follistatin, 13, 14
  and FSH secretion, 12–15
  inhibins, 13
  reproductive function and, 15
  Smads, 12–15
Adipose tissue and testosterone, 216
Adrenal hypoplasia congenita (AHC) and the
    DAX1 gene, 90–91
Adrenal rest tumors
  and CAH, 132
  fertility and, 132, 134
  morphology, 129, 130
  treatment, 132–133
Adrenocorticotropic hormone (ACTH), 249
AIDS. *See* Human Immunodeficiency Virus (HIV)
Allbright, Fuller, 160
Androgens
  biosynthesis, 26–27
  deficiency
    chronic renal failure and, 231–232
    and HIV, 207–208
    malnutrition and, 211
    mechanisms/symptoms of, 264
    testicular function, 232
  leutinizing hormone (LH), 10, 11
  and LH synthesis, 10
  replacement therapy
    benefits/risks of, 356–360
    bone mineral density and, 358
    contraindications, 355
    coronary artery disease, 358–359
    and EPO, 238
    implants and, 363–364
    and Klinefelter's Syndrome, 166
    monitoring, 364
    muscle function in HIV infection, 212–218
    polycythemia and, 238, 360
    preparations available, 360–364
    and the prostate gland, 239, 355, 359
    recipients, determining, 353–355
    renal failure and, 227–228, 232–233, 235,
        236–237

and sexual dysfunction, 356
  spermatogenesis, 360
  testing for, 355–356, 360
  testicular descent and, 178
Andropause, 106. *See also* Hypoandrogenemia,
    aging-related
Anemia, 236–239
Aneurysms and tumors, 154
Anorexia nervosa, 71
Approximate entropy (ApEn) secretion analysis,
    276, 278, 279
Arachnoid cyst defined, 154
Arterial endothelium dysfunction, 339
α subunit expression
  biochemical structure, 102
  control of, 5
  mutations in, 106–107
Atherosclerosis, measures of, 338–340
Athletic training, 71
Azoospermia and FSH-R mutations, 117

B

Bone mineral density and androgen replacement
    therapy, 358

C

Cabergoline treatment, hyperprolactinemia, 142–143
CAH. *See* Congenital adrenal hyperplasia (CAH)
Cancer
  adrenocorticotropic hormone (ACTH), 249
  and chemotherapy, 249–252, 258
  cyclophosphamide, 249–250, 251, 258
  and Hodgkin's Disease, 248
  hypogonadism and cancer treatments, 247–259
  procarbazine, 258
  radiation therapy, 247, 252–255
  tumors, testicular and germ cell cancer, 298–
      299
Cardiovascular disease
  and anabolic steroids, 321–322
  lipoprotein(a) (LPa), 342
  SHBG, 331–332
  testosterone and, 337–338, 341–343
Castration
  and atherosclerosis, 340
  gonadotropin response to, 14, 229
Catarrhini, taxonomy of, 45